Immunohematology
PRINCIPLES AND PRACTICE

THIRD EDITION

Eva D. Quinley

MS, MT(ASCP)SBB, CQA(ASQ)

Senior Vice President, Quality and Regulatory Affairs

American Red Cross

Washington, DC

Wolters Kluwer | Lippincott Williams & Wilkins
Health

Philadelphia · Baltimore · New York · London
Buenos Aires · Hong Kong · Sydney · Tokyo

Acquisitions Editor: John Goucher
Product Manager: Meredith L. Brittain
Vendor Manager: Kevin Johnson
Design Coordinator: Stephen Druding
Compositor: MPS Limited, A Macmillan Company

Third Edition

Library of Congress Cataloging-in-Publication Data
Immunohematology : principles and practice / [edited by] Eva D. Quinley.—3rd ed.
       p. ; cm.
  Includes bibliographical references and index.
  ISBN 978-0-7817-8204-3 (alk. paper)
  1. Immunohematology. 2. Blood banks. I. Quinley, Eva D.
  [DNLM: 1. Blood Transfusion—methods. 2. Blood Banks. 3. Blood Group Antigens. 4. Blood Grouping and Crossmatching. 5. Hematologic Diseases—immunology. WB 356 I323 2011]

  RM171.I43 2011
  615'.39—dc22

                                                      2009036981

DISCLAIMER

Care has been taken to confirm the accuracy of the information present and to describe generally accepted practices. However, the authors, editors, and publisher are not responsible for errors or omissions or for any consequences from application of the information in this book and make no warranty, expressed or implied, with respect to the currency, completeness, or accuracy of the contents of the publication. Application of this information in a particular situation remains the professional responsibility of the practitioner; the clinical treatments described and recommended may not be considered absolute and universal recommendations.

The authors, editors, and publisher have exerted every effort to ensure that drug selection and dosage set forth in this text are in accordance with the current recommendations and practice at the time of publication. However, in view of ongoing research, changes in government regulations, and the constant flow of information relating to drug therapy and drug reactions, the reader is urged to check the package insert for each drug for any change in indications and dosage and for added warnings and precautions. This is particularly important when the recommended agent is a new or infrequently employed drug.

Some drugs and medical devices presented in this publication have Food and Drug Administration (FDA) clearance for limited use in restricted research settings. It is the responsibility of the health care provider to ascertain the FDA status of each drug or device planned for use in their clinical practice.

To purchase additional copies of this book, call our customer service department at (800) 638-3030 or fax orders to (301) 223-2320. International customers should call (301) 223-2300.

Visit Lippincott Williams & Wilkins on the Internet: http://www.lww.com. Lippincott Williams & Wilkins customer service representatives are available from 8:30 am to 6:00 pm, EST.

This edition of **Immunohematology: Principles and Practice** *is dedicated to my family for their support and encouragement, to all the wonderful individuals who work in this great profession, and with special thoughts of Dr. Breanndan Moore, one of the finest blood bankers and most wonderful human beings I have ever known.*

PREFACE

Immunohematology has always been one of the most fascinating and challenging fields in clinical laboratory medicine. *Immunohematology: Principles and Practice* provides clinical laboratory scientists and other health care professionals with a working knowledge of immunohematology. Because the information is presented in a clear and concise manner and is comprehensive and thorough, the text is a useful reference for any individual who desires knowledge of current immunohematology theory.

The third edition of *Immunohematology: Principles and Practice* incorporates the successful elements of the first two editions while expanding on them. Each chapter includes learning objectives, key words, boxes highlighting important concepts, and review questions. A comprehensive glossary and a section of color plates are included for reference as well. These elements serve as aids to increase understanding of the material presented, benefiting both the learner and the instructor.

As with the previous editions, it is the desire of the editor and contributors of this book to provide an excellent resource for those who seek knowledge in immunohematology—one that is written in a manner that is readable, interesting, and easily understood. It is also our hope that the pages of this text will become well worn, having been used time and time again by students, practicing blood bankers, and others who want to know more about this fascinating subject.

ORGANIZATIONAL PHILOSOPHY

This edition of *Immunohematology: Principles and Practice* begins with an overview of blood collection and component practices in Unit 1, "Blood and Blood Components." This unit includes a chapter devoted to apheresis (Chapter 2), one of the fastest growing and most promising methods of blood collection and component harvesting. In Unit 2, "Genetic and Immunologic Principles," chapters on basic concepts of genetics (Chapter 4) and immunology (Chapter 5) provide a foundation for understanding antibody detection and identification (Chapter 6) and the blood group systems (discussed in Unit 4, Chapters 9 through 12).

A thorough discussion of current transfusion practices in Unit 5 (Chapter 13) allows the reader to understand the indications and contraindications for transfusion of various blood components. In Unit 6, "Clinical Conditions Associated with Immunohematology," the importance of transfusion-transmitted diseases is presented (Chapter 15), including etiologic agents, prevalence, pathology, testing, and prevention. This section also includes specific pathologic conditions in which blood banking practices play an important role, such as hemolytic disease of the newborn (Chapter 16) and autoimmune hemolytic anemias (Chapter 17), so that the reader can understand the pathology involved and the interventional role the blood bank plays.

Because regulatory issues have become one of the most important topics in the field of blood banking, Unit 7, "Quality Assurance and Regulatory Issues," includes a chapter devoted to quality assurance and safety issues (Chapter 18) and a chapter on issues related to regulation and accreditation of blood banks (Chapter 19). Unit 8, "Additional Topics of Interest," includes two chapters that are new to this edition: Information Technology (Chapter 20) and Principles of Project Management (Chapter 22). The chapter on process management (Chapter 21) has been expanded to discuss Six Sigma and Lean Principles.

ADDITIONAL RESOURCES

Immunohematology: Principles and Practice, Third Edition, includes additional resources that are available on the book's companion website at thePoint.lww.com/Quinley3e. Students who have purchased the book have access to an online study guide, which includes basic to advanced case studies and questions that are organized to be used as supplements to each chapter. Written with a practical working knowledge of immunohematology, the case studies provide the opportunity to put learned information into practice.

In addition, purchasers of the text can access the searchable Full Text On-line by going to the *Immunohematology: Principles and Practice,* Third Edition website at thePoint.lww.com/Quinley3e. See the inside front cover of this text for more details, including the passcode you will need to gain access to the website.

Patricia Arndt, MSMT, MT(ASCP)SBB
Senior Research Associate
American Red Cross Blood Services
Immunohematology Research Laboratory
Pomona, CA

Suzanne Butch, MA, MT(ASCP)SBB
Administrative Manager
University of Michigan Hospitals & Health Centers
Blood Bank—Pathology
Ann Arbor, MI

Tony Casina, BS, MT(ASCP)SBB
Marketing Manager
Worldwide Marketing
Ortho-Clinical Diagnostics
Raritan, NJ

Ann Church, MS
Director of Change Integration
American Red Cross
Biomedical Services
Washington, DC

Susan Connor, MT(ASCP)SBB, MBGM
Clinical & Therapeutic Apheresis Manager
Gambro BCT
Sales & Marketing
Lakewood, CO

Kay Crull, MS, MT(ASCP)SBB
Vice President, Manufacturing
American Red Cross
Biomedical Services
Washington, DC

Julie Cruz, MD
Associate Medical Director
Indiana Blood Center
Indianapolis, IN

Helene De Palma, MT(ASCP)SBB, CQA(ASQ)
Director of Operations
New York Blood Center
Laboratory of Immunohematology
New York, NY

Theresa Downs, BS, MT(ASCP)SBB
Laboratory Supervisor
University of Michigan Health System
Pathology—Blood Bank & Transfusion Service
Ann Arbor, MI

Steve Gregurek, MD
Assistant Professor
Department of Pathology and Laboratory Medicine
Indiana University School of Medicine

Sandra Hedberg, BS, MT(ASCP)
Partner
SoftwareCPR
Clinton, TN

Susan Hsu, PhD
Director, Histocompatibility / Molecular Genetics
American Red Cross
Histocompatibility/Molecular Genetics
Philadelphia, PA

Regina Leger, MSQA, MT(ASCP)SBB, CMQ/OE(ASQ)
Research Associate
American Red Cross Blood Services
Immunohematology Research Laboratory
Pomona, CA

Mary Lieb, BS, MT(ASCP)SBB, CQA(ASQ)
Quality Consultant
Quality Source by Blood Systems Inc.
Scottsdale, AZ

Sandra Taddie Nance, MS, MT(ASCP)SBB
Adjunct Assistant Professor
University of Pennsylvania, Philadelphia, PA
Senior Director
American Red Cross Biomedical Services
Operations and Heritage Division
Philadelphia, PA

Eva D. Quinley, MS, MT(ASCP)SBB, CQA(ASQ)
Senior Vice President, Quality and Regulatory Affairs
American Red Cross
Washington, DC

Marion Reid, PhD, FIMLS
Director of Immunohematology
New York Blood Center
Laboratory of Immunohematology
New York, NY

Scott Schifter, RPh, BS, MBA
Senior Director
American Red Cross
Client Services and Account Management—Biomedical
Information Management
Washington, DC

Daniel Smith, MD
Professor
Director of Transfusion Medicine
Pathology and Laboratory Medicine
Indiana University
Indianapolis, IN

Jean Stanley, MT(ASCP)SBB, CQA(ASQ)
Consultant
Quality Focus
Moraga, CA

Margaret Stoe, BSMT(ASCP)SBB
Senior Administrative Specialist Healthcare Quality
Corporate Quality Improvement
University of Michigan Hospital and Health System
Ann Arbor, MI

Susan Stramer, PhD
Executive Scientific Officer
American Red Cross
Scientific Support Office
Gaithersburg, MD

Marla Troughton, MD
Associate Medical Director
BioLife Plasma Services
Birmingham, AL

Dan Waxman, MD
Executive Vice President/Chief Medical Officer
Indiana Blood Center
Indianapolis, IN

Connie M. Westhoff, MT(ASCP)SBB, PhD
Adjunct Assistant Professor
Pathology and Laboratory Medicine
University of Pennsylvania, Philadelphia, PA
Scientific Director
American Red Cross
Molecular Blood Group and Platelet Antigen Testing
Philadelphia, PA

TABLE OF CONTENTS

UNIT 4
RED BLOOD CELL GROUPS AND HLA   119

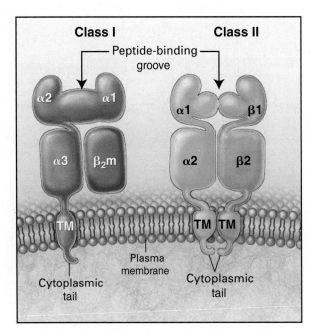

COLOR PLATE C-1 Structures of HLA class I and class II molecules. β_2-Microglobulin (β_2 m) is the light chain of the class I molecule. The α chain of the class I molecule has two peptide-binding domains (α1 and α2), an immunoglobulin-like domain (α3), the transmembrane region (TM), and the cytoplasmic tail. Each of the class II α and β chains has four domains: the peptide-binding domain (α1 or β1), the immunoglobulin-like domain (α2 or β2), the transmembrane region, and the cytoplasmic tail. (Reproduced with permission from Klein J, Sato A. The HLA system: first of two parts. *N Engl J Med.* 2000;343:704.)

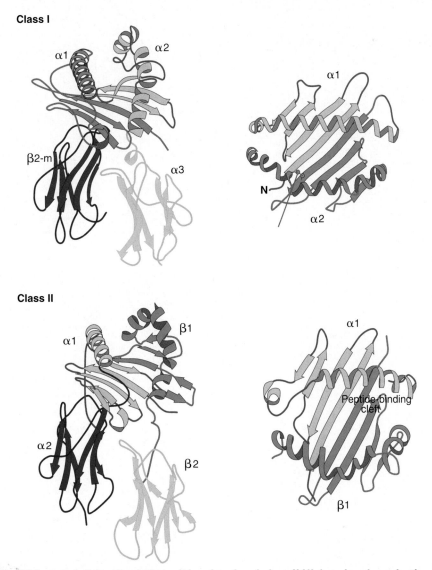

COLOR PLATE C-2 Ribbon structure simulation of the class I and class II HLA molecule and a three-dimensional view of the peptide groove of an HLA class I and class II molecule (Adapted with permission from Macmillan Publishers Ltd. Bjorkman PJ, Saper MA, Samraoui B, et al. The foreign antigen binding site and T cell recognition regions of class I histocompatibility antigens. *Nature.* 1987;329:506).

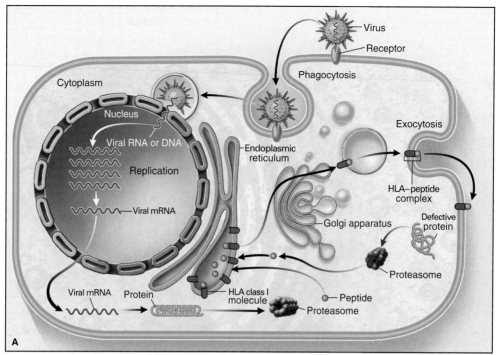

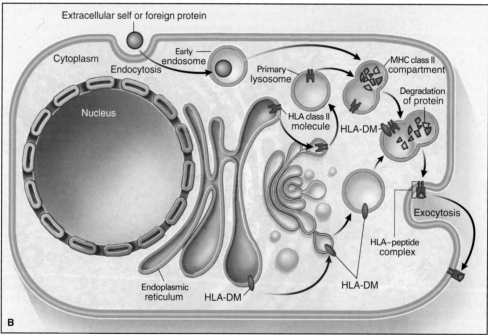

COLOR PLATE C-3 Antigen processing. Panel A shows the principal pathways of generating peptides for loading onto HLA class I molecules. Worn-out or defective proteins in the cytosol are degraded into peptides in proteasomes. Selected peptides are then transported into the endoplasmic reticulum, where they are loaded onto newly synthesized class I molecules. The HLA–peptide complexes are exported by way of the Golgi apparatus to the surface of the cell. In tissues infected with a virus, viral particles are taken up by cells and uncoated. The viral DNA or RNA enters the nucleus and replicates within it. The viral messenger RNA (mRNA) then enters the cytosol and is transcribed into proteins. Some of the proteins are subsequently degraded in proteasomes, and the peptides are delivered into the endoplasmic reticulum, where they are loaded onto class I molecules for export to the surface of the cell. Panel B shows the processing of extracellular proteins. Self or foreign proteins are taken up by endocytosis (or phagocytosis) and sequestered into endosomes. Class II molecules synthesized in the endoplasmic reticulum are delivered by way of the Golgi apparatus into primary lysosomes, which fuse with the early endosomes to form the major histocompatibility complex (MHC) class II compartment. Enzymes brought into this compartment by the lysosomes degrade the engulfed proteins into peptides. HLA-DM molecules synthesized in the endoplasmic reticulum and delivered into the MHC class II compartment by transport vesicles help load the peptides onto the class II molecules. The HLA–peptide complexes are then exported to the surface of the cell. (Reproduced with permission from Klein, J. The HLA system: first of two parts. *N Engl J Med.* 2000;343:705.)

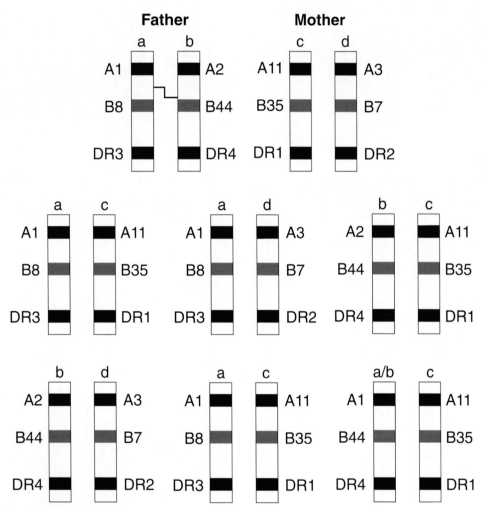

COLOR PLATE C-4 The inheritance of HLA haplotypes. a and b denote paternal haplotypes, and c and d denote maternal haplotypes. a/b denote a paternal recombinant haplotype derived from a recombination event occurring between the HLA-A and HLA-B locus.

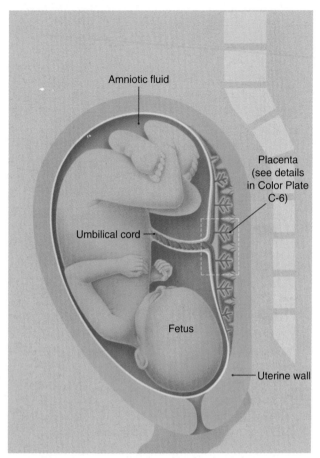

COLOR PLATE C-5 Fetus and placenta. (From *Blood Group Antigens and Antibodies as Applied to Hemolytic Disease of the Newborn*. Raritan, NJ: Ortho Diagnostics, Inc.; 1968, with permission.)

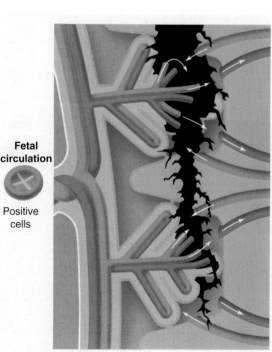

COLOR PLATE C-6 Scheme of placental circulation. White arrows depict separate routines of fetal and maternal circulations within the placenta. Dotted lines represent oxygen nutrient and waste exchange through the placental barrier. (From *Blood Group Antigens and Antibodies as Applied to Hemolytic Disease of the Newborn*. Raritan, NJ: Ortho Diagnostics, Inc.; 1968, with permission.)

COLOR PLATE C-7 Separation of placenta following delivery. Diagram portrays the rupture of placental vessels (villi) and connective tissues allowing escape of fetal blood cells. Prior to complete constriction of the open-end maternal vessels, some fetal blood may enter maternal circulation. (From *Blood Group Antigens and Antibodies as Applied to Hemolytic Disease of the Newborn*. Raritan, NJ: Ortho Diagnostics, Inc.; 1968, with permission.)

BLOOD COLLECTION AND PROCESSING

JEAN STANLEY

OBJECTIVES

After completion of this chapter, the reader will be able to:

1. List information necessary for registration of a donor.

2. Discuss the importance of the uniform donor history questionnaire and the accompanying documents for prospective donors.

3. Define the importance of a medical history and physical examination for determining donor acceptability.

4. Explain the procedure for phlebotomy of a donor.

5. Describe various types of donor reactions and appropriate steps to follow to aid the donor.

6. List the testing requirements for donor processing.

7. Discuss the preoperative autologous donation procedure, including testing and labeling requirements.

8. Describe the other methods of collecting autologous donations.

KEY WORDS

Allogeneic
Autologous
Chagas
Confidential unit exclusion
Dedicated donor
Deferral
Directed donor
Donor processing
Good manufacturing practices

Hematocrit
Hemoglobin
High-risk donor
Infectious disease markers
Intraoperative salvage
ISBT 128
Mobile operation
Nucleic acid testing
Paid donor
Postoperative salvage

Standard operating procedures
Surrogate markers
Syncope
Therapeutic phlebotomy

Traceability
Uniform donor history questionnaire (UDHQ)
Volunteer blood donors
Window period

*B*lood is a scarce resource, with its availability dependent upon the altruistic nature of *volunteer blood donors*. All blood in the United States collected for the transfusion of others or *allogeneic* donations comes from volunteer blood donors. With the addition of numerous screening questions and sophisticated tests to ensure the safety of the blood supply, it is estimated that only 38% of the U.S. population is eligible to donate blood.[1] Volunteer blood donors provide red blood cells (RBCs), plasma, and platelets, each an important component in helping to save lives through blood transfusions. With the diminishing pool of available blood donors, blood centers and blood banks have the responsibility to provide a safe and pleasant environment to recruit and retain donors so that blood and blood components will be available for the patients requiring transfusions.

The donation process is guided by requirements or standards AABB, formly known as American Association of Blood Banks, a professional organization with expertise in standard setting and accreditation in blood banking and transfusion medicine, and the Department of Health and Human Services, U.S. Food and Drug Administration (FDA). These stringent requirements must be followed by facilities collecting and distributing blood and blood components, ensuring the donation process is safe for the donor as well as the blood received for transfusion is safe for the recipient.

To ensure the safety of both parties, *good manufacturing practices* **(GMPs)** must be incorporated into an organization's operations. GMPs are a set of regulations enforced by the FDA to ensure that each step in the manufacturing process is controlled, from the beginning to the end.[2] Every operational department in a facility must have *standard operating procedures* (SOPs) that describe instructions to staff on how to perform each step in the blood collection and manufacturing process.[3] The SOPs should reflect any local, state, and federal regulations pertaining to blood bank operations.

RECRUITMENT OF DONORS

The donation process begins with the recruitment of volunteer donors and scheduling of appointments, which may occur via telephone calls, electronically on a blood organization's web site or by email, or through presentations at company businesses. Many businesses support on-site donations often referred to as a *mobile operation*. Collection staff travels to the business and sets up a mobile collection site to collect blood from the employees during business hours. This type of operation is ideal as a win-win partnership where businesses can support blood donations by allowing their employees to take time from work to donate with minimal impact on their daily business operations.

Access to the Internet has provided another venue for blood facilities to recruit donors. Today donors can schedule a donation appointment online, update contact information, and even earn points toward thank you gifts on their blood organization's web site. Another technique that takes advantage of technology includes sending text messages to donors on their cell phones to remind them of donation appointments. Many blood facilities also offer promotional items for recruiting donors; however, this practice must be carefully monitored to ensure that the items are not considered as a payment for blood donations. The FDA requires that blood collected from a donor who receives a monetary incentive or an incentive that can be converted to cash must be labeled as coming from a *paid donor*.[4]

DONOR REGISTRATION

Allogeneic donors who present may donate whole blood, platelets, and/or plasma depending on certain eligibility requirements; however, the registration process and medical history evaluation are the same for all allogeneic donors. The donation process begins with the proper identification of the potential donor to

---

> ## BOX 1-1
>
> ### Donor Identification Information
>
> Full name: Last, first (middle name or initial is optional)
> Date of birth
> Address
> Home and/or work telephone number
> e-mail address
> Sex
> Ethnic group

---

ensure *traceability* of the collected blood beginning with the donor through the processing and component preparation, to distribution, and final transfusion of the blood to the recipient. Many collection facilities require a photograph for identification, although this is not necessary. FDA regulations require that enough information is available to accurately relate a blood component to a donor, and AABB standards require that a donor's identity be confirmed and whether a repeat donor is linked to existing records.[5] At some collection facilities, computer software includes the incorporation of donor photographs and fingerprints as methods for verifying donor identity. Traceability is important in the event that if an adverse reaction occurs from the blood transfusion, it may require notification of the donor for further investigation. Donor verification is also important in identifying donors whose name is on a temporary or permanent *deferral* list. Identification must occur before the components prepared from that donor's blood are labeled for distribution.[3,6]

A list of information often obtained from the potential donor on the day of donation is found in Box 1-1. In general donors must be in good health and at least 16 years of age or as applicable by state law.[5] Donors can donate a unit of whole blood once every 8 weeks or two units of RBCs collected by automation once every 16 weeks.[5,6]

UNIFORM DONOR HISTORY QUESTIONNAIRE

On the day of donation, the eligibility of a donor is determined by a medical history and physical assessment to ensure that the donor is in good health, that the donation process is safe for the donor, and to identify risk factors for diseases transmissible by blood and blood components.[7] Many blood centers in the United States use the AABB *Uniform Donor History Questionnaire (UDHQ)*, which was developed by a multiorganizational task force at the request of the

FDA.[8] The goal of the task force was to develop questions that would increase the comprehension by donors and by doing so, the accuracy of answering the questions would increase the safety of the blood supply. The task force developed four documents that are meant to be used together.[9]

- Donor education material is an informational sheet designed to be read by the donor prior to completing the questionnaire. The material provides information about the donation process; the importance of answering the questions truthfully and accurately; risks and conditions that would defer an individual from donating blood; defines sexual contact; and explains information on the human immunodeficiency virus (HIV) and acquired immunodeficiency syndrome (AIDS). Figure 1-1 is an example of the donor education material.
- UDHQ simplifies capture questions on a broad basis and triggers follow-up questions if an unacceptable answer is given. The questions are also grouped and listed chronologically to help donors recall information and events that occurred in the past. Figure 1-2 is an example of the UDHQ.
- Medication deferral list is a list of medications that may initiate a deferral and includes rationale for the deferral in language understandable to the donor. Figure 1-3 is an example of the medication list.
- Donor history questionnaire brochure details how the questionnaire should be administered and includes a glossary, flow charts, and suggestions for follow-up questions.

The UDHQ can be self-administered by the donor or be completed as a staff-assisted questionnaire whereby collection staff orally interviews the donor. If self-administered, collection staff will review the donor's answers asking follow-up questions as necessary to further define a donor's eligibility. Many blood centers are implementing automated processes for both the questionnaire and physical assessment. The benefit of computer-assisted programs is that data are captured directly from the donor instead of transcribing donor information by the interviewer. Removing the need to transcribe assists in accurate documentation, which increases the quality and safety of the donation process.

PHYSICAL ASSESSMENT

Following the medical evaluation, the donor must undergo a physical assessment. The primary purpose of

TABLE 1-1	Tests for Assessing Donor Eligibility of Allogeneic Donors
Test	**Minimum Acceptable Value**
Copper sulfate (CuSO$_4$)	1.053 specific gravity
Hemoglobin	$\geq$12.5 g/dL
Hematocrit	$\geq$38%
Temperature	$\leq$37.5°C
Pulse	50–100 beats/min without pathologic irregularities
	<50 beats/min if otherwise healthy athlete
Blood pressure	
Systolic	$\leq$180 mmHg
Diastolic	$\leq$100 mmHg

the physical assessment is to ensure that the donor is in good health and that the donation process will be safe for the donor. Table 1-1 lists the tests used to evaluate the donor and the ranges for acceptability of allogeneic donors. The reader is also referred to the latest edition of the AABB Standards for Blood Banks and Transfusion Services for specific requirements for allogeneic donor qualification.[5] Any exceptions to routine findings must be approved by the blood bank physician and may require an individual evaluation. These should be addressed in the facility's policies and procedures.

Hemoglobin/Hematocrit

The *hemoglobin* concentration or *hematocrit* must be determined before donation with a sample of blood obtained by a finger stick or venipuncture. The purpose of this test is to determine that the donor's packed cell volume is acceptable and that the donor is not anemic. A simple screening method is performed by determining the minimum acceptable density of a drop of blood. A sample of whole blood is dropped into a solution of copper sulfate with a specific gravity of 1.053. If the drop of blood sinks within 15 seconds, the donor's blood volume is equal to or greater than the specific gravity and is acceptable. If the drop of blood floats or drops to the bottom of the container after 15 seconds, another method of determining acceptability may be used to determine the hemoglobin or hematocrit. There are several instruments commercially available for determining either the donor's hemoglobin or hematocrit. The hemoglobin must be a

BloodSource
Sacramento, CA

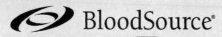 **BloodSource**

Donor Education Sheet, Version 1.1

Making Your Blood Donation Safe

Thank you for coming in today! This information sheet explains how YOU can help us make the donation process safe for yourself and patients who might receive your blood. **PLEASE READ THIS INFORMATION <u>BEFORE</u> YOU DONATE! If you have any questions now or anytime during the screening process, please ask blood center staff.**

Accuracy and Honesty are Essential!

Your **complete honesty** in answering all questions is very important for the safety of patients who receive your blood. **All information you provide is confidential.**

Donation Process

<u>To determine if you are eligible to donate we will:</u>
- Ask questions about health, travel, and medicines
- Ask questions to see if you might be at risk for hepatitis, HIV, or AIDS
- Take your blood pressure, temperature and pulse
- Take a small blood sample to make sure you are not anemic

<u>If you are able to donate we will:</u>
- Cleanse your arm with an antiseptic
- Use a new, sterile, disposable needle to collect your blood

Donor Eligibility – Specific Information

<u>Why we ask questions about sexual contact:</u>
Sexual contact may cause contagious diseases like HIV to get into the bloodstream and be spread through transfusions to someone else.

<u>Definition of "sexual contact":</u>
The words "have sexual contact with" and "sex" are used in some of the questions we will ask you, and apply to <u>any</u> of the activities below, whether or not a condom or other protection was used:
1. Vaginal sex (contact between penis and vagina)
2. Oral sex (mouth or tongue on someone's vagina, penis, or anus)
3. Anal sex (contact between penis and anus)

HIV/AIDS Risk Behaviors and Symptoms

AIDS is caused by HIV. HIV is spread mainly through sexual contact with an infected person OR by sharing needles or syringes used for injecting drugs.

DO NOT DONATE IF YOU:
- **Have AIDS or have ever had a positive HIV test**
- Have ever used needles to take drugs, steroids, or anything not prescribed by your doctor
- Are a male who has had sexual contact with another male, even once, since 1977
- Have ever taken money, drugs or other payment for sex since 1977
- Have had sexual contact in the past 12 months with anyone described above
- Have had syphilis or gonorrhea in the past 12 months
- In the last 12 months have been in juvenile detention, lockup, jail or prison for more than 72 hours
- Have any of the following conditions that can be signs or symptoms of HIV/AIDS:
    - Unexplained weight loss or night sweats
    - Blue or purple spots in your mouth or skin
    - Swollen lymph nodes for more than one month
    - White spots or unusual sores in your mouth
    - Cough that won't go away or shortness of breath
    - Diarrhea that won't go away
    - Fever of more than 100.5°F for more than 10 days

Remember that you <u>CAN</u> give HIV to someone else through blood transfusions even if you feel well and have a negative HIV test. This is because tests cannot detect infections for a period of time after a person is exposed to HIV. **If you think you may be at risk for HIV/AIDS or want an HIV/AIDS test, please ask for information about other testing facilities. *<u>PLEASE DO NOT DONATE TO GET AN HIV TEST!</u>***

Travel to or Birth in Other Countries

Blood donor tests may not be available for some contagious diseases that are found only in certain countries. If you were born in, have lived in, or visited certain countries, you may not be eligible to donate.

What Happens after Your Donation

To protect patients, your blood is tested for hepatitis B and C, HIV, certain other viruses, and syphilis. If your blood tests positive it will not be given to a patient. You will be notified about test results that may disqualify you from donating in the future. **Please do not donate to get tested for HIV, hepatitis, or any other infections!**

Thank You
for Saving a Life Today!

HOTLINE 1-800-821-6277   24 hours a day, 7 days a week

If you donate today, but are concerned for any reason that your blood may not be suitable for transfusion, please call as soon as possible. If you have developed fever, chills, or diarrhea within 24 hours, jaundice at any time, or a diagnosis of West Nile Virus within 2 weeks after donating, please call the BloodSource hotline number.

www.bloodsource.org

Yes, you do save lives.

NRS.des.001 (30336) (BOOK VI – FORMS)
02/24/06 – Page 1 of 2

FIGURE 1-1   Donor education material. (Used with permission of BloodSource, Sacramento, California.)

I have reviewed and understand the blood donor eligibility information and agree not to donate blood or blood components for transfusion to another person or for further processing if I know that I have AIDS or have tested positive for the AIDS virus or if I believe that I may have been exposed to the AIDS virus.

I understand that it is a felony in California for a person with AIDS or who has tested positive for the HIV (AIDS virus) to knowingly donate blood.

I know that I can decide not to donate blood or I may call the blood center's confidential Hotline number and ask that my blood not be used for transfusion without specifying the reason.

I am 16 years of age or older and I am voluntarily donating my blood to BloodSource for use as it deems advisable.

I understand that the primary use of my blood donation will be for transfusion purposes, but may also include further processing and/or research.

I understand that my blood will be tested for evidence of infections that can be transmitted by blood transfusion including, but not limited to, viral hepatitis, HIV (AIDS virus), HTLV, syphilis and other infectious agents. Should there be any circumstance(s) preventing an acceptable quality or amount in my test tubes, I understand that my blood will not be tested.

I understand that blood positive for any test or infections will not be used for transfusion. I will be notified of test results that are confirmed positive, important to my health, or affect my eligibility to donate blood. **However, notice of test results for the HIV (AIDS virus) may be delayed for 50 days.**

I understand any positive tests will be reported to county or state health agencies as required by law. If my blood tests are not clearly negative, my blood will not be used.

The donation process has been explained to me and all questions have been answered to my satisfaction. I understand that blood donors may experience reactions including, but not limited to, light-headedness, fainting, or bruising at the needle site.

I have answered all questions truthfully and to the best of my knowledge, to provide protection for me as a donor and for the safety of the person who receives my blood.

SIGNATURE: _____ DATE: _____

INTERVIEWER SIGNATURE: _____ INITIALS: _____ DATE: _____

Are you YES NO

1. Feeling healthy and well today? (AK)
2. Currently taking an antibiotic? (AO)
3. Currently taking any other medication for an infection? (AO)

Please read the Medication Deferral List.

4. Are you now taking or have you ever taken any medications on the Medication Deferral List? (AQ)
5. Have you read the educational materials?

In the past 48 hours

6. Have you taken aspirin or anything that has aspirin in it? (AP)

In the past 6 weeks

7. **Female donors:** Have you been pregnant or are you pregnant now? (AJ) **(Males: check "I am male.")** ☐ I am male

In the past 8 weeks have you

8. Donated blood, platelets or plasma? (AG)
9. Had any vaccinations or other shots? (AM)
10. Had contact with someone who had a smallpox vaccination? (AM)

In the past 16 weeks

11. Have you donated a double unit of red cells using an apheresis machine? (AG)

In the past 12 months have you

12. Had a blood transfusion? (AI)
13. Had a transplant such as organ, tissue, or bone marrow? (AI)
14. Had a graft such as bone or skin? (AI)
15. Come into contact with someone else's blood? (AI)
16. Had an accidental needle-stick? (AI)
17. Had sexual contact with anyone who has HIV/AIDS or has had a positive test for the HIV/AIDS virus? (BD)
18. Had sexual contact with a prostitute or anyone else who takes money or drugs, or other payment for sex? (BD)
19. Had sexual contact with anyone who has ever used needles to take drugs or steroids, or anything not prescribed by their doctor? (BD)
20. Had sexual contact with anyone who has hemophilia or has used clotting factor concentrates? (BD)
21. **Female donors:** Had sexual contact with a male who has ever had sexual contact with another male? (BD) **(Males: check "I am male.")** ☐ I am male
22. Had sexual contact with a person who has hepatitis? (AF)

In the past 12 months have you YES NO

23. Lived with a person who has hepatitis? (AF)
24. Had a tattoo? (AI)
25. Had ear or body piercing? (AI)
26. Had or been treated for syphilis or gonorrhea? (AD)
27. Been in juvenile detention, lockup, jail, or prison for more than 72 hours? (BX)

In the past 3 years have you

28. Been outside the United States or Canada? (AL)

From 1980 through 1996,

29. Did you spend time that adds up to three (3) months or more in the United Kingdom? (Review list of countries in the UK.) (DB)
30. Were you a member of the U.S. military, a civilian military employee, or a dependent of a member of the U.S. military? (DB)

From 1980 to the present, did you

31. Spend time that adds up to five (5) years or more in Europe? (Review list of countries in Europe.) (DB)
32. Receive a blood transfusion in the United Kingdom? (Review list of countries in the UK.) (DB)

From 1977 to the present, have you

33. Received money, drugs, or other payment for sex? (BP)
34. **Male donors:** Had sexual contact with another male, even once? (BQ) **(Females: check "I am female.")** ☐ I am female

Have you EVER

35. Had a positive test for the HIV/AIDS virus? (BS)
36. Used needles to take drugs, steroids, or anything not prescribed by your doctor? (BO)
37. Used clotting factor concentrates? (BV)
38. Had hepatitis? (AA)
39. Had malaria? (AL)
40. Had Chagas' disease? (BK)
41. Had babesiosis? (BK)
42. Received a dura mater (or brain covering) graft? (BJ)
43. Had any type of cancer, including leukemia? (BB)
44. Had any problems with your heart or lungs? (AC/AB)
45. Had a bleeding condition or a blood disease? (BV)
46. Had sexual contact with anyone who was born in or lived in Africa? (BZ)
47. Been in Africa? (BZ)
48. Have any of your relatives had Creutzfeldt-Jakob disease? (BJ)

Comments: _____

BloodSource, Sacramento, CA 95816-7089 BC.002 (Rev. 02/07) Version 1.1a

FIGURE 1-2 Uniform donor history questionnaire form. (Used with permission of BloodSource, Sacramento, California.)

MEDICATION DEFERRAL LIST

Please tell us if you are now taking or if you have <u>EVER</u> taken any of these medications:

- **Proscar© (finasteride)** – usually given for prostate gland enlargement
- **Avodart© (dutasteride)** – usually given for prostate enlargement
- **Propecia© (finasteride)** – usually given for baldness
- **Accutane© (Amnesteem©, Claravis©, Sotret©, isotretinoin)** – usually given for severe acne
- **Soriatane© (acitretin)** – usually given for severe psoriasis
- **Tegison© (etretinate)** – usually given for severe psoriasis
- **Growth Hormone from Human Pituitary Glands** – used usually for children with delayed or impaired growth
- **Insulin from Cows (Bovine, or Beef, Insulin)** – used to treat diabetes
- **Hepatitis B Immune Globulin** – given following an exposure to hepatitis B*
    - *This is different from the hepatitis B vaccine which is a series of 3 injections given over a 6-month period to prevent future infection from exposures to hepatitis B.
- **Unlicensed Vaccine** – usually associated with a research protocol

If you would like to know why these medicines affect you as a blood donor, please keep reading:

- If you have taken or are taking **Proscar, Avodart, Propecia, Accutane, Soriatane, or Tegison**, these medications can cause birth defects. Your donated blood could contain high enough levels to damage the unborn baby if transfused to a pregnant woman. Once the medication has been cleared from your blood, you may donate again. Following the last dose, the deferral period is one month for Proscar, Propecia and Accutane, six months for Avodart and three years for Soriatane. Tegison is a permanent deferral.

- **Growth hormone from human pituitary glands** was prescribed for children with delayed or impaired growth. The hormone was obtained from human pituitary glands, which are found in the brain. Some people who took this hormone developed a rare nervous system condition called Creutzfeldt-Jakob Disease (CJD, for short). The deferral is permanent.

- **Insulin from cows (bovine, or beef, insulin)** is an injected material used to treat diabetes. If this insulin was imported into the US from countries in which "Mad Cow Disease" has been found, it could contain material from infected cattle. There is concern that "Mad Cow Disease" is transmitted by transfusion. The deferral is indefinite.

- **Hepatitis B Immune Globulin (HBIG)** is an injected material used to prevent infection following an exposure to hepatitis B. HBIG does not prevent hepatitis B infection in every case, therefore persons who have received HBIG must wait 12 months to donate blood to be sure they were not infected since hepatitis B can be transmitted through transfusion to a patient.

- **Unlicensed Vaccine** is usually associated with a research protocol and the effect on blood transmission is unknown. Deferral is one year unless otherwise indicated by Medical Director.

EUROPEAN COUNTRIES LIST

European Countries List is used for deferral of donors based on geographic risk of bovine spongiform encephalopathy (BSE), commonly known as "mad cow disease".

Albania	Federal Republic of	Italy	Romania
Austria	Yugoslavia	Liechtenstein	Slovak Republic
Belgium	Finland	Luxembourg	Slovenia
Bosnia-Herzegovina	France	Macedonia	Spain
Bulgaria	Germany	Netherlands	Sweden
Croatia	Greece	Norway	Switzerland
Czech Republic	Hungary	Poland	United Kingdom*
Denmark	Republic of Ireland	Portugal	

*The United Kingdom should be taken to include all of the following:

England	Northern Ireland	Scotland	Wales
Isle of Man	Channel Islands	Gibraltar	Falkland Islands

THANK YOU for Saving a Life Today!

NRS.des.001 (30336) (BOOK VI – FORMS)
02/24/06 – Page 2 of 2

FIGURE 1-3   Medication deferral list. (Used with permission of BloodSource, Sacramento, California.)

minimum of 12.5 g/dL and the hematocrit a minimum of 38% for allogeneic donors.[6]

Temperature

The donor's oral temperature should not exceed 37.5°C or 99.5°F.[5] Higher temperatures may be an early indication of a fever due to a cold, flu, or other infection.

Blood Pressure

The systolic blood pressure should be no higher than 180 mm Hg and the diastolic pressure should be no higher than 100 mm Hg.[5] Prospective donors with higher readings may have their blood pressure evaluation repeated if it appears that the donor is anxious or recent activity indicates a possible cause for a high reading. In such case it may be advisable for the donor to rest for a few minutes before repeating the blood pressure evaluation.

Pulse

The prospective donor's pulse rate should be counted for a minimum of 15 to 30 seconds and should not reveal any pathologic cardiac irregularities. Acceptable pulse rates should be between 50 and 100 beats/min although some donors who are athletic or exercise regularly may present with an acceptable pulse rate lower than 50 beats/min.[5] Such exceptions should be addressed in each facility's policies and procedures.

CONFIDENTIAL UNIT EXCLUSION

All donors must be given the opportunity to indicate confidentially whether their blood is safe for transfusion.[10] Some facilities provide a second opportunity to prevent use of a unit from a *high-risk donor* through a process called *confidential unit exclusion* (CUE). The CUE may occur during or after the donation process, allowing the donor another chance to indicate whether the unit is suitable for transfusion. One such method involves giving donors a ballot labeled with the bar-coded unit number corresponding to the donation. The donor is asked to mark the appropriate box to determine whether his or her unit is safe to transfuse. The ballot is deposited into a ballot box when the donor leaves the phlebotomy area.

Another method is to use a bar-coded CUE sticker (Fig. 1-4). The donor is asked to apply the appropriate barcode sticker of "yes" or "no" to either the donor card or the blood bag. The sticker is read by a barcode scanner before the processing of the unit is complete.

Confidential *safety check* Instructions

As a final check to assure a safe blood supply, please place one of these labels in the space indicated on your medical history form.

THIS IS AN IMPORTANT PART OF THE DONATION PROCESS – CONSIDER YOUR CHOICE CAREFULLY. REGARDLESS OF YOUR CHOICE, ALL DONATIONS ARE TESTED.

USE	DON'T USE
YOU BELIEVE YOUR DONATION IS SAFE TO GIVE TO A PATIENT	YOUR DONATION TODAY WILL BE THROWN AWAY.

FIGURE 1-4 Confidential unit exclusion (CUE) sticker.

If the scan indicates the unit is unsuitable for transfusion, it is discarded.

A third method which is used most often is to provide the donor with instructions to call a toll-free telephone number if the donor believes that their unit should not be used for any reason. Although the intent is to offer a high-risk donor a way to anonymously request that their unit not be used, most often calls are from donors reporting an illness such as a cold or flu.

In all cases, a mechanism must be in place to allow retrieval and disposal of the unit. The donor must be informed whether testing will be performed and, if so, that notification will occur with any positive tests.[5] The donor should also be told whether a deferral is associated with the self-exclusion.

CONSENT

Following the medical evaluation and physical assessment, the donor's consent must be obtained prior to the donation process. The collection procedure should be explained in a manner that is understandable to the donor, including risks of the procedure and any testing performed to reduce the risk of transmission of infectious diseases.[5] The donor should also be apprised that there may be circumstances when infectious disease testing may not occur. Prior to signing the consent, the donor must have the opportunity to ask questions and to agree to or refuse consent.

BLOOD COLLECTION

Whole-blood donations remain the primary method for collecting blood, although advances in technology provide increased opportunities for blood centers to collect specific components. Automation has advanced from collecting just platelets and plasma to include automated collection of whole blood, which can be processed into separate RBC and plasma components during the collection process. Alternatively, the equivalent of two units of packed RBCs can be collected from one donor. The reader is directed to Chapter 2 to learn more about hemapheresis or automated procedures.

AABB standard states that a maximum of 10.5 mL of whole blood can be collected per kilogram of donor weight, including samples and the blood collection container.[5] Allogeneic donors must weigh a minimum of 110 lb or 50 kg; therefore, a maximum volume of 525 mL of whole blood can be collected from this minimum weight.

Blood is collected in a special container approved by the FDA. Blood bags must be sterile, pyrogen-free, and identified by a lot number.[6] In addition blood bags must contain enough anticoagulant proportional to the amount of blood collected. Most blood centers collect blood in either a 450-mL or 500-mL blood bag, which contains 63 mL of anticoagulant. Depending on the type of anticoagulant, additive solutions may be added to red cells to extend their expiry date. The type of anticoagulant or additive chosen determines the shelf life of the RBCs after collection as listed in Table 1-2. The reader is directed to Chapter 3 for more information on component preparation. Blood bags are also available in a variety of configurations. Most commonly, a blood bag set consists of a primary bag that contains the anticoagulant with one or more satellite bags attached to the primary bag as a closed system which complements the various blood components that can be made from the unit of whole blood.

Labeling and Identification

Proper labeling of the unit is essential for identifying it back to the individual donor from whom the blood was collected. A unique identification number is assigned to the unit at the time of collection and will follow the unit and its components throughout the processing and distribution of its components for transfusion.

TABLE 1-2	Anticoagulants in Whole-blood Containers
Anticoagulant	**Shelf Life (Days)**
Citrate phosphate dextrose (CPD)	21
Citrate phosphate dextrose adenine (CPDA-1)	35
Adenine-saline	42

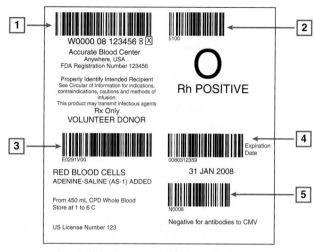

1 **Donation Identification Number**
2 **ABO/Rh Groups**
3 **Product Code**
4 **Expiration Date and Time**
5 **Special Testing**

FIGURE 1-5   ISBT 128 base label. (Used with permission of ICCBBA, San Bernardino, California.)

Effective May 1, 2008, the United States Industry Consensus Standard for the Uniform Labeling of Blood and Blood Components using ***ISBT 128*** (International Society of Blood Transfusion) replaced the 1985 FDA Uniform Labeling Guidelines that were based on the Codabar format.[11] The advantages of ISBT 128 is a labeling scheme that ensures a unique identification number and includes a center prefix that identifies the collecting blood center. In addition product codes are standardized that can be recognized internationally. Another advantage is the check digits in the barcode that can be used for detecting scanning errors, which will increase the safety of identifying the correct unit to the intended recipient.[11] Figure 1-5 is an example of a base ISBT label. The label is made up of four quadrants with the upper left containing the unique barcode identification number of the unit and information about the collecting facility. The upper right quadrant holds the blood type, the lower left quadrant displays the product code and the lower right quadrant displays the expiration date and any special attributes such as CMV antibody status.[12]

Selection of Vein and Arm Preparation

Prior to the collection of blood, both arms of the donor are inspected to select a suitable vein for phlebotomy as well as to ensure the venipuncture site is free of signs of infection or evidence suggestive of "track" marks or sclerotic veins that may indicate intravenous drug use.[6] If the donor's arms are questionable, the donor should be deferred from donating.

Blood is normally drawn from a vein in the antecubital area of the arm. A tourniquet or blood pressure cuff inflated to approximately 40 mm Hg may be used to make the vein more prominent. Once the vein is selected, the venipuncture site must be thoroughly cleansed in preparation for phlebotomy. Aseptic technique must be used throughout the procedure to minimize the risk of bacterial contamination.[5] The venipuncture site is vigorously cleansed with alcohol or an iodine preparation for a minimum of 30 seconds. Once the arm is cleansed, the vein must not be repalpated and sterility must be maintained.

Phlebotomy and Collection of Samples

Before the actual venipuncture, a final check must be made to verify the donor's identification. The donor's name is verified against the donor history record by asking the donor his or her name and verifying the assigned unit number on the donor history record with the numbers attached to the blood set, including all satellite bags and sample tubes.

The blood collection set for phlebotomy is prepared by placing the primary bag on a scale to measure the amount of blood to be drawn. The tubing is clamped with a hemostat at a point selected between the primary bag and the needle. The tourniquet should be reapplied or the blood pressure cuff reinflated to approximately 40 mm Hg. The donor may be asked to make a fist or to squeeze the hand around a squeeze grip several times. Just before needle insertion, the skin at the phlebotomy site should be pulled taut with care taken not to touch the preparation site. With a one-step, smooth action, the venipuncture is accomplished. The hemostat should be released and blood allowed to flow freely into the blood collection bag. The donor should be asked to squeeze his or her fist every few seconds to enhance the flow of the blood into the bag. The hub of the needle can be secured to the donor's arm with tape to prevent dislodging of the needle during the phlebotomy.

Although the actual phlebotomy usually takes less than 10 minutes, the donor should never be left unattended. The primary blood bag should be gently swirled or rocked from side to side to ensure adequate mixing of the blood and the anticoagulant. This mixing must take place at the beginning of the procedure and several times throughout the donation. When the approximate amount of blood has been collected, the tubing should be clamped with a hemostat or by some other suitable technique. Some facilities use automatic scales, which also mix the blood and anticoagulant in the blood bag. When the expected volume of blood is collected, the scale automatically stops mixing and pinches the tubing to prevent further collection of blood from the donor.

Specimen or sample tubes of blood to be used for laboratory testing must be obtained at the time of collection. AABB standards require that the tubes be properly labeled prior to or at the time of collection and must be re-identified with the unit of blood immediately after filling the tubes.[5]

There are a couple of methods for filling the sample tubes. Some blood collection bags have an attached sampling site in the tubing of the blood bag that uses an attached vacutainer holder with a needle that punctures the cork of the tube when the tube is pushed into the holder. Multiple tubes can be filled by this method since the blood is coming directly from the donor's vein. At the end of collection, the bottom of the vacutainer holder is closed to prevent exposure to the sampling needle. Another method includes a pouch attached to the blood bag tubing. Following the venipuncture, the blood is diverted to a pouch. Once the pouch is filled, it is clamped so that the blood can then continue flowing into the collection bag. The objective of filling a diversion pouch prior to filling the blood bag is to minimize the risk of bacterial contamination. Even though the venipuncture site has been thoroughly cleaned if any residual skin bacteria exist it will be diverted to the pouch instead of the blood bag. The blood in the diversion pouch can be used to fill the sample tubes. If platelets are to be prepared from whole-blood collections, the blood bag must include a draw line or inlet diversion pouch as a method of protection against bacterial contamination.[5]

Once the sample tubes have been filled, the needle can be removed from the donor's vein. Sterile gauze is applied over the venipuncture site and the donor is asked to raise the arm and apply pressure to the site. The needle should be detached from the tubing and discarded into a biohazardous waste container. It may be necessary to "strip" the tubing attached to the blood bag. Stripping is a procedure that pushes the blood in the tubing back into the primary bag. The bag is mixed and anticoagulated blood flows back into the tubing. The tubing is sealed in approximately 2-inch increments or segments. These segments must remain attached to the unit throughout processing and are used for compatibility testing of the unit for the intended recipient.[5]

Care of the Donor

The donor's venipuncture site should be inspected to ensure that the bleeding has ceased. Once bleeding has stopped, the arm is wrapped with a bandage and the donor is instructed in postphlebotomy care. The donor is also provided written instruction, and usually a toll-free number for the blood center is provided should the donor have any questions regarding the donation. The donor is allowed to rest a few minutes before proceeding to the refreshment area. The donor should be helped to sit up slowly and observed to make sure that his or her condition appears satisfactory. The donor may be ushered into the refreshment area where further observation can take place. While the donor relaxes and enjoys something to drink and a light snack, staff should be alert to watch for any signs of an adverse reaction.

The donor should be thanked for his or her valuable contribution and encouraged to return to donate again. All of the staff from registration through the donation process should impress upon the donor that he or she is very special. Special effort should be taken to ensure the donation visit has been a pleasurable experience.

DONOR REACTIONS

Most donors tolerate the withdrawal of a unit of blood quite well, but occasionally some donors experience adverse reactions. Donor room staff must be alert to recognize early symptoms of reactions and should be trained to prevent them or minimize them if possible. Studies have shown that first-time donors; donors with elevated pulse, low diastolic or high systolic blood pressure, or a history of previous reactions; and donors obviously nervous or apprehensive are more likely to experience a reaction to phlebotomy.[13] The collection facility must have a process for treating donor reactions and for providing emergency care if needed.[5]

The most frequent reactions are mild and are usually due to psychologic factors such as nervousness about donating or the sight of blood, but may also be due to unexplained causes. The usual symptoms are sweating, unnatural paleness, weakness, dizziness, nausea, rapid breathing, possible twitching or muscle spasms, and occasional fainting (*syncope*). If the donor is in the process of phlebotomy, the needle and tourniquet should be removed. See Box 1-2 for other measures to be taken with syncope reactions.

BOX 1-2

Actions to Take with Syncope Reactions

Elevation of the feet higher than the head
Removal or loosening of tight clothing
Placement of cold compresses on the forehead or behind the neck
Use of ammonia capsules
Allowing the donor to breathe into a paper bag (in case of hyperventilation)
Note: If the donor becomes unconscious, an adequate airway must be ensured.

If a donor feels nauseated or begins to vomit, the donor's head should be turned to the side to prevent possible aspiration. Cold compresses should be applied to the head and/or neck of the donor, and the donor should be instructed to breathe slowly and deeply.

The donor's blood pressure, pulse, and respiration should be monitored until the donor recovers. All information and actions taken should be documented on the donor record. Often, talking to the donor in a continuous, relaxing, calm voice takes the donor's mind off the donation process and may help provide the donor with the psychologic support to prevent the progression of a reaction.

Severe reactions are defined as any or all symptoms previously described with the addition of any or all of the following: involuntary muscle contractions, suspended respirations, cyanotic color, dilated and fixed pupils, excessive salivation, urinary or fecal incontinence, lip and inside-cheek biting, and convulsions. Immediate steps must be taken to prevent injury to the donor or those around the donor. All of the previously stated actions—discontinuing the phlebotomy, making sure the donor does not fall from the donor chair or bed, and making sure the donor's airway is adequate—should be followed. The blood bank physician should be notified as soon as possible. In some cases it may be necessary to call 911. Donor room personnel should be trained and prepared to administer cardiopulmonary resuscitation, if needed.

After the donor has recovered, he or she must be observed for a prolonged period of time before being released. The nature and treatment of the reaction should be recorded on the donor history record or on a separate incident form. This information should be evaluated to determine whether the donor should be accepted for future donations.

DONOR UNIT PROCESSING

All allogeneic units of blood are processed in the laboratory using FDA-licensed reagents. Policies and procedures must be available for the staff and strict compliance with regulatory requirements must be followed. Meticulous records must be kept of all steps, from component preparation and testing to final disposition, and these must allow for traceability and trackability.

In addition to testing the unit of blood, there must be a procedure in place to prevent the release of unsuitable blood.[2] Before the labeling process of the final component, all applicable records must be reviewed to ensure that blood and all components from unsuitable donors are quarantined and not issued for transfusion.[5]

Tests performed on donated blood are described in the following sections.

ABO

At the time of donation, each unit must be tested to determine the ABO group. This is determined by testing the donor red cells with commercial anti-A and anti-B sera and testing the corresponding serum against known A_1 and B reagent cells. The results of the forward and reverse tests must match. In addition, if the donor has donated previously, current records must be checked and compared against prior donations.[2] Blood cannot be released until any and all discrepancies are resolved.

Rh

The donor's red cells must be tested with anti-D sera. If the Rh test is positive, the donor is considered Rh positive. If the initial Rh test is negative, then the cells must be tested by a method to detect a weak D expression. If a weak D is determined, the donor is still considered Rh positive. If the cells test negative for weak D, the donor is considered Rh negative. Routine testing for additional red cell antigens is not required. Methods for determining ABO group and Rh blood type may use tubes, microplate, solid-phase adherence, gel, or automated instrumentation.

Detection of Unexpected Antibodies to Red Cell Antigens

The antibody screen is performed to identify donors with clinically significant unexpected antibodies in the plasma. Although the AABB standards require the performance of this test only on donors with a history of transfusions or pregnancy, most facilities find it easier to test all units collected.[5] Units identified with a positive antibody must be processed so that there is a minimal amount of plasma to avoid possible reactions with a recipient's red cells. Such units should be labeled to indicate the antibody detected. Techniques for performing the antibody screen include tube, microtiter, solid-phase red cell adherence and gel techniques.

Serologic Test for Syphilis

Although the FDA and AABB require a serologic test for syphilis (STS), the likelihood of syphilis transmission is remote; the spirochete is not able to survive in blood stored for more than 72 hours at 1°C to 6°C. However, it is believed that donors with a positive test for syphilis may be at greater risk for the transmission of other sexually transmitted diseases, such as HIV and hepatitis. There is currently a 12-month deferral for donors with a confirmed positive STS or a history of syphilis or gonorrhea. The most common methodologies used in screening for syphilis are the rapid plasma reagin test and an automated treponemal screening test.

Infectious Disease Testing

In addition to the test for syphilis, a sample of blood from each donation is tested for other *infectious disease markers*. These include hepatitis B surface antigen (HBsAg), antibody to hepatitis B core antigen (anti-HBc), antibody to hepatitis C virus (anti-HCV), HCV RNA, antibody to HIV-1 and 2 (anti-HIV1/2), HIV RNA, antibody to human T-lymphotrophic virus (anti-HTLV I/II) and West Nile Virus (WNV). Most recently with advances in molecular testing assays have been developed that detect the genetic material of viruses or *nucleic acid testing* (NAT). NAT has been developed for HIV RNA, HCV RNA, hepatitis B DNA (HBV) and WNV. Since NAT detects the actual virus, the *window period* or the time that an individual is infected with the virus to the time of detection is narrowed considerably as compared to traditional assays of antibody detection in the serum.

Other than NAT the most commonly used testing methods for screening in the United States are enzyme immunoassays (EIAs) or enzyme-linked immunosorbent assays (ELISAs). These methods use a solid support such as bead or microplate coated with an antibody or antigen. The general principle is that serum or plasma is incubated with the solid support coated with antigen or antibody. If the corresponding antigen or antibody is present in the serum or plasma, it binds to the solid support forming an antigen–antibody complex. Excess serum or plasma is washed away, and a conjugate which is enzyme labeled is added that has the ability to bind to the antigen–antibody complex. A substrate appropriate to the enzyme is then added and a color reaction develops that is read on a spectrophotometer. The reactivity or nonreactivity of a sample is determined by comparison of the optical density reading with a calculated cutoff. Samples that test initially positive must be repeated again in duplicate on another run. On repeat, if two of the three total results are reactive, the unit is considered to be positive for the specific test and must be discarded. Some tests have further supplemental or confirmatory testing to determine if the screening test was a true-positive or a false-positive reaction. A newer methodology uses microparticles for the substrate and chemiluminescence for detecting the antigen–antibody reaction.

Hepatitis B Surface Antigen

Until 1985, and except for the STS, routine donor screening for HBsAg was the only required test for infectious disease. Inclusion of this test in 1972 and the requirement for a volunteer donor base dramatically reduced the transmission of hepatitis B through blood transfusion. The sensitivity of HBsAg has increased with a new generation of assays. The FDA requires that HBsAg detection assays to test whole blood and blood components have a lower limit of detection capability of 0.5 ng HBsAg/mL or less in order to adequately reduce the risk of transmission of communicable disease.[14]

Antibody to Hepatitis B Core Antigen

In 1984, before the implementation of the test for hepatitis C, the test for antibody to hepatitis B core (anti-HBc) was added to the *donor processing* profile as *surrogate markers* for non-A, non-B hepatitis. If an individual has a positive test for anti-HBc and a negative HBsAg, it may mean that the person once had hepatitis B, but has recovered from the infection. Currently donors who test positive for anti-HBc on two different donations are indefinitely deferred from donating blood; however, some donors have never been exposed to hepatitis B and are considered to have a false-positive test result. With the licensure of HBV NAT, the FDA is considering an algorithm for re-entry of such donors based on current negative test results with HBsAg, anti-HBc, and HBV NAT.[15]

Antibody to Hepatitis C Virus

It is believed that hepatitis C accounts for most of the non-A, non-B transfusion-transmitted hepatitis cases. Most donors who test positive for the antibody are asymptomatic and have no recollection of a previous exposure to hepatitis C. It is recommended that these donors seek medical evaluation because hepatitis C infection may lead to long-term liver disease.

Antibody to Human Immunodeficiency Virus 1 and 2

In 1985, the first test for anti-HIV-1 was licensed. In 1992, a combination anti-HIV-1/2 test was licensed that detects antibody to both HIV-1 and 2.[16] HIV-1 is more common in the United States and HIV-2 in western Africa. In 1994, a new strain of HIV, HIV-1 group O, was discovered that could jeopardize the blood supply, and the FDA mandated that all manufacturers of test kits for anti-HIV enhance the sensitivity of their kits to detect HIV-1, group O viruses.[17]

Antibody to Human T-lymphotrophic Virus I and II

Human T-lymphotrophic virus I (HTLV-I) is a retrovirus that is transmitted in cellular components and is associated with adult T-cell leukemia in some individuals. There is also an association with cases of tropical spastic paraparesis or HTLV-I-associated myelopathy. HTLV-II is usually associated with intravenous drug use, especially with individuals who share needles and syringes.

West Nile Virus

Since the 1980s, the focus in blood banking has been on increasing the safety of the blood supply. Advances in technology have provided increased sensitivity in screening tests and earlier detection of blood-borne diseases including vector-borne infectious agents such as WNV and *Trypanosome cruzi*.

WNV is primarily a seasonal epidemic in North America, which occurs from summer to early fall.[18] WNV is transmitted by a bite from a mosquito and can cause transfusion-transmitted infections through blood transfusion or organ transplantation. Potential donors who are infected with WNV are deferred from donating for 120 days from diagnosis or if their blood was implicated in a transfusion-transmitted infection.

Testing for WNV is by NAT both in mini-pools (MP-NAT) and as individual tests (ID-NAT). AABB has provided recommendations for WNV testing including triggering criteria for determining when to convert from MP-NAT to ID-NAT and back to ID-NAT.[18] The three minimum criteria recommended are (1) the number of positive reactions within a defined period; (2) a rate of greater than 1 reactive donation per 1,000 donations; and (3) the defined geographic area for the first two criteria. In addition AABB has established on their web site a WNV Biovigilance Network reporting tool for reporting WNV activity.

Chagas Disease

Chagas disease is caused by the parasite *T. cruzi*. Humans are usually infected through a bug bite caused by the triatomine bugs also known as the kissing or reduvid bug. Transmission occurs when the feces of the bug are rubbed into the bug bite wound. The parasite is found in the continental Americas, usually Latin America but is finding its way in North America with the change in population demographics. There have been rare cases reported of transmission through transfusion and organ transplantation in the United States and Canada.[19]

An ELISA test for the detection of the parasite was licensed in 2007.[19] Although the test is not required, many blood centers have implemented the assay. Different approaches have been discussed with some centers screening all donors at each and every donation and others screening only one time. Donors who test reactive are deferred indefinitely.

Cytomegalovirus

Most people who are positive for the antibody to **cytomegalovirus** (CMV) probably do not even know when the infection occurred. In most cases, the infection is mild, with few if any complications. The prevalence of the antibody in most donor populations is 40% to 60% or more. CMV, however, can cause serious illness in patients such as premature infants, bone marrow or organ transplant patients, or others who may be immunosuppressed. For these patients, it is important to provide CMV antibody-negative units for transfusion. There is no deferral associated with CMV reactivity.

SPECIAL DONATIONS

Autologous Donation

Perhaps the safest donation that an individual can receive is a unit of his or her own blood. This is called an *autologous* donation and is donated by an individual for his or her own use, most often for an elective surgery. Autologous donations can also occur during a surgical procedure. There are five categories of autologous blood donations:

- Preoperative: One or more units of blood are donated before an elective surgery and are stored until needed. The actual collection of whole-blood units is done in the same way as for allogeneic donors.
- Normovolemic hemodilution: One or more units of blood are collected from the surgery patient within 24 hours or immediately before the start of surgery. The patient's blood volume is returned to normal with fluids, and autologous blood may be returned to the patient after the surgery is complete.
- *Intraoperative salvage*: Blood is collected from the operative site or from an extracorporeal circuit, is centrifuged or washed, and reinfused through a filter to the patient.
- *Postoperative salvage*: Blood is collected from the surgical site from body cavities, joint spaces, and other closed operative or trauma sites in the postoperative period, filtered, and returned to the patient within 6 hours of collection.

- Long-term storage: Autologous blood may be stored frozen for 10 years with or without a definite need. Patients requiring more blood than they can donate before surgery may use this option. Another reason for long-term storage would be for an individual who is known to lack a public antigen or who has developed rare or multiple clinically significant antibodies that make it difficult to find compatible blood if needed.

Autologous Blood Collection

Blood collection for later autologous transfusion requires the consent of the donor patient's physician. Because of the special circumstances surrounding the requirements for an autologous transfusion, the criteria for donor selection are not as rigid as for allogeneic donors.[5] Once the unit is collected, it must be segregated and used solely for autologous transfusion unless it meets allogeneic criteria and procedures are in place to change its designation. Written policies and procedures must be available for all autologous donor selection and blood collection. Any deviations must be approved by the blood bank physician.[20] Some guidelines are that the hemoglobin must be a minimum of 11 g/dL and the packed cell volume no less than 33%. The frequency of phlebotomy must be determined by blood bank policy and the donor's physician. Iron supplements often are given before beginning of and during the donations as an aid to increasing the donor's hematocrit. Occasionally erythropoietin is used to stimulate erythrocyte production. Blood should not be drawn within 72 hours of the anticipated surgery or transfusion, to allow for the replenishment of an adequate blood volume.

Contrary to allogeneic donors, autologous donors do not have a weight limit. For patients weighing less than 50 kg, there should be a proportional reduction in the volume of blood collected and a proportional reduction in the anticoagulant solution used.

Another limiting factor is that donors must not be accepted who are being treated for bacteremia or have a significant bacterial infection that can be associated with bacteremia.[5] Bacteria or bacterial products in the blood might reach dangerous levels in a short storage period and cause adverse reactions when reinfused.

Testing of Blood

The FDA does not require the same testing for autologous blood as for allogeneic units (see Box 1-3). Testing is to be performed on an autologous unit prior to shipping on at least the first unit shipped during each 30-day period.[20,21] If all units collected for a

BOX 1-3

Tests Required by the FDA on Allogeneic
Donations

ABO	Anti-HTLV-I/II
Rh	HCV RNA
HBsAg	HIV-1 RNA
Anti-HBc	STS
Anti-HCV	WNV RNA (seasonal)
Anti-HIV-1/2	

series are shipped together, testing may be performed on the most recently donated unit. Most blood centers incorporate autologous units into their routine donor processing and do not differentiate testing from allogeneic units. Provisions are made, however, if a unit is collected at the same site at which it will be used, such as at a hospital-based blood bank. In such cases, only the ABO and Rh testing need be performed and infectious disease testing is not required.[22]

If a unit tests positive for one of the required infectious disease markers and the unit is to be shipped to another facility, the shipping facility must notify the receiving transfusion service. In addition, the patient's physician and the patient must be informed of any medically significant abnormalities.[5]

Labeling Requirements

In addition to routine labeling requirements, the following information must appear on a label or tag attached to the blood container: the donor classification statement "Autologous Donor"; "For Autologous Use Only" (if the unit does not meet routine allogeneic criteria for transfusion); the patient's name; the name of the facility where the patient is to be transfused (if available); and the patient's hospital registration number (or social security number, birth date, or similar identifying information). If tests are repeatedly reactive for infectious disease markers or if confirmatory testing is positive, a "Biohazard' label must be placed on each unit from the donor. If the unit is untested the phrase "Donor Untested" is applied or "Donor tested within the last 30 days."[22]

Directed Donation

With the heightened awareness of AIDS and HIV infection in the 1980s, many recipients of blood and their families demanded units drawn from family and friends. Emotionally, it was felt that the blood from

these *directed donors* was safer than the blood from the general blood supply. Evidence, however, has shown that directed donors are no safer than volunteer blood donors. In recent years, the number of directed donors has decreased dramatically in the United States.

Directed donors in general present at a blood center or blood bank with the intent that their blood will be given to a specific recipient but there is no guarantee. If a donor's blood is ABO and Rh type incompatible or if the CMV status is incompatible, the unit is returned to the general inventory. In addition the donor must meet all of the same donor qualifications of an allogeneic donor including full testing of the unit.

Often, directed donors are immediate family members of the intended recipient. Because of this familial connection, there may be a higher risk of graft-versus-host disease (GVHD). This condition occurs when immunocompetent donor lymphocytes engraft and multiply in a recipient. The engrafted donor cells then react against the recipient's cells and destroy the tissues. To reduce the risk of GVHD, all cellular blood components from blood relatives of the intended recipient are irradiated with a minimum of 25 Gy.[23]

Dedicated Donors

Dedicated donors are another category similar to directed donors. The difference, however, is that dedicated donors are individuals who donate specifically for a single recipient. Donated units must be tested as for allogeneic units with the exception if multiple donations are made for the same recipient testing may occur on the first donation within a 30-day period. Units must be labeled with "Donor Tested Within the Last 30 Days" label and must have a label with intended recipient information containing the name and identifying information of the recipient.[22]

Therapeutic Phlebotomy

A *therapeutic phlebotomy* is when a unit of blood is withdrawn from an individual on a periodic basis as treatment for an underlying medical condition. Therapeutic phlebotomies must be prescribed by a patient's physician and approved by the blood bank physician. The prescription must indicate the amount of blood to be withdrawn, the frequency, and the desired hematocrit level postdonation. The blood should not be used for allogeneic transfusion unless the indication for the therapeutic phlebotomy is for hereditary hemochromatosis; the phlebotomy is performed at no expense to the individual; and the program has received a variance from the FDA.[24] If the unit is crossed over for allogeneic use, the donor must meet all other donor qualifications.

SUMMARY

The process of collecting blood and maintaining the blood supply is complex. The standard in blood banking has changed tremendously with public awareness and demands to increase the safety of the blood supply. The blood banking community is more proactive in identifying potential risks to the blood supply and has taken steps to implement a biovigilance network for monitoring new infectious disease such as WNV and Chagas.

Today, with the intense screening procedures that are in place, including the medical history questionnaire and donor screening tests, the current blood supply is safer than it has ever been. However, the future supply of blood is uncertain. With the addition of new regulatory requirements and new deferrals, the pool of eligible donors continues to shrink. The implementation of new tests and regulations, as well as general changes in health care, all affect how blood banks and blood centers must operate. Resource sharing, affiliations, mergers, and competition will affect the collection of blood and how it is processed. Equipment is becoming more sophisticated to accommodate testing and development of new technology continues. State-of-the-art technology will continue with the application of molecular genetics for the detection of infectious agents.

Whatever the changes, blood will still be needed for patients requiring a transfusion. Blood banks and blood centers must continue to meet the needs of their customers, both the patients and the donors who provide the blood.

Review Questions

1. The minimum hemoglobin concentration for an autologous donor is:
   a. 11 g/dL
   b. 12 g/dL
   c. 2.5 g/dL
   d. 13 g/dL

2. Which documents are to be used for the medical history assessment?
   a. Medication deferral list
   b. Uniform donor history questionnaire
   c. Donor history questionnaire brochure
   d. Donor education material
   e. All of the above

3. With the addition of sample tubes, donors who weigh 50 kg may donate the following maximum amount of whole blood:
   a. 450 mL
   b. 475 mL
   c. 500 mL
   d. 525 mL
   e. 575 mL

4. To ensure traceability and trackability of a collected unit, a unique identifying number should be applied to:
   a. Donor history record
   b. Primary collection bag
   c. All pilot tubes
   d. CUE ballot
   e. All of the above

5. Which of the following tests is not required with routine donor unit processing?
   a. HBsAG
   b. Serologic test for syphilis
   c. CMV
   d. ABO/Rh
   e. None of the above

6. Which of the following is required to help ensure a safe blood supply?
   a. Trained, qualified personnel
   b. Written policies and procedures
   c. Documentation of all steps to ensure traceability and trackability
   d. Accurate and truthful information from a donor
   e. All of the above

7. Which of the following blood pressures is unacceptable for donation?
   a. 120/70
   b. 145/90
   c. 190/60
   d. 110/80
   e. All are acceptable

8. Which of the following steps should be taken in the event of a donor reaction?
   a. Elevate feet
   b. Apply cold compresses
   c. Ensure adequate airway
   d. Use ammonia capsule
   e. All of the above

9. Which test is not required on an allogeneic donation?
   a. HIV-1/2 antibody
   b. HCV NAT
   c. HBc antibody
   d. STS for syphilis
   e. Chagas

REFERENCES

1. Riley W, Schwei M, McCullough J. The United States' potential blood donor pool: estimating the prevalence of donor-exclusion factors on the pool of potential donors. *Transfusion*. 2007;47(7):1180–1188.

2. Food and Drug Administration. *Guideline for Quality Assurance in Blood Establishments, July 11, 1995*. Rockville, MD; Docket No. 91N-0450.

3. *Code of Federal Regulations*. Title 21 CFR, Part 606. Washington, DC: US Government Printing Office; 2007.

4. HHS, FDA. Compliance Policy Guidance for FDA Staff and Industry, Blood Donor Incentives. Sec. 230.150. ORA web site. Available at: http://www.fda.gov/ICECI/ComplianceManuals/CompliancePolicyGuidanceManual/ucm122798.htm.

5. Price TH, ed. *Standards for Blood Banks and Transfusion Services*. 25th ed. Bethesda, MD: AABB; 2008.

6. *Code of Federal Regulations*. Title 21 CFR, Part 640. Washington, DC: US Government Printing Office; 2007.

7. Food and Drug Administration. *Guidance for Industry: Implementation of Acceptable Full-length Donor History Questionnaire and Accompanying Materials for Use in Screening Donors of Blood and Blood Components*. Rockville, MD; October 2006.

8. Fridey JL, Townsend MJ, Kessler DA. et al. A question of clarity: redesigning the American Association of Blood Banks blood donor history questionnaire—a chronology and model for donor screening. *Trans Med Rev*. 2007;21(3):181–204.

9. AABB. *Association Bulletin #04-05: Uniform Donor History Questionnaire*. Bethesda, MD; June 2004.

10. Food and Drug Administration. *Memorandum: Revised Recommendations for the Prevention of Human Immunodeficiency Virus (HIV) Transmission by Blood and Blood Products*. Rockville, MD; April 1992.

11. AABB. *Association Bulletin #05-12: ISBT 128 Implementation*. Bethesda, MD; October 2005.

12. Ashford P, ed. (2006). *ISBT 128: An Introduction*. 3rd ed. York, PA: ICCBBA, Inc.

13. AABB. *Association Bulletin #08-04: Strategies to Reduce Adverse Reactions and Injuries in Younger Donors*. Bethesda, MD: AABB; August 2008.

14. Food and Drug Administration. *Guidance for Industry: Adequate and Appropriate Donor Screening Tests for Hepatitis B; Hepatitis B Surface Antigen (Bag) Assays Used to Test Donors of Whole Blood and Blood Components, Including Source Plasma and Source Leukocytes*. Rockville, MD; November 2007.

15. Food and Drug Administration. Center for Biologics Evaluation and Research. Frequently Asked Questions. Available at: http://www.fda.gov/cber/faq/bldfaq.htm. Accessed February 25, 2008.

16. Food and Drug Administration. *Memorandum: Revised Recommendations for the Prevention of Human Immunodeficiency Virus (HIV) Transmission by Blood Ban Blood Products*. Rockville, MD; April 1992.

17. Food and Drug Administration. *Memorandum: Interim Recommendations for Deferral of Donors at Increased Risk for HIV-1 Group Infection*. Rockville, MD; December 1996.

18. AABB. *Association Bulletin #07-02: West Nile Virus—Recommendations for Triggering Individual Donation Nucleic Acid Testing and Developing a Communication Plan*. Bethesda, MD; April 2007.

19. AABB. *Association Bulletin #06-08: Information Concerning Implementation of a Licensed Test for Antibodies to Trypanosoma cruzi*. Bethesda, MD; December 2006.

20. Food and Drug Administration. *Memorandum: Guidance for Autologous Blood and Blood Components*. Rockville, MD; March 1989.

21. Food and Drug Administration. *Memorandum: Autologous Blood Collection and Processing Procedures*. Rockville, MD; February 1990.

22. *Code of Federal Regulations*. Title 21 CFR, Part 610. Washington, DC: US Government Printing Office, 2007.

23. Food and Drug Administration. *Memorandum: Recommendations Regarding License Amendments and Procedures for Gamma Irradiation of Blood Products*. Rockville, MD; July 1993.

24. Food and Drug Administration. *Guidance for Industry: Variances for Blood Collection from Individuals with Hereditary Hemochromatosis*. Rockville, MD; August 2001.

AUTOMATED COLLECTION OF BLOOD PRODUCTS

SUSAN M. CONNOR

OBJECTIVES

After completion of this chapter, the reader will be able to:

1. Explain what the term "apheresis" means.
2. Describe the history of hemapheresis.
3. Explain separation by centrifugation.
4. Discuss the various apheresis technologies available and the basic principles of separation for each technology.
5. Explain separation by membrane filtration.
6. Explain separation by adsorption.
7. List the components that may be collected by apheresis.
8. Discuss the role of apheresis in therapeutic applications.
9. List the types of therapeutic cytapheresis procedures that can be performed.
10. Discuss the diseases that are treated by therapeutic apheresis.

KEY WORDS

Apheresis	Membrane filtration
Erythrocytapheresis	Plasmapheresis
Hemapheresis	Plateletpheresis
Hematopoietic progenitor cells	Surge
Immunoadsorption	Therapeutic apheresis
Leukapheresis	Thromocytapheresis
Lymphocytapheresis	

*A*pheresis means "to remove" and *heme* refers to "blood." In *hemapheresis*, whole blood is removed from a donor or patient and separated into components. One or more of the components is retained, with the remaining portion recombined and returned to the donor or patient. This technology has made it possible to just select the component needed or to automate the production of multiple components. Blood cells, platelets, plasma, and/or granulocytes may be collected using automated blood collection devices based on apheresis technology.

Apheresis is also used as a treatment modality. Although there are difficulties in the documentation of benefit, there is general agreement that therapeutic apheresis is effective treatment for certain disease conditions. The following is a list of diseases that are treated by therapeutic apheresis:[1,2]

- Hematology/oncology conditions
- Paraproteinemias
- Hyperleukocytosis
- Thrombocythemia
- Thrombotic thrombocytopenic purpura/ hemolytic uremic syndrome
- Sickle cell disease
- Posttransfusion purpura
- Neurology conditions
- Acute Guillain–Barré syndrome
- Chronic inflammatory polyneuropathy
- Myasthenia gravis
- Cryoglobulinemia
- Rapidly progressive glomerulonephritis associated with antibody to neutrophil cytoplasmic antigen
- Homozygous type II familial hypercholesterolemia
- Refsum disease

BRIEF HISTORY ON THE SEPARATION OF BLOOD

Throughout history, blood has been seen as a crucial element of disease and health. In the past, the practice of eliminating disease or unwanted elements was accomplished by bloodletting. This was used as a therapeutic technique for many centuries and is still sometimes used today. The practice of bloodletting eventually led to *plasmapheresis*, first described by Abel and coworkers in 1914. This was followed by donor and therapeutic *hemapheresis*, which later combined centrifugal force technology to fractionate on a much larger scale. The use of centrifugal force marked the beginning of semiautomated, large-scale *plasmapheresis* of donors for the collection of plasma.

The development of sterile plastic containers later allowed manual separation of plasma from whole blood using a series of interconnected disposable bags. This system allowed separation of platelets, the first cellular element harvested by apheresis. Up to this time, all procedures were manual because automated systems were not available. In the late 1950s and early 1960s, two centrifugation systems were developed that permitted, for the first time, the automated harvesting of granulocytes, platelets, and plasma. In addition, therapeutic plasmapheresis and cytapheresis, the removal of cellular elements, became a means of direct therapeutic treatment. In recent years, the refinements and improvements made to centrifugation technology, including additional automation, have increased safety to the donor, reduced time to perform the procedures, and improved yields for component collections.

SEPARATION BY CENTRIFUGATION (INTERMITTENT OR CONTINUOUS FLOW)

Many automated collection devices use centrifugal force to separate the blood into its various components. Separation is based on the differences in component density. A controlled amount of anticoagulant solution is added to the whole blood as it is drawn from the donor. This mixture of anticoagulant and blood is then pumped into a rotating bowl, chamber, or tubular rotor, and it is here that the whole blood is separated into layers of components based on each component's density. In component harvest, the desired layer of component is collected and the remaining portions of the blood are returned to the donor.

Automated centrifugal separation of blood components is performed by either intermittent- or continuous-flow cell separation. In the intermittent-flow method, the centrifuge container is alternately filled and emptied, and the same venous access line is used for both withdrawal and return of the blood. In the continuous-flow method, two venous access sites are used. One access site is used for removal of the whole blood from the donor or patient and the other site is used for return of the "unwanted" portion back to the donor. Some instruments can be used in either continuous- or intermittent-flow mode.

All automated separation devices require prepackaged sets of sterile bags, tubing, and centrifugal devices. Most of these are specifically designed for use on instruments of a particular manufacturer.

The IBM 2997 cell separator, which was a continuous-flow machine, set a high standard for low cross-contamination when the instrument was introduced in the late 1970s. It also offered a shorter procedure time than existing technology. This technology has now been replaced with systems that automate the procedure, further reduce cross-cellular contamination, and enhance efficiency. The first automated cell separation device to use a closed system for platelet storage (CS-3000) was introduced in the 1980s by the Fenwal Division, Baxter Healthcare Corporation (Deerfield, IL).[3]

BOWL TECHNOLOGY

The separation technology based on the work of Dr. Jack Latham uses a disposable bowl with a rotating seal and discontinuous flow. The blood to be processed enters the bowl through the inlet port and feed tube (Fig. 2-1). When the blood meets the base of the bowl, it is redirected to the angular velocity of the bowl. Centrifugal force causes the blood to migrate out to the space between the body and the outer core, which is the separation chamber. It is here, in the separation chamber that the blood separates into its components. The plasma is forced out of the separation chamber and into the upper assembly from which it enters the effluent tube. The plasma leaves the bowl through the effluent tube and outlet port and goes into the effluent line. Platelets and white blood cells follow, leaving the red blood cells (RBCs) in the bowl. RBCs and plasma are then returned separately through a reinfusion bag.

A technology known as *"surge"* was introduced by the Haemonetics Corporation (Braintree, MA). "Surge" is a Haemonetics term for the elutriation (washing) of platelets away from the buffy coat. In surge technology, plasma is recirculated through the bowl at a high-enough velocity to pull platelets out but leave white and RBCs behind. This potentially increases platelet yields and reduces white blood cell contamination. Haemonetics used surge elutriation and Latham bowl technology to create a small machine, the MCS+ 3P Mobile Collection System. This

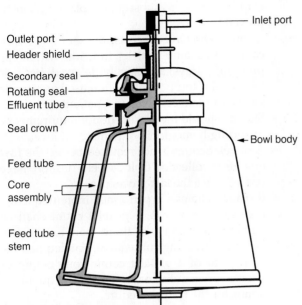

FIGURE 2-1 Latham bowl technology. (From Smit Sibinga H: Fluid dynamics in a bowl: A modeling approach for separation of blood in a bowl. Braintree. MA, Haemonetics Corp., 1991. This is a copyrighted work of Haemonetics Corporation and is used by permission of Haemonetics Corporation.)

was the first-generation device developed. The MCS+ 9000 (Fig. 2-2) is dedicated to blood component collection, specifically platelets, red cells, and plasma.[4]

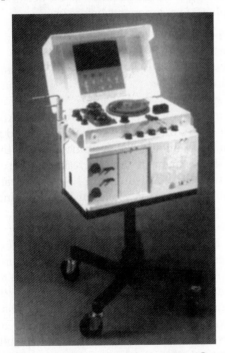

FIGURE 2-2 Mobile Collection System. (Courtesy Haemonetics Corporation. This is a copyrighted work of Haemonetics Corporation and is used by permission of Haemonetics Corporation.)

Whenever components intended for transfusion are collected by automation, the donor must give informed consent. Although the collection and preparation processes are different from those used for whole-blood–derived components, storage conditions, transportation requirements, and some quality control steps are essentially the same. The facility must maintain written protocols for all procedures used and must keep records for each procedure as required by AABB Standards for Blood Banks and Transfusion Services.[5]

Automated Blood Products

Blood components collected by automation for transfusion include:

- Plasma
- Platelets
- Red blood cells
- Granulocyte concentrates
- *Hematopoietic progenitor cells* (stem cells)

Plasma

Plasma for transfusion, fresh frozen plasma (FFP), or plasma for source plasma for further manufacturing can be collected by automation. Large plasma collection facilities use pheresis to harvest source plasma that is further manufactured into pharmaceuticals.

Selection of the Donor

Plasma donations may be classified as either "occasional plasmapheresis" or "serial plasmapheresis." The procedure is classified as occasional plasmapheresis when the donation of plasma is made no more often than once in 4 weeks. Serial plasmapheresis occurs when the donation is more frequent than every 4 weeks.

Donor selection and monitoring for the "occasional" donor are the same as for whole-blood donations. Donor selection and monitoring for the "serial" donor have additional requirements. These include:

- Donors must provide informed consent and be observed closely during the procedure, and emergency medical care must be available.
- The red cell loss, including samples collected for testing, must not exceed 25 mL/wk, so that no more than 200 mL of red cells are removed each 8 weeks. If the donor's red cells cannot be returned during the procedure, the donor must be deferred from donating hemapheresis or whole blood for 4 weeks.

- At least 48 hours should elapse between successive procedures and donors should not, ordinarily, undergo more than two procedures within a 7-day period.
- At the time of initial plasmapheresis and at 4-month intervals thereafter, serum or plasma must be tested for total protein and immunoglobulin G (IgG) and immunoglobulin M (IgM) content. Results must be within normal limits.
- A qualified, licensed physician, well trained in all aspects of hemapheresis, must be responsible for the program.

Testing of the Component

Plasma units collected as FFP intended for transfusion require the same testing as for red cell components. Plasma collected as source plasma for manufacturing of plasma derivatives has different requirements for viral testing. The requirements depend on whether the donation is occasional or serial.

Platelets

Large numbers of platelets can be obtained from a single donor using automated collection or apheresis. Single-donor plasma helps to limit the number of different donor exposures patients receive when large doses of platelets are required. Crossmatch-compatible or human leukocyte antigen (HLA)-matched platelets from an apheresis platelet donor may be the only source of platelets for alloimmunized patients, who have become refractory to random allogeneic platelets. Advances in technology now offer leukoreduction during the automated collection of platelets. This eliminates the need for filtration to remove the unwanted white blood cells before transfusion.

Selection of the Donor

Donors for *plateletpheresis* may donate more frequently than whole-blood donors; however, they must meet all other donor criteria. The AABB has written standards on the collection of apheresis platelets. These standards include the following:[5]

- There must be at least 48 hours between donations.
- The donor should not have a plateletpheresis procedure performed more than twice in a week or 24 times in a year.
- If the donor donates a unit of whole blood or if it is impossible to return the donor's red cells during plateletpheresis, at least 4 weeks should

elapse before a subsequent plateletpheresis procedure.
- Donors who have taken aspirin, or other medications that alter platelet function within the previous 3 days, are usually deferred, because the platelet component is often used as a single source of platelets given to a patient.
- Donors should meet usual donor requirements, including hemoglobin or hematocrit level.
- A platelet count is not required before the first apheresis collection or if 4 weeks or more have passed since the last procedure.
- If plateletpheresis is performed more frequently than every 4 weeks, a platelet count shall be obtained and must be more than $150,000/\mu L$ before performing subsequent plateletpheresis.
- The result of a platelet count done before or after a procedure may be used to qualify a donor for the next procedure.

The U.S. Food and Drug Administration (FDA) requires that the total volume of plasma collected should be no more than 500 mL (or 600 mL for donors weighing more than 80 kg [176 lb]). The platelet count of each unit should be determined and kept on record, but it does not have to be recorded on the product label.

Testing of the Component

The following tests are required to be performed on plateletpheresis components before use:[3]

- ABO and Rh type
- Test for unexpected alloantibodies
- Tests for markers for transfusion-transmitted diseases

Testing requirements differ between the AABB and the FDA. The AABB requires each unit be tested unless the donor is undergoing repeated procedures for the support of a single patient. In this case, testing for the disease markers need be repeated only at 10-day intervals. The FDA requires testing only once at the beginning of a donation period not to exceed 30 days.

If the unit from plateletpheresis contains visible red cells, a hematocrit should be determined. The FDA guidelines require that if the unit contains more than 2 mL of red cells, a sample for compatibility testing must be attached to the platelet container. AABB standards require a crossmatch be performed if the component contains more than 5 mL of red cells.

Plasma for use as FFP may also be collected concurrently during plateletpheresis procedures. If the collection of concurrent plasma is performed more often than once every 8 weeks, additional testing of the donor is required. These tests are the same as those required for frequent plasma donors, described in the section on Plasma.

Red Blood Cells

Both AABB standards and FDA-approved protocols address the removal of two allogeneic or autologous red blood cell units every 16 weeks by an automated apheresis method.[5] Saline infusion is used to minimize volume depletion, and the procedure is limited to persons who are larger and have higher hematocrits than current minimum standards for whole-blood donors.

Selection of the Donor

Donors for automated red cell collections must meet all criteria for the donation of whole blood but the minimum requirements for weight and hematocrit are higher. The donation interval is also longer (112 days as opposed to 56 days).

Testing of the Component

Testing of red cells collected by automated methods is the same as for whole blood.

Granulocyte Concentrates

Through automated collections, granulocytes for transfusion may be collected. This process is called *leukapheresis*. (For drugs used in leukapheresis, see Box 2-1.) This product is a suspension of granulocytes, plasma, and RBC contaminants. The indications for granulocyte transfusion are controversial. In general, there is agreement that effectiveness depends on an adequate dose ($>1 \times 10^{10}$ granulocytes/day) and crossmatch compatibility (no recipient antibodies to granulocyte antigens). There is renewed interest in granulocyte transfusion therapy for adults because much larger cell doses from donors who receive colony-stimulating factors are available. Some success

---

BOX 2-1

Drugs Used in Leukapheresis

Hydroxyethyl starch: Sedimenting agent that allows enhanced granulocyte harvest

Corticosteroids: Drugs (i.e., prednisone, dexamethasone) that mobilize granulocytes from the marginal pool, thus increasing the harvest

Growth factors: Drugs (colony-stimulating factor) that increase granulocyte yields

---

with granulocyte transfusions has been observed in the treatment of septic infants.[6]

Selection of the Donor

Donors must meet the AABB and FDA standards for blood donation. Additionally donors/recipients should be ABO compatible due to the large number of red cells in the concentrate. Cytomegalovirus (CMV)-seronegative patients, particularly if immunocompromised, should receive granulocytes only from CMV-seronegative donors. For an adequate yield, the donor's granulocyte count must be increased. Stimulation with 60-mg prednisone or 8-mg dexamethasone is well tolerated and will raise the donor's granulocyte count two-to threefold.

In the nonalloimmunized patient, it is not necessary to select donors on the basis of leukocyte compatibility. However, alloimmunized recipients are more likely to experience transfusion reactions if transfused with incompatible granulocytes, and the transfusion will be ineffective. Reliable detection of alloimmunization requires a panel of sophisticated tests, not available in most institutions. Alternatively, the likelihood of alloimmunization may be estimated by the patient's history of transfusion reactions, response to random donor platelets, and results of antibody screens.

Testing of the Component

The testing required on granulocyte concentrates collected by apheresis include:

- ABO and Rh types
- Antibody screen
- Testing for infectious disease markers

If possible, testing should be performed during the donation to avoid delay in administration of the granulocyte concentrate. RBC contamination of the granulocyte concentrate does occur. Therefore, the red cells should be ABO compatible with the recipient of the concentrate, and if more than 5 mL of red cells are present, a crossmatch must be performed with the recipient's serum before transfusion.

Because granulocyte function deteriorates during storage, concentrates should be transfused as soon as possible after preparation. The AABB standards state a storage temperature of 20°C to 24°C for no longer than 24 hours. Agitation is not suggested during storage.

Hematopoietic Progenitor Cells (Stem Cells)

Hematopoietic progenitor cells, also referred to as peripheral blood stem cells, collected by automated collections are used for both autologous and allogeneic purposes. Autologous progenitor cells are collected for bone marrow reconstitution in patients with cancer, leukemia in remission, and various lymphomas. In allogeneic collections, the progenitor cells are collected from the circulating blood of healthy donors.

Selection of Donors

The selection criteria of these donors are similar to the requirements of apheresis donors, with allowances for the special importance of HLA matching of the donors to the patient for bone marrow reconstitution.[7]

Testing of the Component

The testing recommended on the donor's blood is identical to the testing required on whole blood. When repeated collections are performed on a single donor to support a single recipient, testing is performed at least every 10 days.

The AABB has standards for labeling, storage, and record keeping of the progenitor cells. Progenitor cells that are intended for reconstitution of the bone marrow must not be irradiated. They may be further processed and cryopreserved for future use.

Impacts of Automated Blood Collections

The collection of multiple components from a single donor through automated blood collections has many impacts. The areas of larger impact include:

- The blood supply
- Donor recruiting process
- Blood center and transfusion services operations

At any one time, the United Sates needs a cushion of a million units of blood available to meet the nation's blood needs. Meeting this need must be managed through blood collection strategies to obtain more of the components needed by patients. Collections based on what is needed currently means maximizing your precious raw material, the donor, to meeting the needs of the patient. Moving to a component-driven collection strategy involves changing the way a blood center manages blood inventory, donor recruitment, and blood collections.

Donor Recruiting

Recruiting and maintaining an adequate number of blood donors is one of the most challenging aspects of managing a blood center. With more and more potential donors being deferred, meeting the collection goals with the current donor population is a challenge. Automated blood collections also have benefits to the donor, which can be used to enhance the donor recruitment, retention, and recognition efforts. Donor satisfaction as well as selective product collection can also result in increased donation frequency. With automated collection technology, the donor experiences advantages and increased comforts including a smaller needle for the collection, rehydration, and the gratification of giving multiple transfusable products per donation experience.

Operations

Blood Collection Facilities

The collection of blood components by automation also impacts the blood center and transfusion service operations. In addition to the decrease in eligible donors, more regulatory requirements add to the cost of producing blood components. The reimbursement for the blood products also has not historically kept pace with the expense associated with providing blood components. For the blood center, automated collections change the way the blood inventory is managed, how the donors are scheduled and with that staff scheduling, staff training, and job satisfaction. Training of the staff requires knowledge of the device and a competence in operating the technology, in addition to donor and product care and management. This can provide opportunity for staff development and job advancements with additional responsibilities in operating the various automated collection devices.

Automated blood collection offers improved collections planning and logistics. It provides the flexibility to make short-notice adjustments in component collections to better fit with the inventory needs. With the use of automated collection technology, you can collect the specific components in multiple combinations from a single donor, returning the blood components not collected back to the donor. This results in more products needed from few donors.

Transfusion Facilities

For the transfusion service, blood components prepared from automation offer all the benefits that blood components derived from whole blood with the addition of even more consistent product dosing or yield. Automation allows the collection to be controlled to offer a more consistent end product, given the variations in the raw material, that is, the individual donors and their varying hematologic characteristics.

THERAPEUTIC USES OF APHERESIS

Methodologies

Separation by Membrane Filtration

Filtration technology, which has been widely used in hemodialysis and hemofiltration for many decades, has also been introduced for both donor and *therapeutic apheresis*. Filtration methods use microporous membranes that are made up of a wide variety of materials and hollow fibers, arranged either in parallel plates or a flat membrane. In these instruments, whole blood flows across a membrane containing pores of a defined size. Higher pressure in the blood phase than in the filtrate pushes plasma constituents smaller than the pore size through the membrane and into the filtrate. Surface properties of the inner membrane surface repel cellular elements in the laminar flow of blood so that platelets are not activated and RBC survival is not shortened. The plasma then passes through the membrane matrix and escapes at right angles to the stream of flow. A degree of selection to the type of plasma protein removed is made possible by varying the pore size of the membrane.

Separation by Immunoadsorption

Selective extraction of pathologic materials in the plasma or blood cells has theoretical advantages over the depletion of all plasma constituents. Both centrifugal devices and *membrane filtration* can be adapted to allow selective removal of specific soluble plasma constituents using the principles of affinity chromatography. In affinity chromatography, a substance with a specific binding affinity is linked to an insoluble matrix specifically to bind its complementary substance from a mixture of materials in suspension or solution. The sorbent, or ligand, coupled to the matrix can be a chemical compound such as heparin, charcoal, dextran sulfate, protein, antigen, or antibody.

Immunoadsorption uses an antigen or antibody as the ligand, or a protein capable of removing immune reactants or complementary substances by a mechanism of immunochemistry. The ability to absorb a specific undesirable substance is made possible by the specificity of the immune reaction.

Therapeutic Plasmapheresis

Therapeutic plasmapheresis (also referred to as therapeutic plasma exchange) is the removal of abnormal cells, plasma, or plasma proteins and their replacement with either crystalloid, albumin or, in some cases, FFP. This technique is useful in the treatment of a number of disease states.

Therapeutic Cytapheresis

Therapeutic cytapheresis is the removal or harvesting of cellular elements and includes:

- *Thrombocytapheresis* (plateletpheresis)
- *Leukapheresis* (white blood cell reduction)
- *Thrombocytapheresis* (also known as therapeutic plateletpheresis)
- *Lymphocytapheresis* (lymphocyte reduction)
- *Erythrocytapheresis* (RBC exchange/reduction)

Thrombocytapheresis

Thrombocytapheresis is the removal of abnormal amounts of platelets, with the accompanying risk of hemorrhage or thrombosis.

Leukapheresis

Therapeutic leukapheresis is intended significantly to reduce the peripheral count of leukemic cells and therefore reduce leukostasis and leukemic infiltration. The treatment is often done in conjunction with the use of chemotherapy and radiation therapy to control the leukocyte count.

Lymphocytapheresis

The purpose of lymphocytapheresis is to remove large quantities of lymphocytes, and therefore generate immunosuppression or immune modulation. It is used for the direct therapeutic manipulation of the patient's cell-mediated immunity, in contrast to plasma exchange that would primarily affect humoral immunity.

Erythrocytapheresis

This therapeutic procedure is most often used in sickle cell disease. It removes abnormal red cells, aids in the correction of anemia, and exchanges the abnormal sickle cells with normal cells.

SUMMARY

The collection of blood components through automation has evolved from the early work of plasmapheresis in the early 1900s, which was performed manually, to the introduction of automated and "closed-systems," which allowed for the storage of the blood components collected. Automated collection of blood components has made rapid and impressive progress over the past decade. Dramatic growth has been seen in automated red cell collections, as shown in the following chart.

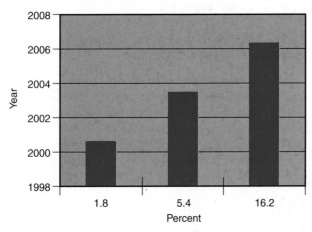

Most of this increase in automated red cell collections has been in the double red cell collections. John Zeman, President, Zeman & Company, Inc., predicts that blood centers will continue to utilize this technology to help maximize their donor base as well as red cell collections. The projection is that automated red cell collections will reach as high as 30% to 35% of total collections and plateau, until blood centers determine if they are going to proceed into the next level of automated collections.

Continued refinement and improvements have been made through the efforts of research and development. The technology has been exponentially advanced to provide improvements to the separation principles, adding more automation, increased safety and comfort for the donor, reduction in the time to perform the collections, and improvements to the blood product yields.

Review Questions

1. Most apheresis equipment uses which of the following methods for separation?
   a. separation by centrifugation
   b. separation by membrane filtration
   c. separation by adsorption
   d. separation by osmosis
2. "Surge" elutriation and the Latham bowl technology are used by which system?
   a. COBE Spectra
   b. Haemonetics MCS
   c. Baxter CS-3000
   d. Fresenius AS 104
3. Cellular components for transfusion that may be collected by apheresis include:
   a. platelet concentrates
   b. granulocyte concentrates
   c. hematopoietic progenitor cells
   d. all of the above
4. AABB standards allow plateletpheresis procedures on a donor up to _____ times in 1 year.
   a. 12
   b. 18
   c. 24
   d. 34
5. If a donor donates a unit of whole blood or if it is impossible to return the donor's red cells during plateletpheresis, at least _____ weeks should elapse before a subsequent plateletpheresis procedure.
   a. 2
   b. 4
   c. 6
   d. 8
6. If a unit of plateletpheresis component contains visible red cells, a hematocrit should be determined. The FDA guidelines require a sample for compatibility be attached to the platelet container if more than _____ mL of red cells are present.
   a. 2
   b. 3
   c. 4
   d. 5
7. If collection of concurrent plasma is performed on a plateletpheresis donor more often than once every _____ weeks, additional testing of the donor is required.
   a. 4
   b. 6
   c. 8
   d. 12
8. AABB standards require that granulocyte components collected by apheresis contain a minimum of _____ granulocytes in about 75% of units tested.
   a. 1.0×10^{10}
   b. 5.5×10^{10}
   c. 3.0×10^{10}
   d. 1.5×10^{10}
9. Therapeutic cytapheresis includes:
   a. thrombocytapheresis
   b. leukapheresis
   c. erythrocytapheresis
   d. all of the above
10. The collection of blood components through automated blood collections has an impact on:
    a. the blood supply
    b. the donor recruiting process
    c. the blood center and transfusion services operations
    d. all of the above

REFERENCES

1. AABB Extracorporeal Therapy Committee. *Guidelines for Therapeutic Hemapheresis.* Bethesda, MD: American Association of Blood Banks; 1992.
2. Strauss RG, Ciavarella D, Gilcher RO, et al.; Haemonetics Corporation. An overview of current managements. *J Clin Apheresis.* 1993;8:189.
3. Baxter Healthcare Corporation. *Operator's Manual CS-3000 Plus Blood Cell Separator.* Deerfield, IL: Baxter Healthcare Corporation Fenwal Division; 1991.
4. *Haemonetics Mobile Collection System Owner's Operating and Maintenance Manual.* Braintree, MA: Haemonetics Corporation; 1991.
5. *Standard for Blood Banks and Transfusion Services.* Bethesda, MD: AABB; May 1, 2008.
6. Strauss RG. Granulocyte transfusion. In: Rossi EC, Simon TL, Moss GS, Gould SA, eds. *Principles of Transfusion Medicine.* 2nd ed. Baltimore, MD: Williams & Wilkins; 1995:321.
7. Read EJ, ed. Standard for Bone Marrow and Peripheral Blood Progenitor Cells. Excerpted from *Standards for Blood Banks and Transfusion Services.* 16th ed. Bethesda, MD: American Association of Blood Banks; 1995.

ADDITIONAL READINGS

Aubuchon JP, Dumont LJ, Herschel L, et al. Automated collection of double red cell units with a variable-volume separation chamber. *Transfusion.* 2007;48:147–152.

Brecher ME, ed. *Technical Manual.* 15th ed. Bethesda, MD: AABB; 2005.

Moog R, Zeiler T, Heuft H, et al. *Revised Guideline for the Collection of Platelets, Pheresis.* Coded FDA Memorandum. Food and Drug Administration; October 7, 1988.

Moog R, Zeiler T, Heuft HG. Collection of WBC-reduced single-donor PLT concentrates with a new blood cell separator: results of a multicenter study. *Transfusion.* 2003;43:1107.

Simon T. The collection of platelet by apheresis procedure. *Transfus Med Rev.* 1994;8:133.

Strauss RG. Granulocyte transfusion. In: Rossi EC, Simon TL, Moss GS, et al., eds. *Principles of Transfusion Medicine.* 2nd ed. Baltimore, MD: Williams & Wilkins; 1995:321.

BLOOD COMPONENTS: PREPARATION, STORAGE, AND TRANSPORT

KAY CRULL

OBJECTIVES

After completion of this chapter, the reader will be able to:

1. List the elements of whole blood anticoagulant and the purpose of each element.
2. Describe the characteristics of blood collection sets and the various components that can be prepared from whole blood.
3. Describe the preparation process for each blood component and the clinical indications for their use.
4. Describe the approved uses of a sterile connection device and their advantages.
5. Discuss the indications for irradiated blood components.
6. Describe the storage and transportation temperature requirements for each blood component.

KEY WORDS

Additive solution
Anticoagulant
Blood component
Closed system
Deglycerolization
2,3-Diphosphoglycerate
Graft-versus-host disease
Irradiation
Open system

Rejuvenation
Sterile connecting devices

STANDARD ABBREVIATIONS

2,3-DPG: 2,3-Diphospho-glycerate

AABB: AABB (formerly American Association of Blood Banks)

ATP: Adenosine triphosphate

CFR: Code of Federal Regulations

DEHP: Di-(2-ethylhexyl) phthalate

FDA: Food and Drug Administration

GMPs: Good manufacturing practices

GVHD: Graft-versus-host disease

HLAs: Human leukocyte antigens

ISBT: International Society of Blood Transfusion

SOPs: Standard operating procedures

TRALI: Transfusion-related acute lung injury

Various **blood components** can be harvested from a single donation of whole blood by differential centrifugation or automated separation devices. The purpose of the separation is to supply the specific blood component needed to provide treatment for the patient. One unit of whole blood, separated into its various components, can thus benefit multiple patients. An efficient system must be in place to ensure proper component production, as well as proper storage and transport of the blood products within the allowed time frame and at the correct temperature.

Multiple regulatory bodies produce standards and requirements for the preparation of blood components. These various agencies are described in other chapters. Blood is considered a drug and is dispensed by prescription to treat patients. As such, all steps in the collection and processing of blood must conform to good manufacturing practices (GMPs) as established in the Code of Federal Regulations (CFR). Records of all identification or lot numbers of collection bags, equipment, and disposable supplies utilized in component production must be maintained according to regulations (GMPs and CFR) and standard operating procedures (SOPs). This chapter describes the production, storage, and transportation of blood and blood components from whole blood in accordance with regulations and standards.

ANTICOAGULANTS

Anticoagulants are provided by the manufacturer in the whole blood collection set and mixed with donor blood during the collection process. Blood will clot during the collection process unless mixed with anticoagulant contained within the container. The primary anticoagulants used are citrate-phosphate-dextrose (CPD), citrate-phosphate-2-dextrose (CP2D), and citrate-phosphate-dextrose plus adenine (CPDA-1). The composition of each anticoagulant is described in Table 3-1. All of the anticoagulants contain citrate, which chelates calcium in the blood, thus inhibiting the calcium-dependent steps in the coagulation cascade. The anticoagulants also contain sodium biphosphate that maintains the pH of the component during storage. Maintaining the pH level is necessary to maintain adequate levels of **2,3-diphosphoglycerate (2,3-DPG)**. Red blood cells (RBCs) deliver oxygen (O$_2$) from the lungs to body tissues using a differential affinity for the O$_2$ molecule. In areas of high partial pressure like the lungs, the affinity of the RBC for O$_2$ is increased. As the RBCs travel to the tissues and the partial pressure decreases, the affinity for oxygen decreases and the oxygen molecules are released from the RBCs to the tissues. The amount of 2,3-DPG in the blood modulates the affinity of the RBC for oxygen. Though the level of 2,3-DPG decreases during the first 2 weeks of storage, the levels within the transfused RBC regenerates within 12 to 24 hours of transfusion.[1,2]

Dextrose is added to the collection set as a substrate for adenosine triphosphate (ATP) production needed for cellular energy. When adenine is also provided in the anticoagulant solution (CPDA-1) for ATP production, the RBCs have better viability than in anticoagulant solutions that do not contain adenine, such as CPD or CP2D. This improved viability is reflected in the shelf life of the RBCs per anticoagulant type. Despite the chemicals in the anticoagulant, the environment within the blood bag is different from the environment in the body. The impact of this altered environment on the blood product is referred to as the storage lesion. It is these biochemical changes within the blood container that determine the maximum length of storage time for each component. The changes include progressively increasing hemolysis, progressively decreasing levels of ATP and 2,3-DPG, and ultimately reduced posttransfusion survival. All of these changes are captured in Table 3-2. Blood collected in CPD or CP2D has a shelf life of 21 days when stored at 1°C to 6°C. Blood collected in CPDA-1 has a shelf life of 35 days when stored at 1°C to 6°C.[3] Expiration time is generally at midnight on the date of expiration unless the product is altered and requires a time of expiration.

TABLE 3-1	Summary Chart of Anticoagulants					
Anticoagulant/Preservative	Trisodium Citrate (g/L)	Citric Acid (g/L)	Monobasic Sodium Phosphate (g/L)	Dextrose (g/L)	Adenine (g/L)	Shelf Life (days)
A(ACD-A)[a]	22.0	8.0	0	24.5	0	21
CPD	26.3	3.27	2.22	25.5	0	21
CP2D	26.3	3.27	2.22	51.1	0	21
CPDA-1	26.3	3.27	2.22	31.9	0.275	35

[a]A(ACD-A) is used as a preservative for apheresis components as recommended by the manufacturer.
Source: Circular of Information, 2002.

TABLE 3-2   **Biochemical Changes of Stored Red Blood Cells**

Variable	CPD		CPDA-1				AS-1*	AS-3*	AS-5*
	Whole Blood	Red Blood Cells	Whole Blood	Red Blood Cells	Whole Blood	Red Blood Cells	Red Blood Cells	Red Blood Cells	Red Blood Cells
Days of storage	0	21	0	0	35	35	42	42	42
% Viable cells (24 h posttransfusion)	100	80	100	100	79	71	76	83	80
pH (measured at 37°C)	7.20	6.84	7.55	7.60	6.98	6.71	6.6	6.5	6.5
ATP (% of initial value)	100	86	100	100	56	45	60	58	68.5
2,3-DPG (% of initial value)	100	44	100	100	<10	<10	<5	<10	<5
Plasma K^+ (mmol/L)	3.9	21	5.10	4.20	27.30	78.50	50	N/A	45.6

*Based on information supplied by the manufacturer.

CPD, citrate-phosphate-dextrose; CPDA-1, citrate-phosphate-dextrose-adenine; AS, additive solution.

Source: Roback JD, et al., eds. *Technical Manual.* 16th ed. Bethesda, MD: American Association of Blood Banks; 2008:289.

ADDITIVE SOLUTIONS

Additive solutions were developed to further extend the shelf life of the RBCs. The additive solution contains saline, adenine, and dextrose for enhanced ATP generation, and other minor substances that improve RBC viability in the blood bag. The expiration date of the RBCs is extended to 42 days.[3] The absolute composition of the additive solution varies by blood collection set manufacturer. The additive solution is added to the RBCs after the plasma is separated/expressed into the satellite bag. The final hematocrit of RBCs containing the additive solution is between 55% and 65% compared to RBCs without an additive solution which must be less than 80%.[4] The decreased hematocrit and viscosity of an additive RBC facilitates improved flow of the blood during transfusion. The additive solution must be added to the RBCs within 72 hours of collection or per manufacturer's instructions.

BLOOD COLLECTION SETS

Blood collection sets must be approved by the Food and Drug Administration (FDA) or the appropriate governing body. The sets must be sterile, uncolored, transparent, and hermetically sealed. Key properties for the containers are flexibility, pliability, and toughness. They should be kink and scratch resistant. They should allow adequate gas exchange of O_2 and CO_2, but prevent evaporation of the liquid. The base label applied by the manufacturer and any other label added to the collection set must utilize an FDA-approved adhesive that will not leach into the container and adversely affect the blood component. The whole blood collection set is a sterile *closed system* with a primary blood bag and one or more satellite containers. The collection set may have a leukoreduction filter integrally incorporated into the set to filter the white blood cells out of either whole blood or RBCs. The primary blood bag is used for the whole blood collection. It contains a standard premeasured volume of anticoagulant for the amount of blood collected as established for the container by the manufacturer. After collection is completed, the blood bag can be processed and separated into components. Blood centers carefully evaluate the number and type of each component to produce from the collected whole blood to eliminate any wastage of a limited resource. The number of satellite bags on a collection set depends on what blood components need to be prepared (Table 3-3).

A closed system collection set maintains the sterility of the blood. During component production, no external air is introduced into the system; instead an internal access port or cannula allows the transfer of components from bag to bag. If for any reason the seal is broken or compromised, the expiration date and time must be changed and the set is now considered an *open system*. For an open system, if a product is stored from 1°C to 6°C, it must be transfused within 24 hours after the system is opened. If a product has an assigned storage temperature of 20°C to 24°C, then the unit must be transfused within 4 hours after the system becomes

TABLE 3-3	Examples of Bag Types and Components That Can Be Made in a Closed System	
Bag Type	**Number of Satellite Bags**	**Components**
Single	0	Whole blood
Double	1	Red blood cells/plasma
Triple	2	Red blood cells/platelets/plasma or red blood cells/cryoprecipitate/plasma
Quadruple	3	Red blood cells/platelets/cryoprecipitate/plasma

open.[3] These reduced times are required to prevent the possibility of bacterial contamination and subsequent growth.

Sterile connecting devices (SCDs) are available that allow the connection of one bag to another without exposure to air by sterilely welding compatible tubing together. Examples of use are listed in Table 3-4, although this list is not exhaustive. When an SCD is utilized, the component set is still considered to be a closed system and the original expiration date and time of the component remains the same.[5] An inspection of each weld must be performed; if the integrity of the weld is suspect, the container must be considered to be an open system.

Most blood bags are produced of polyvinyl chloride (PVC) plastic. The addition of the plasticizer di-(2-ethylhexyl) phthalate (DEHP) allows many different PVC configurations to be produced ranging from very rigid to soft and highly flexible materials.[3] It also enables the containers to be transparent. Everyone is exposed to DEHP in small amounts but medical patients may receive higher levels of exposure because DEHP can leach out of plastic medical devices into solutions. Exposure to DEHP has produced a range of adverse effects in laboratory animals, particularly on the development of the male reproductive system. No reports of these adverse effects in humans have been reported, but there have been no studies to rule them out. The FDA does suggest precautions to limit the exposure of developing males to DEHP and has advocated not using medical bags or devices that can leach DEHP when an alternative is available.[6] The European Union has performed a risk assessment and stated that DEHP poses no general risk to human health; however, a scientific review is also being undertaken to determine if there is risk to select patients, such as children and neonates, undergoing long-term blood transfusion.[7] Because of these purported adverse effects of prolonged exposure to DEHP, many manufacturers are responding with alternative products.

TABLE 3-4	Use of Sterile Connecting Devices for Modification of Collection Containers
Use	**Comment**
To prepare components	Some examples include adding a bag to make cryoprecipitate, adding solution to the RBC unit, or adding an in-line filter
To pool blood products	Appropriate use of a sterile connecting device (SCD) to pool platelets or cryoprecipitate prepared from whole blood collection may obviate potential contamination from the spike and port entries commonly used
To prepare an aliquot for pediatric use and divided units	FDA provides specific guidance if this activity is considered to be manufacturing new products
To attach processing solutions	Examples include washing and freezing RBCs
To add an FDA-cleared leukocyte reduction filter	To prepare prestorage leukocyte-reduced RBCs
To remove samples from blood product containers for testing	Label may need revision if cell count of the product is affected

Source: Roback JD, et al. eds. *Technical Manual.* 16th ed. Bethesda, MD: American Association of Blood Banks; 2008:192.

WHOLE BLOOD

The use of whole blood for transfusion has greatly decreased over the last 30 years as the ability to prepare and store each component separately to maximize its specific therapeutic properties increased. Though whole blood contains all of the cellular and plasma components of blood, the labile coagulation factors diminish over time and the platelets become nonfunctional at the 1°C to 6°C storage temperature. The average unit of collected whole blood is usually either 450 or 500 mL of blood (±10%) plus the appropriate premeasured anticoagulant. The clinical indications for whole blood are few and whole blood transfusions should be reserved for those few patients who need both volume replacement and oxygen-carrying capacity. Fully tested fresh whole blood can be used for neonatal exchange transfusion. Alternatively, whole blood for exchange transfusions may be reconstituted by combining RBCs and fresh frozen plasma (FFP) to a predetermined hematocrit level. Documentation and labeling of this reconstituted product should be in full accordance with regulations, standards, and SOPs.

RED BLOOD CELLS

The three major blood components—RBCs, platelets, and plasma—are prepared from whole blood through a differential centrifugation process to separate the various components. Varying the centrifuge spin time and spin speed (rpm) produces different components based on optimal yield parameters and product requirement of the patient. This centrifugation process is primarily a manual process, though automated and semiautomated equipment is now approved by the FDA for use in the United States and eliminates many of the manual steps in whole blood processing.

Once the whole blood unit is centrifuged, the plasma is expressed from the RBC through the internal access port into one of the satellite bags attached to the collection set. Maintaining a closed system is essential. If an additive solution is not used, enough plasma must remain with the RBCs to ensure a hematocrit of less than 80%. If the hematocrit of the RBCs without additive is greater than 80%, an adequate supply of nutrients and preservatives may not remain for the RBCs to remain viable for the entire storage period.[8] Routine quality control testing is required to verify proper preparation of the RBCs, including hematocrit value. When additive solution is added to the RBCs, the maximum amount of plasma can be expressed into the satellite bag. The plasma is removed prior to the addition of the additive solution. The additive solution must be added to the RBCs within 72 hours of collection or according to the manufacturer's specifications. Each RBC unit has tubing attached that is divided into 13 to 15 segments for crossmatching or other investigations.[3] A segment from each blood unit should have the unique donation identification number attached and can be reserved at the blood center for a period of time defined in the SOPs.

RBC transfusions are indicated for those patients needing additional red cell mass for oxygen-carrying capacity due to blood loss or a disease process that reduces RBC count. One unit of RBCs will typically increase the hematocrit of a nonbleeding patient by approximately 3% and the hemoglobin by approximately 1 g/dL.

Red Blood Cells Leukocytes Reduced

Red cells are often prepared in a method that will reduce the white blood cell or leukocyte mass. There are multiple reasons to remove the white blood cells: to reduce the number of febrile nonhemolytic transfusion reactions, to reduce the incidence of human leukocyte antigen (HLA) or granulocyte alloimmunization, to minimize the transmission of transmissible diseases such as cytomegalovirus (CMV), and to reduce the number of adverse transfusion reactions to stored blood from the enzymes and cytokines released by the leukocytes as they deteriorate and fragment.[8] Several methods are available to prepare leukoreduced RBCs for transfusion. Leukocytes can be filtered out of the RBCs at the patient's bedside through the use of a special leukoreduction filter attached to the transfusion set. One disadvantage of this technique is that it does not have a quality control mechanism to evaluate the effectiveness of the filter. This technique also does not prevent all adverse reactions and alloimmunization to the white blood cell fragments that accumulate in stored red cell units.[9]

Leukocytes can also be removed from either whole blood or RBCs during component production. One method uses a collection set that has an integral in-line leukoreduction filter in the set, allowing the whole blood or RBC to be filtered during the component preparation process. Filtering during component preparation ensures that most leukocytes are still intact and are removed before they fragment with age and storage. When an in-line filter is used with whole blood, the whole blood is passed through the leukoreduction filter resulting in leukoreduced whole blood, which is then processed into components. If an in-line integral filter is used with RBCs after plasma removal, the RBCs are passed through the filter into an attached satellite bag and the bag is sealed. This is a closed system and the red cells maintain their original expiration date. Integral filters require filtration within 72 hours of collection, or per manufacturer's instructions.

A third method for producing leukoreduced RBCs involves using a leukoreduction filter that is connected to the RBCs utilizing an SCD which attaches to the filter while maintaining a closed system. This method allows blood centers to only use a leukoreduction filter on acceptable units after full testing and processing. This method is labor intensive and has significant documentation requirements. Filtration must occur within 120 hours of collection to ensure that most leukocytes are filtered intact.

A leukoreduced RBC must contain 85% of the original RBCs and the final leukocyte count must be less than 5×10^6.[4] The most common reason for filter failure is blood from a donor with sickle cell trait. The cells will either incompletely filter or the filter will remove an inadequate number of leukocytes to qualify as a leukoreduced unit. A robust quality control program must be in place with a sampling strategy that ensures a leukoreduced product is prepared in accordance with all regulations and standards. RBCs and leukoreduced RBCs can also be collected via apheresis technology as described in Chapter 2 of this text. Quality control requirements for leukoreduction are the same for apheresis collections and leukoreduced units prepared from whole blood or RBCs. The RBC collected by automation also has a specific weight and hemoglobin or hematocrit requirement, depending on the instrument.

Red Blood Cells Washed

A clinician may order washed RBCs for a patient who is IgA deficient when an IgA-deficient cellular component is not available, or if the patient is experiencing multiple and progressively worse allergic reactions to transfused units. Washing RBCs is not considered to be an effective method to achieve leukoreduced RBCs. Washed cells are usually prepared with an automated cell washing device, though they can be prepared by a manual batch centrifugation process. The automated cell washer adds 0.9% saline to the RBCs, centrifuges the product, and then expresses the supernatant plasma and saline mixture into a waste bag. This process is repeated several times using 1 to 2 L of saline solution. Because the closed blood bag system is compromised and because all the anticoagulant and plasma nutrients are also washed away, the expiration date of a prepared washed RBC is 24 hours from the time the system is opened. Storage temperature remains at 1° C to 6° C.

Red Blood Cells Frozen or Red Blood Cells Deglycerolized

RBCs may be frozen for later use under specific circumstances. These cells without additive solution must be frozen within 6 days of collection. RBCs with additive solution may be frozen any time before the expiration date. Frozen RBCs are stored at $-65°C$.[4] The primary reasons for freezing RBCs are for special transfusion circumstances, such as autologous use, and to store very rare units based on their specific phenotype. The frozen RBCs have an expiration date of 10 years. The process to freeze and subsequently thaw and deglycerolize RBCs for patient use is time-consuming, expensive, and loses valuable red cell mass. Once the cells are prepared for transfusion, the open system process leads to a short shelf life of 24 hours. This makes frozen red cells impractical as a routine inventory item, although interest in frozen blood has increased because of the strategic importance of a frozen blood reserve to military planning.

A cryoprotective agent must be used for the red cells to protect the RBC membrane from rupture due to ice crystals that would form within the RBCs while freezing. Glycerol is the most commonly used cryoprotective agent. The RBCs and the glycerol are each warmed to 25°C to 37°C as the first step in preparation. Approximately 100 mL of glycerol is added to the warmed RBCs and the unit is gently mixed, then allowed to equilibrate undisturbed for at least 10 to 30 minutes. This process allows the glycerol to be transported across the RBC membrane. The remaining glycerol is transferred to a special polyolefin bag that is more resistant to breaking than the usual PVC bag. The glycerolized RBCs are then added with slow agitation. The unit is placed into a canister to protect it during freezing. The canister and the blood must be labeled in accordance with all regulations and standards to reflect the correct product name, "Red Blood Cells Frozen." The canister is placed into a $-65°C$ freezer. The time from the removal of the original RBC from the refrigeration storage until the unit is placed into the freezing environment cannot exceed 4 hours.

As donor tests for new infectious diseases may be added, it is important to freeze a sample of serum or plasma from the donor of the frozen unit for future testing since these units are placed into long-term storage (up to 10 years). Rare units that have not been tested for new infectious disease markers, and where no sample is available, should be used only if no other units are available and medical approval is documented. Product labeling must clearly reflect the missing test. A device has been FDA approved for closed system freezing and subsequent *deglycerolization* of RBCs within 6 days of collection. The red cells can be frozen for 3 years. Because this device processes the RBCs in a closed system, the RBCs outdate 14 days after thawing.[10]

Red Blood Cells Rejuvenated and Red Blood Cells Rejuvenated Deglycerolized

On occasion, an RBC unit may have outdated or missed the time limit for freezing, but they are either very rare, unique to a specific patient, or are for autologous use. *Rejuvenation* solutions are approved by the FDA for specific anticoagulants per manufacturer's instructions. Depending on the anticoagulant of the original RBC, the rejuvenation can occur after the expiration date of the RBC. The solutions replenish depleted ATP and 2,3-DPG levels in the RBCs to nearly that of fresh blood through the addition of an adenine, inosine, pyruvate, and sodium phosphate mixture.[1] The rejuvenation solution is mixed with the RBCs for 60 minutes and then washed to remove the inosine prior to transfusion. The rejuvenated RBCs can also be frozen with glycerol for future use. In either approach, the rejuvenating solution must be removed by deglycerolization or washing prior to transfusion. This is an open system process and the product must be transfused within 24 hours.

PLASMA

Plasma is the liquid portion of whole blood and consists of water, electrolytes, clotting factors, and other proteins, primarily albumin and globulins, most of which are stable at room temperature. Factors V and VIII, however, will deteriorate if the plasma is not stored at $-18°C$ or lower.[3] Plasma can be prepared from whole blood by centrifugation or sedimentation—the heavier cellular components will fall to the bottom of the collection container and the plasma remains as a supernatant. It is extracted from the RBCs by opening the internal access port or cannula to express the plasma into the attached empty satellite bag. The two components can then be separated by sealing the connection tubing with a heat-sealing device. Differential centrifugation is the method of varying the centrifuge speed or length of centrifugation. This technique either allows the plasma to be cell free or to retain the platelets. The following section describes the further processing of this plasma component into products specifically adapted to patient need. Platelets are addressed in a separate section.

Fresh Frozen Plasma or Plasma Frozen within 24 Hours after Phlebotomy

Plasma is frozen after separation from whole blood to preserve the coagulation factors. Though many of the coagulation factors are stable at refrigerator temperatures, the two labile factors V and VIII in plasma are not stable and the plasma must be frozen to maintain their potency levels over time. To maintain the maximum levels of these labile factors, the plasma should be placed into a freezing environment within 8 hours of collection. Quick freezing can be accomplished with a blast freezer, dry ice, a mixture of dry ice with ethanol or antifreeze, or a mechanical freezer. This product is labeled as FFP and can be stored up to 1 year after collection at $-18°C$ or lower.[4] If the plasma is frozen within 24 hours after collection, it can be labeled for transfusion as "Plasma Frozen Within 24 Hours after Phlebotomy." This product contains all the stable coagulation factors. Though the factor V and VIII levels are slightly reduced (15%) in comparison to FFP,[8] many transfusion services successfully utilize this product when the physician needs plasma for therapeutic treatment as it is clinically efficacious. Either product can be used for replacement of coagulation factors in a severely bleeding patient or if a therapeutic plasma exchange is needed. Other solutions, such as albumin or saline, should be used for volume or protein replacement and commercially available factor preparations should be used for a specific coagulopathy.

If the storage unit is not equipped with continuous temperature monitoring, the plasma unit must be frozen by a method that will detect thawing and subsequent refreezing. Methods may include freezing with a rubber band around the product or with a piece of tubing that will create an impression in the frozen product. After freezing and before storage, the rubber band or piece of tubing is removed so that thawing and refreezing is detectable. Another method is to freeze the plasma horizontally but store it upright so that the air bubble migration, if thawed, is readily apparent.

Plasma is thawed between 30°C to 37°C.[4] An FDA-approved microwave thawing device may be used or alternatively a water bath may be used. A rigorous equipment program must be in place to ensure that the temperature restrictions are met with either method of thawing. After thawing, the component should be used immediately or transfused within 24 hours if stored at 1°C to 6°C. If the thawed plasma is not transfused within that storage period, it may be relabeled as "Thawed Plasma" and stored for transfusion for another 4 days, provided it was collected in a closed system.

Plasma collected from some multiparous women or from donors who have received a blood transfusion can potentially contain donor leukocyte antibodies.

Substantial circumstantial evidence exists that these antibodies, if transfused into susceptible recipients, can be one of the mechanisms causing transfusion-related acute lung injury (TRALI).[11] The AABB issued Guidance on TRALI recommending that blood centers take steps to reduce the potential to transmit TRALI by minimizing the preparation of high-volume plasma components from donors known to be or at high risk of being leukocyte alloimmunized. High-volume plasma components include frozen plasma from whole blood or apheresis, apheresis platelets, buffy coat platelets, and whole blood.[12] Several options are currently being utilized by blood centers to meet the Guidance recommendations, including HLA testing of selected donors or preferentially utilizing male plasma for transfusion and sending female plasma to fractionators for further manufacture into transfusable derivative products.

Recovered Plasma

Not all of the plasma collected from volunteer donors is needed for transfusion. This plasma is labeled as "Recovered Plasma" and shipped to a plasma derivative manufacturer for further manufacture by fractionation into transfusable derivative products such as albumin, immune globulins, and specific coagulation factors. This plasma component has no expiration date so records need to be retained indefinitely; however, most manufacturers require shipment within a certain period based on their short supply agreement with the collecting facility.

Plasma, Cryoprecipitate Reduced

In the process of making cryoprecipitate, described in a later section, a residual plasma product is created that has had the cryoprecipitate removed. This plasma product can be shipped to a plasma derivative manufacturer for further manufacturing or labeled as "Plasma Cryoprecipitate Reduced." This plasma can be frozen for up to 12 months at $-18°C$.[4] The labeled product is primarily used as a plasma replacement fluid in the therapeutic treatment of Thrombotic Thrombocytopenic Purpura. Though the cryoprecipitate has been removed, it contains normal levels of many of the coagulation factors and other key proteins for therapeutic plasma exchange.

CRYOPRECIPITATE

Cryoprecipitate is prepared from FFP, that is, plasma that is frozen within 8 hours of collection. When the plasma is thawed in a 1°C to 6°C circulating waterbath or allowed to thaw slowly in a refrigerator, the cold-insoluble proteins that precipitate out of the plasma can be collected by centrifugation at 1°C to 6°C. The plasma supernatant over the cryoprecipitate "pellet" is removed via the internal access port into a second satellite bag, maintaining the closed system. Approximately 5 to 15 mL of plasma is retained on the cryoprecipitate. The "cryo-reduced" plasma can be sent to a manufacturer for further manufacturing or labeled as "Plasma, Cryoprecipitate Removed" as described above. The remaining cold-insoluble proteins are labeled as "Cryoprecipitated AHF" and must be refrozen within 1 hour of being removed from the cold environment. Once refrozen, it must be stored at -18°C or lower for up to 12 months from the collection date.[4] Cryoprecipitate contains factors VIII and XIII, as well as fibrinogen, von Willebrand factor, and fibronectin. A quality control program must regularly verify that a sampling of cryoprecipitate units contains at least 80 IU of factor VIII and 150 mg of fibrinogen per unit in accordance with AABB standards.[4]

Once thawed for use at 30°C to 37°C, the cryoprecipitate must be stored at room temperature and transfused as quickly as possible as factor VIII levels begin to decline 2 hours after thawing. Several units of ABO-identical cryoprecipitate can be pooled after thawing with the addition of a small amount of sterile 0.9% saline to flush each bag and enhance the recovery of the small volumes of cryoprecipitate. The number of cryoprecipitate in a pool varies by institution but is generally between 4 and 10 units. Because the seal is broken and the saline is added, this product expires 4 hours after pooling.

Alternatively, cryoprecipitate can be pooled in small groups of 4 to 10 units prior to refreezing. The addition of saline and pooling can be done with an SCD and a multilead closed system set, thus preserving the original outdate. The pooled product is then refrozen and is available for transfusion immediately after thawing. It must be assigned a unique pool identification number.[4] The pooling facility must retain a record of all products contained within that pool. Storage and transfusion requirements remain the same as individual cryoprecipitate units. The product quality control requirements are the same except that the pooled container must contain the minimum amount of factor VIII and fibrinogen multiplied by the number of units in a pool.[4]

PLATELETS

Platelets can be prepared from a whole blood unit or collected from an apheresis donor. Platelets are primarily used in preventing or treating bleeding in thrombocytopenic patients or patients whose platelets are adequate in number but dysfunctional. Platelets collected by apheresis are addressed in Chapter 2 of this book.

In the United States, platelets from whole blood are produced by a two-step differential centrifugation process. The whole blood after collection is stored to cool toward 20°C to 24°C and the platelets must be separated from the whole blood within 8 hours of collection.[3] The first spin is sometimes referred to as a "soft" spin as the whole blood is centrifuged at a speed that will sediment the RBCs but retains the platelets suspended in the supernatant plasma. This platelet-rich plasma is expressed from the RBCs via the internal access port into a satellite bag. The RBCs and the platelet-rich plasma are then separated by applying a heat seal to connecting tubing. Additional centrifugation of the platelet-rich plasma to sediment the platelets and the removal of most of the supernatant plasma into a second satellite bag results in a concentrate of platelets suspended in a small volume of plasma. An average of 40 to 70 mL of plasma remains on the platelets to provide nutrients and a balanced pH to optimize the platelets' survival.

In Europe, platelets are prepared using a buffy coat method. Following a hard spin, the supernatant plasma is removed to a satellite bag from the top of the bag and the RBCs are removed from the bottom of the bag through a separate cannula. The buffy coat that remains in the primary bag contains the platelets. The single centrifuge step induces less platelet activation but up to 13% of the RBCs are retained in the buffy coat, resulting in RBCs with a lower hematocrit.[3] Both methods provide an acceptable platelet product for transfusion.

The two-step centrifuge process can cause the platelets to aggregate, and current practice recommends an hour of "resting" time before platelets are placed into storage. Platelets must be stored at 20°C to 24°C with gentle agitation to maintain their viability and adhesive properties.[3] The combination of the gas-permeable bag, room temperature storage, and continual agitation ensures maximum platelet survival prior to transfusion. Platelets expire 5 days after collection, although research is under way to extend this to 7 days.

Collection sets are available with integral leukoreduction filters for either the whole blood prior to the first spin or the platelet-rich plasma depending on the bag manufacturer. Both methods reduce the leukocyte count to less than 8.3×10^5.[4] Platelets may also be leukoreduced at the patient's bedside with a leukoreduction filter. Leukoreduced platelets should be considered for transfusion when a patient has become refractory to platelet transfusion and no longer responds with an improved platelet count.

Alloimmunization to HLAs or platelet-specific antigens is a major cause of patients becoming refractory.[2] Utilizing leukoreduced platelets for patients anticipating multiple platelet transfusions can delay or prevent alloimmunization. Once a patient has been established as refractory, HLA-compatible or cross-matched platelets should be transfused.

Multiple platelets of the same ABO group can be pooled manually in an open system with a 4-hour expiration date. They can also be pooled using an SCD and a special closed system bag with multilead tubing. When platelets are pooled with this closed system, they can be stored for the full 5-day shelf life of the original product. A sample of this pooled product can be tested for the presence of bacteria. Without pooling, the bacterial detection test requires too large an inoculum from a single unit of whole blood–derived platelets. Single platelets are generally tested for the presence of bacteria in the transfusion service setting immediately prior to manual pooling or transfusion.

Apheresis platelets are considered a high-volume plasma component, and AABB Guidance recommends methods be implemented to reduce the incidence of TRALI.[12] The suggested methods are similar to those described in the section above on plasma components.

A quality control program is required that tests a sampling of platelets for pH, platelet count, and leukocyte count (if leukoreduction was performed). This testing should be done at either outdate or at time of distribution to ensure the processing and storage environments in a facility are in a state of control and retaining the platelet viability.

An increasing number of blood transfusion authorities around the world are adopting a policy of routine bacterial testing of all platelet concentrates prior to transfusion, and AABB has created a standard to that effect. Testing can be performed at the collection center or at the bedside.

GRANULOCYTES

Granulocytes can be prepared from whole blood collections, but the most common collection technique is leukapheresis as described in Chapter 2. Granulocytes are most commonly used as a treatment for bacterial sepsis in a neutropenic patient when no other therapeutic intervention has been successful. Their usage is in decline, especially those collected from whole blood. To prepare granulocytes, use a freshly collected, unrefrigerated whole blood to which 60 mL of hydroxyl ethyl starch (HES) has been added. Rest the unit for 1 hour and then centrifuge. The buffy coat contains the granulocytes layered between the plasma and the RBCs. The plasma and buffy coat are expressed from the RBCs through the cannula into a satellite bag. A second centrifugation step sediments the white cells and then 90% of the supernatant plasma is removed into a second satellite bag. The granulocytes are stored at 20°C to 24°C without agitation and expire 24 hours after collection.[3] They have an average hematocrit of 4% and must be ABO and crossmatch compatible.

ALIQUOTING

In some clinical situations, the standard volume of RBCs and plasma exceeds what should be safely transfused into a patient. Examples include pediatric patients or patients with circulatory overload. In these cases, the products can be divided into smaller volumes either using attached satellite bags or using an SCD to add an additional multilead transfer pack or syringe set. Syringe sets expire 4 hours after aliquoting, but products stored in FDA-approved bags retain their original expiration date.[3] Platelets require very specialized bags for gas exchange, so they may only be divided and stored in bags approved for platelet storage.

IRRADIATION OF BLOOD COMPONENTS

The cellular components of blood contain viable lymphocytes that can cause *graft-versus-host disease* (GVHD) in patients who are not immune competent. Plasma and cryoprecipitate do not contain lymphocytes as they are considered cell free. Though GVHD is very rare, to prevent GVHD in susceptible patients, cellular blood products are irradiated to inactivate the lymphocyte and prevent it from attacking the host. *Irradiation* is the only approved method to prevent GVHD.[13] GVHD can be caused by incomplete histocompatibility between the donor and the recipient (host) when the product contains lymphocytes and the host is unable to defend against them. The donor lymphocytes engraft and multiply and attack the host. GVHD is an extremely serious disease of significant mortality with symptoms that include fever, skin rash, and severe diarrhea. GVHD has been noted in transfusions among family members because they may share the same HLA haplotype and fail to recognize the donor cells as foreign. Transfusion of cellular components to the following groups should be irradiated:

- Neonates, especially those receiving intrauterine transfusions
- Selected immunocompromised or immunoincompetent recipients
- Blood relatives of the donor of the component
- Bone marrow or peripheral blood progenitor cell transplant recipients
- Recipients whose donor is selected for HLA compatibility

There are two irradiation sources currently in use: (i) γ-rays from either Cesium-137 or Cobalt-60 and (ii) x-rays produced by linear accelerators or stand-alone units. Either has been shown to successfully inactivate lymphocytes. The irradiation dose is measured at the center of the field and must be at least 2,500 cGy and no more than 5,000 cGy.[13] The minimum dose delivered to any portion of the container must be 1,500 cGy when the canister is filled to maximum. Dose mapping is required to monitor performance of the irradiator at regular intervals as defined by the device manufacturer and after major repair or relocation. In addition to the routine required dosimetry testing, irradiation-sensitive labels are applied to each product prior to irradiation. If the irradiator successfully delivered the correct dose, the label will indicate that the product was irradiated. RBC membranes can be slightly damaged by irradiation and cause some potassium leakage into the supernatant plasma. Though RBCs can be irradiated throughout their shelf life, there is a 28-day allowable shelf life after irradiation. Thus, irradiated RBCs can be stored for up to 28 days after irradiation or until the original expiration date, whichever comes first. Platelets are not damaged by irradiation and retain their original expiration date. SOPs should clearly define the correct expiration date for the irradiated red cells and any required documentation.

Recently the Nuclear Regulatory Commission (NRC) has imposed a number of controls on the license holder of a gamma source irradiator because of the radioactive material. The intent of the restrictions is to prevent the radioactive material from falling into the wrong, unauthorized hands. Controls include extensive background checks to verify that employees with irradiator access are trustworthy and reliable; restricted physical access including locked, reinforced, or barred doors, ceilings, and windows to prevent unauthorized break-ins; and recently fingerprinting of all employees with access to the irradiator.[14,15] Some blood banks are considering switching from a gamma source irradiator to a stand-alone x-ray irradiator because of the increasing regulations. The blood bank is still challenged to decommission the gamma source and move it to a secure government facility.

Records must be maintained of all required maintenance and dosimetry mapping. A radiation safety officer must be appointed for any facility with a gamma source irradiator. Records should be kept of all steps in the irradiation process to include operator identification, blood component identification, date, time, and documentation of the acceptability of the irradiation indicator label. Products are labeled with the blood component product code and the word "Irradiated."

LABELING REQUIREMENTS

The FDA has very specific requirements for the labeling of blood components detailed in the CFR and Guidance documents.[13,16] Both machine-readable (bar coded) and eye-readable labels are applied and a verification step is required to ensure the proper labels were used. The standard label requirements for all blood products are usually preprinted on the primary base label and the satellite bags by the bag manufacturer. The FDA has published guidelines for the uniform labeling of blood products.[17] At a minimum, the following information is required on the label:

- The proper name of the blood component, including an indication of any qualification or modification such as irradiation
- Method of collection—by whole blood collection or apheresis
- Expiration data and time if applicable
- The donor category—paid, volunteer, or autologous
- Volume of blood components if other than the standard volume assumed in the Circular of Information
- The anticoagulant or preservatives used in the preparation of the component
- Test results, for example, CMV
- Storage temperature requirements of the blood component
- Autologous donor/recipient information or special handling instructions
- Statements regarding the necessity to properly identify the recipient, the Circular of Information,[13] infectious disease risks, and the requirement for a prescription to dispense

An additional labeling requirement was added in 2006.[18] The following information must be applied to the final container in both machine- and eye-readable format. This requirement adds a significant layer of safety in the transfusion setting to allow information systems to track and dispense the product.

- The unique facility identification number (registration number), name, address, and U.S. License number (if applicable) of the collecting and processing facility

- The donor identification number
- The component product code
- ABO group and Rh type, if applicable

If units are pooled, such as platelets or cryoprecipitate, the following additional information must be included on the label:

- The name of the pooled component (machine and eye readable as required above)
- The number of units in the pool
- Final volume of the pooled component
- Identification of the facility pooling the component
- A unique identification number for the pool

There is other information relevant to the product that may be applied to a tie tag attached to the unit. This tie tag is considered an extension of the label and all verification requirements apply. Examples of information included on tie tags include autologous or directed unit recipient information and antigen or antibody results. The Circular of Information is jointly produced by the AABB, America's Blood Centers, and the American Red Cross. The Circular provides important prescribing and transfusing information about each component and should be readily available for reference to all practitioners involved in blood collection, processing, and transfusion including physicians and nurses.[13]

ISBT 128

A new bar code symbology was created in 1994 to attempt to standardize blood component labeling worldwide. This new symbology is called ISBT 128 and provides a common system for identifying, naming, and bar coding blood components. ISBT is the abbreviation for International Society of Blood Transfusion. The FDA approved ISBT 128 for use in the United States in 2000. AABB has required its members to implement ISBT 128 by May 2008.[19] The benefits of a standard labeling symbology include uniform look of labels for all blood components, better traceability of components, fewer misreads, an expanded number of product codes, improved self-checking features embedded in the bar codes, and a unique donor identification number specific to the year and collecting facility which avoids duplicate numbers for 99 years.[20] This is just a small listing of all the benefits of this symbology. The reader is referred to the ISBT website, or the ICCBBA website (formerly International Council for Commonality in Blood Banking Automation).

STORAGE OF BLOOD COMPONENTS

Monitoring the temperature of blood components is critical to maintaining their quality. Failing to adhere to the storage requirements will threaten the viability of the component and its clinical effectiveness. Though technology has evolved from a simple thermometer and recorder chart to an electronic thermometer or probe with a data logger, either is acceptable. The AABB standards require that the temperature is monitored continuously and recorded. These requirements apply anywhere blood is stored—from the laboratory to an operating room.

The storage equipment must alarm to notify personnel to take immediate and corrective action. The alarm needs to be tested at periodic intervals that are clearly defined in the facility SOPs. The high- and low-set points for the storage equipment should be at a temperature that will allow adequate time to respond before the storage temperature limits are violated. Any variance from acceptable storage range must be thoroughly investigated and documented. The storage units should be maintained clean and should have sufficient capacity to store blood products in an orderly manner. Storage areas should be clearly labeled and segregate unfinished products from finished products, allogeneic products from autologous products, and contain a restricted quarantine area for suspect or biohazardous products if needed.

If a piece of equipment fails and cannot be recovered to maintain the proper storage temperature of the product, written SOPs must be in place to relocate the products to another unit or into validated storage boxes. In the event of a power failure, a back-up generator may be used. The generator must be evaluated for adequate reserve capacity to operate the essential equipment; it must have SOPs for its use and a regular testing program to ensure it will respond in the event of a failure.

The storage temperature for RBCs is 1°C to 6°C. The refrigerator must be designed with an internal fan to circulate air and maintain an even distribution of temperature throughout the unit. The storage temperature of platelets and granulocytes is 20°C to 24°C. Whether they are stored on an agitator in an open room or an incubator designed to hold the agitator, the temperature must be continuously monitored to ensure the platelets are maintained at 20°C to 24°C at all times. Platelets must be stored on an agitator to ensure a free exchange of gases within and around the bags. Platelet agitation helps maintain optimal pH for maximum viability. An alarm system should be utilized to detect motion failure as well as temperature failure. If the platelets are stored in an incubator, the user should be able to inspect the contents and operation without opening the door to minimize temperature changes. Frozen plasma products are stored in a freezer at −18°C or lower. Frozen RBCs must be stored at −65°C or lower. See Table 3-5 for storage and transport temperatures.

All blood components must be examined/inspected for acceptability during production, storage, and at time of distribution or issue or reissue and receipt. The inspection should be documented. The inspection should evaluate the component for integrity of the seals, hemolysis or any other abnormal color, clots or any flocculant material, cloudiness or any other abnormal appearance. For RBCs, at least one integral segment should be attached to the bag. Though the color of the segment is not completely representative of the bag contents, they should be examined as part of the visual inspection as an indicator. If a product's appearance is questionable, it should be removed and quarantined pending a decision on final disposition.

TRANSPORT OF BLOOD COMPONENTS

An efficient system must be in place to ensure all blood components are received in the blood center after collection within the allowed time frame and proper temperature as established by a validation protocol. Whole blood should be transported in a container cooling toward 1°C to 10°C. An exception would be whole blood extended for platelet production; in that case the whole blood should be cooled toward 20°C to 24°C but no colder.[3]

For RBCs, the recommended refrigerant is wet ice in leakproof containers such as a plastic bag. The ice must be placed on top of the units as cold air moves downward. RBCs must be kept at a temperature of 1°C to 10°C during transport as opposed to 1°C to 6°C during storage. Ice that has not started to melt should not be used because the super cold ice can create pockets of low temperature that can cause RBCs or integral segments to freeze and subsequently hemolyze. Ice should not come into direct contact with the RBCs.

Frozen plasma products and frozen red cells must be shipped at or below the storage temperature of −18°C/−65°C, respectively. Dry ice is the usual coolant to maintain this temperature and should be placed on the bottom and top of the container or in accordance with the validation protocol. The plasma products become very brittle at this temperature and can be protected from breakage with a plastic bubble wrap or other dry packing material.

TABLE 3-5   Requirements for Storage, Transportation, and Expiration for Select Components

Component	Storage	Transport	Expiration	Additional Criteria
Whole blood	1–6°C	Cooling toward 1–10°C If intended for room temperature components, cooling toward 20–24°C	CPD: 21 days CPDA-1: 35 days	
Red blood cells Red blood cells, leukocytes reduced	1–6°C	1–10°C	CPD: 21 days CPDA-1: 35 days Additive solution: 42 days Open system: 24 h	
Deglycerolized RBCs	1–6°C	1–10°C	Open system: 24 h Closed system: 14 days or as FDA approved	
Frozen RBCs	≤65°C	Maintain frozen state	10 yr	
RBCs irradiated	1–6°C	1–10°C	Original expiration or 28 days from date of irradiation, whichever is sooner	
Rejuvenated RBCs	1–6°C	1–10°C		Follow manufacturer's written instructions
Washed RBCs	1–6°C	1–10°C	24 h	
Platelets Platelets pheresis Platelets irradiated	20–24°C with continuous gentle agitation	20–24°C	5 days in a closed system	Maximum time without agitation 24 h
Pooled platelets	20–24°C with continuous gentle agitation	20–24°C	Open system: 4 h Closed system: original outdate	Maximum time without agitation 24 h
Granulocytes	20–24°C	20–24°C	24 h	Transfuse as soon as possible
Cryoprecipitated AHF Pooled cryoprecipitate (closed system)	≤18°C	Maintain frozen state	12 mo from original collection	Thaw the FFP at 1–6°C Place cryoprecipitate in the freezer within 1 h
Cryoprecipitated AHF or pooled cryoprecipitated AHF, after thawing	20–24°C	20–24°C	Open system: 4 h Single unit: 6 h	Thaw at 30–37°C
Fresh frozen plasma Plasma frozen within 24 h after phlebotomy Plasma, cryoprecipitate reduced	≤18°C	Maintain frozen state	12 mo from collection	Place plasma in freezer within 8 or 24 h and label accordingly
Thawed plasma	1–6°C	1–10°C	5 days from when original product was thawed	Closed system: 5 days

Source: Price TH, ed. *Standards for Blood Banks and Transfusion Services.* 25th ed. AABB; 2008.

Platelets or granulocytes must be transported at 20°C to 24°C. Shipping times should not exceed 24 hours because of the interruption in agitation. A chemical pack to moderate the internal temperature under various shipping conditions is often used and validated as part of the packaging procedure.

Shipping Containers

Boxes or containers for blood product transport should be well insulated and should undergo an especially designed validation study to ensure they can reliably maintain the required temperature during transport for each product type. The validation protocol should be written and should test all the different transit times, transport modes, climactic conditions that the container could be exposed to, etc. Any discrepancies should be immediately investigated and results documented. Because the coolant is placed in specific places in a box, the proper orientation of the container should be clearly evident by the external markings. Shipping boxes should also be tested for robustness—the resistance of the container to breakage when repeatedly dropped to simulate potential actual use.[21]

SUMMARY

Preparing whole blood into various components provides lifesaving therapy targeted at the patient's need. RBCs are available to assist with oxygen-carrying capacity and can be modified as leukoreduced, washed, deglycerolized, or irradiated depending on the therapeutic demand. Plasma products such as FFP, plasma cryoprecipitate reduced, and cryoprecipitate all can be used to assist in massive transfusions or other clinical situations when there is a specific coagulation deficiency. Platelets are prepared and made available for the treatment of patients that are bleeding due to a decreased number or dysfunctional platelets. Component preparation isolates each component, then prepares and stores it in a way that maximizes its life span and effectiveness until transfused. Facilities that prepare blood components must adhere to all standards and regulations, and have written procedures for the preparation of each product.

Review Questions

1. Which of the following is not an action of the chemicals contained in common whole blood anticoagulants?
   a. chelates the calcium to prevent blood from clotting
   b. maintains the pH level at optimal levels
   c. provides a substrate for ATP generation
   d. prevents ATP production to increase viability of red cells

2. Which of the following are useful features of adding an additive solution to red cells?
   a. further extends the life of the red blood cells
   b. facilitates improved flow during transfusion
   c. provides additional adenine and dextrose for ATP generation
   d. all of the above

3. The following are characteristics of blood collection sets:
   a. sealed, sterile, and pyrogen free
   b. transparent, flexible, and pliable
   c. one or more satellite bags are attached
   d. allow gas transfer
   e. all of the above

4. Finished red blood cells may be transported at what temperature range?
   a. 1°C to 10°C
   b. 2°C to 12°C
   c. 35°C to 37°C
   d. 20°C to 24°C

5. Which of the following is not an approved use for a sterile connecting device?
   a. extend the life span of an open system product
   b. pool blood components
   c. aliquot blood products into smaller doses
   d. add a leukoreduction filter
   e. to remove samples for testing

6. Which of the following is not a step in platelet production?
   a. soft spin to sediment red blood cells
   b. hard spin to separate platelets from platelet-rich plasma
   c. separation of all but 40 to 70 mL of plasma from platelets
   d. resting phase at 1°C to 6°C
   e. resting phase at 20°C to 24°C

7. Irradiated blood components are indicated for the following patients except:
   a. neonate requiring an exchange transfusion
   b. a 25-year-old immunocompromised man receiving platelets after chemotherapy
   c. a patient receiving a directed donor unit from a blood relative
   d. a 43-year-old woman receiving a knee replacement

8. Frozen plasma products must be stored at what temperature?
   a. 1°C to 6°C   b. -18°C or lower
   c. 20°C to 24°C   d. 2°C to 8°C

(continued)

REVIEW QUESTIONS (continued)

9. Leukocyte-reduced red cells can be prepared by the following methods:
   a. in-line whole blood or red blood cell filter
   b. sterile connected leukoreduction filter
   c. bedside filter
   d. all of the above
10. A blood product storage unit should have the following:
    a. a system to monitor temperature continuously
    b. an alarm to alert personnel if temperature limits are exceeded
    c. sufficient capacity to store products in an orderly manner
    d. SOPs to recover products in the event of a failure
    e. all of the above

11. A red blood cell component prepared in an open system unit has what outdate?
    a. 4 hours
    b. 12 hours
    c. 24 hours
    d. 35 days
    e. 42 days
12. Which of the following are required to be on the label of all blood products?
    a. the proper name of the blood component
    b. expiration date and time if applicable
    c. donor category—paid, volunteer, or autologous
    d. storage temperature requirements of the product
    e. all of the above

REFERENCES

1. Yoshida T, AuBuchon JP, Dumont LJ, et al. The effects of additive solution pH and metabolic rejuvenation on anaerobic storage of red cells. *Transfusion.* 2008;48:2096–2105.
2. McPherson RA, Pincus MR, eds. *Henry's Clinical Diagnosis and Management by Laboratory Methods.* 21st ed. Philadelphia: Saunders; 2007.
3. Roback JD, Combs MR, Grossman BJ, et al., eds. *Technical Manual.* 16th ed. Bethesda, MD: AABB; 2008.
4. Price TH, ed. *Standards for Blood Banks and Transfusion Services.* 25th ed. Bethesda, MD: AABB; 2008.
5. Food and Drug Administration. *Use of an FDA Cleared or Approved Sterile Connecting Device (STCD) in Blood Bank Practice.* FDA Memorandum; August 5, 1994.
6. Food and Drug Administration. *FDA Public Health Notification: PVC Devices Containing the Plasticizer DEHP.* FDA Advisory; July 12, 2002.
7. Joint Research Centre European Commission. *BIS (2-Ethylhexyl) Phthalate (DEHP) Summary Risk Assessment Report.* European Communities; 2008.
8. Beutler E, Lichtman MA, Coller BS, et al., eds. *Williams Hematology.* 6th ed. New York: McGraw-Hill; 2001.
9. Food and Drug Administration. *Recommendations and Licensure Requirements for Leukocyte Reduced Blood Products.* FDA Memorandum; May 29, 1996.
10. Bandarenko N, Hay SN, Holmberg J, et al. Extended storage of AS-1 and AS-3 leukoreduced red blood cells for 15 days after deglycerolization and resuspension in AS-3 using an automated closed system. *Transfusion.* 2004; 44:1656–1662.
11. Middelburg RA, van Stein D, Briet E, et al. The role of donor antibodies in the pathogenesis of transfusion-related acute lung injury: a systematic review. *Transfusion.* 2008; 48:2167–2176.
12. Transfusion-Related Acute Lung Injury. *Association Bulletin No. 06-07.* Bethesda, MD: AABB; 2006. Available at http://www.aabb.org/content>Members Area>Association Bulletins. Accessed October 13, 2008.
13. AABB, American Red Cross, and America's Blood Centers. *Circular of Information for the Use of Human Blood and Blood Components.* Bethesda, MD: AABB; 2002.
14. U.S. Nuclear Regulatory Commission. *EA-05-090 Enforcement Action: Order Imposing Increases Controls (Licensees Authorized to Possess Radioactive Material Quantities of Concern).* Rockville, MD: NRC; November 14, 2005.
15. U.S. Nuclear Regulatory Commission. RIS 2007-14. *Fingerprinting Requirements for Licensees Implementing the Increased Control Order.* Rockville, MD: NRC; June 5, 2007.
16. U.S. Department of Health and Human Services, Food and Drug Administration. *The Code of Federal Regulations, 21 CFR 600.* Washington, DC: US Government Printing Office; 2002.
17. Food and Drug Administration. *Guidelines for Uniform Labeling of Blood and Blood Components.* Rockville, MD: CBER Office of Communication, Training, and Manufacturers Assistance; August 1985.
18. Food and Drug Administration. *Bar Code Label Requirements for Human Drug Products and Biological Products.* FDA Guidance; February 26, 2004.
19. ISBT 128 Implementation for Blood Banks and Transfusion Services. *Association Bulletin No. 08-02.* Bethesda, MD: AABB; 2008. Available at http://www.aabb.org/content>Members Area>Association Bulletins. Accessed October 13, 2008.
20. Food and Drug Administration. *Guidance: Industry Consensus Standard for the Uniform Labeling of Blood and Blood Components Using ISBT 128.* Version 2.0.0. November 2005. Rockville, MD: CBER Office of Communication, Training, and Manufacturers Assistance; September 22, 2006.
21. World Health Organization. *Manual on the Management, Maintenance and Use of Blood Cold Chain Equipment.* Geneva; 2005.

GENETICS

EVA D. QUINLEY

OBJECTIVES

After completion of this chapter, the reader will be able to:

1. Understand the importance of blood group genetics as it relates to the overall field of genetics.
2. Understand the basics of inheritance of blood group traits.
3. Describe the role of DNA and RNA in inheritance.
4. Understand inheritance patterns and pedigree charts.
5. Understand the processes of mitosis and meiosis.
6. Explain dominant versus recessive codominant traits.
7. Explain the difference between phenotype and genotype.
8. Describe the role of population genetics in calculating gene frequencies.
9. Understand crossing-over and linkage.
10. Differentiate public versus private genes.
11. Understand the use of blood group genes as genetic markers.

KEY WORDS

Alleles	Genotype
Amorph	Heterozygous
Autosome	Homozygous
Chromosome	Linkage
Crossing-over	Meiosis
DNA	Mendelian
Dosage	Mitosis
Genes	Parentage testing

Pedigree chart	Public genes
Phenotype	RNA
Polymorphic	Trait
Population genetics	X-linked
Private genes	

Just as genetic information determines the color of one's eyes, it also plays an important role in determining the blood groups expressed. Blood groups are inherited in *Mendelian* fashion. Each parent contributes half of the inheritance. The genetic information is carried on double strands of deoxyribonucleic acid (*DNA*) known as *chromosomes*. DNA is composed of the sugar deoxyribose, the purine bases adenine and guanine, and the pyrimidine bases thymine and cytosine. The strands of DNA are held together by specific pairings of the bases, and they twist around each other to form the classic double-helix configuration. Figure 4-1 shows a simplified sketch of a DNA molecule. Normal humans have 23 pairs of chromosomes, comprising 22 pairs of *autosomes* and 1 pair of sex chromosomes. The autosomes are alike, whereas the sex chromosomes are different in size and composition.

The units that code for various expressions of inherited genetic information are known as *genes*. Genes are found in specific places along the chromosomes. These specific places are called loci. Table 4-1 shows the location of some of the more common blood group genes.

For each locus, there may be several different forms of a gene, which are known as *alleles*. For example, one may inherit *K* (Kell) gene or *k* (Cellano) gene in the Kell blood group system at a particular Kell system locus. Because two genes are inherited,

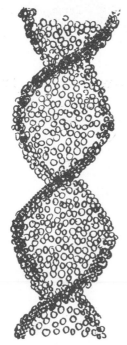

FIGURE 4-1   Diagram of human DNA molecule. Note double-helix configuration.

one from each parent, a person could be *KK, Kk,* or *kk,* depending on which genes were passed on from the parents.

TABLE 4-1	Location of Some of the Most Common Blood Group Genes

Blood Group Locus	Chromosome
Rh	1
Duffy	
MNSs	4
Chidc	6
Rogers	
ABO	9
Kidd	18
Lewis	19
Secretor	
Lutheran	
H	
XG	X
XK	
XS	

When both the inherited alleles are identical, the person is *homozygous* (*KK* or *kk*). If the inherited genes differ, the person is *heterozygous* (*Kk*). Sometimes, homozygous inheritance produces a stronger expression of the gene than would be seen in a heterozygous individual. This stronger expression is known as *dosage* and is important to blood bankers because some blood bank antibodies react more strongly with red blood cells (RBCs) homozygous for a particular blood group inheritance than with those with heterozygous inheritance.

A Punnett square can be used to diagram the possibilities for the offspring of two people.[1] For example, if two people of the *genotypes Kk* and *kk* mate, the offspring would be as shown in the following square:

	K	k
k	*Kk*	*kk*
k	*Kk*	*kk*

Half of the children would be heterozygous (*Kk*) and the other half would be homozygous (*kk*). Obviously, the more genes that are added to consider, the more complicated this diagram would become.

MITOSIS AND MEIOSIS

There are two kinds of cell division: mitosis and meiosis. To truly understand blood group inheritance, it is necessary to have a basic knowledge of these processes. *Mitosis* is a process whereby a cell divides into two cells that are identical. For this to occur, the pairs of chromosomes in the original cell must separate and then replicate; the 23 pairs of chromosomes become 46 pairs. When the original cell divides, half of the pairs go to one daughter cell and half to the other. The result is two identical cells, each having the original 23 pairs of chromosomes. The stages of mitosis are diagrammed in Figure 4-2. Interphase is the stage in which cells are resting and various metabolic activities are occurring. Toward the end of interphase, the DNA content of the cell doubles. Once the nucleus begins to change and the chromosomes become visible, the cell has entered the second phase of division, known as prophase. During this phase, each chromosome has doubled and now consists of a pair of long, thin strands (chromatids) that are held together at a spot known as the centromere.

At this point, the nuclear membrane disappears, and the centriole, an organelle outside the nuclear membrane, duplicates. The centriole pair then

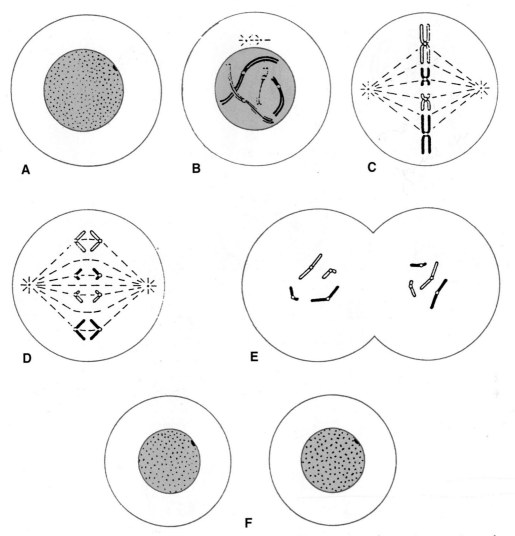

FIGURE 4-2   Mitosis. Only two chromosome pairs are shown. Chromosomes from one parent are shown in outline and from the other parent in black. A: Interphase; B: prophase; C: metaphase; D: anaphase; E: telophase; F: interphase.

separates, and each centriole moves toward opposite poles of the cell. The chromosomes then center between the two centrioles, and the cell is now in metaphase. A spindle forms that connects the centrioles to the centromeres of the chromatids. The centromeres now divide, and the paired chromatids become chromosomes. This stage is known as anaphase. The fibers of the spindle contract and draw the daughter chromosomes toward opposite poles. Once the chromosomes have separated, the cell is in telophase. At this point, the cytoplasm of the cell begins to divide, and eventually a membrane develops that results in the formation of two identical cells, both with identical chromosomal content. The nuclear membrane reappears as the chromosomes become invisible, and the cells return to interphase. This is a simplification of the process, but should be sufficient for basic understanding. Most cells of the body are formed through the process of mitosis.

Meiosis is a process in which the result is four daughter cells that have only 23 chromosomes each instead of 46. Meiosis is the way eggs and sperm are formed. The chromosome pairs duplicate just as in mitosis, but in meiosis, instead of separating, they remain together, and a pair of daughter cells is formed that has 23 pairs of chromosomes each. A second division then occurs in which the chromosome pairs separate from each other. Note that there is no replication of the chromosome before this division. The result is four daughter cells, each with 23 chromosomes. These cells are known as gametes (eggs and sperm). As with mitosis, there are various stages to meiosis, which are outlined in Figure 4-3.

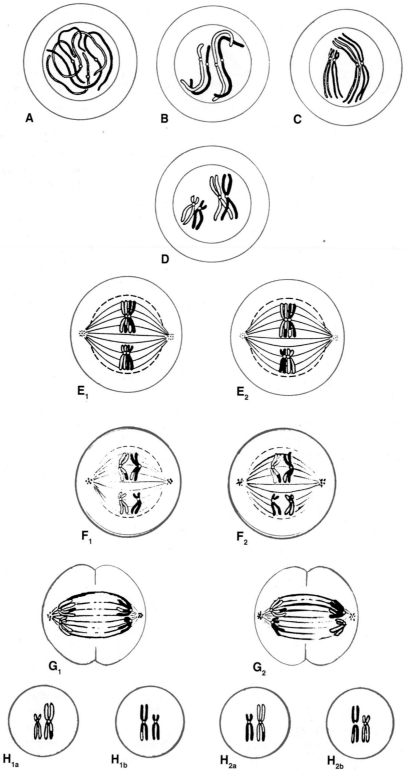

FIGURE 4-3   The first meiotic division. Only 2 of the 23 chromosome pairs are shown; chromosomes from one parent are shown in outline; chromosomes from the other parent are in black. A: Leptotene; B: zygotene; C: pachytene; D: diplotene; E_1 and E_2: metaphase; F_1 and F_2: early anaphase; G_1 and G_2: late anaphase; H_{1a}, H_{1b}, H_{2a}, H_{2b}: telophase. One possible distribution of the two parental chromosome pairs is shown in illustrations (E_1 to H_1); the alternative combination is in illustrations (E_2 to H_2).

The sex chromosomes, X and Y, determine a person's sex. Females inherit an X chromosome from each parent, whereas males inherit an X from the mother and a Y from the father. Some blood group system genes are located on the X chromosome and are referred to as *X-linked*. At this time, three blood group genes have been assigned to the X chromosome: Xg^a, Xk, and XS; none have been assigned to the Y chromosome.

PHENOTYPES AND GENOTYPES

Normally, genes produce detectable products known as *traits*; a few do not and are known as *amorphs*. The observation of these detectable traits determines a person's *phenotype*. For example, in the laboratory, reagents can be used to detect the product of an inherited *D* gene. If no reaction is obtained, it is assumed that the *D* gene must not have been present because its product was not found. If the reagent does produce a reaction, it is assumed that the *D* gene was present. Phenotypes are much easier to determine than genotypes. To determine a genotype, it may be necessary to study inheritance patterns in a family for several generations. A genotype is composed of the actual genes inherited from each parent. In Figure 4-4, the individual to whom the arrow points is noted as being group A. Group A individuals can inherit an *A* gene from both parents or an *A* gene from one parent and an *O* gene from the other. (The *O* gene was considered to be an amorph until recently because a detectable product had not been discovered; people who are group O have the genotype *OO*.) The individual in the figure has inherited the *A* gene from at least one parent, but without looking at the diagram, it is not known whether she received the gene from both parents. After examining the diagram, it is evident that her genotype must be *AO* because one of her parents was O and could only contribute an O gene.

The diagram is referred to as a *pedigree chart*. Pedigree charts are discussed later in this chapter. Here, the chart simply indicates that the person under study did not get an *A* gene from both parents.

Genetic expression is determined by whether the trait produced by a gene is dominant, recessive, or codominant to other allelic products. A trait that is dominant is expressed to the exclusion of the expression of the product of its allele(s). The gene can be inherited in double dose, a homozygous condition, or in single dose, a heterozygous condition. A recessive gene trait, however, is detected only if a person is homozygous for the gene or, in males, if the gene is X-linked (i.e., carried on the X chromosome). Codominant genetic traits are detectable, and neither overshadows the expression of the other. Most blood group genes produce traits that are codominant.

INHERITANCE PATTERNS

Pedigree charts can be used to study the inheritance patterns of dominant versus recessive traits in relation to whether the genes are on autosomes or are X-linked. Pedigree charts make use of symbols, as seen in Figure 4-5. Most pedigree charts follow this design. Figure 4-6A–D demonstrates the use of pedigree charts to show various inheritance patterns. These charts are somewhat more complicated than the

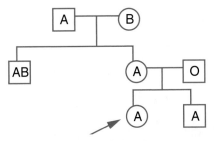

FIGURE 4-4 Inheritance of blood group genes. The ABO group of the individual is found within the symbol. The propositus, indicated by the arrow, must have a genotype of *AO* because her father has an obligate genotype of *OO*.

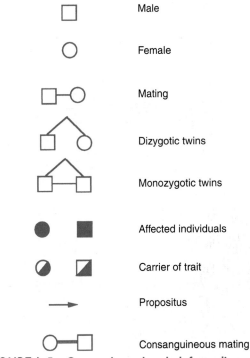

FIGURE 4-5 Commonly used symbols for pedigree charts.

example previously shown. The individual for whom a pedigree study is initiated is known as the propositus or index case and is usually indicated by an arrow. Pedigree charts can be useful in determining inheritance in families.

An autosomal dominant or codominant trait, as seen in Figure 4-6A, is easy to recognize. The expression of the gene is found whenever it is inherited and occurs equally in males and females. As previously stated, most blood groups' genes are inherited in this pattern.

An autosomal recessive trait also is seen in an equal number of males and females. Only people homozygous for the gene express the trait. Note that in Figure 4-6B, one of the parents of the propositus carries the gene for the trait but does not express it, whereas the other parent expresses the trait fully. A carrier is heterozygous for a gene, the presence of which is not phenotypically apparent. Recessive traits (those resulting from genes with a frequency of <1 in 10,000) are usually seen only in one generation and not in preceding or successive generations.

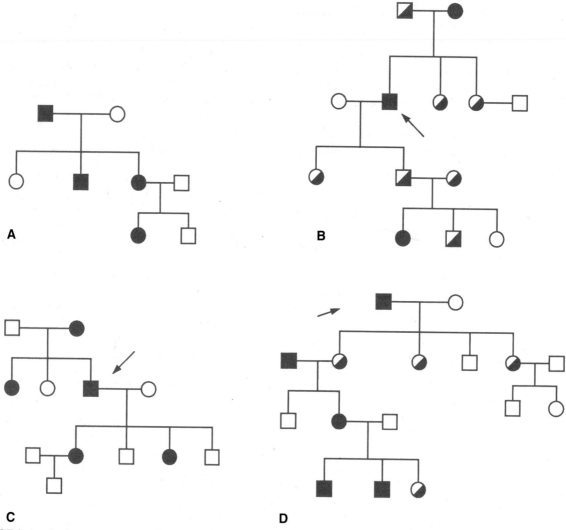

FIGURE 4-6 A: Autosomal dominant or codominant inheritance. The trait is expressed in an equal number of males and females. B: Autosomal recessive inheritance. The father of the propositus is a heterozygous carrier to the recessive trait, whereas the mother is homozygous and fully expresses the trait. Note that all her children either express the trait or are carriers. Also note that the mating of the two carriers produced a female child who neither expresses nor is a carrier of the trait. C: X-linked dominant inheritance. All daughters of the affected male express the trait, whereas none of the sons do. D: X-linked recessive trait. Note the propositus passes the gene for the recessive trait to all daughters but not to his son. The daughters do not express the trait. The affected female's sons express the trait, but her daughter is a carrier.

Such recessive traits usually are seen only when blood relatives mate (a consanguineous mating) because rare genes are more likely to be seen in related people.

An X-linked dominant or recessive trait (Fig. 4-6C,D) is not passed from male to male. This is because a male must pass the Y chromosome to a male offspring. In the case of an X-linked dominant trait, all daughters of a male with the trait express the trait. If it is X-linked recessive, all daughters of a male with the trait are either carriers of the trait or fully express the trait if they inherit the recessive allele from their mother as well. All sons of a male with an X-linked recessive trait do not carry the gene for the trait because they have received a Y chromosome from their father.

CONTRIBUTION OF BLOOD GROUP GENETICS TO THE FIELD OF HUMAN GENETICS

For a genetic trait to be useful as a genetic marker, it must possess certain characteristics:

- A simple and unequivocal pattern of inheritance
- Classification of phenotypes by reliable techniques
- A relatively high frequency of each of the common alleles at a particular locus
- Absence of effect of environmental factors, age, interaction with other genes, or other variables on the expression of the trait

Blood group genetics has resulted in many contributions to the field of human genetics. Multiple allelism was first demonstrated in humans by the ABO blood group genes. The *linkage* of the secretor gene to the Lutheran gene was the first example of autosomal linkage in humans, and *population genetics* has made extensive use of blood group genes.[2]

POPULATION GENETICS

Phenotype frequencies are determined by randomly testing RBCs from a large number of individuals of a particular population. The percentage of those positive (or negative) for a particular trait is then calculated. This percentage is the frequency of a particular phenotype and may be written as a percentage or as a decimal (33% or 0.33 of the population). Once the individual frequencies of traits are known, it is possible to calculate the frequency of multiple traits by multiplying the frequencies of each trait, as in the following example:

Thirty percent of the population is negative for C. Ninety-one percent of the population is negative for K.

Thirty-three percent of the population is negative for Fy[a].

The percentage of the population negative for all three is found by multiplying the three individual frequencies.

$$0.3 \times 0.91 \times 0.33 = 0.09(9\%)$$

The frequency of individual alleles may be calculated by using the phenotype frequencies. The sum of the frequencies at a given locus on a chromosome must equal 1. When two alleles are involved, it is possible to use the Hardy–Weinberg equation to determine the frequency of each allele.[2] This equation states the following:

$$p^2 + 2pq + q^2 = 1$$

p represents the frequency of the allele p; q represents the frequency of the allele q; p^2 represents the frequency of the homozygous phenotype pp; q^2 represents the frequency of the homozygous phenotype qq: and $2pq$ represents the frequency of the heterozygous phenotype pq.

The frequency of an allele in the population is represented by the sum of the frequency of the allele in the homozygous state plus the frequency of the allele in the heterozygous state.

$$\text{Frequency of } p = p^2 + 2pq$$

From the Hardy–Weinberg equation, it is derived that

$$q^2 = 1 - (p^2 + 2pq)$$

Then,

$$q = \sqrt{[1 - (p^2 + 2pq)]}$$

Using a numerical example, if the frequency of p in a population is known to be 0.75 (75% of the population are positive for p), then

$$p^2 + 2pq = 0.75$$

and

$$q^2 = 1 - (p^2 + 2pq)$$

or

$$q^2 = 1 - 0.75 = 0.25$$

Then,

$$q = \sqrt{0.25} = 0.5$$

Because the frequency of the alleles must equal 1

$$p = 1 - q$$

$$p = 1 - 0.5 = 0.5$$

LINKAGE

According to Mendelian genetics, genes that are not allelic assort independently of one another, a statement of the law of independent assortment. There is, however, an exception to this law. This phenomenon is known as linkage; if two genes are linked, they do not assort independently. Linked genes are located close to each other on the same chromosome, and there is a 50% or greater chance that they will remain together and be passed to the same gamete. Several blood group genes have been found to be linked to other genes. The linkage of the locus for the Lutheran blood group trait to the locus for the secretor trait was the first known example of autosomal linkage in humans, reported by Mohr in 1951.[2] Another example of genes being linked to each other is found in the MNSs blood group system in which the M and N loci are closely linked to the locus controlling expression of S and s. The approximate frequencies of the alleles follow:

M = 0.53
N = 0.47

S = 0.33
s = 0.67

If the genes segregated independently, the observed frequencies would be the product of the frequencies of each allele. However, the observed frequencies are not those expected.

Expected frequency	Observed frequency
MS = 0.53 × 0.33 = 0.17	0.24
Ms = 0.53 × 0.67 = 0.36	0.28
NS = 0.47 × 0.33 = 0.16	0.08
Ns = 0.47 × 0.67 = 0.31	0.39

Because the genes are not inherited independently of each other, they are not in equilibrium. This is known as linkage disequilibrium.

CROSSING-OVER AND RECOMBINATION

Crossing-over is a random event that occurs after the chromosome pairs have replicated during meiosis. Genes that are closely linked on the chromosomes usually are not affected by this process, whereas genes that are not closely linked are likely to cross over and exchange genetic information. As shown in Figure 4-7, this recombination results in two new and different chromosomes. The rate at which crossing-over occurs is determined by the distance between two loci and by chance.

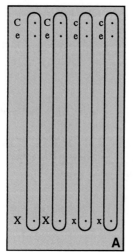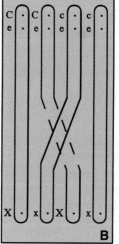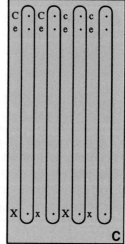

FIGURE 4-7   Crossing-over. Genetic material has been exchanged after the crossing-over of the chromosomes in frame (B). Two new chromosomes now exist, as seen in frame (C).

POSITIONAL OR MODIFIER EFFECTS OF GENES

Sometimes genes can interact with each other depending on their location on the chromosome pair. When two genes are located on the same chromosome, they are said to be in *cis* position. If the genes are located on homologous chromosomes (paired), they are said to be in *trans* position. For example, *C* and *D* are genes in the Rh system. It has been found that *C* exerts an effect on *D* in the *cis* and *trans* states, which results in a weakened expression of *D*. Some genes can modify or suppress the expression of other genes, although in most cases the exact mechanism for this action is not understood. Genes that are known to modify or suppress include *In(Lu)*, which suppresses the expression of Lutheran genes, and $X^\underline{o}r$, which suppresses the conversion of Rh precursor into detectable Rh traits.

GENE ACTION

Genetic information is found in the double strands of DNA. The sequence of base pairs that make up the DNA determines the particular protein that is produced. The base pairs are arranged in codons, each composed of three base pairs. Sixty-four codons have been identified. Most of these codons code for 1 of the 21 amino acids; some are known as terminator codons and signal that the protein synthesis is complete.

The DNA, through a process called transcription, assembles a protein known as messenger *RNA* (mRNA), which carries a code for the production of the protein to be made within a cell. RNA is similar to a single strand of DNA. Ribose, however, replaces deoxyribose, and uracil is the base instead of thymine. An enzyme, RNA polymerase, allows the DNA double strands to separate. The mRNA is formed using one of the DNA strands as a template. The process is somewhat complicated, and the reader is referred to genetic texts for a complete explanation.

Once the mRNA is formed, it moves to the cell's cytoplasm, where it attaches to ribosomal RNA (rRNA). The rRNA reads the mRNA and attaches a third type of RNA known as transfer RNA (tRNA). Each tRNA is composed of three base pairs. This attachment continues until a termination code is encountered. This process is known as translation and results in the production of detectable proteins that differ according to the sequence of amino acids forming them. This is how protein blood group traits differ. However, not all blood group traits are protein in nature; some are carbohydrate. In these cases, blood group genes work to produce enzymes called transferases. Specifically,

TABLE 4-2 Transferases and Their Corresponding Sugars Added by the ABH Genes

ABH Gene	Transferase	Sugar
H	L-fucosyltransferase	L-fucose
A	*N*-acetylgalactosamine transferase	*N*-acetylgalactosamine
B	Galactosaminyltransferase	D-galactose

the transferases are known as glycosyltransferases. These have the specific job of adding sugars to basic precursor substances, resulting in the expression of carbohydrate-based blood group antigens. Therefore, the carbohydrate blood group differs according to the sugars added to the precursor substances. Table 4-2 lists the transferases for which the ABO genes code. A brief discussion of the basic biochemistry of the blood group systems is found in the chapters dealing with each system.

SILENT GENES

In some blood group systems, as stated previously, certain genes are considered silent because they do not produce a detectable product. Such silent alleles are known as amorphs. Table 4-3 gives a list of some of the silent genes of interest to blood bankers and the phenotypes they produce when inherited in the homozygous state.

Sometimes genes are considered silent because another gene (suppressor gene) is inhibiting the expression of their products. An example of this is

TABLE 4-3 Silent Genes

Blood Group Gene	Blood Group System	Homozygous Phenotype
h	ABO	O_n or Bombay
=	Rh	Rh_{null}
r		
K^0	Kell	$Kell_{null}$ or K_0
Lu	Lutheran	Lu(a− b−)
Jk	Kidd	Jk(a− b−)
Fy	Duffy	Fy(a−b−)

found in the Lutheran blood group system. People who inherit the *In(Lu)* gene in the homozygous state fail to express the products of Lutheran genes they may have inherited because of the inhibitory effect of *In(Lu)*.

BLOOD GROUP NOMENCLATURE

Some attempts have been made to standardize blood group nomenclature, but these attempts have not been completely successful. For example, in typical Mendelian genetics, dominant genes are usually capitalized, and recessive genes are lowercase. In blood group genetics, expression is not standardized. In the ABO system, for example, a person who is group A and inherits an *A* gene from one parent and an *O* gene from the other is genotypically noted as *AO*. Both *A* and *O* are capitalized, even though *A* is considered dominant to *O*. In the Rh system, a person who is heterozygous at the *Cc* locus is genotypically noted as *Cc*. Although the *c* is lowercase, it is not recessive to *C* but rather codominant with it. Many methods are used to denote various blood group genotypes and phenotypes. These are discussed in detail in a 1990 review article by Issit and Crookston.[3]

Some blood group genes are denoted by single letters such as M, K, and I. The phenotype resulting from these genes can be written using a plus symbol (+) to indicate the presence of the trait (detected by using antibody directed toward the trait) or a minus symbol (−) to indicate its absence. For example, RBCs reacting with anti-M, anti-K, and anti-k but not with anti-N would be phenotypically M+N−K+k+. This designation is not used in the ABO system, however, because RBCs reacting with anti-A but not with anti-B are designated group A, not A+B−.

Sometimes the genes of a blood group system are denoted by two letters with different superscripts to differentiate the alleles. Genes of the Duffy system fall into this category. The letters "Fy" indicate the Duffy system, and a superscript "a" or "b" is placed with the Fy to indicate alleles. Phenotypes in this system are written using the same symbols in a format that uses pluses and minuses to indicate the presence or absence of traits. RBCs that react with Fy[a] and not with Fy[b] are phenotypically Fy(a+b−). This mode of nomenclature is used in the Lutheran, Kidd, Scianna, and Gerbich systems as well.

Numeric nomenclature has been developed for most blood group systems. In this instance, each gene is written with a letter and a number (e.g., the Kell trait is K1). Phenotypes are written using a letter followed by a colon and a positive number if the particular trait represented by the number is present or a negative number if the trait represented by the number is absent (i.e., K: −1 would be written for

RBCs failing to react with antibody to K1). Genes are written using the letter and a superscript number (K[1]); K1 is the product of K[1].

The Rh system is even more confusing for the student of blood group systems because several different nomenclatures are used. Chapter 10 discusses the nomenclature used in this system in detail.

PUBLIC AND PRIVATE GENES

Certain genes and their resulting traits are found in most of the population. These genes are referred to as *public genes*. Other genes are exceedingly rare and are sometimes referred to as *private genes*. These can be found in few people, often only in a particular race or family.

BLOOD GROUP GENES AS GENETIC MARKERS

Because blood group genes are *polymorphic*, they can be useful in detecting several types of genetic problems. Disputed parentage is perhaps the most common problem. Box 4-1 lists some of the blood group systems that are commonly used in *parentage testing*. The histocompatibility or human leukocyte antigen (HLA) system and RBC enzyme studies, in addition to detection of the product of red cell genes, are useful in such testing.

By using blood group genetics, it is possible to exclude people from parentage. Such exclusions are either direct or indirect. In a direct exclusion, the offspring possesses a trait that neither the mother nor the alleged father possess, as in the following example:

> Mother *AA*
> Father *OO*
> Child *AB*

BOX 4-1

Blood Group Systems Commonly Used in Paternity Testing

ABO
Duffy
HLA
Kell
Kidd
MNSs
Rh

The alleged father is directly excluded on the basis that the child possesses a group B gene that he or she could not have received from the mother or the alleged father. The gene, therefore, must have been contributed by another person.

Indirect exclusion refers to a case in which an offspring does not possess a gene that should have been inherited. In the case shown below, the child should possess the *c* gene because the alleged father is homozygous and should pass *c* to any of his offsprings. The child, however, does not possess this gene; therefore, an indirect exclusion is established.

Mother *CC*
Alleged father *cc*
Child *CC*

SUMMARY

Blood group genetics is extremely important to the entire field of genetics. The study of inheritance in the blood group systems has added to our knowledge and understanding of how traits are inherited.

For the student of blood banking, a basic understanding of genetics is crucial. An understanding of the production of detectable blood group traits and the interaction of genes in relation to those traits is necessary to understand many basic blood banking concepts. Further insight into the various blood group systems is presented with the discussion of each system. The interested reader is referred to the references for further reading.

Review Questions

1. The normal human cell contains _____ pairs of chromosomes.
   a. 12
   b. 23
   c. 46
   d. 92
2. A gamete would contain _____ chromosomes.
   a. 23 pairs of
   b. 46 pairs of
   c. 23
   d. none of the above
3. Eggs and sperm are formed through the process of
   a. mitosis
   b. meiosis
   c. linkage
   d. crossing-over
4. With which of the following would an anti-K showing dosage react most strongly?
   a. a red cell of the genotype *Kk*
   b. a red cell of the genotype *kk*
   c. a red cell of the genotype *KK*
   d. none of the above
5. If the frequency of gene *Y* is 0.4 and the frequency of gene *Z* is 0.5, one would expect they should occur together 0.2 (20%) of the time. In actuality, they are found together 32% of the time. This is an example of
   a. crossing-over
   b. linkage disequilibrium
   c. polymorphism
   d. linkage equilibrium
6. A gene that produces no detectable product is referred to as
   a. an amorph
   b. a trait
   c. an allele
   d. a polymorph

7. Alternate forms of a gene that can occur at a single chromosome locus are referred to as
   a. traits
   b. alleles
   c. chromosomes
   d. phenotypes
8. Which of the following describes the expression of most blood group genes?
   a. dominant
   b. recessive
   c. codominant
   d. corecessive
9. For a trait to be useful as a genetic marker, which of the following is important?
   a. a simple and unequivocal pattern of inheritance
   b. lack of polymorphism
   c. regular interaction with other genes that alter its expression
   d. none of the above
10. A gene found only in a few individuals, usually in a particular race or family, is referred to as:
    a. an amorphic gene
    b. a public gene
    c. a private gene
    d. a genetic aberration
11. True or false? A standard nomenclature used uniformly for all blood group systems exists.
12. True or false? An individual who is group A cannot product a child who is group B.
13. True or false? Genes located far apart on the chromosome are more likely to cross over, resulting in changed genetic information.
14. True or false? In a direct exclusion, the child has failed to inherit a gene that should have been passed by the alleged father.
15. True or false? Some genes can inhibit the expression of other genes.

REFERENCES

1. Campbell N, Reece J. *Biology*. 7th ed. San Francisco: Benjamin-Cummings Publishing Company; 2004.
2. Brecher ME, ed. *AABB Technical Manual*. 15th ed. Bethesda, MD: AABB; 2005.
3. Issit PD, Crookston MC. Blood group terminology: current conventions. *Transfusion*. 1984; 24: 2.

ADDITIONAL READINGS

Burns G. *The Science of Genetics: An Introduction to Heredity*. 2nd ed. New York: Macmillan; 1972.

Issit PD. *Applied Blood Group Serology*. 3rd ed. Miami: Montgomery Scientific Publications; 1985.

BASIC IMMUNOLOGIC PRINCIPLES

EVA D. QUINLEY

OBJECTIVES

After completion of this chapter, the reader will be able to:

1. Describe cellular and humoral immunity, including clonal selection theory.
2. Describe the constituent cells of the immune system and their functions.
3. Describe the interrelationship between inflammation and specific acquired immunity.
4. Discuss the distinctive properties of antigens.
5. Describe structure and functions of each immunoglobulin type.
6. Describe an antigen-antibody reaction.
7. Explain the complement activation cascade in the classic and alternate pathways.

KEY WORDS

Activation	Clone
Alternate pathway	Complement
Anamnestic response	Cytokines
Anaphylatoxin	Cytotoxic T lymphocyte
Antibody	Disulfide bonds
Antigen	Epitope
Antigen presentation	Fc receptor
B lymphocyte	Haptens
Cell-mediated immunity	Heavy chains
Cell surface receptors	T-helper cell
Classic pathway	Hinge region
Clonal selection theory	Humoral immunity

Hypervariable	Nonspecific inflammation
Idiotype	Perforin
IgG, IgM, IgA, IgD, and IgE	Phagocytosis
Immunization	Plasma cell
Immunogen	Primary immune response
Immunoglobulin	Properdin pathway
Killer cell	Recognition
Leukocyte	Secondary immune response
Light chains	Self
Lymphocyte	Specific, acquired immunity
Macrophage	T lymphocyte
Memory cell	Variable and constant regions
Nonself	Zeta potential

The term "immune" is derived from the Latin word *immunis*, which meant "exempt from charges" (i.e., taxes or expenses). Today, of course, immunity refers to the body's ability to resist infection by pathogenic microorganisms.

Much of what is known about immune function in humans and the function of cells in the immune system comes from concepts presented by Metchnikoff and Ehrlich. Metchnikoff was a brilliant Russian biologist who in 1880 first described *phagocytosis* and cellular immunity as he studied the role of motile cells in starfish larvae that surrounded and engulfed a rose thorn.[1] Metchnikoff proposed correctly that inflammation included enzymatic digestion of intruders engulfed by motile cells capable of moving into tissues in a process he termed "diapedesis."

In the early 1900s, Ehrlich stated his side-chain theory that represented an attempt to explain the formation of antibodies in the blood.[2] It was Ehrlich's idea that cells in the blood had "side chains" or specific receptors on their surfaces. Once the side chain on a cell was bound by a foreign substance, the cell produced more side chains, which entered the blood as antibodies.

It is a safe assumption that Metchnikoff and Ehrlich were familiar with the foundation that had been laid a century earlier by the English physician Jenner, who had performed and published on the first *immunization* procedures. He called these procedures "vaccination" from the Latin vacca, meaning "cow," because he injected his volunteers with cowpox as a way to immunize against smallpox.

Since these pioneering discoveries, an immense and diverse body of information has been developed in the area of biology we now call immunology. It will be necessary to condense, simplify, and restrict this chapter to the fundamentals of immunology that are essential for the immunohematologist. These areas of knowledge include cellular and *humoral immunity*, cells of the immune system and their development, structure and function of *antigens* and antibodies and their serologic behavior, the mechanisms of antigen reactions and agglutination, and the role of *complement*.

CELLULAR AND HUMORAL IMMUNITY

The immune system has evolved to allow recovery from infectious disease and to provide the host organism protection from infection. This system, made up of the *leukocytes* (also known as the white blood cells) and various organs like the spleen, lymph nodes, lymphatic channels, and the thymus, relies on complex interactions between cells located in the blood, the lymph, and in body tissues. The spleen and lymph nodes of the immune system are composed of a lattice or meshwork of tissue. When leukocytes travel through these organs, the cells are trapped by the lattice formation, and effective cell–cell interaction can occur. These interactions may lead to the production of antibodies or activated cells capable of destroying pathogens, virus-infected cells, or cancer cells.

The first step in launching a protective immune response is the *recognition* that something foreign has invaded the body. The immune system must be able to distinguish *self* from *nonself*, and it relies on the leukocytes to do so. Under certain circumstances, the foreign, nonself substance that leads to an immune response is known as "antigen," abbreviated Ag. In humans, the ability to distinguish self from nonself is

developed during embryonic growth, although how the recognition occurs is not completely understood. Once immune competence is established (usually by 4 to 6 months after birth in the human), external substances encountered in the body by leukocytes will be regarded as nonself, and an immune response may be triggered. In the period before immune competence is established, the immune system is immature and relatively unresponsive to antigens.

The response to antigenic challenge can be categorized into two types based upon the primary actor in the response: humoral immunity and *cell-mediated immunity*. Humoral immunity may be defined as an immune response that leads to the production of *antibody*. Cell-mediated immunity is conferred by activated leukocytes known as *T lymphocytes*, as well as another class of lymphocytes called *killer cells*. Most immune responses to pathogenic microorganisms include both a humoral and a cell-mediated component.

Looked at another way, most immune responses include a nonspecific inflammatory arm as well as an arm that includes *specific, acquired immunity*. When we speak of specific, acquired immunity, we are referring to an immune response that includes antigens binding to antibodies or structures on the surface of *lymphocytes* very specifically, with a lock-and-key type of fit. Inflammation, generated by *macrophages* and neutrophils, does not require this sort of specific binding to destroy microorganisms. These distinctions cannot be fully appreciated without some knowledge of the cells involved in the immune system and their function.

LEUKOCYTES: CELLS OF THE IMMUNE SYSTEM

All cellular elements of blood (red cells, leukocytes, and platelets) derive from a pluripotent stem cell, including those that are relevant to immune responses. During early fetal development, these stem cells migrate from the embryonic yolk sac into the fetal liver, spleen, and bone marrow. It is in these sites that the lymphoid stem cells that will eventually produce the specific cells of the immune system, the lymphocytes, undergo additional differentiation. Some of these cells migrate to and mature in the thymus and are referred to as thymus derived, or T lymphocytes. T lymphocytes manifest cellular immunity but also play a "helper" role in humoral immunity.

Other lymphoid stem cells influenced by the fetal liver, bone marrow, or gut-associated lymphoid tissue (GALT) differentiate to become *B lymphocytes* or bone marrow–derived cells. The B lymphocytes mature during immune responses and become the antibody-producing *plasma cells*.

The immune response also involves three other types of immunocompetent cells: macrophages, K cells (killer cells), and natural killer (NK) cells. Some authors group K and NK cells into a single category, killer cells.

Macrophages

The macrophages, neutrophils, and mast cells make up the inflammatory arm of the immune response. The macrophage is a mononuclear cell with a nonlobulated nucleus that may be found fixed in tissues (sessile), or motile. Motile macrophages are mature forms of the peripheral blood monocytes. The fixed tissue macrophages include the Kupffer cells in the liver, connective tissue histiocytes, and other fixed cells that make up the so-called reticuloendothelial system. Macrophages may also be found in the lining of sinusoid tissues of the spleen, lymph nodes, and bone marrow.

Functionally, the macrophage is a *nonspecific, phagocytic* cell. The phagocytic macrophages engulf and destroy their targets, attracted to particles in the body when these particles are "opsonized" (i.e., coated with either antibody or activated complement). The macrophages find antibody- or complement-coated particles very palatable because the macrophages have nonspecific *cell surface receptors* for antibody that has bound to its antigen. This receptor is called the *Fc receptor*. Macrophages also have a receptor for activated complement on their surface. The engulfment of particles like bacteria is performed when the macrophage extends some of its cell contents to surround the particle. The cell extensions are called "pseudopodia," meaning "false feet." These cells, as well as other cells of the immune system, are drawn to the site of infection by inflammatory chemicals called "chemotaxins."

Macrophages do not bind their targets specifically. In other words, the macrophage does not care if it is engulfing a virus or a fungal particle or a sliver of wood. In fact, it is able to phagocytize all three at once!

In addition to removing particles, pathogens, damaged white and red blood cells (RBCs), and foreign organic matter from the blood, the macrophages also serve to "process" antigens and "present" the processed antigen to T and B cells. Once the macrophage phagocytoses an antibody or complement-coated particle, it uses proteolytic enzymes located inside the cell to kill and then degrade the engulfed particle into fragments. The degraded proteins or polysaccharides derived from the engulfed particle are displayed on the macrophage surface in combination with a self-protein called human leukocyte antigen (HLA) class II, in the process called *antigen presentation*. The T lymphocytes of the specific, acquired side of immunity now try to bind the displayed fragment in their specific (lock-and-key type) cell surface receptor. If the T lymphocyte receives a specific antigen in its receptor, and receives a chemical signal from the macrophage, or if it interacts with the appropriate molecule on the surface of the macrophage, it becomes activated and begins generating specific, acquired immunity. These steps are shown in Figures 5-1 and 5-2.

In addition to this primary function, many other functions of macrophage have been identified, among

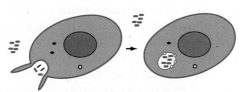

1. Macrophage drawn to infection site by chemotaxis. Pseudopodia.

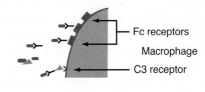

2. Attachment of Ab or C opsonized bacteria to Fc receptors. C3 receptors on macrophage pseudopod.

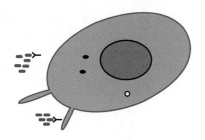

3. Endocytosis. Ingestion. Vacuolization.

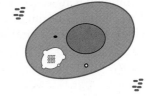

4. Granule release. Killing. Digestion to peptides.

FIGURE 5-1   Phagocytosis and antigen presentation.

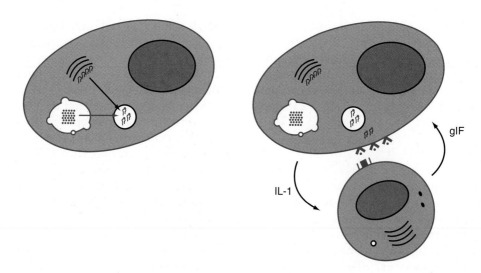

5. HLA Class II made in the ER moves to
   Golgi. Bacterial peptides move to Golgi.
   Combination made.

6. Ag presentation to the specific T-helper cell
   Ag receptor. Cytokines exchanged. Specific
   immune response is launched.

FIGURE 5-2   Phagocytosis and antigen presentation, continued.

them is the ability to produce and secrete enzymes that activate plasminogen, denature collagen, and produce complement components.

Lymphocytes and Specific Antigen Binding by Cell Surface Receptors

The B and T lymphocytes have cell surface receptors capable of *specifically* binding a single antigen. It is the physical shape of these cell surface receptor proteins that allows the binding of one antigen and not another. Think of it this way: if you hold your hands in such a way that an orange fits snugly between them, the shape that your hands form will not hold onto a banana very tightly. A different shape is required to hold the banana, and that shape will not hold the orange. This is an example of specific binding. Of course, the lymphocyte cell surface receptors and antibodies do not need to bind oranges or bananas, but staphylococcal bacteria, cytomegalovirus, and the like. The cell surface receptor that binds the staphylococcus does not fit tightly with the virus, and vice versa. All of the cell surface receptors on a single lymphocyte, and all of the antibodies made by a single plasma cell have the same shape. Thus, all of the cell surface receptors on a single lymphocyte bind to only one antigen.

T Lymphocytes

The thymic-derived lymphocytes originate in the bone marrow and are believed to migrate early in embryonic life to the thymus, where they mature under the influence of thymosin and other thymic hormones. Later they move through the lymphatic system and bloodstream to reside in the lymph nodes and spleen. Some remain in the bloodstream. T lymphocytes are morphologically indistinguishable from B lymphocytes in preparations made with Wright stain. To characterize the T cells, supravital techniques or mitogen stimulation is required.

T cells comprise 70% to 80% of the peripheral blood lymphocyte population and are durable; they have an average half-life of more than 2 years, and some survive as long as 20 years. Functionally, the T cell is important in providing protection against infections by viruses, fungi, and, particularly, facultative microorganisms. A number of subpopulations or subsets in the T-lymphocyte population have now been recognized.

T-Helper Lymphocytes

T-helper cells account for approximately 40% to 60% of the peripheral blood T-lymphocyte population. The T-helper cell may be distinguished from other cells of the immune system because they carry a protein on their surface called CD4. The CD4 protein assists the T-helper cell bind its *specific* surface antigen receptor to antigen being presented by a macrophage, as shown in Figure 5-3. The T-cell receptor is made up of two protein chains, and the presented antigen fits in the groove between these two chains. Once the T-helper cell has bound its specific antigen and received a signal from

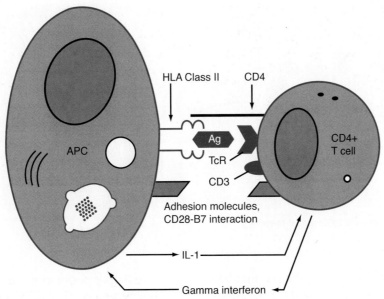

FIGURE 5-3 CD4 + T-cell activation: launching the immune response. (Source: Garratty G, ed. *Red Cell Antigens and Antibodies.* Arlington, VA: American Association of Blood Banks; 1986.)

the macrophage, it amplifies the immune response by producing proinflammatory proteins called *cytokines* that act as growth factors and help to activate other immune system cells, as shown in Figure 5-4. It is through the production of a mixture of cytokines that CD4-positive T-helper cells help to activate B cells. If a B cell has recognized its specific antigen using its specific cell surface antigen receptor (which for the B cell is actually antibody molecules) and has received a cytokine signal from the T-helper cell, it divides and differentiates to become a plasma cell, which gushes antibody for 3 to 4 days. The antibody produced by the plasma cell has the same antigen-binding specificity as the cell surface antigen receptor.

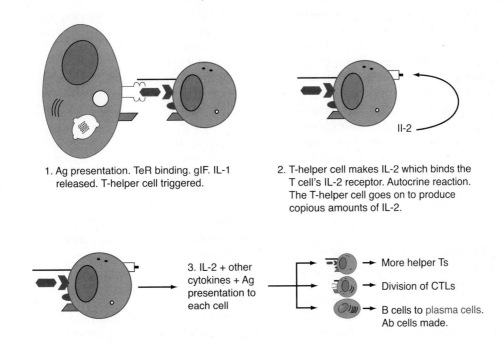

FIGURE 5-4 CD4 + T-cell activation; launching the immune response. (Source: Garratty G, ed. *Red Cell Antigens and Antibodies.* Arlington, VA: American Association of Blood Banks; 1986.)

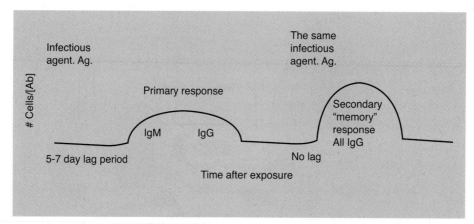

FIGURE 5-5   Specific immunization and memory.

T-helper cells also play a role in the cell-mediated immune response and participate in the graft-versus-host reaction. The T-helper cell's CD4 surface protein is the site on the cell to which the human immunodeficiency virus attaches.

The first time a T-helper cell interacts with its antigen, its response is relatively slow. This *primary immune response* may take 5 to 7 days to generate antibodies and appreciable numbers of activated cells. That is why we often become ill during our first exposure to a pathogen; the microorganisms have about a week to grow in our bodies before an immune response can destroy them. The immune response we generate to our first exposure to a disease may allow us to recover, but it usually will not prevent infection. However, as part of the primary immune response, our immune systems generate *memory cells*, which may circulate in our blood for years. If we are reexposed to a pathogen to which we have generated memory cells in the past, these cells become activated very quickly. There is very little lag between exposure and immunity. These *secondary immune responses* may actually prevent disease, and this concept is the basis of immunization or vaccination (Fig. 5-5). All of the lymphocyte populations can generate "memory," but the nonspecific inflammatory cells, like the macrophages or neutrophils, do not.

Cytotoxic Suppressor T Cells

A second subpopulation of T lymphocytes bears a surface protein called CD8. The CD8-positive T-cell population is capable of carrying out two vastly different functions. These cells can downregulate immune responses through their suppressor function and can also kill virus-infected cells, tumor cells, or transplanted tissue through their cytotoxic capacities. The CD8 cytotoxic suppressor T cells, like the CD4-positive helper population, carry antigen-specific cell surface receptors. The CD8 cells become activated when their antigen receptor binds specifically to a target, and the cell also receives a cytokine signal from the T-helper cell. Once activated, the *cytotoxic T lymphocytes* (CTLs) kill virus-infected cells when their antigen receptor binds specifically to viral antigen on the surface of the infected cell. The CD8 protein stabilizes the interaction of the antigen receptor and the viral antigen by recognizing HLA class I molecules on the infected cell surface. Cytokines help turn on the CTL, which activates granules in the cytoplasm that contain a protein called *perforin*. Perforin kills virus-infected cells by establishing nonspecific calcium channels in the target cell. The rapid, uncontrolled influx of calcium into the virus-infected cell poisons it, preventing further virus replication. These steps are displayed in Figures 5-6 and 5-7. The cytotoxic suppressor T cells produce memory as part of the primary immune response.

Killer Cells

Killer cells are large, granular lymphocytes that appear to have the ability to destroy tumor cells. The nature of the antigen receptor on these cells is not well characterized, although it is known that K cells have Fc receptors on their surfaces. Thus, the K cell may be drawn to an antibody-coated tumor cell target, just as a macrophage is drawn to antibody-coated particles.

Natural Killer Cells

The NK cells are thought to have widespread cytotoxic ability against a variety of virally infected and tumor cells. Their antigen receptor and method of killing are not well understood (Fig. 5-8).

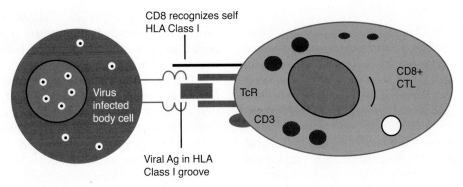

FIGURE 5-6   Specific cells of the immune response.

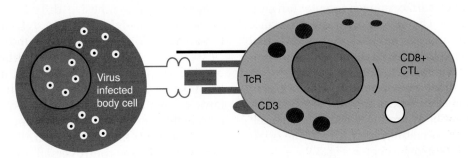

1. CTL binds target with TcR. Granules move into area. Perforin released.

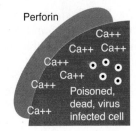

2. Perforin sets up ion channels which allow unlimited Ca++ to enter the cell, poisioning it.

FIGURE 5-7   CD8 + cytotoxic T-lymphocyte antiviral activity.

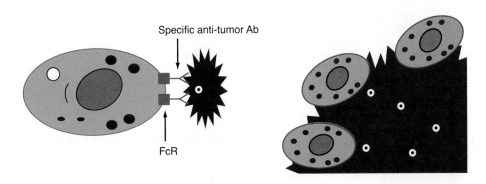

Killer cells have Fc receptors that bind Ab already bound to the tumor target.

NK cells bind their tumor targets by an unknown mechanism. Kill with perforin.

FIGURE 5-8   Killer and natural killer cells. Large granular lymphocytes that carry neither T- nor B-cell markers. Kill tumor cells using the perforin mechanism.

B Lymphocytes

The remaining 5% to 15% of peripheral blood lymphocytes can be classified as B lymphocytes on the basis of their surface antigen receptors, which are actually antibody molecules. After migration from the bone marrow, B lymphocytes reside in the germinal centers and medullary areas of the lymph nodes and spleen, where they lose some cytoplasm and become smaller. More than 50% of the lymphocytes in the spleen and tonsils are B lymphocytes. The immature B lymphocyte may be thought of as the precursor to the antibody-producing and morphologically recognizable plasma cell, which is differentiated by exposure to antigen and interaction with T-helper cells.

If a B cell has recognized its specific antigen using its specific cell surface antigen receptor (an antibody molecule, which may also be called surface *immunoglobulin*) and has received a cytokine signal from the T-helper cell, the B cell divides and differentiates to become a plasma cell. The plasma cells, which are large and full of protein-producing machinery (called the endoplasmic reticulum), gush antibody for 3 to 4 days. The antibody produced by the plasma cell has the same antigen-binding specificity as the original B cell's surface antigen receptor (Fig. 5-9).

Groups of B cells or plasma cells that produce antibody with the same specificity are said to be members of the same B cell *clone*. Not all B cells are transformed into plasma cells and produce antibody. Some become memory cells capable of rapid antibody production on reexposure. The antibodies produced during this so-called *anamnestic response* are very high-quality antibodies said to belong to the immunoglobulin G or IgG subclass.

The preceding discussion described the *clonal selection theory* in its basic form. This theory postulates that a given B lymphocyte is triggered by contact with an antigen for which it carries specific cell surface receptors. The activated cell proliferates and synthesizes antibody with the same binding specificity as the surface antigen receptor. The theory also states that all of the progeny of that activated lymphocyte produce antibody of identical structure and specificity. Although the cells in the B-lymphocyte population have many features in common, they synthesize different classes of immunoglobulin—*IgM, IgG, IgA, IgD,* and *IgE.* Additional variation has led to subdivision of the classes into subclasses, the importance of which becomes apparent in the section on immunoglobulin subclasses later in this chapter. It is also important to realize that antibody synthesis is an extremely complex process under the control of genes beyond those that control diversification. Many aspects are controversial and under intense investigation.

Keep in mind that most immune responses are a combination of *nonspecific inflammation* (caused predominantly by macrophages, neutrophils, and mast cells) and specific, acquired immunity (conferred

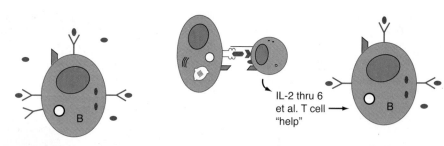

1. B cells surface Ig Ag receptor binds free Ag or receives Ag from APCs.

2. B cells are stimulated to divide and differentiate by Ag binding and cytokines.

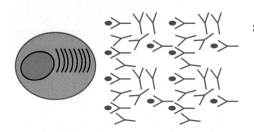

3. Plasma cells gush Ab for 3-4 days. The Ab specificity is the same as the sIg (same variable regio AA sequence). The Ab produced helps to destroy the Ag. Thus the Ag has selected the B cell clone producing Ab that eventually led to the destruction of Ag. Immunization, memory.

FIGURE 5-9   Antibody production: the antigen selection hypothesis.

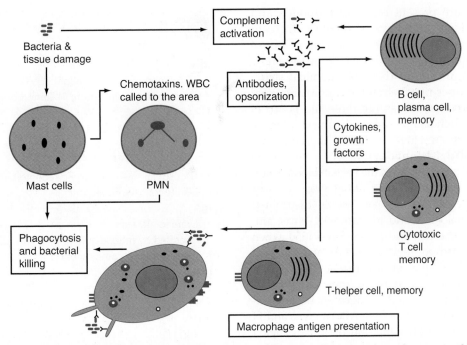

FIGURE 5-10   An immune response consists of both nonspecific inflammation and specific acquired immunity.

by lymphocytes). The complex interactions and cooperation demonstrated by these cell populations are shown in diagrammatic fashion in Figure 5-10. This example describes the cells that work together to fight off a bacterial infection.

IMMUNOGENS VERSUS ANTIGENS

An *immunogen* is a substance that causes a detectable immune response. Frequently, the terms "immunogen" and "antigen" are used interchangeably, although they are not, in the strictest sense of their definitions, the same thing. An antigen is a substance that is capable of reacting with the product of an immune response. Antigen combines with antibody (i.e., "antigen–antibody reaction" is used instead of "immunogen–antibody reaction").

Introduction of nonself immunogens present on human RBCs, white blood cells, and platelets may elicit antibody production. On a biochemical level, an immunogen is a substance with a molecular weight of 10,000 D or more. Substances with a molecular weight of less than 5,000 D seldom cause antibody formation. If coupled with larger carrier molecules, however, these substances, known as *haptens*, can become immunogenic (able to stimulate an immune response). Once an immune response has been initiated by the hapten–carrier complex, the hapten alone can react with the product of the immune response (i.e., antibody). Complex biochemical compounds, especially those containing proteins or polypeptide–carbohydrate combinations, are highly immunogenic. The more diverse the molecule is, the more immunogenic it becomes. As previously indicated, the structure must be recognized by the cells of the recipient's immune system to be nonself.

Route of Administration

Intravenous and intraperitoneal injection of immunogen is highly effective in producing an immune response. Intradermal, subcutaneous, or intramuscular routes are less effective.

Shape and Charge

It is now recognized that molecular shape and charge are the most important features affecting immunogenicity and antigenicity (the ability of a substance to react with the product of an immune response). Antigens on human RBCs protrude from the cells' membrane in a steric (three-dimensional) configuration and carry ionic charges. These immunogens are proteins coupled with carbohydrate molecules (glycoproteins) or lipids (lipoproteins). Although the immunogen is large, the antigenic determinant, known also as the *epitope*, is a small portion that may be composed of as few as five or six amino acids or sugars. This small epitopic region is responsible for specificity, meaning that the region contains the molecular configurations that allow recognition by the corresponding antibody.

Many epitopes are present on an immunogen and multiple antibodies that have somewhat different specificity and reactivity may be formed in response to a single, large immunogen. Because of the steric or spatial configuration of these biochemical structures, some epitopes may be rendered nonfunctional or unable to combine unless the molecule is structurally altered (such as may occur during deliberate modification with enzymes or during the combination of antigen with its antibody).

The chemical composition of the human blood group substances has been studied for many years. Similar macromolecular configurations are widely distributed throughout the biologic world in mammals, birds, amphibians, reptiles, bacteria, and plants. Since 1950, when the carbohydrate composition of the A, B, and H blood group substances became known, the new science of immunochemistry has added much knowledge to our understanding of the structural arrangement of the component sugars. The structures of the ABO, Lewis, and H antigens are better understood than any of the other blood groups. Also, the Rh antigens have a lipoprotein structure. Because the task is complicated by the isolation of antigens from the red cell, much remains to be learned about many of the other blood group antigens.

The lipoprotein immunogens (antigens) are probably even more complex than the carbohydrate structures. Antigens expressed on human red cells are developed under the control of genes. The names for the genes and the antigens each defines are the same for most of the blood groups (i.e., A gene codes for the A antigen).

ANTIBODIES

The terms "antibody" and "immunoglobulin" are commonly used interchangeably, though there is a semantic difference between the two terms. Immunologists call a molecule an antibody if its binding specificity is known—for example, an antimeasles virus antibody. Immunoglobulin refers to a collection of different antibodies with no single binding specificity, such as a preparation of intravenous immunoglobulin.

Antibodies may be thought of as substances produced in response to immunogenic stimulation that are capable of specific interaction with the provoking antigens. The immunoglobulins that function as antibody may be divided into five classes based on their different physical, chemical, and biologic properties: *IgG, IgM, IgA, IgD, and IgE.* Each of these classes can bind antigens. Box 5-1 summarizes some of the properties of these immunoglobulins, and Figure 5-11 shows the simplified structure of IgG, dimeric IgA, and pentameric IgM.

BOX 5-1 Properties of the Immunoglobulin Classes

IgG
- Monomer; molecular weight 180,000 D
- Most abundant in serum; 1^0 immune response, class shift
- "Maternal Ab"; crosses placenta
- Binds complement to destroy antigens which have been bound
- Is opsonic; macrophage Fc receptors have high affinity for IgG Fc regions

IgA
- Dimeric, 400 kD
- Secreted by mucous membranes, in mother's milk
- Does not bind complement

IgM
- Pentameric, 900 kD
- Primary immune response Ab; binds complement

IgD
- 180 kD
- B cell surface Ig?

IgE
- Monomeric, 180 kD
- In allergy or anaphylaxis, binds mast cell and allergen

Immunoglobulins are the product of plasma cell protein production, and these protein–carbohydrate moieties (glycoprotein) bind to their antigens in a highly specific fashion. Each immunoglobulin molecule is made of 82% to 96% protein (polypeptide) and 4% to 18% carbohydrate. Human blood group antibodies are generally of two types, IgM or IgG, although IgA forms also exist. Within the five classes of immunoglobulins, there exist differences in each single type that have resulted in the further division into subgroups or subclasses. For example, IgG has four identified subclasses: IgG1, IgG2, IgG3, and IgG4.

Structure and Physiochemistry

Each immunoglobulin molecule may be thought of as consisting of two identical polypeptide *heavy chains* (H) and two identical polypeptide *light chains* (L) (Fig. 5-12). Each of the heavy chains contains a sequence of approximately 440 amino acids with a molecular weight between 50,000 and 70,000 D that is identical within each molecule. The light chains are also identical to each other within the same molecule, although different from the heavy chains. The light chains contain about 220 amino

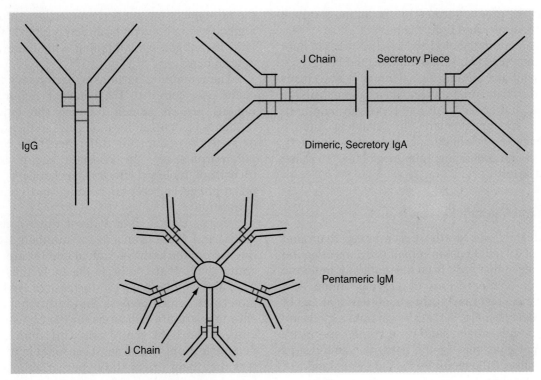

FIGURE 5-11 Simplified structures of IgG, IgA, and IgM.

acids with a weight of 20,000 to 25,000 D. These two pairs of chains are held together covalently by molecular bridges called **disulfide bonds** (S–S) and noncovalent forces. The interaction of disulfide bonds holds together loops of folded polypeptide chains known as domains. The disulfide bonds also allow the antibody molecule to flex, and to change shape in three-dimensional space. Antigens are

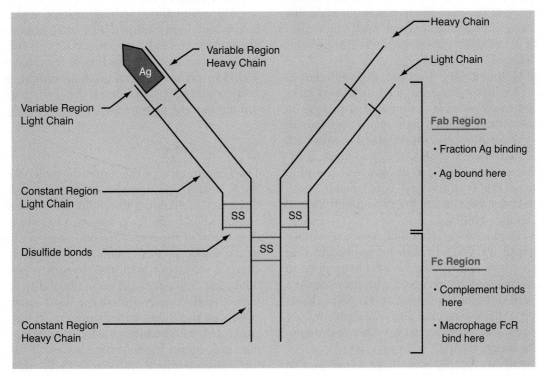

FIGURE 5-12 Basic structure of the immunoglobulin molecule.

bound in the groove formed by the amino-terminal ends of the heavy and light chains.

Human immunoglobulins have two types of light chains, known as kappa and lambda, and both types can form antigen-binding sites. Human heavy chains are found in five variations known as gamma, alpha, mu, delta, and epsilon. All five types can bind antigens. An immunoglobulin (Ig)-containing gamma heavy chains is called immunoglobulin gamma, or IgG, whereas a mu-containing immunoglobulin is called IgM, and so forth.

Variable and Constant Regions

Approximately one fourth of each heavy chain and one half of each light chain contains regions of amino acid sequence that vary from one antibody molecule to another. These regions of varying amino acid sequence may be found at the amino-terminal end of the molecule (see Fig. 5-12). The variable regions are concerned with antigen binding and confer specificity on the molecule; that is, the particular amino acid sequence allows the molecule to bind or not bind to a particular antigen.

There are about 20 different amino acids that are used to make up human proteins, and each amino acid has its own unique shape. Therefore, the amino acid sequence of the variable region determines the three-dimensional shape of the antibody-binding site. Thus, this sequence determines which antigen is bound by that antibody molecule. If the amino acid sequence of the variable region is changed, the shape of the antibody-binding site and which antigen will fit in the groove between the H and L chains are also changed.

Actually, the ability to bind one antigen as opposed to another is believed to be controlled more precisely by *hypervariable* amino acid sequences in these regions, three in each light chain and four in each heavy chain. More specifically, the shapes of both are complementary and dictate the "goodness of fit" and whether the antibody and antigen will complex. The analogy of the "lock and key" supplemented with positive and negative charges is a good description of antibody–antigen binding.

(The principle of *variable and constant regions* described here for the formation of antibodies that bind their antigen specifically can also be applied to the T-cell surface antigen receptor, with the exception that the T-cell receptor is made of two protein chains with one antigen-binding site. Antibodies are constructed of four protein chains with two antigen-binding sites per molecule.)

The sequence of amino acids in the hypervariable regions of the heavy and light chains is referred to as the *idiotype* of the antibody molecule. Anti-idiotype antibodies can prevent the antibody from complexing with its antigen by combining with these idiotypic determinants.

The remaining portions of each heavy and light chain pair comprise the constant regions. These regions are so named because the amino acid sequence is identical for molecules in the same class or subclass (except for differences due to genetic polymorphisms). The constant regions function to control biologic effector mechanisms, such as macrophage Fc receptor binding and complement *activation*.

Heavy chains have at least three constant regions, and these domains are numbered consecutively from the amino-terminal end (as are all of the amino acids that comprise the molecules) as C_H1, C_H2, and C_H3 (and C_H4 in the case of IgM and IgE molecules, which possess this additional domain). Although specific functions for the C_L (constant region of the light chain) and C_H1 domains elude demonstration, it is at least reasonable to suppose that they help orient the hypervariable sequences for antigen binding. The C_H2 domain has been shown specifically to activate complement by binding the Clq molecule. The C_H3 domain is the C region responsible for binding to macrophages. In addition, the constant region is involved in placental transfer, which confers passive immunity to the newborn. IgG constant and variable domains are shown in Figure 5-13.

These functions of the constant regions of the heavy and light chains are of vital importance and should not be considered secondary to the essential "antigen recognition" function of the amino-terminal end. The primary interactions of antigen with antibody would be insignificant if these effector functions did not become manifest.

The Hinge Region

The *hinge region* of the antibody molecule between the C_H1 and C_H2 domains is the area that provides flexibility in allowing the molecule to combine with antigen (Fig. 5-13). As is apparent from the previous discussion of the hypervariable sequences, the electric charges present, with positive and negative charges attracting and like charges repelling each other, the molecule must have the ability to conform three-dimensionally and shape itself spatially to fit closely or widely separated antigens. It has also been suggested that the molecule in the unbound state, as normally occurs in the serum, is in a "T" shape with the amino-terminal ends maximally distant from each other. When combined with antigen, these ends

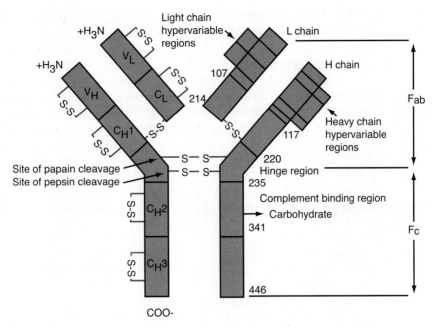

FIGURE 5-13   IgG molecule.

flex to become "Y" shaped, and the arms swing inward. This flex change may also allow the C_H2 and C_H3 effector domains more accessibility for complement binding by reducing steric hindrance. The lengths and flexibility of the hinge have been found to vary with each of the IgG subclasses, and this variability is reflected in the ability to trigger the biologic or effector functions.

Fragment, Antigen-binding and Fragment, Crystallizable

In 1959, the research of Rodney Porter showed that the IgG molecule could be split in the hinge region by the use of proteolytic enzymes. Different products also are obtained when the enzymes pepsin and papain are used. When papain is used, the molecule is split into three fragments, two of which are identical and capable of antigen binding (although not capable of causing red cell agglutination or precipitation reactions). These two fragments are referred to as fragment, antigen-binding (Fab) because they bind antigen, and each is composed of one light chain and roughly half of its heavy chain (Fig. 5-12).

The remaining portion of the molecule split by papain is referred to as the fragment, crystallizable (Fc) region. This is composed of the two remaining carboxy-terminal end halves of the heavy chains. Enzyme treatment has allowed these two portions to be studied independently, and the functions of

complement activation (C_H2), placental transport, and macrophage binding (C_H3) were assigned to the Fc fragment. Treatment with pepsin results in a slightly different type of Fab fragment, called F(ab')2, which in addition to retaining its antigen-binding ability, is capable of causing agglutination and precipitation reactions. F(ab')2 is roughly the top half of the molecule, including the disulfide bonds holding the two heavy chains together. Pepsin splits the heavy chains just below the disulfide bonds: papain splits them above these bonds. Pepsin also splits the remaining Fc pieces into many small fragments.

IgG Subclass and Function

Immunoglobulins help to protect from disease by specifically binding with the nonself substance that elicited their production. After antigen binding, the immunoglobulin molecule promotes phagocytosis, because macrophage and other cells have a receptor on their surface that binds to the Fc region of the molecule. This function allows for the destruction of potentially harmful bacteria and the neutralization of toxic substances. The Fc regions of antibodies, which have bound their antigen, also activate complement. For the immunohematologist, these basic functions extend to and include the nonself antigens present on allogeneic transfused RBCs, white blood cells, and platelets. Through the action of antibody, elimination of transfused cells may occur extravascularly (outside the blood vessels) in the reticuloendothelial system (a system of fixed-tissue phagocytic cells in organs like the liver), or intravascularly (within the blood vessels) through the mechanism of complement activation.

Of the total amount of serum immunoglobulin in a normal adult, fully 80% is constituted by IgG: its level is approximately 600 to 1600 mg/dL of serum. Within this class, approximately 60% to 70% is IgG1, 20% to 30% is IgG2, 4% to 8% is IgG3, and 1% to 6% is IgG4. The level of each is influenced by genetics, age, race, and sex and may vary considerably from one individual to another. The main interest in subclasses lies in the differences in their biologic properties.

In humans, IgG is the only immunoglobulin class capable of crossing the placenta. IgG also fixes complement with unequal facility within the subclasses, in the order IgG3 > IgG1 > IgG2, with IgG4 possibly activating only in the *alternate pathway*. This difference in complement-binding ability derives from differences in subclass hinge region flexibility, as previously described, but it is influenced by the length of the hinge region and the number of interchain disulfide bonds (which varies among each of the subclasses).

IgG1 and IgG3 molecules also complex with macrophages through Fc receptors. At least three different receptor types have now been studied: FcRI, FcRII, and FcRIII. The interaction between these receptors and the IgG molecule is integral to the processes of phagocytosis and immune complex clearance.

Hybridomas and Monoclonal Antibodies

Since the mid-1980s, the use of monoclonal antibodies has expanded considerably. A monoclonal antibody is a very specific preparation. All molecules produced are identical, unlike what would be seen in a normal immune response. In the normal immune response, many clones of lymphocytes produce antibody directed toward many different epitopes. The heterogeneous antibodies produced by many lymphocyte clones are known as polyclonal, and they represent the normal immune response.

The proliferation of a single lymphocyte clone producing antibody of identical specificity and having identical heavy and light chains results in a monoclonal antibody. This situation is abnormal and often pathologic, as in cold hemagglutination disease, in which the monoclonal antibody is IgM and may be anti-I or anti-i.

In 1975, it was shown that mouse myeloma cells grown in culture could be fused with lymphocytes from immunized animals to produce a cell, called a hybridoma, that would grow continuously and secrete antibody specific for the immunizing antigen. The advantages of this new technology were at once clear. The synthesized antibodies made from the single-cell clone are structurally identical to each other and therefore are monospecific, capable of binding a single epitope. Further, cell lines can be maintained continuously in a culture and may be frozen and recovered. Hybridomas provide a highly reproducible, well-defined, and replenishable supply of homogeneous antibody. The application of monoclonals has had a profound effect in immunology. They have made diagnostic testing more sensitive and specific. This is true for the monoclonal reagents used in blood banking.

ANTIGEN–ANTIBODY REACTIONS

The structural framework comprising the typical mammalian cell membrane is a bilayer of lipid and phospholipid molecules, approximately 4.5 nm thick, arranged with the hydrophilic heads forming the outer and inner membrane surfaces. The hydrophobic tails meet at the center of the membrane. Many other molecules are also present in this membrane structure, including, on RBCs, the carbohydrate molecules comprising the A, B, and H antigens, the lipoprotein structures of the Rh system antigens, and other essential membrane molecules, such as cholesterol and *N*-acetylneuraminic acid (also called sialic acid) and other blood group system molecules. In transfusion, these molecules may act as antigens.

The Zeta Potential

The microenvironment of the red cell and the ions that may be present in human plasma or serum can dramatically influence whether an antibody is able to attach to RBCs, or whether the red cells themselves spontaneously aggregate. In 1965, the work of Pollack[3–5] and others showed that the red cell carries a net negative charge that results from the ionization of carboxyl groups of the essential membrane constituent, *N*-acetylneuraminic acid. The negatively charged RBC attracts positively charged cations in an ionic environment such as human serum. The red cell then travels in a cloud of positive cations, the density of which decreases as the distance from the cell increases. The zone separating the most dense layer surrounding the cell from the remainder of the cationic environment is referred to as the slipping plane of plane of shear. The *zeta potential* is the force expressed at this boundary that results from the difference in electrostatic potential at the red cell surface and the boundary. Any increase in the ionic strength of the microenvironment (or suspending medium) results in an increase in the charge density and a decrease in the thickness of the cation cloud and the zeta potential.

Hydration and Surface Tension

Zeta potential theory is not the entire story concerning the physics of red cell–antibody binding. Steane[6] have also investigated the ability of IgG molecules to cause agglutination. They concluded that the degree of hydration at the red cell surface also contributes to the agglutination phenomenon. These investigators found that the hydrophilic heads of phospholipids comprising the red cell membrane attract and orient water molecules. Phospholipid structures in the membrane are not static, but move more or less freely in a dynamic shifting and reorienting of water, creating a surface tension effect at the water–lipid interface. Many other factors, including the number, size, and distribution of antigen sites and van der Waals forces, also contribute. Artificial alteration of the normal ionic environment through the use of intravenous solutions in patients who have lost blood and as in vitro suspending media, such as low–ionic-strength saline (LISS), causes complex problems for the blood banker when determining the presence and compatibility of IgG alloantibody.

IMMUNE RESPONSE TO BLOOD PRODUCTS AND SUBSEQUENT HEMAGGLUTINATION

The immune response has already been described in some detail, with specific reference to antigen presentation and the formation of antibodies. The chapter has described the concepts of the primary and secondary immune responses and the regulation of these responses.

The blood banker may be primarily concerned with the B-cell antibody product made in response to antigenic material such as allogeneic ("foreign": from a donor other than the transfusion recipient) red cells and sometimes white blood cells, platelets, and drugs. Immunization, or sensitization (exposure to foreign antigens resulting in immune response) to these substances, occurs through transfusion or pregnancy. Cellular elements from the donor or fetus contain antigens recognized by the immune system of the recipient as nonself. When presented to the recipient, these antigens are processed by the recipient's immune system and may result in the formation of detectable antibody. This occurs in 30% to 70% of all people transfused with blood products that contain leukocytes (nonleukoreduced). The antibodies made in response to foreign blood products may be of the IgG or IgM subclasses. IgM antibodies are usually the result of the primary immune response, are of a relatively low concentration, and are detectable within 3 to 4 weeks. On reexposure to a nonself antigen, a secondary response may occur, with typical IgG antibody production in 1 to 2 days and in much larger amounts than the IgM response. This secondary response is known as the anamnestic response.

Many factors, known and unknown, affect the primary and secondary responses. Among the most important are the immunogenicity of the antigen, its survival in the circulation, and the strength of the immune system of the recipient. The immune response of the recipient depends on factors such as age, nutritional status, and prior exposure.

Mechanisms of Agglutination

Antigen–antibody reactions follow the law of mass action[7] in a simple combination reaction (Ab + Ag $\rightleftharpoons$ AbAg complex) that is followed by secondary and tertiary reactions. The reactions are reversible and depend on many factors, the most important of which are goodness of fit of antibody-binding site and antigen, complementarity of charge, the concentration of antigen and antibody, the pH of the suspending medium, temperature, and ionic strength.

Antibody Binding to Red Blood Cells

For red cell–antibody binding to form a visible agglutination reaction, a minimum number of antibody molecules must be bound to antigen. It follows that the larger the number of antibodies bound on each red cell, the stronger the observed reaction will be. Also, increasing the serum-to-cell ratio has a desirable effect regarding the appearance of observable agglutination; the test sensitivity is increased. Conversely, increasing the antigen concentration by increasing the strength of the red cell suspension in a test system results in lower sensitivity, and fewer antibody molecules are bound per red cell.

The law of mass action also allows for a description of binding in several stages. The primary reaction may be viewed simply as one of recognition in which an antigen and its specific antibody possess complementary structures that enable them to come into very close apposition to each other. They then are held together by weak intermolecular noncovalent bonds. The weakness of these intermolecular bonds may or may not be sufficient to hold the complex together. Several types of noncovalent bonds have been described. The simplest ionic bonds arise from electrostatic attraction of positive and negative charges, which are dramatically influenced by the distance between the charges.

Weak hydrogen bonds result from the sharing of hydrogen atoms between protons and contribute to bonding. van der Waals forces are normally present from the shifting in the ionic environment of various positive cations and the resultant attraction of negative ions. (Remember that electrons are in constant motion around the atomic nucleus.) Hydrophobic bonds are extremely weak and result from water molecule exclusion from the antigen–antibody complex formation. Figure 5-14 describes the binding of an antibody to its antigen.

Hemagglutination

The second stage of a red cell antigen–antibody reaction involves agglutination, or, more precisely, hemagglutination. Hemagglutination as an observable reaction may or may not occur as a consequence of a patient becoming immunized to allogeneic red cell antigens, and depends on many variables, including the amount and type of antibody present; the size, number, and location of available antigen sites; and the pH, temperature, and ionic strength of the test system.

Although much progress has been made in the biochemical characterization of blood group antigens, their location over the surface of the red cell membrane, and their approximate numbers, many problems must be resolved before a more complete picture emerges.

Essentially, however, the membrane surface should be thought of as a fluid moiety of phospholipids and glycolipids with antigen molecules having the ability to move around and reorient themselves. Furthermore, the antigens protrude from the membrane bilipid layer. The reaction of specific antibodies largely depends on the pH of the medium in which they are suspended. Most blood group antibodies react within a relatively narrow pH range, 6.5 to 7.5, but there are many exceptions to this range. For example, pH-dependent forms of anti-M and anti-Pr (Sp$_1$) can be encountered.

Blood group antibodies, depending on their class, may react in the range of 4°C to 37°C. The rate at which antibody complexes with antigen increases with temperatures up to 37°C, and the rate of dissociation increases as the temperature is increased above that temperature. This principle is used in all antigen–antibody tests, from the compatibility test to the antibody elution procedure that uses heat to remove the antibody from the red cell surface. The clinical significance of antibodies reacting throughout this range is discussed later, but as an example of the influence of temperature, it has been demonstrated that the binding of anti-D is 20 times more efficient at 37°C than at 4°C.

The important findings of Hughes-Jones[7] and Hughes-Jones et al.[8] revealed that reducing the ionic strength of the suspending medium results in an increase in the antigen–antibody association rate. In other

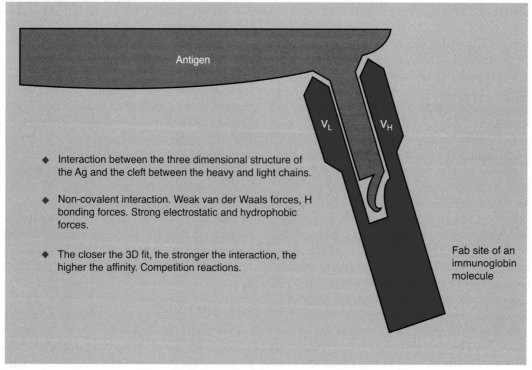

FIGURE 5-14   Binding of antigen to its corresponding antibody.

words, the zeta potential is increased when the ionic strength is decreased. Although, at face value, these facts are the basis of modern blood bank technology, they were problematic for many years because of other variables. Included in these variables is the fact that immunoglobulins undergo changes that result in the activation of complement at decreased ionic strength. Low and Messeter are credited with resolving these difficulties using an ionic strength of 0.031 in antibody tests, which becomes 0.091 with the addition of one volume of serum. Confirmation by Moore and Mollison in 1976[9] that unwanted positive reactivities were due to complement activation, and the elimination of the use of polyspecific antihuman serum, led to the use of a standardized LISS suspension medium for routine compatibility tests. It seems inevitable that with other media in use, such as polyethylene glycol and polybrene, the compatibility test will undergo additional charges.

No single serologic method is useful for the detection of all blood group antibodies. Because a single method fails to demonstrate reactivity, it should not be inferred that a serum does not contain a specific antibody, only that it has failed to be demonstrated by a particular technique, at a particular temperature or pH. Agglutination or clumping reactions observed in vitro result from the bonding of antigen and antibody with all the attendant variables influencing the character and amount of observable reactivity.

Tertiary Reactions

The final steps in red cell–antibody binding, which leads to the destruction of the red cell target, include complement activation, phagocytosis, opsonization, chemotaxis, immune adherence, and cellular degranulation.

COMPLEMENT

Shortly after the discovery of antibody, between 1880 and 1890, came the discovery that another constituent of normal human serum, complement, was necessary for the final inactivation and removal of foreign antigen. Pfeiffer discovered complement in 1894, and in 1898 Bordet confirmed this with a description of immune hemolysis. These discoveries represent milestones in the development of our understanding of these proteins. Without complement, red cell surface binding (sensitization) and agglutination by antibody would be incomplete and ineffectual. Both antibody and complement function as opsonins, molecules that when bind to a cell surface promote phagocytosis by cells that bear receptors for immunoglobulin Fc or

activated complement. Complement may also lead to the lysis of the red cell.

Complement activation may be thought of as a tertiary or third-stage reaction, completing the task started by antibody and resulting in cell lysis. For the immunohematologist, the importance of these reactions is clear. Antigen–antibody reactions involving the activation of complement may result in hemolysis if the reaction proceeds into the final stages. If it does not, those earlier-acting components of complement participating in the initial phases of activation may be detected on the red cell by anticomplement antibodies present when a broad-spectrum or polyspecific antiglobulin reagent is used.

The individual glycoproteins of the complement system, which constitute 10% to 15% of the plasma globulin fraction and 4% to 5% or approximately 300 mg/dL of total serum proteins, are usually functionally inactive molecules that become biologically "self-assembling" when the cascade sequence is activated. They differ and are distinguishable in their biologic activity from immunoglobulins and other serum proteins in several ways: complement functions in immune cytolysis after a specific antigen–antibody reaction; however, not all cells are equally susceptible to complement-mediated destruction. In general, the most susceptible cells are white blood cells, RBCs, platelets, and gram-negative bacteria, whereas yeasts, fungi, gram-positive bacteria, and most plant and mammalian cells are resistant to complement-mediated cytolysis.

Complement proteins are labile and are degraded by heat. Studies by Garratty indicate that 60% of normal levels (the level necessary for weak complement-binding antibodies to be detected) are still present after 2 weeks at 4°C or 2 months at -20°C. However, storage at room temperature for 48 to 72 hours results in only approximately 0% to 40% being detectable. Complement is inactivated entirely or destroyed after 30 minutes at 56°C.

The immunoglobulins IgG and IgM are the only antibody classes that bind or activate complement. IgG subclasses, however, do not do so with equal facility, as previously mentioned. Complement proteins are normally present in all mammalian sera, and some of the components function in various effector roles, such as promoting histamine release from mast cells, virus neutralization, and direct mediation of inflammatory processes by directed migration of leukocytes.

Current data indicate that for certain isolated complement components, namely C1, C3, and C4, the site of production is the macrophage. More specifically, C1 is thought to be produced by the macrophages of the intestine and peritoneum, whereas C3 may be synthesized in many organs, including the liver, lymph nodes, bone marrow, gut, and epithelial organs.

Components of the Complement System

The complement system proteins make up a highly complex system involving as many as 24 chemically and biologically distinct entities that form two interrelated enzyme cascades, the ***classic pathway*** and the ***alternate*** or ***properdin pathway***. In basic terms, once a complement protein has been activated, it activates the next protein in the pathway until all have been activated. The final step in complement activation usually includes water rushing into a cellular target and subsequent cell lysis.

The symbol for complement is C and the native precursor components are numbered from 1 to 9, with subcomponents receiving letters from a to e when cleaved by proteolysis. Each of the components must be assembled under appropriate conditions in a sequential order for the reaction to progress. The activation of complement should be thought of as a series of sequential assemblages of these various units and subunits. In some cases, active enzymes are formed, and these are designated by a bar placed over the compound that has become an active enzyme, such as C3 convertase, $\overline{C4b2a}$. Further, decay products are present as the result of activation and are indicated by the use of a lowercase "i" after the component (e.g., C4i)

when the fragment loses activity. The two different pathways of complement activation involve independent but parallel mechanisms converging at the C5 reaction. The reactions from C5 through C9 are common to both pathways. Figure 5-15 attempts to simplify these complicated schemes.

The Classic Pathway Reaction

Activation of complement in the classic pathway can be initiated by a number of immunologic and nonimmunologic substances. The participation of IgG3, IgG1, IgG2, and IgM has been mentioned. Activation by these antibody molecules occurs by direct binding of C1 to the Fc regions of two antibody molecules that have bound their targets and are spatially near each other. The C1q protein actually bridges the gap between two Fc regions. As early as 1965, it was suggested that only one IgM molecule on the red cell membrane or two IgG molecules with a proximity of 25 to 40 nm were necessary to activate C1. Such nonimmunologic substances as trypsin-like enzymes, plasmin, plant and bacterial polysaccharides, lysosomal enzymes, endotoxins, lymphocyte membranes, and low–ionic-strength conditions also may initiate activation by direct attachment on the C1 molecule.

It is convenient to think of the classic pathway as occurring in three stages: recognition by the C1

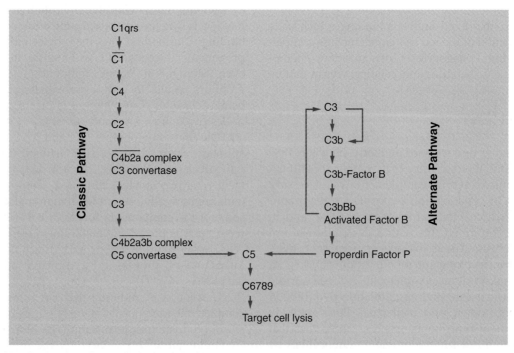

FIGURE 5-15   Pathways of complement activation.

component; activation by C4, C2, and C3; and membrane attachment by C5 through C9.

C1 Recognition

The first component of complement, C1, is a trimolecular macromolecule consisting of three distinct proteins called C1q, C1r, and C1s, held together by a calcium-dependent bond (Ca^{2+}). Removal of calcium by chelating agents, such as the commonly used anticoagulant ethylenediaminetetraacetic acid (EDTA), causes dissociation into the three subunits. Recalcification can be accomplished using calcium chloride, because free calcium ions cause reassociation into the trimeric form.

The C1q subunit is the largest of the three subunits and has a molecular weight of approximately 410,000 D, large enough to be seen with the electron microscope. It appears as a six-globed structure, and strings or shafts appear to be fused into a single base. It is believed that the globe ends serve as the recognition unit that binds to the Fc region of the immunoglobulin molecule, specifically to the C_H2 and C_H4 domains of the IgG and IgM antibody molecules, respectively. Evidence for this globe function of binding is found in the fact that six immunoglobulin molecules can bind to one C1q molecule. For C1q to initiate the cascade sequence, it must attach to two Fc fragments. Therefore, IgG is less efficient at complement binding because the molecules must attach at adjacent sites and be in close-enough proximity for C1q to attach. IgM molecules are pentametric and therefore have five Fc pieces available. One molecule of IgM is independently capable of C1q binding.

The C1r and C1s subunits are much smaller molecules with molecular weights of approximately 190,000 and 87,000 D, respectively. C1r is known to activate C1s enzymatically if the C1 macromolecule is intact. C1s acquires proteolytic enzyme activity after partial cleavage by C1r. The complement sequence can proceed unimpaired once this new enzyme status is achieved. The other reactants, including antigen and antibody, are no longer necessary for the cascade to continue.

C4 Activation

Activated $\overline{C1}$ and $\overline{C1s}$ esterase serve to activate the next two complement components: C4 and C2; C4 in a progenitor form is synthesized by macrophages and has a normal serum level of approximately 400 mg/mL. It consists of three peptide chains (subunits) joined by disulfide bonds: C4a, C4b, and C4c. The activated $\overline{C1s}$ causes the subunit C4a to be split from the molecule. It is free to float in the serum and plays no further part in the sequence, although it does function

as an *anaphylatoxin* by binding to mast cells and causing degranulation. The $\overline{C4}$b has the ability to bind directly to the RBC surface, bacterial cell membranes, and other antigens. However, not all $\overline{C4}$b actually complexes with the red cell surface, owing in part to its rapid decay. Likewise, the C4c subunit is released into the body fluids.

C2 Activation

Once $\overline{C4}$b activation has occurred, C2 activation is accomplished. C2 has a molecular weight of approximately 30,000 D and is cleaved into the fluid phase. C2a is known to activate C3 and C5. The activated product is the $C\overline{4b2a}$ complex and is also known as C3 convertase. The C4b subunit has been bound to the red cell surface, and the $C\overline{4b2a}$ complex formation has resulted from a collision with C2a.

C3 Activation

C3, originating again in precursor form from macrophages, consists of two polypeptide chains (subunits), C3a and C3b. It is the complement component with the highest concentration in the serum, approximately 1250 mg/mL. The C3 convertase ($C\overline{4b2a}$) previously formed has the ability to split C3 into its subunits. C3a is known to be an anaphylatoxin, causing smooth muscle contraction and histamine release from mast cells and platelets. This action results in increased vascular permeability through dilation of capillaries. C3a no longer contributes to the activation sequence at the cellular level. The remaining C3b portion attached to the $C\overline{4b2a}$ complex is still present on the cell membrane and leads to the formation of the final enzyme in the classic pathway, $C\overline{4b2a3b}$, also known as C5 convertase, which activates C5.

The mechanisms of recognition (by C1) and activation (by C4, C2, and C3) are unique to the classic pathway and result in the formation of C5 convertase. From this point, the mechanism of membrane attack ensues, and the sequence of the cascade is identical in the alternate and the classic pathways. The foregoing discussion is a deliberate simplification of a highly complex and detailed system of reactions and reactants, some omitted to present the material in a readily accessible and comprehensible form to the student. A wealth of excellent literature exists for detailed study.

C5 Membrane Attack

C5 is the complement component acted on by $C\overline{4b2a3b}$ (C5 convertase). C5 is also a precursor derivative of the macrophages and is structurally similar to C3. It is composed of two peptide chains, C5a and C5b, which are split by C5 convertase; C5a released into body fluids acts as an anaphylatoxin that mediates inflammation and is a chemotaxin for granulocytes. The remaining C5b portion can be further split into C5c and C5d. Intact C5b activates C6 and C7. Although not specifically active as an enzyme, C5b adsorbs C6 and C7, which may stabilize the cell-bound complex. Once stabilized, the C5b67 complex is further able to adsorb C8 and C9, which is responsible for hemolysis of the RBC. The C566789 complex is not enzymatically active but may undergo steric or configurational changes on the membrane surface and has a molecular weight of approximately 1 million daltons. The lesions formed in the cell membrane by this final complex are approximately 100 nm in diameter and allow rapid passage of ions. The lesions seem to be consistently of this size regardless of the initial perpetrating antibody; they are funnel shaped with the large end toward the membrane surface. The cell on which complement has been activated is no longer capable of maintaining its intracellular contents because of this lesion, and lysis and cell death result from osmotic pressure changes.

The Alternate Pathway

The significant difference between the classic and alternate systems of complement activation is that the alternate, or properdin pathway does not require the presence of specific antibody for activation. In addition, since the description of the properdin, may other plasma factors functioning within this system have been identified.

Properdin has been isolated and found to be a glycoprotein with a molecular weight of 220,000 D. It reacts with a number of polysaccharides and lipopolysaccharides that may be found in the cell membranes of bacteria, and even erythrocytes. Five other plasma factors also react in this system: factor A, which is actually C3; factor B, also called C3 proactivator; factor D; factor H; and factor I. Each of these factors represents proteins that have a unique molecular weight and structure, electrophoretic mobility, defined plasma concentration, and function. The initial reactant in the alternate pathway is C3b, which is continuously generated in the circulation in small amounts. C3b is formed from the interaction of a number of activators. These activators comprise a variety of substances, including polysaccharides found in the cell walls of bacteria and fungi, endotoxins, and aggregates of IgA and probably IgG as well.

A combination of C3b and factor B, the C3 proactivator of the coagulation system, results in C3b being inactivated through cleavage by factors I and H. Factor D cleaves factor B from the foregoing complex, releasing a fragment Ba and resulting in activated C3bBb or activated factor B, which in turn activates large amounts of C3 molecules. The formation of additional activated C3 molecules results in the formation of more C3b. Activated factor B then functions to enhance or amplify the formation of additional C3b. It also functions as a C5 activator. Properdin acts at this point in the sequence to stabilize the activated C3bBb complex, rendering it more functionally efficient by slowing its dissociation.

Several of the factors mentioned in the alternate and classic pathways have analogous physiochemical properties. For example, C1s cleaves C4 and C2; each of the larger fragments is then incorporated into a new enzyme in the presence of magnesium. Factor B, similar to C2, is cleaved by factor D in the presence of C3b, which is similar to C4b.

Effects of Complement Activation

Activation of complement may result in fixation or binding to cell membranes and the generation of components free in the fluid phase that have important biologic functions, whether this activation is by the classic or alternate pathway. These biologic functions are not considered here, although the student is encouraged to read the wealth of excellent material written on this subject. For the immunohematologist, the most obviously significant result of complement fixed to the red cell membrane is cell lysis or hemolysis. Most frequently this occurs through the classic antibody-mediated activation mechanism. The alternate pathway mechanism, however, was shown by Gotze and Muller-Eberhard in 1972[10] to be responsible for the hemolysis of red cells in patients with paroxysmal nocturnal hemoglobinuria.

Although the attack sequence components from C5 through C9 have well-defined functions, less is known about them from a functional standpoint; however, C5 is known to cause membrane lesions, although apparently not cytolysis. When C8 and C9 are activated, the lesions are increased, and these are lethal. The experienced blood banker will have realized how quickly in vitro hemolysis can occur, when O serum is mixed with A- or B-incompatible cells. Issitt[11] has reported that major contributing factors to the ability of antibody to cause hemolysis include not only the amount of bound C3, which eventually leads to C8 and C9 activation, but possibly the presence of inhibitors in the serum, the molecular structure of the antibody rather than the amount, and the variability of the amount of complement that may be present in an individual serum.

SUMMARY

Immunohematology as a science depends on the field of immunology. The immunohematologist's primary goal is to detect antigen and antibody reactions that could be potentially harmful to a recipient of blood components. Knowledge gained from immunologic research related to antigens and antibodies has led to the development of sensitive techniques that ensure that transfused blood is as serologically safe as possible. As advances occur in the field of immunology, they will surely benefit the science of immunohematology. As reagents become more sensitive and specific, blood-banking techniques will become more streamlined and cost effective.

Review Questions

1. Antibody is produced by
   a. B cells differentiated into plasma cells
   b. T cells under the influence of thymosin
   c. B cells, T cells, and macrophages
   d. the pluripotent stem cell
2. The clonal selection theory
   a. indicates that clones of T cells react with antigen of certain composition
   b. states that antigenic exposure to T cells results in antibody formation
   c. postulates that stimulated pluripotent stem cells develop into B cells, T cells, and macrophages
   d. indicates that identical and specific antibody is produced by progeny of B cells after stimulation
3. The following does not influence immunogenicity:
   a. shape and charge of the antigen molecule
   b. sterility
   c. route of administration
   d. size of molecule
4. The immunoglobulin molecule consists of
   a. two heavy and two light chains
   b. identical heavy and identical light chains
   c. four heavy and four light chains separated by disulfide bonds
   d. carbohydrate sequences that confer subclass specificity in the variable regions
5. Which of the following is least likely to activate complement?
   a. IgG1
   b. IgG2
   c. IgG3
   d. IgG4
6. Complement activation occurs in the disulfide bond regions of
   a. the hinge region
   b. the variable regions of the heavy chains
   c. the constant regions of the light chains
   d. the Fab fragment
7. Hemagglutination in antigen–antibody reactions is influenced by
   a. ionic strength of the test system
   b. pH
   c. incubation time
   d. all of the above
8. Complement activation in vitro
   a. does not result in observable hemolysis
   b. is possible if EDTA plasma is used
   c. is not observed in EDTA plasma
   d. is detected only if polyspecific antihuman globulin is used
9. Antibody binding is controlled from
   a. the hypervariable sequences in the V regions
   b. the invariable region of the heavy chain
   c. the Fc fragment
   d. the carboxy-terminal end
10. Most immune responses include
   a. both a cellular and humoral component
   b. inflammation and specific acquired immunity
   c. recognition of a nonself substance and cell activation
   d. all of the above
11. Macrophages are
   a. phagocytic and nonspecific
   b. phagocytic and specific
   c. capable of generating memory
   d. the source of complement and antibody
12. The immune system has evolved to
   a. protect microorganisms from the sun's rays
   b. protect the host against infection and prevent reinfection through generation of memory
   c. prevent us from paying higher taxes
   d. protect a host's memory and generate infection

REFERENCES

1. Metchnikoff E. *L'Immunite dans les Maladies Infectieuses.* Paris: Massom; 1901.
2. Ehrlich P. *Gesammelte Arbeiten zur Immunitatsforschung.* Berlin: August Hirschwald; 1904.
3. Pollack W. Some physicochemical aspects of hemagglutination. *Ann N Y Acad Sci.* 1965;127:892.
4. Pollack W, Hager JH, Reckel R, et al. Study of the forces involved in the second stage of hemagglutination. *Transfusion.* 1965;5:158.

5. Pollack W, Reckel R. The zeta potential and hemagglutination with Rh antibodies. A physiochemical explanation. *Int Arch Allergy Appl Immunol.* 1970;38:482.

6. Steane EA. *Antigen–Antibody Reactions Revisited.* Washington, DC: AABB; 1982:67.

7. Hughes-Jones NC. Nature of the reaction between antigen and antibody. *Br Med Bull.* 1973;19:171.

8. Hughes-Jones NC, Gardner B, Telford R. The effect of pH and ionic strength on the reaction between anti-D and erythrocytes. *Immunology.* 1964;7:72.

9. Moore HC, Mollison PL. Use of a low ionic strength medium in manual tests for antibody detection. *Transfusion.* 1976;16:291.

10. Gotze O, Muller-Eberhard HJ. *J Exp Med.* 1972;134:91.

11. Issitt PD. *Applied Blood Group Serology.* 3rd ed. Miami: Montgomery Scientific Publications; 1985.

RED CELL ANTIBODY DETECTION AND IDENTIFICATION

SANDRA NANCE

OBJECTIVES

After completion of this chapter, the reader will be able to:

1. Discuss red cell antigen and antibody reactions.
2. Discuss the purpose and use of the antibody screen in the compatibility test.
3. Describe the phases of antibody identification.
4. Identify critical information in the interpretation of antibody identification testing.
5. Describe the use of automated test results and the next testing for positive antibody screens in patients when first panels performed using automation do not resolve the specificity of the reactivity.
6. Describe techniques useful in complex antibody resolution.
7. Describe process flows for antibody identification.
8. Describe differences in results of investigation of allo- versus autoantibodies.
9. Discuss use of serologic methods for diagnostic testing.
10. Discuss the application of molecular testing in complex antibody resolution.
11. Discuss antibodies of potential clinical significance.
12. Differentiate antibodies that are potentially clinically relevant from those that are generally not clinically relevant.
13. Discuss methods for determination of clinical relevance.
14. Discuss unexpected reactivity that may yield positive test results not due to red cell alloantibodies.
15. Discuss critical steps in determination of validity of serologic tests.
16. Discuss troubleshooting of testing errors.

KEY WORDS

Alloadsorption
American Rare Donor Program
Antibody detection
Antibody screening
Antiglobulin
Autoadsorption
Autoantibody
Autocontrol
Autoimmune hemolytic anemia
Clinically significant
Cold agglutinin disease

Diamond-Blackfan anemia
Direct antiglobulin test
Dithiothreitol
Drug solution addition test method
Monocyte monolayer assay
Monospecific
Paroxysmal cold hemoglobinuria
Polyspecific
Screening cells
Zygosity

RED CELL ANTIGEN AND ANTIBODY REACTIONS

An understanding of how red cell antigens and antibodies react is basic to the field of immunohematology. Such reactions are seen as *agglutination* or *hemolysis*. Agglutination, or *hemagglutination* as it refers to red cells, occurs in two ways: sensitization, where antibody attaches to the antigens on the red cells, and visible agglutination. Hemolysis is caused by complement activation and resultant breakdown of the red cell membrane.

Hemagglutination, hemolysis, and the factors affecting these reactions are discussed in more detail in Chapter 5.

SELECTION OF METHOD FOR DETECTION OF ANTIBODIES

The selection of the method for *antibody detection* is critical. It is dependent on the activity level of the laboratory, the education and experience of the technical staff, and the caseload of patients served by the facility. If the laboratory has a very high volume of samples or has peak times of workload higher than staff can perform manually, the facility might be best served by high-throughput automation rather than increasing staffing, particularly if there are space constraints in the facility. Similarly, if the staff education and experience level is low or the facility uses a rotation method for staffing the transfusion service laboratory (especially on nonroutine work shifts), then an automated method which may not need to be high throughput may be desired. The complexity of the samples submitted is also a consideration in selection of test methods. For example, in a children's hospital, the number of positive screens may be lower than that of a facility serving oncology and/or sickle cell patients receiving chronic transfusions. Likewise, a small community hospital with a lower caseload may need to weigh the benefits of consistency in testing with automation with rotating staff activity against the cost and number of samples tested.

Most manufacturers of blood bank automation provide a panel that can also be tested on their instrument when a positive *antibody screening* test is obtained. This panel is usually designed to resolve single specificity antibody cases. If the sample contains multiple antibodies or is not an antibody to a common antigen, then the automated test method is abandoned for manual methods. This transition to another test method may lead to differences in test results.

PRINCIPLES OF THE ANTIGLOBULIN TEST

The *antiglobulin* test depends on the following basic premises:

- Antibodies are globulins.
- The antihuman antibodies bind to the Fc portion of sensitizing antibodies and form bridges between antibody-coated red cells, resulting in visible agglutination.

The Indirect Antiglobulin Test

The first use of the antiglobulin test was in the detection and identification of IgG anti-D. Red cells were sensitized with IgG anti-D during an incubation period.

Then AHG was added. The antiglobulin test was successful in agglutinating D-positive red cells that had been sensitized but not agglutinated by IgG anti-D. This test to detect bound antibody indirectly became known as the **indirect antiglobulin test**, or IAT.

In traditional IAT procedures, serum is incubated with red cells which will allow the red cells to become sensitized if antibody(ies) to antigen(s) on the red cells is(are) present. The red cells are then washed to remove any unbound antibody whose presence could inactivate the AHG. After this washing, AHG is added. Agglutination indicates a positive reaction between the serum antibody and antigen present on the red cells.

Factors Affecting the Indirect Antiglobulin Test

The IAT can be affected by anything that alters the tenacity with which antibody attaches to red cells or that affects the amount of antibody that attaches to red cells. Factors that can affect the IAT include:

- Incubation time and temperature
- pH
- Ionic concentration
- Affinity constant of the antibody
- Proportion of antigen and antibody

Incubation Time and Temperature

In general, antibodies that are not detected in the 37°C incubation phase or IAT are not thought to be clinically relevant.

pH

The optimal pH for red cell antigen–antibody interactions is usually considered to be in the physiologic range of pH 6.8 to 7.2.

Ionic Concentration

Reducing the ionic concentration of the environment in which antigens and antibodies react allows the rate of binding to increase. This occurs as the natural shield effect from positive and negative ions is weakened. The use of a low–ionic-strength saline (LISS) solution reduces the time needed for suitable levels of antibody to be bound in vitro for detection and identification. When using LISS reagents, it is important to follow the manufacturer's instructions, especially in volumes of sera and LISS used. The effectiveness of an LISS solution is adversely affected if the final ionic concentration of the reaction mixture is not appropriate.

Affinity Constant of the Antibody

Every red cell antibody has characteristics that are peculiar to that antibody. One of those characteristics is the affinity constant, also called the equilibrium constant. The affinity constant is partly responsible for the amount of antibody that binds to red cells at the point of antigen–antibody equilibrium. As a general rule, the higher the affinity constant, the higher the level of antibody association during the sensitization phase of antigen–antibody reactions.

Proportion of Antigen and Antibody

The speed with which antigen–antibody reactions occur depends on the amount of antibodies present and the number of red cell antigens available. Increasing the serum-to-red cell ratio may increase the test sensitivity because more antibodies are available to combine with the red cell antigen sites.

Applications of the IAT

IAT procedures can be used to detect either red cell antigens or red cell antibodies. The IAT application that focuses on the detection of red cell antigens is phenotyping of patient's and donor's red cells. IAT applications that detect red cell antibody are:

- Unexpected antibody detection
- Unexpected antibody identification
- Antibody titration
- Red cell eluate testing for detection and identification
- Crossmatch

ANTIBODY SCREENING

Selection of Screening Cells

In the United States, most antibody screens are performed using commercial sources of group O reagent red cells. The FDA requires the following antigens on antibody detection cells: D, C, c, E, e, K, k, Jk^a, Jk^b, Fy^a, Fy^b, M, N, S, s, P$_1$, Le^a, and Le^b. There is no requirement regarding *zygosity* of cells. For patient testing, the antibody *screening cells* must be nonpooled and it is best if the manufacturer can provide screening red cells from donors that are homozygous for C, c, E, e, K, Fy^a, Fy^b, Jk^a, Jk^b, M, N, S, and s. Because red cells of the perfect antigen mix may not be available to make a configuration of only two reagent red cell bottles, the number of vials needed may be three or four to get double-dose cells. Selecting antibody-screening red cells with a single dose (from a donor heterozygous for the antigen) of some antigens should be a conscious decision and usually made because a more sensitive test method is being used in the antibody screen. It is best if the zygosity of the donor is determined by molecular tests, since there may be deletions of genes that make the donor's cells

appear to be double dose in serologic testing when they are not.[1] For example, a donor's cells may test Jk(a−b+), but instead of the donor possessing two genes for Jk^b, they may have one Jk^b gene and a deletion gene. Serologically, this donor would appear as double-dose Jk^b Jk^b, but due to the deleted gene, the red cells would have the Jk^b antigen strength seen in a Jk(a+b+) cell which has a single dose of Jk^b.[1]

Role of Antibody Screening Tests in Compatibility Testing

The ***compatibility test*** encompasses ABO/Rh determination, *antibody screen* and ***crossmatch***. The antibody screen is used to detect antibodies in the patient that are directed toward common or high-prevalence antigens. It will not detect antibodies to antigens of low prevalence, nor will it detect antibodies bound to the red cells of the patient if an ***autocontrol*** is not tested in parallel with the antibody screen. Detection of red cell–bound autoantibodies will be covered later in this chapter. There are many methods for detection of red cell antibodies in patients and donors. See Table 6-1.

Although this chapter does not discuss crossmatching in detail, there is a trade-off that has been implemented in some centers in the United States whereby the crossmatch is abbreviated to an immediate spin for detection of ABO incompatibility only, and no antiglobulin phase is performed. Therefore, if a patient had an antibody to a low-prevalence antigen reactive only at the antiglobulin phase, it would not be detected. This is an extraordinarily rare occurrence, but if it is of concern to transfusionists, then consideration should be given to retaining the antiglobulin phase of the crossmatch. For a broader discussion of the topic, please see the articles by Garratty[2] and Judd.[3]

There are situations where the antibody screen will be positive and crossmatches negative that are due to the selection of cells. One example exists when the antibody screening cells are double dose and the crossmatched cells are single dose. This exemplifies the importance of performing antibody screening and not just a crossmatch. Another example is when a

TABLE 6-1	Methods for Antibody Detection
Saline	Gel
Albumin	Solid phase
LISS	Automated gel
Polyethylene	Automated solid
glycol	phase

low-prevalence or moderate-prevalence antigen is present on the screening cells such as Lu^a, Yt^b, and Co^b. Cells with these antigens are not usually the optimal selection, but there are occasions when the manufacturers do not have other cells available.

Conversely, there are scenarios when the crossmatch is positive and the antibody screen is negative. Listed below are some examples of when this could occur:

- The incorrect ABO group donor is selected for crossmatch. For example, the patient is group O and crossmatched cells are erroneously selected that are group A. The crossmatch will be positive and the antibody screen (type O cells) negative.
- The donor cells are subgroups of A or B and this was not detected in grouping. If anti-A,B is not used for donor screening, the anti-A,B, for example, in a group O patient might detect a subgroup of A donor who had an anti-A1 and was therefore grouped as O.
- Passive transfusion of ABO antibodies as in the case of an A patient receiving O platelets. The anti-A, B from the donor plasma in the platelet product may react in a crossmatch.
- The crossmatched cells contain an antigen not on the screening cells. This commonly occurs with antigens of low prevalence like Lu^a, V, Wr^a, but can also occur with f, a frequent antigen not present on screening cells sold in two-vial sets (R_1R_1 and R_2R_2).
- The screening cells are single dose, and the crossmatched cells contain a double dose of the antigen.
- The age of the red cells is a factor in reactivity. Some red cell antigen strengths decrease with storage and thus if the antibody screening cells are at the end of their lifespan, they may be less reactive than red cells from fresh units, especially when tested with weak examples of the antibody.

Selection of Test Method

As seen in Table 6-1, there are quite a few common methods for red cell antibody screening. The first four are performed by manual tube methods, the next two by manufacturer-provided test methodologies, and the last two by automated instruments. This chapter is not intended to be a decision-making toolkit, but judgments need to be made in the selection of test method that will provide certainty that red cell antibodies capable of destroying red cells in vivo are detected reliably. In general, saline methods are not employed routinely because a 60-minute incubation is needed to ensure appropriate sensitivity in the detection of clinically relevant antibodies. Methods other than those in this table are used in antibody identification but are not appropriate for antibody detection as some antibody specificities have been reported to not be detected. Those include methods that utilize ficin and polybrene.

There are a few must-read articles regarding antibody screening methods, two of which are from Peter Issitt.[4,5] In the 1993 article, seeking the significance of antibodies reactive with only enzyme-treated cells, the authors chronicle a study of 10,000 patients' samples that were tested by LISS antiglobulin screen and were negative, then transfused with immediate spin-compatible products. In subsequent testing after transfusion, there were 35 patients whose serum contained enzyme-only antibodies. The transfused red cells were typed for the corresponding antigens and of the 35 patients, 19 had received 32 antigen-positive units. Only one (an anti-c) yielded a clinical transfusion reaction. In the others, there was no evidence that there was a reaction or further alloimmunization against the antigens. The study supported the concept that enzyme-only red cell antibodies were not clinically relevant. In the study, in addition to antibodies with specificities thought to be clinically relevant, there was a host (321) of other positive reactions requiring investigation that were not clinically relevant and would have used valuable resources to evaluate.[4] In a review article from 2000[5], Issitt clearly summarizes the controversy elicited with the selection of a sensitive method that may not yield the specificity (i.e., detection of only clinically relevant antibodies) desired. This topic was further discussed by Combs and Bredehoeff[6] in 2001 when they described the Duke University Hospital Transfusion Service selection of antibody screening method. The article describes test method use and detection of antibodies in sequential years (not parallel studies) for polyethylene glycol and Gel (Ortho MicroTyping System, Raritan, NJ). No hemolytic transfusion reactions and fewer delayed serologic transfusion reactions (not detected clinically, only through subsequent serologic testing) were reported in the Gel testing year. In 2006, a review by Casina[7] looked at the various manual and automated test methods available. The summation was that manual and automated test methods are not substantially different in detection of significant antibodies. In addition, there continue to be reports of method-dependent antibodies, which do not appear to have changed with the advent of automated methods.[8] In a review by the College of American Pathologists (CAP) of proficiency survey participants in 2005, the majority were using Gel tests (45%).[9] The list of methods and percent of participants using each method is in Table 6-2.

Some of the method papers in the literature that may be of interest to the reader are included in "Additional Readings" section of this chapter.

TABLE 6-2	CAP Survey Participants' Methods for Antibody Detection 2005	
Saline 2%		Polyethylene glycol 8%
Albumin 5%		Gel 45%
LISS 37%		Solid phase 2%

Selection of Incubation Phase

In general, commercially available reagents are distributed with a package insert that determines the test method that will be used. This should be explicitly followed. In some cases, there are multiple methods in the package insert, meaning that the manufacturer has determined that the methods are essentially equivalent, but it is important to read the entire package insert noting the limitations. Most antibody detection methods used in the United States do not include an immediate spin or room temperature incubation phase for antibody detection. Thus many clinically insignificant cold-reactive antibodies will not be detected. Most antibody detection methods do include a 37°C phase and it is important to adhere to the incubation times prescribed in the package insert as these times may vary from manufacturer to manufacturer.

Selection of Antiglobulin Sera

When not prescribed by the method manufacturer, *antiglobulin* sera must be selected for use in the antibody screen method, usually for the first four methods in Table 6-1. In the United States, most laboratories use **monospecific** anti-IgG instead of *polyspecific* antiglobulin sera for the antibody screen. This limits detection of nonspecific and for the most part, clinically insignificant reactivity. Most anti-IgG sera are from monoclonal sources and include antibodies to human IgG subclasses 1, 2, and 3. Antibodies to IgG4 are not usually included and red cell antibodies that are solely IgG2 or IgG4 are very uncommon. Most clinically relevant red cell antibodies are of the IgG1 or IgG3 subclass.

ANTIBODY IDENTIFICATION

Steps in Antibody Detection and Identification—Preanalytic Phase

When the antibody detection test is positive, the preanalytic phase of antibody identification requires examination of the patient's history as well as knowledge of the volume of sample provided. See Table 6-3. Of primary importance is information regarding the need for blood products. This drives the urgency of the entire process for identification of the antibody(ies) present and may be the difference in simultaneously performing multiple test methods, and resource (both human and reagent)-intensive work. If the transfusion is urgently needed, then the rate-limiting factors need to be known and controlled. The first critical factor being, whether there is sufficient sample to complete the evaluation. In many cases, an urgent sample evaluation will consume more samples because more tests are performed simultaneously instead of sequentially after technical analysis. Most referral laboratories have a minimum suggested volume of sample to be submitted to complete an evaluation. This is to minimize occasions of sample size restricting or causing cessation of an evaluation. Figure 6-1 shows a process flow for evaluation of samples. The flow chart is formatted such that the performance responsibilities are shown in horizontal "swim lanes" that describe the relative order of events for the screening laboratory, the identification laboratory (which can be off-site or on-site), and the reviewing staff person. For laboratories operating under good manufacturing practices (GMP), the reviewer must be a second person not involved in the testing.

TABLE 6-3	Antibody Identification Analytic Steps
Preanalytic Information	
Transfusion need	Race
Sample volume	Diagnosis
Previous antibody identification	Prior transfusions
Analytic Information	
DAT	Initial panel
Rh phenotype	Case-specific testing
Postanalytic Information	
p-values met	Correct interpretation
Controls tested and valid	Report reflects results
Equipment QC performed	
Equipment QC reviewed	
Reagent QC performed and reviewed	
Double dose antigen [positive cells used for rule out of antibodies]	

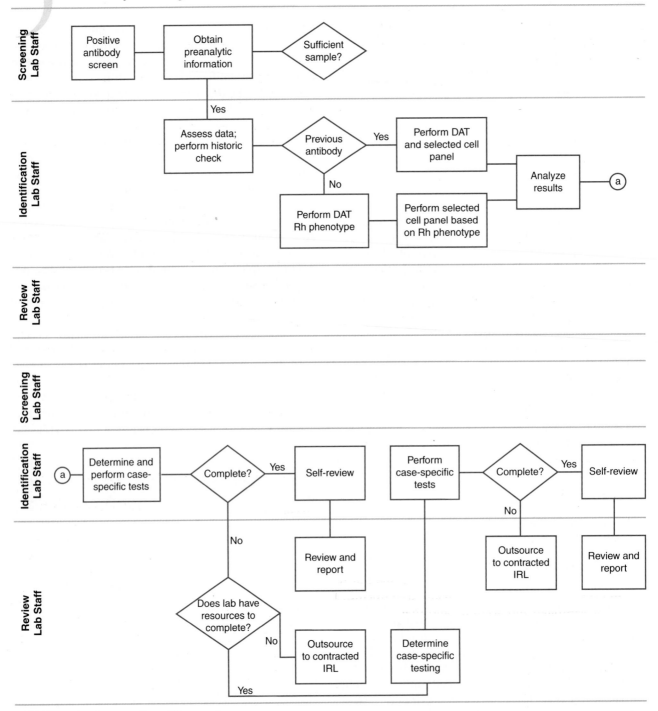

FIGURE 6-1   Process flow: IRL sample.

With urgent samples, the initial testing may be increased and overlap with other testing. The information gathering happens simultaneously and is critical to the correct evaluation and is usually completed by the identification laboratory (or later by the screening laboratory).

In a review of critical steps in antibody evaluations and evaluating the risk if a particular step fails, one of the most critical steps in the preanalytic phase is the check for historic antibody information and knowledge of previous transfusion, especially recent transfusion. These two items impact the course of the evaluation and, if incorrect, can lead to selection of the wrong test methods and incorrect recommendations for transfusion. The reason for requiring a check for previous antibodies is that antibodies do not always persist for the person's lifetime. Rosse et al. found a surprising number of antibodies (35%) were undetectable only a year from identification in a study of patients with sickle cell anemia.[10]

Checking for recent transfusions is also a critical step. For example, patients with *autoantibodies* require adsorption to look for underlying alloantibodies. *Autoadsorption* can be performed if the patient has not been recently transfused (in the preceding 3 to 4 months). *Alloadsorption* must be used if the patient has been recently transfused. If the laboratory is not informed of a recent transfusion and autoadsorption is performed, it is possible the persisting transfused antigen-positive cells could adsorb alloantibody making it undetectable in tests of the adsorbed sera.

Knowing the patient's history where it relates to previous antibodies and transfusion is critical and thus, it is important to have a robust process for obtaining this information.

As with any testing, it is important in the preanalytic phase to ensure laboratory qualification processes for reagents and equipment, including preventive maintenance, are completed before the first sample is processed for the day. This ensures all equipment and reagents are within compliance standards.

Within a single antibody identification, as shown by the process flow, the tester may return to the preanalytic step in the determination of the next testing to perform. In looking at steps to perform after initial routine testing, the results of the testing, along with historical information, must be considered to determine how to proceed.

Steps in Antibody Detection and Identification—Analytic Phase

Once the appropriate information is obtained (for nonurgent samples) or as the testing begins (for urgent samples), the tester must ensure that documentation is complete and accurate and that the sample used in all testing is the correct one. While some facilities may have only one sample evaluation being performed by a technologist at a given time, this does not likely happen often. Thus, it is critical to be diligent in reidentification of tubes, cards, or plates in this process.

Direct Antiglobulin Test Negative Samples

If the direct antiglobulin test (DAT) is negative, often a different course of testing is pursued than if the sample is DAT positive. When the DAT is negative, concentration on alloantibody identification is the course of testing. In general, most immunohematology reference laboratories (IRLs) have an initial test process that is followed with all samples to ensure consistency and efficient case evaluations.

Single Alloantibody

A single specificity can usually be resolved with one panel especially if the Rh phenotype results are used to determine selected panel cells to test. For example, if the Rh phenotype results show the patient is likely c−E−, the productivity of a random panel that contains only two c− cells is limited. However, if a panel is constructed that contains two c+E− and two c−E+ cells and the rest of the red cells as c−E− to rule out other specificities, it is much more productive. This approach allows the technologist to "name that antibody" in as few panels as possible, thus preserving resources for other evaluations. There is commercial software available that allows computer selection and printing of the selected cell panels that can expedite this activity. AABB IRL standards require that to confirm specificity, two antigen-positive and two antigen-negative cells must be tested and react appropriately to identify an antibody.[11] Many laboratories require three positive and three antigen-negative cells, and that the antigen must be in double dose for the specificity to be ruled out, including the rare K+k− cell. Some laboratories require that to rule out a specificity, multiple antigen (two or three)-positive cells including at least one double-dose cell be tested and negative. Once the specificity has been identified, the patient's cells should be tested for the corresponding antigen(s) if the patient has not recently been transfused. If the antibody specificity is clinically relevant, antigen-negative blood should be recommended. After the antibody has been identified, it may be useful to determine if the antibody reacts at 37°C to know whether antigen-negative blood should be provided. This can be helpful in cases with antibodies in the Lewis and MN systems. Prewarmed testing is used to determine if such antibodies are *clinically significant*. This test, however, should only be performed if the antibody has been identified and not as a way to "make antibodies go away." This topic has been the subject of pro and con articles and much discussion.[12,13] It is important to perform both the 37°C settle technique and prewarmed anti-IgG technique[14] to avoid the outcome of a case described by Storry et al. of an anti-Vel that was reactive at 37°C but nonreactive in prewarmed tests performed only at the antiglobulin phase.[15] There is an article by Endoh et al. that suggests 30°C as a prewarmed temperature instead of 37°C where a loss in reactivity of some antibodies has been reported.[16,17] Prewarmed testing can be advantageous when there is specificity like anti-M in that if the prewarmed tests are negative, random blood products can be given. Typically, these antibodies present with strongest reactivity in room temperature tests (either immediate spin or incubation phase) and weaker reactivity at 37°C or antiglobulin phase. The reactivity at 37°C and antiglobulin phases may represent carryover agglutination; thus if 37°C-only incubation is used, the reactivity will not be seen.

Once the specificity is resolved, the attention turns to provision of blood products. If it is a common antigen, it is not difficult to find compatible blood in the facility's inventory or from the local blood center. Resolution of antibodies to antigens of high prevalence is covered later in the chapter.

Multiple Alloantibodies

Multiple specificities may be identified if a patient has received multiple transfusions. As the patient is transfused, one or more may be identified in each subsequent sample. If the facility has no historic record of antibodies, it is valuable to determine if the patient has been seen elsewhere to ensure all specificities are known. As with single specificities, it is helpful to perform initial testing with most cells matching the patient's Rh phenotype and if there are known antibodies, red cells negative for those should be included as well. One of the things to keep in mind is that patients whose cells are R_1R_1 are likely to form both anti-c and anti-E. If the testing reveals one specificity, the tester or reviewer should be mindful the other may be present.[18] There is little value in reidentifying antibodies to clinically relevant antigens already identified in your facility. Most IRLs will confirm historic specificities identified elsewhere the first time the patient's sample is referred so as to be prepared if in the future, a rare blood request is needed.

If the evaluation is very complex, it is useful to phenotype the patient, by serological testing if untransfused or by molecular methods if the patient has been transfused.[19–22] If all red cells tested are reactive but the strengths of reactivity or phases of testing vary, then it may be helpful to use alloadsorption techniques to separate the specificities. This method is commonly used to remove autoantibodies and to adsorb antibodies to high-prevalence antigens to determine underlying specificities, but it can also be used to identify multiple specificities especially when the combination of alloantibodies precludes the availability of reagent red cells. For example, if a patient has anti-e, -s, -N, -Jk^b, -Fy^a, finding antigen-negative cells can be very difficult. If adsorbing cells are utilized where one adsorbs the anti-e and another cell the anti-s, then the identification is less complex. Additionally, if nontreated cells are used for the first adsorption, then an eluate can be made to confirm the specificity(ies) adsorbed.

Once the multiple specificities have been determined and all other specificities ruled out, the patient's red cells should be tested for the corresponding antigens if the patient has not been transfused. If this is desired in a transfused patient, the testing can be done using molecular methods, reticulocyte separation, or in sickle cell disease patients, a hypotonic wash technique.

In cases involving multiple antibodies to common antigen, there are times when the resolution indicates that rare blood is needed. One of the categories of rare blood in the **American Rare Donor Program** (the program that coordinates rare blood needs in the United States) is that of multiple common antigens. This category is defined as type A or O, R_0, R_1, R_2, or rr and K:−1 and negative for one of the antigens in each of the three systems: Fy^a or Fy^b, Jk^a or Jk^b, and S or s. See Table 6-4 for definition of R_0, R_1, R_2, and rr, and Table 6-5 for rare blood categories for the American Rare Donor Program.[23]

Antibody to High-prevalence Antigen

While the antibody to an antigen of high prevalence is a single specificity, identification can be highly resource intensive, often utilizing all the skills in the arsenal of the immunohematologist. Generally, the evaluation results include that the reactivity with all cells is consistent in strength and phase, and red cells that are similar in common antigen phenotype to the

TABLE 6-4	Rh Phenotypes
R_0	D+C−E−c+e+
R_1	D+C+E−c−e+
R_2	D+C−E+c+e−
rr	D−C−E−c+e+

TABLE 6-5	American Rare Donor Program Categories

Multiple common antigen negative

Type A or O R_0, R_1, R_2 or rr and K:−1 and Fy(a−) or Fy(b−) and Jk(a−) or Jk(b−) and S− or s−

Type A or O R_1, R_2, or rr and K:−1 and Fy(a−b−)

All ABO groups negative for high incidence antigen (1 in 10,000) such as K₀, U−, Js(b−), Kp(b−), Yt(a−), McLeod

TABLE 6-6	Commonly Encountered Serologic Reactivity[a]
Enzyme—ficin or papain sensitive	Plasma neutralized
Fy^a, Fy^b, M, N, S, s, Ch, Rg	Ch, Rg
Ge2, Ge4, In, JMH, En^a FS	
DTT sensitive (200 mM)	Nonreactive with cord cells
k, Kp^b, Js^b, LW, Yt^a	I, Sd^a, Ch, Rg, AnWj
Do, JMH, Sc, Jr, Cr,	
Some Di	

[a]Not all blood group antibodies or antigens will react as expected.

patient's cells are reactive. This is the time when different methods, knowledge of the race of the patient, and a large inventory of aliquots of rare cells lacking antigens of high prevalence are needed. Table 6-6 details key features of some antigens that may allow quicker identification; techniques such as enzyme treatment of cell, *dithiothreitol (DTT)* treatment of cell, plasma neutralization, or testing cord cells are available. One unique item is that loss of S antigen has been reported in red cells exposed to very low concentrations of sodium hypochlorite.[24,25] If S is involved, this might be used as a tool in identification.

Since red cells negative for high-prevalence antigens are rare, it may be difficult to find compatible blood and it may have to come from far away. Some specificities that are particularly difficult to locate are McLeod, K_0, hr^S−, hr^B− often found with other common antibody specificities. One test that has proven its value over 20 years is the *monocyte monolayer assay (MMA)*. This in vitro test is used to predict the clinical significance of red cell alloantibodies. Originally described in 1987 by Nance, the assay continues to be used for practical decision making.[26–28] One note on the MMA is that it is critical that this assay be performed as close to the transfusion as possible as antibody specificities may change in their clinical significance.[29]

Presence of a Positive Direct Antiglobulin Test

When the *direct antiglobulin test* (DAT) is negative, the immediate focus is on identification of alloantibody. However, DAT-positive samples are much more efficiently evaluated if the specificity of the antibody causing the positive DAT is known. Since most antibody screening methods do not include an autocontrol, especially the automated methods, it is useful to perform a DAT when the Rh phenotype is performed. Once the DAT-positive result is known, it is helpful to

determine if the red cells are coated with IgG or C3d. Patient samples that are reactive with all cells, including the autocontrol, at 37°C and antiglobulin phases usually yield a positive DAT with anti-IgG, but a proportion, 13% according to Petz and Garratty,[30] will only be positive with anti-C3d. Still, it is an advantage to know the results of the anti-IgG and anti-C3 to prepare for evaluation of a cold versus a warm reactive *autoantibody*. When performing an evaluation with only the results of a positive gel or solid phase panel with all cells reactive, workers may find it beneficial to start with an antibody screen with autocontrol using a method that includes 37°C reading as well as antiglobulin, with a room temperature saline phase to define the preferred temperature of reactivity.

Steps in Antibody Identification—Postanalytic Phase

It is in the postanalytic phase of testing where experience and knowledge rule the day. It is advised to review all work submitted by the referring institution prior to reviewing the current local work. One of the difficult, experience-driven decisions is how to recognize when the testing is complete, and it is one of the critical decisions in a case. Too much testing wastes resources and limits the number of other samples that can be tested; too little testing and wrong answers may be obtained. See Box 6-1 that lists the things that

---

BOX 6-1

Results Suggesting Further Investigation Is Needed

- Transfusion reaction
- Hemolyzed serum noted
- Hemolysis seen in testing
- Cephasporins (or other drugs known to cause drug-induced hemolytic anemia) listed in medication list
- Mixed-field DAT
- D-negative patients that are C or E positive
- R_1R_2 phenotype
- All cells tested are positive including pheno-similar in a DAT-negative case
- Autoantibody conclusion in a DAT 1+ with serum 3+
- Anti-e in an e+ patient
- Anti-D ruled out on an R_0 cell
- Anti-U (vs. anti-U/GPB)
- African American reagent red cells giving unexplained negative or positive reactions
- P_1-negative patients

should elicit a need for more caution in interpretation. Not all cases pan out to be worthy of further testing, but if a case has been referred to a referral laboratory, caution is indicated.

Box 6-1 is a list of the author's hot spots in a review that cause increased scrutiny in the case and may render a case as needing more testing. As readers review the list, they may think these are not commonly encountered. This may be true, even in a large IRL, but it is the experience of having found these before and knowledge of the circumstances of the cases, that make these valuable pearls in the review of a case. The list is in the likely order seen by the technologist resolving the case or by the reviewer.

First ask if the sample is referred for a transfusion reaction evaluation. This is always important because the patient has had a clinical reaction around the time of blood product administration and it means that there is a potential presence of new or previously undetected alloantibody. If the evaluation shows no apparent cause for the reaction, attention should be given to using test methods with increased sensitivity, performing a complete phenotype for common antigens on the patient's pre- and posttransfusion reaction samples along with the units that the patient received, and looking for mixed field reactions as evidence of transfused cell survival.

Concentration would be given to negative results from the pretransfusion reaction sample and mixed field reactions in the posttransfusion reaction serum, which indicates differences in antigens between patient's and donor's blood. An investigation of the phenotype of the units for those particular antigens may reveal the antibody specificity. The second and third topics on the list are also indicative of potential cell destruction and should be regarded as a reason to investigate further if patient history or routine tests do not indicate an explanation for the hemolysis noted.

Fourth is a drug history that includes any of the cephalosporins. Keeping in mind that it is rare to have a drug-induced hemolytic anemia, cephalosporins often are the cause of drug-induced immune hemolytic anemia. If the patient has one of the cephalosporins listed in the drug history, it would prompt a review of the DAT for reactivity. If the DAT were positive, reflexing to perform an eluate would be a good idea. If the eluate was negative, an investigation of immune hemolysis due to drug should be pursued.

Fifth is a mixed-field DAT. In transfused patients with no antibodies, there should be a negative DAT. If the DAT is positive and noted to have mixed-field agglutination, with no explanation, an eluate should be performed. This is an especially important finding if transfusion has not been indicated in the patient's history. A finding of a DAT that is mixed field in a case

where the patient is reported as not being recently transfused should prompt a call to investigate this with the patient or the caregiver. The mixed field is evidence that tests involving phenotyping or autoadsorption should not be utilized as alloantibodies may be missed.

Sixth, a donor or patient who is D− and C+ or E+ may have a variant D or e antigen and should be reviewed carefully for evidence of those antibodies. Seventh, a patient whose red cells type as D+ C+ c+ E+ e+ (R_1R_2) should be reviewed carefully for evidence of an anti-f. Although an uncommon antibody in most patients, anti-f may be the first antibody response in R_1R_2 patients.

Items 8 through 13 are items noted on review of antibody panel testing. In number 8, all cells are positive including ones with a phenotype similar to the patient's phenotype (phenotypically similar) in a case with a negative DAT. This indicates there may be an antibody to an antigen of high prevalence and the patient's serum should be tested with rare red cells known to lack high-prevalence antigens. Alternatively, the patient's red cells can be typed with antisera to antigens of high prevalence. Number 9 involves an autoantibody where the serum/plasma reacts stronger than the DAT. This should not happen and is indicative of an alloantibody possibly underlying the autoantibody, if indeed an autoantibody is present in the serum/plasma at all. The finding of anti-e in an e+ patient, for example, number 10, should always lead to the recommendation for molecular testing to ensure the antibody reactivity is not an alloantibody. In number 11, ruling out D on a red cell that is D+ C− E− (Ro) should always cause concern for the tester and reviewer. Not only is this D+ cell one of the weakest D antigens expressions, it is also more likely to be a partial D antigen cell. If the patient's other antibodies make the use of an Ro cell mandatory unless adsorptions are done, as a general rule, at least four Ro cells should be tested and negative prior to ruling out anti-D. Besides anti-U being an antigen of high prevalence, number 12 in the list, it is also an antibody made by people with at least two different genetic backgrounds. The first is those who lack the U antigen only, and these patients can receive blood known commonly as U^{VAR}. Other people are U/GPB (glycophorin B) negative and require blood of the same type, commonly referred to as true U negative or U/GPB negative. This distinction is critical in ensuring compatible blood is ordered. Item 13 indicates a need for review for African American red cells [Le(a−b−), Fy(a−b−)] that are unexpectedly negative or positive in looking at unexplained reactivity. It may indicate an antibody to a high-prevalence antigen like Hy or an antibody to a low-prevalence antigen like V.

Finally, number 14, if in the course of an investigation to an antibody reactive with all reagent cells tested, it is noted that the patient's cells are P_1 negative, then the rare cells in the Globoside system should be tested as most people who make antibodies to the high-prevalence antigens in this system are P_1 negative.

Besides the review of the reactions, is also important to perform the review for validity and completeness. Many reference laboratories are particularly demanding of perfection in documentation. A missing check cell documentation means that the test must be invalidated and repeated if needed in the evaluation. A review by a second person provides a measure of confidence that the interpretation is based on meeting minimum criteria required by the laboratory. This review includes but is not limited to, reviewing previous reports, ABO/Rh and DAT testing and interpretation, performance of an eluate in appropriate circumstances, including a test of the last wash for wash effectiveness, performance of required routine tests, meeting the p values for antibody identification testing established by the laboratory, resolving all unexplained reactivity, recommendation of appropriate products based on current and historic information, and ensuring that all testing is correctly documented by labeling paperwork with testing phases and samples used to obtain results. This assures that prior to result release, the case contains the information to support the recommendations.

SEROLOGIC TESTING FOR PROVISION OF BLOOD PRODUCTS

In investigating a patient's sample with a positive DAT, often the serum/plasma reactivity is weaker than the DAT. If the serum/plasma is stronger than the DAT, the suspicion is that there may be an alloantibody present. In theory, the patient's own cells should adsorb the antibody preferentially, filling all available sites prior to "spilling over" to the serum. There are situations when this may not be true as with depression of autologous antigen, which then makes the sample reactivity appear to be due to alloantibody. Cases like this may show severe clinical hemolysis.

In the case of a positive DAT with serum/plasma reactivity, it is important to determine if underlying alloantibodies are present. Adsorption techniques can be used to remove the panreactive autospecificity and leave any alloantibody(ies) in the adsorbed serum/plasma. It is preferred to use autologous cells to perform the adsorption, but this is not possible when the patient has been recently transfused. For an autoadsorption, the patient's cells may be treated with heat, an enzyme solution, or with a solution that

TABLE 6-7	Adsorbing Cells[a]
R_1	D+C+c−E−e+ K− Jk(a−) S−
R_2	D+C−c+E+e− K− Jk(b−) s−
rr	D−C−c+E−e+ K−

[a]Enzyme treated therefore Fy(a−b−) M− N−.
Adsorbing cells are not usually typed for Lewis or P_1 antigens.

contains both enzyme and DTT (known as ZZAP).[31] This acts to reduce the amount of autoantibody on the cells and allows subsequent adsorption from the serum/plasma. It should be remembered that ZZAP also removes red cell–bound complement as well as IgG.[32] An aliquot of the patient's serum/plasma is incubated with the first aliquot of the pretreated washed packed patient's cells. It is important to pack the adsorbing cells well prior to starting the adsorption to remove extra saline that could dilute the final adsorbed serum. After the incubation, the mixture is centrifuged and the adsorbed serum/plasma removed and added to the next, fresh aliquot of the patient's pretreated cells, incubated and so on for the number of adsorptions needed. The larger the volume of red cells, the more efficient the adsorption. There are times when the patient's sample volume does not allow the preparation of different aliquots of cells. In those cases, the patient's cells may be washed, retreated, and used again. This makes the adsorption technique considerably longer to perform, but may be necessary in cases of limited pretransfusion cells. There is controversy in the literature regarding use of polyethylene glycol to aid in the adsorption process. Some authors have indicated that alloantibodies may be adsorbed onto antigen-negative cells, thus giving false-negative tests when the adsorbed serum is tested.[33–39] It has also been reported that LISS may assist in adsorption studies.

When the patient has been recently transfused, and an adsorption is needed, a few phenotyped type O cells predetermined to lack common antigens are used to adsorb the serum. Typically a set of three cells is used, and the serum is adsorbed sequentially onto aliquots of cells (usually pretreated with enzyme or enzyme/DTT combination). Table 6-7 shows a typical configuration of adsorbing cells. Table 6-8 shows the potential alloantibody specificities that would remain (if present) in using the cells in Table 6-7. This trio of red cells lacks the all common, clinically relevant antigen specificities; therefore, if any antibodies to common antigens are present, they will be detected in the adsorbed serum/plasma that lacked the antigen on the adsorbing cells. Studies have shown the incidence of alloantibodies underlying an

TABLE 6-8	Adsorption Outcomes Using Allogeneic Red Cells in Table 6-7	
Serum Adsorbed with:	**Common Antibodies Potentially in Adsorbed Sera**
R_1 cells	$-c$, $-E$, $-K$, $-Jk^a$, $-S$, $-Fy^a$, $-Fy^b$, $-M$, $-N$
R_2 cells	$-C$, $-e$, $-K$, $-Jk^b$, $-s$, $-Fy^a$, $-Fy^b$, $-M$, $-N$
rr cells	$-D$, $-C$, $-E$, $-K$, $-Fy^a$, Fy^b, $-M$, $-N$

autoantibody to be 30% to 40%.[40] This makes it important to reevaluate samples after transfusion to detect newly formed antibodies.

There are publications that describe mimicking and "like" antibodies.[41] This is a complex subject and has been observed in many blood group systems. These antibodies may represent cross-reactivity of antigens with newly forming antibodies and must be differentiated from allospecificities that are associated with partial antigen status (e.g., anti-hr^B). Issitt reported a case of a patient with an anti-E who then received E-negative blood for a year. During that year, the DAT was positive on every sample, and the eluates yielded anti-E. The antigen typing was E− the entire time. The patient had no clinical signs of cell destruction. Further studies showed that the anti-E adsorbed onto E+ and E− red cells. Thus the antibody specificity, although stronger with E+ red cells, was unlikely to be solely alloanti-E and more likely a mimicking (or cross-reactive) antibody.[42]

An inherent risk of using allogeneic cells for adsorption is that an antibody to a high-prevalence antigen will be adsorbed onto the adsorbing cells and be undetected in the adsorbed serum/plasma. One method to evaluate if a sample contains an autoantibody is to completely remove the antibody coating the patient's autologous red cells and test those cells against the patient's serum/plasma. If there is an antibody to a high-prevalence antigen and no autoantibody, this test will be negative. This is also useful, if after repeated autoadsorption, the adsorbed serum/plasma is still reactive with all cells tested, to determine if there is an antibody to a high-prevalence antigen as well as an autoantibody in the sample. If there is an antibody to a high-prevalence antigen and the autoantibody is adsorbed completely, the test with autoadsorbed serum/plasma would be negative with the treated patient's red cells. An example of this is a warm autoantibody with an underlying anti-Kn^a.

In looking at the results of testing alloadsorbed serum/plasma using the cells in Table 6-7, if the patient had a warm autoantibody with underlying anti-c and anti-K, the anti-c would be detected in the R_1-adsorbed serum/plasma and the anti-K in all three adsorbed serum/plasmas, assuming the auto and allo specificities were adsorbed completely in the procedure. One point that some laboratories miss is that it is not sufficient to do a phenotype (serologically) and use phenotypically matched cells for an alloadsorption. If this is the approach, then all cases involving patient's cells with variant antigens, such as hr^S or hr^B or partial D, would not have the appropriate cells used for the adsorption to detect if there is an alloantibody. For example, if the patient's cells were hr^B negative (one form of variant or "partial" e), the patient's cells type e+; therefore when the phenotypically similar adsorbing cell is selected, it would be e+. If anti-hr^B were present, it would be adsorbed by the e+ cell and go undetected when the adsorbed serum is tested. To avoid this pitfall, use the trio of adsorbing cells as described earlier. The anti-hr^B would be detected in the R_2 (e−) adsorbed sera.

Technologists often wonder how many adsorptions will be enough to remove the autoantibody. Some laboratories perform DATs after adsorption onto the adsorbing cells and adsorb until negative and others use a rule of performing one more adsorption than the initial strength of reactivity in the serum/plasma. The first way may result in one more adsorption than needed and thus waste time and resources, the second may result in incomplete autoadsorption in rare cases. For a Lean approach and conservation of resources, the second method seems a reasonable approach.

LEAN APPROACH

Lean approaches to laboratory work are of special interest in cases involving extensive testing. In new cases involving allogeneic adsorption where alloantibodies are not expected, it may be helpful to test the adsorbed serum/plasma against the screening cell set and a K+k−. Alternatively, a more time-consuming approach is to select reagent red cells for each adsorbed serum/plasma for which the adsorbing cells were negative. In looking further down the line to providing crossmatch-compatible products, there has been a report in the literature suggesting that it may not be necessary to perform more than an immediate spin crossmatch to detect ABO incompatibility in patients with only autoantibodies or with clinically insignificant antibodies.[43] It is an interesting and totally

Lean concept in that the result of an IAT crossmatch will be positive, so why do it at all? Challenges have come from the conservative thought process that chronically transfused patients may be more likely to form antibodies to low-prevalence antigens and the antiglobulin phase although it may be positive, might be positive to a greater strength of reactivity if an alloantibody were present. In the study by Lee, there were no adverse reactions reported in 222 *autoimmune hemolytic anemia* cases or in 40 patients with HTLA-like antibodies where this approach was used.

DIAGNOSTIC TESTING FOR AUTOIMMUNE DISEASE

When there is a suspicion of autoimmune hemolytic anemia, a complete serologic evaluation should be pursued. If a positive DAT is discovered in the course of an evaluation, the report should describe the reactivity, and the physician should be notified if the sample shows hemolytic activity in vitro in case there is an undetected autoimmune process in the patient. The incidence of autoimmune hemolytic anemia in the general population was reported in 1969 to be 1 in 80,000.[44] Many patients whose positive DATs are discovered in the laboratory are not clinically affected with autoimmune hemolytic anemia. The DAT is the start of the investigation with anti-IgG and anti-C3. Some of the diagnostic testing includes a serum screen with neat (undiluted) and acidified serum incubated at room temperature and 37°C with untreated and enzyme-treated cells with and without fresh complement added. An evaluation for hemolysis and agglutination is done to determine warm versus cold immune hemolytic anemia.[30] There are also tests like thermal amplitude studies that include adult O, ABO-compatible cells, I or cord cells, and the autocontrol versus a titration of the patient's serum separated at 37°C to determine reactivity strength and phase for cold agglutinins. An eluate may be helpful if there is blood group specificity and if the result is negative, indicating an evaluation for drug-induced hemolytic anemia may be warranted.

Autoimmune Hemolytic Anemia—Direct Antiglobulin Test Negative

One of the most confounding presentations is a patient with all the clinical hallmarks of hemolytic anemia and a negative DAT. When such a patient presents, it is essential to refer the sample to a laboratory with techniques to evaluate the sample for low levels of immunoglobulin on the red cells and for low-affinity antibodies. Some of these cases are associated with very severe levels of hemolysis. The laboratories that investigate this use a battery of tests to evaluate the possibility that the patient has DAT-negative autoimmune

hemolytic anemia. Some of the tests used by researchers have been developed to detect low levels of immunoglobulin-coated cells. These include flow cytometry and anti-IgG, anti-IgA, and anti-IgM standardized for use with human red cells, enzyme-linked immunosorbent assay, polyethylene glycol autocontrol, and testing a concentrated eluate prepared from the patient's red cells. Additionally, 4°C saline washes and manual polybrene for the detection of low-affinity antibody have been used.[30]

Paroxysmal Cold Hemoglobinuria

Although rare, *paroxysmal cold hemoglobinuria* usually presents in young patients as an acute transient hemolytic anemia with hemoglobinuria. The hallmark test indicated is the Donath Landsteiner test. The autoantibody present in these cases is a biphasic IgG hemolysin acting in the cold (0°C to 4°C) to sensitize the red cells and only hemolyzes when the sample is transitioned to 37°C. Control samples tested solely at 0°C to 4°C or 37°C show no lysis. There also may be some agglutination observed. IgG sensitization can be detected in the antiglobulin phase after the 0°C to 4°C incubation if 0°C to 4°C saline and anti-IgG is used. Antibody specificity is usually anti-P (not the common anti-P_1) and is detected by testing the rare p cells in the Donath Landsteiner test as described before. The samples for the test must be collected and immediately put at 37°C to transport to the testing laboratory. The Donath Landsteiner test can be carried out by incubation of the entire clot tube at the different temperature, or by taking the serum from the tube at 37°C and testing in a test tube. Some cautions are in order. If the patient's specimen is quite hemolyzed in vivo, care must be taken in the evaluation of hemolysis in tube testing to observe the size of the cell button after centrifugation and to compare to a similarly sized aliquot of patient's serum not used in the test for color differences. In this case, the indirect antiglobulin test in the cold (0°C to 4°C) may be useful. Patients with cold agglutinins may yield positive Donath Landsteiner tests. In general these have a high thermal range and show hemolytic activity.[30]

Cold Agglutinin Disease

Since the use of routine room temperature phase incubation is mostly limited to reference laboratories, it is important to recognize the hallmarks of *cold agglutinin disease*. This may be first recognized as cold agglutination by the laboratory investigating a sample reactive with all reagent cells tested and includes a reactive autocontrol. If differential DAT testing is performed, these samples will commonly react with only anti-C3. Often the cold agglutinins will interfere with other tests performed in the laboratory notably those in hematology performed at room temperature with whole blood samples. These samples may be associated with a severe clinical course, or may be benign. There is also the aforementioned 13% of cases of warm autoimmune hemolytic anemia that present with only C3 coating and may have warm and cold antibodies present. Most laboratories are familiar with thermal amplitude testing where the patient's serum (drawn and separated at 37°C) is diluted in a master titration (doubling dilutions from 1:1 to 1:2048) and tested with a variety of red cells (autologous, adult and cord type O, and ABO-matched adult cells) incubated and read successively at four temperatures (prewarmed 37°C, then to 30°C, and then room temperature, and finally 0°C to 4°C). A particularly valuable test is the albumin 30°C test, which is diagnostic of cold agglutinin syndrome. In this test, all ingredients are prewarmed and kept strictly at 30°C. The patient's serum is incubated at 30°C with 30% albumin and the test will invariably be positive in patients with cold agglutinin disease.[30] This test is extremely valuable if other test results are not clear.

Diamond-Blackfan Anemia

Reference laboratories may receive requests for testing to help diagnose *Diamond-Blackfan anemia*. This is a disease recognized in childhood that physicians need to differentiate from transient anemia of childhood. A hallmark of Diamond-Blackfan disease is persistence of the i antigen which is usually waning in strength to not detectable around the age of 2, but there is variation in the levels of i antigen that can be seen as infants age. Patients with Diamond-Blackfan disease have higher than normal strength of i antigen that persists far longer than normal children. The method reference laboratories use is a titration study. First, obtain a control sample from a normal child that is age matched to the patient's samples (within 1 to 2 months difference in birth dates) and test a 4% suspension of the patient's and the control's sample against a serial dilution of anti-i. This will yield a semiquantitative measure of the amount of i antigen present on the red cells. If the patient's cells react at dilutions significantly higher than the control's, this may indicate the disease is present.[45]

Drug-induced Immune Hemolytic Anemia

Drug-induced immune hemolytic anemia is rare. One of the serologic hallmarks, along with a positive DAT due to IgG and/or C3d coating the cells, is a finding that the eluate is negative. Most often, in cases where a non-type O patient's cell has a positive DAT and the eluate is

negative, it is due to transfusion of out-of-group plasma or platelets and the patient has passively acquired anti-A or anti-B. For example, a group A patient receives HLA-matched type O platelets containing anti-A. The anti-A from plasma of the type O donor coats the patient's type A cells. Therefore, a wise practice to do in the laboratory is to test type A and B red cells in cases where non-type O patients have a relatively strong (2+ or more) positive DAT and a negative eluate. If this is performed and is negative, the suspicion should be that the patient has a drug-induced hemolytic anemia. There is also the possibility that an antibody to a low-prevalence antigen is coating transfused antigen-positive red cells in the patient's serum, which would not be detected by a panel of cells that lack the antigen. The most important thing that is needed at this point is the medication history. It is also important to assess if the patient has clinical signs of hemolysis. Not all patients with serologic indications of an immune process are clinically anemic. However, if it has been established that the patient is hemolyzing and the serologic signs point to drug-induced hemolytic anemia, it is important to find the drug causing the symptoms.

Drug-induced hemolytic anemia could be a whole-chapter topic for which there is no room here; thus the concentration will be on the serologic tests and their interpretation. Clearly one of the first steps is the determination of what medications the patient is taking that could cause the hemolytic anemia. The serologist should focus on drugs the patient is taking that are associated with hemolysis and there should be enough serologic testing to support an immune basis for the hemolysis. Such a list of implicated drugs has been kept and updated by George Garratty and appears periodically in *Immunohematology*.[46] An older version of the list with more discussion can be found in the Petz and Garratty's book.[30] When reviewing a list of medications a particular patient is receiving, it is best to use the latest published list. While the medication list is being gathered, the laboratory should be performing a DAT with anti-IgG and anti-C3, as this can help determine what testing should be done. Some drug-induced hemolytic anemias present with cells coated with IgG only, others C3 only, and still others have both. The laboratory should also ensure that it has sufficient sample to complete the battery of tests that may be needed. Throughout the chapter, the use of serum or plasma has usually been synonymous, but here it is important to use serum as tests for hemolytic activity will be performed. As eluate testing will also be done, there must be a sufficient number of patient cells. Often drug investigations require a redraw of patient's blood, so a careful evaluation of the volume of sample remaining should be performed early in the investigation.

Investigation of Drug-induced Autoimmune Hemolytic Anemia

There are several methods for detection of drug antibodies. It would be ideal if there were positive controls for each drug tested, but for the most part, these are not available except to laboratories that have performed many of these tests and for whom large volumes of patient material were submitted. Additionally, if a drug has been well investigated, such as penicillin or cephalosporins, methods have been described that most often resolve the case, but if it is a new drug, this is often not the case. Although some drugs are easy to work with and produce expected results, there are some things to be noted. Not all drugs are easily suspended in solution because they are not soluble in water. There may be manipulations needed such as heating or vortexing, or resuspension with alcohol or other solvents, then dilution or dialysis with saline, adjusting the pH. Some reports of drug-induced immune hemolytic anemia have indicated that it is drug metabolites (breakdown products) and not the whole drug that induces the hemolysis. The technologist may need to obtain serum or urine from other patients on the drug, which would contain the desired metabolites. A practical tip is to obtain the exact drug the patient is receiving from the treating facility so as to decrease variables in the testing.

There are occasions when the presentation of a case can be confusing if there is serum reactivity with all cells tested. In these cases it is thought that the drug present in the patient's serum can interact with reagent red cells, thus forming the hapten–drug complex that may be needed for the patient's antibody to react. A case report in the *Educational Forum of Immunohematology* discusses resolution of such a case.[47]

Test methods for Drug-related Antibodies

There are two common primary approaches to testing for drug-related antibodies, one is coating red cells with the drug and the other is using a suspension of the drug added to the patient's serum and reagent red cell mixture.

Drug coating requires a suspension of the drug at a concentration of 40 mg/mL.[30] The drug the patient is taking may not be that concentrated and in those cases, a request needs to be made of the pharmacy or drug manufacturer for a more concentrated version of the drug. Care needs to be taken in the selection of red cells to coat. If the patient has a red cell alloantibody, cells must be antigen negative. The drug is usually incubated with type O red cells. Next, the red cells are washed and then incubated with the patient's serum and separately with the eluate prepared from the patient's red cells. Testing is performed at 37°C and AHG (with polyspecific antisera) phases. Polyspecific antiglobulin serum is used to detect red cell–bound IgG and C3d. Parallel tests are set up with untreated reagent cells, the same as those used for the drug coating to control for reactivity of the patient's serum in the absence of drug. Normal, inert pooled serum (e.g., from donors that tested negative in antibody screening tests) should be tested with the drug-coated cells to detect nonspecific protein adsorption that some drugs cause, which means the drug-coated cells would be positive with any serum tested and the serum may not contain drug-specific antibody. If the laboratory desires, drug-coated cells can be stored either refrigerated or frozen for future use. Although not always possible, if a positive control (previous patient with proven antibody) is available, it should be tested to ensure the method used resulted in the drug coating the red cells. Table 6-9 shows possible reactions and

TABLE 6-9	Drug-coated Cells Test Method Setup and Interpretation			
Test Milieu Components		**Possible Results**		
Patient's serum	Drug-coated red cells	+	+	+
Patient's eluate	Drug-coated red cells	+	+	+
Normal pooled sera	Drug-coated red cells	−	+	−
Patient's serum	Uncoated red cells	−	−	+
Patient's eluate	Uncoated red cells	−	−	+
Normal sera	Uncoated red cells	−	−	−
Result interpretation		Drug antibody	Invalid—requires dilution studies	Possible auto or alloantibody—likely not drug antibody

TABLE 6-10   Drug Solution Addition Test Method Setup and Interpretations

Test Milieu Components				Possible Results			
Tube Contents: Red Cells Drug or Saline Complement?							
Patient's serum	Untreated cells	Drug solution	None	+	+	+	−
Patient's serum	Untreated cells	Drug solution	Fresh complement	+	+	+	−
Patient's serum	Untreated cells	Saline	None	−	−	+	−
Patient's serum	Untreated cells	Saline	Fresh complement	−	−	+	−
None	Untreated cells	Drug solution	Fresh complement	−	+	−	−
None	Untreated cells	Saline	Fresh complement	−	−	−	−
Patient's serum	Ficin-treated cells	Drug solution	None	+	+	+	−
Patient's serum	Ficin-treated cells	Drug solution	Fresh complement	+	+	+	−
Patient's serum	Ficin-treated cells	Saline	None	−	−	+	−
None	Ficin-treated cells	Saline	Fresh complement	−	−	−	−
None	Ficin-treated cells	Drug solution	Fresh complement	−	+	−	−
None	Ficin-treated cells	Saline	Fresh complement	−	−	−	−
Result interpretation				Drug antibody	Invalid, inert serum reactive in presence of drug solution	Possible auto or alloantibody	No antibody

interpretation of the testing. Important aspects of this test include ensuring that serum (not plasma) is used for the test, reading for agglutination and hemolysis at 37°C, using positive control when possible, using polyspecific antiglobulin serum (containing anti-IgG and anti-C3) and a control of normal, inert pooled serum. If reactivity is present with the normal pooled serum, it will be necessary to repeat the testing using dilutions of the patient and control serum, with a starting point of 1:20 and 1:100 dilutions.

The *drug solution addition method*, formerly known as "immune complex", features using the drug solution at a concentration of 1 mg/mL as an additive to the test, much like albumin or polyethylene glycol is used, and the drug solution being added to the red cells and serum. For this method, the drug also has to go into solution and calisthenics may be needed to make that happen as described previously. For this method, a source of fresh complement should be used. This should be a pool of inert, freshly frozen serum (within 2 days of draw), previously tested and negative against untreated and ficin-treated reagent red cells, since this test involves ficin-treated cells. The washing of the cells for the antiglobulin phase (using polyspecific antiglobulin sera) should be done with the drug solution. For practical purposes and convenience in the laboratory, the pooled serum can be the same as the pooled serum used in the drug-coated cell testing as a control. For setup of the test and possible interpretations, see Table 6-10.

UNEXPECTED REACTIVITY NOT DUE TO RED CELL ANTIBODIES

Rarely, the reactivity seen in immunohematological testing is due to something other than a red cell allo- or autoantibody. This reactivity can be due to other chemicals or drugs in the solutions used for testing or in the red cell diluents used to sustain the red cell during the dating period. There have been observations of reactivity to certain manufacturers' reagents and because of the proprietary nature of commercial manufacturers, the specific substance causing the reactivity may be difficult to determine. In a review article in *Immunohematology* in 1998, George Garratty described what has been reported in the literature and summarizes what is known about the chemicals present in commercial red cell diluents and drugs added to reagents.[48] One way to recognize this is when red cells from different manufacturers are tested and there is a clear demarcation of reactivity between manufacturers' cells. Sometimes this can be resolved by prewashing the red cells prior to testing, but in some cases washing does not resolve the reactivity. One case of this appeared to be caused by sugars (dextrose and lactose) adsorbing to the red cells. Often this phenomenon is recognized in a referral laboratory when cells from the various manufacturers are tested in parallel testing. It is not recognized at the hospital laboratory because commonly only one manufacturer's reagents are purchased and used.

Another cause of nonblood group specificity was recognized to be due to formaldehyde used in the sterilization of dialysis membranes, which may alter red cells; or cause a formaldehyde antibody that resembles anti-N and has come to be known to some as anti-N[form].

It has also been recognized that there are antibodies that react preferentially with stored cells that are likely related to the senescent cell antigen, which is linked to cell clearance at the end of the red cell lifespan.[49,50] There have been other reports of antibodies to stored cells, so this should be considered when reactions are not consistent with red cell antigens.[51]

INTEGRATION OF SEROLOGIC AND MOLECULAR TESTING

A new tool has come to the immunohematology laboratory, molecular testing. This can give a prediction of the red cell phenotype based on DNA and/or RNA test results. This is especially useful in cases where the patient has been recently transfused, or a positive DAT cannot be eliminated by chemicals for antiglobulin testing. The phenotype results along with the antibody test results can be used in tandem to resolve complex cases. It is especially useful in the resolution of variant antigens especially in the Rh system and should be a mandatory part of the resolution of cases thought to be anti-D or anti-e that type serologically as antigen positive. It is also recommended that molecular typing be performed if an anti-e is present in

adsorbed serum from an allogeneic adsorption in a case involving an autoantibody. Often the cause is an auto-anti-e but there is a chance the reactivity represents cross-reactivity or antibody formed in a patient with a variant e antigen. Other applications include testing of fetal cells to predict D types. There is also a potential for complete automation of molecular testing that may make mass donor phenotyping much more available. To date, molecular testing methods are not licensed by any manufacturer and one automated platform is available for testing in a research or prescreening mode.

CLINICAL RELEVANCE OF RED CELL ALLOANTIBODIES

The literature over the ages has discussed the relevance of allo- and autoantibodies,[52–54] and the book references given previously, especially the *Blood Group Antigen Facts Book*[55], detail each antigen and a short summary of the published clinical relevance of the associated antibodies. A discussion of hemolytic disease of the newborn will not be covered here, as it is a full topic on its own, but clearly it is important whether the antibody is clinically relevant. There have also been some excellent reviews in *Immunohematology* that give the reader information regarding action steps when all red cells are incompatible from a serologic and clinical perspective.[56,57] Some have relied on the specificity of the antibody to determine clinical significance, which would means that all Rh, Kell, Kidd and Duffy system antibodies are clinically significant. Often that is correct. The term clinically significant is not well defined. Most would agree that a clinically significant antibody causes hemolysis and cell destruction. But how much cell destruction would be needed to qualify an antibody as clinically significant? Most often the term is variable and dependent on the needs of the patient. In the case of surgery, it is likely that the patient's cells only need to survive long enough for the patient's own cells to restore to a normal hemoglobin level, but in a chronically transfused patient, the longer the survival of the cells, the longer the duration between transfusions and less transfusions are needed. Most rely on no signs of cell destruction clinically or in the laboratory tests and an increment in hemoglobin. The temperature of reactivity has been discussed in reference to prewarming; thus room temperature–only reactive antibodies are considered by most to be benign, and concentration is given to those that react at 37°C (at the 37°C reading phase or antiglobulin phase). There are in vivo and in vitro assays that have been used to determine clinical relevance like the MMA discussed previously. Most serologists rely on knowing the specificity, the temperature of reactivity, and the frequency of antigen-negative blood to drive how much testing is done. If antigen-negative blood can be found easily, as is the case of a patient with anti-E, further studies of temperature of reactivity and MMAs would be more resource intensive than providing the antigen-negative blood. However, when the blood is difficult to find, then these methods are employed to assist in making blood available.

SUMMARY

This chapter was intended to give the reader a sense of the mystery, intrigue, and problem solving inherent in immunohematological case resolutions that an immunohematologist in an IRL encounters on a regular basis. There are longer discussions that could be had on each topic and books have been written on some of them. It is hoped by the discussion and references that the reader is more informed and can make better choices in methods of testing and in case resolution.

Review Questions

1. Which of the following factors affects the indirect antiglobulin test?
   a. pH
   b. ionic concentration
   c. proportion of antigen to antibody
   d. all of the above
2. Antibody screening cells are of which ABO group?
   a. A
   b. B
   c. O
   d. AB
3. True or false? The antiglobulin test is based on the premise that antibodies are globulins.
4. True or false? Most antibodies require an incubation time of approximately 30 minutes at 37 °C if saline or albumin test systems are used.
5. True or false? The FDA places zygosity requirements on red cells used for screening in the United States.
6. True or false? Most antibody detection methods used in the United States do not include an immediate spin or room temperature phase of incubation.
7. Autoadsorption can only be performed if the patient has not been recently transfused. Why?
8. If the antibody identified has clinical significance, what requirement is placed on any red cells used for transfusion?
9. What is the hallmark test for paroxysmal cold hemoglobinuria?

REFERENCES

1. Storry J. Application of DNA analysis to the quality assurance of reagent red blood cells. *Transfusion.* 2007; 47:73S–78S.
2. Garratty G. Screening for RBC antibodies—what should we expect from antibody detection RBCs. *Immunohematology.* 2002;18:71–77.
3. Judd J. Commentary: testing for unexpected red cell antibodies—two or three red cell samples. *Immunohematology.* 1997; 13: 90–93.
4. Issitt PD, Combs MR, Bredehoeft SJ, et al. Lack of clinical significance of "enzyme-only" red cell antibodies. *Transfusion.* 1993;33:284–293.
5. Issitt PD. From kill to over kill: 100 years of (perhaps too much) progress. *Immunohematology.* 2000;16:18–25.
6. Combs MR, Bredehoeft SJ. Selecting an acceptable and safe antibody detection test can present a dilemma. *Immunohematology.* 2001;17:86–89.
7. Casina TS. In search of the Holy Grail: comparison of antibody screening methods. *Immunohematology.* 2006;22:196–202.
8. Rumsey DH, Ciesielski DJ. New protocols in serologic testing: a review of techniques to meet today's challenges. *Immunohematology.* 2000;16:131–137.
9. College of American Pathologists. CAP survey final critique J-B 2005.
10. Rosse WF, Gallagher D, Kinney TR, et al. Transfusion and alloimmunization in sickle cell disease. The Cooperative Study of Sickle Cell Disease. *Blood.* 1990;76:1431–1437.
11. *AABB IRL Standards.* 5th ed. Bethesda, MD.
12. Mallory D. Controversies in transfusion medicine. Prewarmed tests: Pro-why, when and how, not if. *Transfusion.* 1995;35:268–270.
13. Judd WJ. Controversies in transfusion medicine. Prewarmed techniques: Con. *Transfusion.* 1995;35:271–275.
14. Roback JD, Combs MR, Grossman BJ, et al., eds. *AABB Technical Manual.* 16th ed. Bethesda, MD; 2008.
15. Storry JR, Mallory D. Misidentification of anti-Vel due to inappropriate use of prewarming and adsorption techniques. *Immunohematology.* 1994;10:83–86.
16. Endoh T, Kobayashi D, Tsuiji N, et al. Optimal prewarming conditions for Rh antibody testing. *Transfusion.* 2006;46:1521–1525.

17. Leger RM, Garratty G. Weakening or loss of antibody reactivity after prewarm technique. *Transfusion.* 2003; 43:1611–1614.

18. Judd WJ, Dake LR, Davenport RD. On a much higher than reported incidence of anti c in R1R1 patients who present with anti-E. *Immunohematology.* 2005;21:94–96.

19. Garratty G. Where are we, and where are we going with DNA based approaches to Immunohematology? Is serology finished? DNA: a workshop on molecular methods in Immunohematology. *Transfusion.* 2007; 47:1S–2S.

20. Westhoff C. Molecular testing for transfusion medicine. *Curr Opin Hematol.* 2006;13:471–475.

21. Hillyer CD, Shaz BH, Winkler AM, et al. Integrating molecular technologies for red blood cell typing and compatibility testing into blood centers and transfusion services. *Transfus Med Rev.* 2008;22:117–122.

22. Kroll H, Carl B, Santoso S, et al. Workshop report on the genotyping of blood cell alloantigens. *Transfus Med.* 2001;11:211–219.

23. Flickinger C. In search of red blood cells for alloimmunized patients with sickle cell disease. *Immunohematology.* 2006;22:136–142.

24. Rygiel SA, Issitt CH, Fruitstone MJ. Destruction of the S antigen by sodium hypochlorite. *Transfusion.* 1985; 25:274–277.

25. Long A, Tremblay I, Richard L, et al. Nondetection of the S antigen due to the presence of sodium hypochlorite. *Immunohematology.* 2002;18:120–122.

26. Nance SJ, Arndt P, Garratty G. Predicting the clinical significance of red cell alloantibodies using a monocyte monolayer assay. *Transfusion.* 1987;27:449–452.

27. Nance SJ, Arndt PA, Garratty G. The effect of fresh normal serum on monocyte monolayer assay reactivity [letter]. *Transfusion.* 1988;28:398–399.

28. Arndt PA, Garratty G. A retrospective analysis of the value of monocyte monolayer assay results for predicting the clinical significance of blood group alloantibodies. *Transfusion.* 2004;44:1273–1281.

29. Nance S, Scandone P, Fassl L, et al. Monocyte Monolayer Assay (MMA) results are affected by the transfusion of incompatible red cells. *Transfusion.* 1997;37:37S.

30. Petz, LD, Garratty G. *Immune Hemolytic Anemias.* 2nd ed. Philadelphia, PA: Churchill Livingstone; 2004.

31. Branch DR, Petz LD. A new reagent (ZZAP) having multiple applications in immunohematology. *Am J Clin Pathol.* 1982;78:161–167.

32. Leger RM, Garratty G. A reminder that ZZAP reagent removes complement in addition to IgG from coated RBCs. *Immunohematology.* 2006;22:205–206.

33. Liew YW, Duncan I. Polyethylene glycol in autoadsorption of serum for detection of alloantibodies (letter) *Transfusion.* 1995;35:713.

34. Champagne K, Moulds M. Autoadsorptions for detection of alloantibodies—should polyethylene glycol be used? (letter) *Transfusion.* 1996;36:384.

35. Barron CL, Brown MB. The use of polyethylene glycol (PEG) to enhance adsorption of autoantibodies. *Immunohematology.* 1997;13:119–122.

36. Cheng CK, Wong MI, Lee AW. PEG adsorption of autoantibodies and detection of alloantibodies in warm autoimmune hemolytic anemia. *Transfusion.* 2001;41:13–17.

37. Leger RM, Garratty G. Evaluation of methods for detecting alloantibodies underlying warm autoantibodies. *Transfusion.* 1999;39:11–16.

38. Combs MR, Eveland D, Jewet-Keefe B, et al. The use of polyethylene glycol in adsorptions: more evidence that antibodies may be missed. *Transfusion.* 2001;41:30S.

39. Judd WJ, Dake L. PEG adsorption of autoantibodies causes loss of concomitant alloantibody. *Immunohematology.* 2001;17:82–85.

40. Maley M, Bruce DG, Baab RG, et al. The incidence of red cell alloantibodies underlying pan-reactive warm autoantibodies. *Immunohematology.* 2005;21:122–125.

41. Issitt PD, Zellner DC, Rolih S, et al. Autoantibodies mimicking alloantibodies. *Transfusion.* 1977;17:531–538.

42. Issitt PD. Some messages received from blood group antibodies. In: Garratty G, ed. *Red Cell Antigens and Antibodies.* Arlington, VA: American Association of Blood Banks; 1986.

43. Lee E, Redman M, Burgess G, et al. Do patients with autoantibodies or clinically insignificant alloantibodies require an indirect antiglobulin test crossmatch? *Transfusion.* 2007;47:1290–1295.

44. Pirofsky B. *Autoimmunization and the Autoimmune Hemolytic Anemias.* Baltimore: Williams and Wilkins; 1969.

45. Crookston MC. Anomalous ABO, H, and Ii phenotypes in disease. In: Garratty G, ed. *Blood Group Antigens and Disease.* Arlington, VA: American Association of Blood Banks; 1983:67–84.

46. Garratty G, Arndt P. An update on drug induced immune hemolytic anemia. *Immunohematology* 2007;23:105–119.

47. Johnson ST. Warm autoantibody or drug dependent antibody? That is the question! *Immunohematology.* 2007; 23:161–164.

48. Garratty G. In vitro reactions with red blood cells that are not due to blood group antibodies: a review. *Immunohematology.* 1998;14:1–11.

49. Kay MMB. Senescent cell antigen: a red cell aging antigen. In: Garratty G, ed. *Red Cell Antigens and Antibodies.* Arlington, VA: American Association of Blood Banks; 1986:35–82.

50. Easton JA, Priest CJ, Giles C. An antibody against stored blood associated with cirrhosis of the liver and false positive serological tests for syphilis. *J Clin Pathol.* 1965; 18:460–461.

51. Trimble J. An unusual antibody reacting with prediluted 0.8% reagent RBCs and with 0.8% older (aged) RBCs prepared at time of testing [letter]. *Immunohematology.* 2004;20:122–123.

52. Weiner AS, Peters HR. Hemolytic reaction following the transfusion of the homologous group, with three cases in which the same agglutinogen was responsible. *Ann Intern Med.* 1940;13:2306–2322.

53. Vogel P. Current problems in blood transfusion. *Bull N Y Acad Med.* 1954;30:657–674.

54. Engelfriet CP, Pondman KW, Wolters G, et al. Autoimmune hemolytic anemia III. Preparation and examination

of specific antisera against their complement components and products, and their use in serological studies. *Clin Exp Immunol*. 1970;6:721–732.

55. Reid M, Lomas-Francis C. *The Blood Group Antigen Facts Book*. 2nd ed. San Diego, CA: Elsevier Academic Press; 2007.

56. Nance SJ, Arndt PA. Review: What to do when all RBCs are incompatible—serologic aspects. *Immunohematology*. 2004;20:148–160.

57. Meny G. Review: transfusion incompatible RBCs—clinical aspects. *Immunohematology*. 2004;20:161–166.

ADDITIONAL READINGS

Albrey JA, Simmons RT. The use of a papain solution of approximately pH 3.0 in Rh testing and atypical detection. *Med J Aust*. 1960;2:210–213.

Armstrong B, Hardwick, J, Raman L, et al. *Introduction to Blood Transfusion Technology, ISBT Science Series* 2008;3:1–300.

Champagne K, Spruell P, Chen J, et al. Comparison of affinity column technology and LISS tube tests. *Immunohematology*. 1998;14:149–151.

Chanfong SI, Hill S. Comparison of gel technology and red cell affinity column technology in antibody detection. *Immunohematology*. 1998;14:152–154.

Chaplin H. Review: the burgeoning history of the complement system 1888–2005. *Immunohematology*. 2005;21:85–93.

Chiaroni J, Touinssi M, Mazet M, et al. Adsorption of autoantibodies in the presence of LISS to detect alloantibodies underlying warm autoantibodies. *Transfusion*. 2003;43:651–655.

Cid J, Ortin X, Pinacho A, et al. Use of polyethylene glycol for performing autologous adsorptions. *Transfusion*. 2005;45:694–697.

Daniels G. Human Blood Groups. 2nd ed. Oxford, UK: Blackwell Science; 2002.

Derr DA, Dickerson SJ, Steiner EA. Implementation of gel column technology, including comparative testing of Ortho ID-MTS with standard polyethylene glycol tests. *Immunohematology*. 1998;14:72–74.

Duguid JKM, Bromilow IM. New technology in hospital blood banking. *J Clin Pathol*. 1993;46:585–588.

Duran J, Figueiredo M. Antibody screening in 37°C saline. Is it safe to omit it using the indirect antiglobulin (gel) test. *Immunohematology*. 2002;18:13–15.

Fossati-Jimack L, Reininger L, Chicheportiche Y, et al. High pathogenic potential of low affinity autoantibodies in experimental autoimmune hemolytic anemia. *J Exp Med*. 1999;190:1689–1695.

Gammon RR, Lake M, Velasquez N, et al. Confirmation of positive antibody screens by solid phase red cell adherence assay using a tube technique method with polyethylene glycol enhancement. *Immunohematology*. 2001;17:14–16.

Issitt PD, Anstee DS. *Applied Blood Group Serology*. 4th ed. Durham, NC: Montgomery Scientific Publications; 1998.

Judd WJ, Steiner EA, Knafl PC, et al. The gel test: use in the identification of unexpected antibodies to blood group antigens. *Immunohematology*. 1998;14:59–62.

Klein HG, Anstee DJ. *Mollison's Blood Transfusion in Clinical Medicine*. 11th ed. Oxford, UK: Blackwell Publishing; 2005.

Lalezari P, Jiang AF. The manual polybrene test: a sample and rapid procedure for the detection of red cell antibodies. *Transfusion*. 1980;20:206–211.

Lapierre Y, Rigal D, Adam J, et al. The gel test: a new way to detect red cell antigen–antibody reactions. *Transfusion*. 1990;30:109–113.

Lin M. Compatibility testing without a centrifuge: the slide polybrene method. *Transfusion*. 2004;44:410–413.

Low B, Messeter L. Antiglobulin test in low ionic strength salt solution for rapid antibody screening and crossmatching. *Vox Sang*. 1974;26:53–61.

Low KS, Liew Y-W, Bradley PM. Improved detection of weak clinically significant antibodies by supplementation of polyethylene glycol with a low-ionic solution. *Immunohematology*. 1998;14:68–71.

Lown JAG, Barr AL, Davis RE. Use of low ionic strength saline for crossmatching and antibody screening. *J Clin Pathol*. 1979;32:1019–1024.

Lown JAG, Ivey JG. Polybrene technique for red cell antibody screening using microplates. *J Clin Pathol*. 1988;41:556–557.

Mallory D, ed. *Immunohematology Methods and Procedures*. Washington, DC: American National Red Cross; 1993.

Meade D, Stewart J, Moore BPL. Automation in the blood transfusion laboratory: IV ABO grouping, Rh and kell typing, antibody screening, and VD testing of blood donations in the auto analyzer. *Can Med Ass J*. 1969;101:35–39.

Morton JA, Pickles MM. The proteolytic enzyme test for detecting incomplete antibodies. *J Clin Pathol*. 1951;4:189–199.

Nance SJ, Garratty G. A new potentiator of red blood cell antigen–antibody reactions. *Am J Clin Pathol*. 1987;87:633–635.

Petz LD. Review: evaluation of patients with immune hemolysis. *Immunohematology*. 2004;20:167–176.

Roback JD, Barclay S, Hillyer C. Improved method for fluorescence cytometric immunohematology testing. *Transfusion*. 2004;44: 187–196.

Schonewille H, van de Watering LMG, Loomans DSE, et al. Red cell alloantibodies after transfusion: factors influencing incidence and specificity. *Transfusion*. 2006;46:250–256.

Shirey RS, Boyd JS, Barrasso C, et al. A comparison of a new affinity column system with a conventional tube LISS-antiglobulin test for antibody detection. *Immunohematology*. 1999;15:75–77.

Stroncek DF, Njoroge JM, Proctor JL, et al. A preliminary comparison of flow cytometry and tube agglutination assays in detecting red blood cell-associated C3d. *Transfus Med*. 2003;13:35–41.

Tamai T, Mazda T. Evaluation of a new solid phase immunoassay for alloantibody detection using bromelin-treated and untreated red blood cells. *Immunohematology*. 2001;17:17–21.

Tamai T, Mazda T. Enzyme and DTT treatment of adherent RBCs for antibody identification by solid phase immunoassay system. *Immunohematology*. 2002;18: 114–119.

Uhl L, Johnson ST. Evaluation and management of acute hemolytic transfusion reactions. *Immunohematology*. 2007;23:93–99.

MOLECULAR TESTING FOR BLOOD GROUPS IN TRANSFUSION MEDICINE

M. E. REID AND H. DEPALMA

OBJECTIVES

After completion of this chapter, the reader will be able to:

1. Explain the basics of the structure and processing of a gene.

2. Discuss mechanisms of genetic diversity and the molecular bases associated with blood group antigens.

3. Describe applications of PCR-based assays for antigen prediction in transfusion and prenatal settings.

4. Describe some instances where RBC and DNA type may not agree.

5. Delineate the limitations of hemagglutination and of PCR-based assays for antigen prediction.

6. Summarize relevant regulatory issues.

KEY WORDS

Alleles	Molecular testing
Blood group antigens	Prediction of blood groups
DNA to protein	

A blood group antigen is a variant form of a protein or carbohydrate on the outer surface of a red blood cell (RBC) that is identified when an immune response (alloantibody) is detected by hemagglutination in the serum of a transfused patient or pregnant woman. The astounding pace of growth in the field of molecular biology techniques

and in the understanding of the molecular bases associated with most **blood group antigens** and phenotypes enables us to consider the prediction of blood group antigens using molecular approaches. Indeed, this knowledge is currently being applied to help resolve some long-standing clinical problems that cannot be resolved by classical hemagglutination.

Blood group antigens are inherited, polymorphic, structural characteristics located on proteins, glycoproteins, or glycolipids on the outer surface of the RBC membrane. The classical method of testing for blood group antigens and antibodies is hemagglutination. This technique is simple and when done correctly, has a specificity and sensitivity that is appropriate for the clinical care of the vast majority of patients. Indeed, direct and indirect hemagglutination tests have served the transfusion community well for, respectively, over 100 and over 50 years. However, in some aspects, hemagglutination has limitations. For example, it gives only an indirect measure of the potential complications in an at-risk pregnancy, it cannot precisely indicate *RHD* zygosity in D-positive people, it cannot be relied upon to type some recently transfused patients, and it requires the availability of specific reliable antisera. The characterization of genes and determination of the molecular bases of antigens and phenotypes has made it possible to use the polymerase chain reaction (PCR)[1] to amplify the precise areas of deoxyribose nucleic acid (DNA) of interest to detect **alleles** encoding blood groups and thereby predict the antigen type of a person.

This chapter first provides an overview of the processing of DNA to a blood group antigen and then summarizes current applications of molecular approaches for predicting blood group antigens in transfusion medicine practice for patients and donors, especially in those areas where hemagglutination has limitations.

FROM DNA TO BLOOD GROUPS

The Language of Genes

DNA is a nucleic acid composed of nucleotide bases, a sugar (deoxyribose), and phosphate groups. The nucleotide bases are purines (adenine [A] and guanine [G]) and pyrimidines (thymine [T] and cytosine [C]). The language of genes is far simpler than the English language. Compare four letters in DNA or RNA (C, G, A, and T [T in DNA is replaced by U in RNA]) with 26 letters of the English alphabet. These four letters are called nucleotides (nts) and they form "words," called codons, each with three nucleotides in different combinations. There are only 64 (4 × 4 × 4 = 64) possible codons of which 61 encode the 20 amino acids and 3 are stop codons. There are more codons ($n = 61$) than there are amino acids ($n = 20$) because some amino acids are encoded by more than one codon (e.g., UCU, UCC, UCA, UCG, AGU, and AGC, all encode the amino acid called serine). This is termed redundancy in the genetic code.

Essentials of a Gene

Figure 7-1 shows the key elements of a gene. Exons are numbered from the left (5', upstream) to right (3', downstream) and are separated by introns.

Nucleotides in exons encode amino acids or a "stop" instruction, while nucleotides in introns are not encoded. Nucleotides in an exon are written in upper case letters and those in introns and intervening sequences are written in lower case letters. At the junction of an exon to an intron, there is an invariant sequence of four nucleotides (AGgt) called the donor splice site, and at the junction of an intron to an exon is another invariant sequence of four nucleotides (agGT) called the acceptor splice site. The splice sites interact to excise (or outsplice) the introns, thereby converting genomic DNA to mRNA. A single strand of DNA (5' to 3') acts as a template and is duplicated exactly to form mRNA. Nucleotide C invariably pairs with G, and A with T. Upstream from the first exon of a gene, there are binding sites (promoter regions) for factors that are required for transcription (from DNA to mRNA) of the gene. Transcription of DNA always begins at the ATG, or "start," transcription codon. The promoter region can be ubiquitous, tissue specific, or switched on under certain circumstances. At the 3' end of a gene there is a "stop" transcription codon (TAA, TAG, or TGA) and beyond that there is often an untranslated region. Between adjacent genes on a chromosome, there is an "intervening" sequence of nucleotides, which are not transcribed.

After the introns are excised, the resultant mRNA contains nucleotides from the exons of the gene. Nucleotides in mRNA are translated (from mRNA to protein) in sets of three (a codon) to produce a sequence of amino acids, which form a protein. Like transcription of DNA, translation of mRNA always

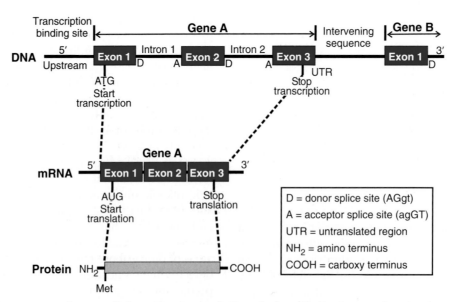

FIGURE 7-1 The anatomy of a gene. Schematic representation of a hypothetical gene, showing transcription of DNA to mRNA and translation from mRNA to the corresponding protein.

begins at the "start" codon (AUG) and terminates at a "stop" codon (UAA, UAG, or UGA). The resultant protein consists of amino acids starting with methionine (whose codon is AUG) at the amino (NH_2) terminus. Methionine, or a "leader" sequence of amino acids, is sometimes cleaved from the functional protein and thus, a written sequence of amino acids (or mature protein) does not necessarily begin with methionine.

DNA is present in all nucleated cells. For the prediction of a blood group, DNA is usually obtained from peripheral white blood cells (WBCs), but also can be extracted from epithelial cells, cells in urine sediment, and amniocytes.

Molecular Bases of Blood Groups

Although many mechanisms give rise to a blood group antigen or phenotype (Table 7-1), the majority of blood group antigens are a consequence of a single nucleotide change. The other mechanisms listed give rise to a small number of antigens and various phenotypes. Figure 7-2 shows a short hypothetical sequence of double-stranded DNA together with transcription (mRNA) and translation (protein) products. The effect of a silent, missense, or nonsense single nucleotide change together with examples involving blood group antigens are illustrated.

Effect of a Single Nucleotide Change on a Blood Group

Due to redundancy in the genetic code, a silent (synonymous) nucleotide change does not change the amino acid and, thus, does not affect the antigen expression. Nevertheless, because it is possible that such a change could alter a restriction enzyme recognition site or a primer binding site, it is important to be aware of silent nucleotide changes when designing a PCR-based assay. In contrast, a missense (nonsynonymous) nucleotide change results in a different amino acid, and these alternative forms of an allele encode antithetical antigens. Figure 7-2 illustrates this where "G" in a lysine codon (AAG) is replaced by "C," which gives rise to the codon for asparagine (AAC). The example of a missense nucleotide change shows that a "C" to "T" change is the only difference between the clinically important blood group antigens k and K. A nonsense

TABLE 7-1   Molecular Events That Give Rise to Blood Group Antigens and Phenotypes

Molecular Mechanism	Example for Blood Group
Single nucleotide changes in mRNA	Multiple (see Fig. 7-2 and Table 7-2)
Single nucleotide change in a transcription site	T > C in GATA of *FY*
Single nucleotide change in a splice site	ag > aa in Jk(a−b−)
Deletion of a nucleotide(s)	Multiple (see Fig. 7-2 and Table 7-2)
Deletion of an exon(s)	Exon 2 of *GYPC* in Yus phenotype
Deletion of a gene(s)	*RHD* in some D-negative people
Insertion of a nucleotide(s)	37-bp insert in *RHDΨ* in some[a] D-negative people (see Fig. 7-2 and Table 7-2)
Insertion (duplication) of an exon(s)	Exon 3 of *GYPC* in Ls(a+)
Alternative exon	Exon 1 in I-negative people
Gene crossover, conversion, other recombination events	Many hybrid genes in MNS and Rh systems
Alternative initiation (leaky translation)	Glycophorin D
Absence/alteration of a required interacting protein	RhAG in regulator Rh_{null} and Rh_{mod}
Presence of a modifying gene	*InLu* in dominant Lu(a−b−)
Unknown	K_{null}, Gy(a−)

[a]Not uncommon in African Americans and Japanese.[2]

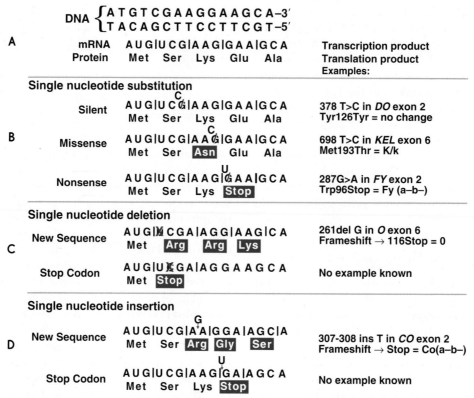

FIGURE 7-2   A hypothetical piece of DNA and the effect of single nucleotide changes. A short hypothetical sequence of double-stranded DNA and the resultant transcription (mRNA) and translation (protein) products are shown. The figure also shows the five amino acids that are determined by the codons in the DNA (**Panel A**). **Panels B** through **D** demonstrate the effect of three different types of single nucleotide changes, substitution (**Panel B**), deletion (**Panel C**), and insertion (**Panel D**), and the effects on the amino acids. Where available, examples of these various types of changes in blood groups are given.

nucleotide change transforms a codon for an amino acid to a stop codon. Figure 7-2 and Table 7-2 give examples relative to blood groups.

Effect of Deletion or Insertion of Nucleotide(s)

A deletion of one nucleotide results in a −1 frameshift and an eventual stop codon (see Fig. 7-2 and Table 7-2). Typically, this leads to the encoding of a truncated protein, but it can cause elongation. For example, a deletion of "C" close to the stop codon in the A^2 allele results in a transferase with 21 amino acids more than in the A_1 transferase.[2] Similarly, deletion of two nucleotides causes a −2 frameshift and a premature stop codon. Deletion of a nucleotide also can cause a stop codon, but there is no known example for a blood group.

An insertion of one nucleotide results in a +1 frameshift and a premature stop codon (see Fig. 7-2 and Table 7-2). Insertion of two nucleotides causes a +2 frameshift and a premature stop codon. Insertion

of a nucleotide can cause a stop codon, but there is no known example for a blood group.

APPLICATIONS OF MOLECULAR ANALYSIS

The genes encoding 29 of the 30 blood group systems (only P1 remains to be resolved) have been cloned and sequenced.[3,4] Focused sequencing of DNA from patients or donors with serologically defined antigen profiles has been used to determine the molecular bases of variant forms of the gene. This approach has been extremely powerful because antibody-based definitions of blood groups readily distinguish variants within each blood group system. Details of these analyses are beyond the scope of this chapter but up-to-date details about alleles encoding blood groups can be found on the *Blood Group Antigen Gene Mutation* database at:

TABLE 7-2	Molecular Bases Associated with a Few Blood Group Antigens		
Antigen/Phenotype	Gene	Nucleotide Change	Amino Acid
Missense nucleotide change			
S/s	GYPB	143T > C	Met29Thr
E/e	RHCE	676C > G	Pro226Ala
K/k	KEL	698T > C	Met193Thr
Fyª/Fyᵇ	FY	125G > A	Gly42Asp
Jkª/Jkᵇ	JK	838G > A	Asp280Asn
Doª/Doᵇ	DO	793A > G	Asn265Asp
Nonsense nucleotide change			
Fy(a–b–)	FY	407G > A	Try136Stop
D–	RHD	48G > A	Trp16Stop
Gy(a–)	DO	442C > T	Gln148Stop
Nucleotide deletion			
D–	RHD	711Cdel	Frameshift → 245Stop
D–	RHD	AGAG	Frameshift → 167Stop
Nucleotide insertion			
Ael	ABO	798-804Gins	Frameshift → Stop
D–	RH	906GGCTins	Frameshift → donor splice site change (I6 + 2t > a)

http://www.ncbi.nlm.nih.gov/projects/gv/mhc/xslcgi.cgi?cmd=bgmut/systems, or by entering "dbRBC" in a search engine. While there are 30 blood group systems, 34 associated gene loci, and 270 antigens, there are close to 1,000 alleles that encode the blood group antigens and phenotypes.

Techniques Used to Predict a Blood Group Antigen

Once the molecular basis of a blood group antigen has been determined, the precise area of DNA can be analyzed to predict the presence or absence of a blood group antigen on the surface of an RBC. Fortunately, as the majority of genetically defined blood group antigens are the consequence of a single nucleotide change, simple PCR-based assays can be used to detect a change in a gene encoding a blood group antigen. Innumerable DNA-based assays have been described for this purpose. They include PCR-restriction fragment length polymorphism (RFLP), allele-specific (AS)-PCR as single or multiplex assay, real-time quantitative PCR (Q-PCR; RQ-PCR), sequencing, and microarray technology. Figure 7-3 illustrates readout formats for these assays. Microarrays use a gene "chip," which is composed of spots of DNA from many genes attached to a solid surface in a grid-like array.[5,6] Microarrays allow for multiple single nucleotide changes to be analyzed simultaneously and overcome not only the labor-intensive nature of hemagglutination but also data entry. This technology has great potential in transfusion medicine for the *prediction of blood groups* and phenotypes.

There are clinical circumstances where hemagglutination testing does not yield reliable results and yet the knowledge of antigen typing is valuable to obtain. Molecular approaches are being employed to predict the antigen type of a patient to overcome some of the limitations of hemagglutination. Determination of a patient's antigen profile by DNA analysis is particularly useful when a patient, who is transfusion dependent, has produced alloantibodies. Knowledge of the patient's probable phenotype allows the laboratory to determine to which antigens the patient can and

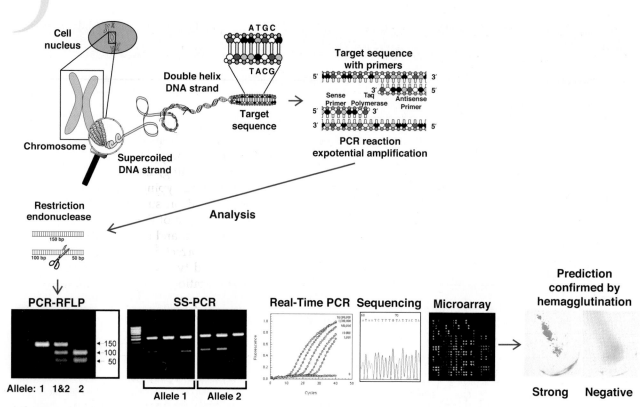

FIGURE 7-3   From DNA to PCR-based assay readouts. Schematic representation of DNA isolated from a nucleated cell, with a particular sequence targeted and amplified in PCR amplification. The readout formats of some of the various techniques available to analyze the results are shown.

cannot respond to make alloantibodies. It is extremely important to obtain an accurate medical history for the patient because with certain medical treatments, such as stem cell transplantation and kidney transplants, typing results in tests using DNA from different sources (such as WBCs, buccal smears, or urine sediment) may differ. DNA analysis is a valuable tool and a powerful adjunct to hemagglutination testing. Some of the more common clinical applications of DNA analyses for blood groups are listed in Box 7-1.

Applications in the Prenatal Setting

The first application of molecular methods for the prediction of a blood group antigen was in the prenatal setting, where fetal DNA was tested for *RHD*.[7] Hemagglutination, including titers, gives only an indirect indication of the risk and severity in hemolytic disease of the fetus and newborn (HDFN). Thus, antigen prediction by DNA-based assays has particular value in this setting to identify a fetus who is *not* at risk for HDFN, that is, antigen negative, so that aggressive monitoring of the mother can be avoided.

Certain criteria should be met before obtaining fetal DNA for analyses: the mother's serum contains an IgG antibody of potential clinical significance and the father is heterozygous for the gene encoding the antigen of interest or when paternity is in doubt. It is helpful to know the ethnic origin and to concurrently test both mother and father, in order to restrict the genes involved and to identify potential variants that could influence interpretation of the test results. DNA analysis can be performed for any blood group incompatibility where the molecular basis is known.

Fetal DNA can be isolated from cells obtained by a variety of invasive procedures; however, the use of amniocytes obtained by amniocentesis is the most common source. Remarkably, free fetally derived DNA can be extracted from maternal serum or plasma[8,9] and *RHD* typing is possible after 5 weeks of gestation.[8,10–13] The *RHD* type is the prime target because, at least in the majority of Caucasians, the Rh-negative mother has a deleted *RHD*, thereby permitting detection of the fetal *RHD* DNA. Furthermore, anti-D is still notoriously clinically significant in terms of HDFN (reviewed in Avent and Reid[14]).

Clinical Applications of DNA Analyses for Blood Group Antigens

- To type patients who have been recently transfused
- To type patients whose RBCs are coated with immunoglobulin (+DAT)
- To identify a fetus at risk for hemolytic disease of the fetus and newborn (HDFN)
- To determine which phenotypically antigen-negative patients can receive antigen-positive RBCs
- To type donors for antibody identification panels
- To type patients who have an antigen that is expressed weakly on RBCs
- To determine *RHD* zygosity
- To mass screen for antigen-negative donors
- To resolve blood group A, B, D, and e discrepancies
- To determine the origin of engrafted leukocytes in a stem cell recipient
- To type patient and donor(s) to determine the possible alloantibodies that a stem cell transplant patient can make
- To determine the origin of lymphocytes in a patient with graft-versus-host disease
- For tissue typing
- For paternity and immigration testing
- For forensic testing
- Prediction of antigen type when antisera is unavailable
- Identify molecular basis of a new antigen

For analysis of single nucleotide changes (e.g., K/k), a source of DNA consisting of mostly fetal DNA, for example, amniocytes, is preferred.

Before interpreting the results of DNA analyses, it is important to obtain an accurate medical history and to establish if the study subject is a surrogate mother, if she has been impregnated with nonspousal sperm, or if she has received a stem cell transplant. For prenatal diagnosis of a fetus not at risk of HDFN, the approach to molecular genotyping should err on the side of caution. Thus, the strategy for fetal DNA typing should detect a gene (or part of a gene) whose product is not expressed (when the mother will be monitored throughout pregnancy), rather than fail to detect a gene whose product is expressed on the RBC membrane (e.g., a hybrid gene).

When performing DNA analysis in the prenatal setting, it is also important to always determine the *RHD* status of the fetus, in addition to the test being ordered. In doing so, if the fetus has a normal *RHD* there is no need to provide Rh-negative blood for intrauterine transfusions.

Applications in the Transfusion Setting

For Transfusion-dependent Patients

Certain medical conditions, such as sickle cell disease, thalassemia, autoimmune hemolytic anemia, and aplastic anemia, often require chronic blood transfusion. When a patient receives transfusions, the presence of donor RBCs in the patient's peripheral blood makes RBC phenotyping by hemagglutination complex, time-consuming, and often inaccurate. The interpretation of RBC typing results of multitransfused patients, based on such things as number of units transfused, length of time between transfusion and sample collection, and size of patient (the "best guess"), is often incorrect.[15] Because it is desirable to determine the blood type of a patient as part of the antibody identification process, molecular approaches can be employed to predict the blood type of patients, thereby overcoming this limitation of hemagglutination.

For Patients Whose RBCs Have a Positive DAT

DNA-based antigen prediction of patients with autoimmune hemolytic anemia, whose RBCs are coated with immunoglobulin, is valuable when available antibodies require the indirect antiglobulin test. Although useful for the dissociation of bound globulins, IgG removal techniques (e.g., EDTA-acid-glycine, chloroquine diphosphate) are not always effective at removing bound immunoglobulin or may destroy the antigen of interest.[2] The management of patients with warm autoantibodies who require transfusion support is particularly challenging, as free autoantibody present in the serum/plasma may mask the formation of an underlying alloantibody. Knowledge of the patient's predicted phenotype is useful not only for determining which alloantibodies he or she is capable of producing, but also as an aid in the selection of RBCs for heterologous adsorption of the autoantibody. This phenotype prediction is extremely valuable for the ongoing management of patients with strong warm autoantibodies. Potentially, the predicted phenotype could be used to precisely match blood types, thereby reducing the need to perform extensive serologic testing.

For Blood Donors

DNA-based assays can be used to predict the antigen type of donor blood both for transfusion and for antibody identification reagent panels. This is particularly useful when antibodies are not available or are weakly reactive. An example is the Dombrock blood group polymorphism, where DNA-based assays[16–18] are used to type donors as well as patients for Do^a and Do^b in order to overcome the dearth of reliable typing reagents. This was the first example where a DNA-based method surpassed hemagglutination. Although some antibodies are not known to cause RBC destruction, such as antibodies to antigens of the Knops blood group system, they are often found in the serum/plasma of patients and attain significance by virtue of the fact that a lack of phenotyped donors makes their identification difficult and time-consuming.[19] DNA-based assays can be useful to predict the Knops phenotype of donors whose RBCs are used on antibody identification panels and thereby aid in their identification.

PCR-based assays are valuable to test donors to increase the inventory of antigen-negative donors. As automated procedures attain fast throughput at lower cost, typing of blood donors by PCR-based assays is rapidly becoming more widespread.[20] With donor typing, the presence of a grossly normal gene whose product is not expressed on the RBC surface would lead to the donor being falsely typed as antigen-positive, and although this would mean the potential loss of a donor with a null phenotype, it would not jeopardize the safety of blood transfusion.

DNA analysis is useful for the resolution of apparent discrepancies, for example, the resolution of ABO typing discrepancies due to ABO subgroups, and for reagent discrepancies that would otherwise potentially be reportable to the FDA. Another example is to classify variants of *RHD* and *RHCE*.[21]

For Patients and Donors

Detecting Weakly Expressed Antigens
DNA analysis can be useful to detect weakly expressed antigens. For example, a patient with a weakened expression of the Fy^b antigen due to the Fy^x phenotype (*FY* nt 265) is unlikely to make antibodies to transfused Fy(b+) RBCs. In this situation, PCR-based assays can help determine which phenotypically antigen-negative patients can be safely transfused with antigen-positive RBCs. It has been suggested that DNA assays can be used to detect weak D antigens in apparent D-negative donors to prevent possible alloimmunization and delayed transfusion reactions[22] or to save true D-negative RBC products for true D-negative patients.

Limitations of DNA Analysis

When recommendations for clinical practice are based on molecular analyses, it is important to remember that, in rare situations, a genotype determination will not correlate with antigen expression on the RBC (see Table 7-3).[23–25] If a patient has a grossly normal gene that is not expressed on his or her RBCs, he or she could produce an antibody if transfused with antigen-positive blood. When feasible, the appropriate assay to detect a change that silences a gene should be part of the DNA-based testing. Examples of such testing include analyses for the GATA box with *FY* typing,[26] presence of *RHD* pseudogene with *RHD* typing,[27] and exon 5 and intron 5 changes in *GYPB* with S typing.[28]

In addition to silencing changes that can impact antigen expression, there are other circumstances, both iatrogenic and genetic, that may impact the results of DNA analysis (see Table 7-4). With certain medical treatments such as stem cell transplantation and kidney transplants, typing results may differ depending on the source of the DNA; therefore, it is extremely important to obtain an accurate medical history for the patient. These medical procedures, as well as natural chimerism, can lead to mixed DNA populations; therefore, the genotyping results will be impacted by the source of the DNA used for testing.

Another limitation of DNA analysis is that not all blood group antigens are the consequence of a single nucleotide change. Furthermore, there may be many alleles per phenotype, which could require multiple assays to predict the phenotype. There are also some blood group antigens for which the molecular basis is not yet known.

OTHER APPLICATIONS FOR MOLECULAR ANALYSES

Molecular biology techniques can be used to transfect cells with DNA of interest and then grow the transfected cells in tissue culture. These cells, which express a single protein, and thus the antigens from only one blood group system, can be used to aid in the identification of antibodies. Indeed, single-pass (Kell) and multi-pass (Duffy) proteins have been expressed in high levels in mouse erythroleukemic (MEL) cells or 293T cells and detected by human polyclonal antibodies.[29] Similar experiments have been performed with antibodies to Lutheran antigens.[30] Thus, it is theoretically possible to produce a panel of cell lines expressing individual proteins for development of an automated, objective, single-step antibody detection and identification procedure. Such an approach would eliminate the need for antigen-matched, short-dated, potentially biohazardous RBC screening and panel products derived from humans. As promising as this approach is, some major hurdles are yet to be overcome; for example, antigens from all blood group

TABLE 7-3   Examples of Molecular Events Where Analyses of Gene and Phenotype Will Not Agree

Event	Mechanism	Blood Group Phenotype
Transcription	Nucleotide change in GATA box	Fy(b−)
Alternative splicing	Nucleotide change in splice site: partial/complete skipping of exon	S− s−; Gy(a−)
	Deletion of nucleotides	Dr(a−)
Premature stop codon	Deletion of nucleotide(s) → frameshift	Fy(a−b−); D−; Rh$_{null}$; Ge: −2, −3, −4; Gy(a−); K$_0$; McLeod
	Insertion of nucleotide(s) → frameshift	D−; Co(a−b−)
	Nucleotide change	Fy(a−b−); r′; Gy(a−); K$_0$; McLeod
Amino acid change	Missense nucleotide change	D−; Rh$_{null}$; K$_0$; McLeod
Reduced amount of protein	Missense nucleotide change	Fy^x; Co(a−b−)
Hybrid genes	Crossover	GP.Vw; GP.Hil; GP.TSEN
	Gene conversion	GP.Mur; GP.Hop; D- -; R$_0^{Har}$
Interacting protein	Absence of RhAG	Rh$_{null}$
	Absence of Kx	Weak expression of Kell antigen
	Absence of amino acids 59–76 of GPA	Wr(b−)
	Absence of protein 4.1	Weak expression of Ge antigens
Modifying gene	*In(LU)*	Lu(a−b−)
	In(Jk)	Jk(a−b−)

systems must be expressed at levels that are at least equivalent to those on RBCs and the detection system should have low background levels of reactivity. Importantly, the highly clinically significant Rh anti-

TABLE 7-4   Limitations of DNA Analysis

Iatrogenic	Stem cell transplantation
	Natural chimera
	Surrogate mother/sperm donor
Genetic	Not all polymorphisms can be analyzed
	Many alleles per phenotype
	Molecular basis not yet known
	Beware of possible silencing changes that can affect antigen expression (Rh and RhAG, Band 3, and GPA dominant Lu(a−b−))
	Not all alleles in ethnic populations are known

gens are proving difficult to express in adequate levels.

Transfected cells expressing blood group antigens also can be used for adsorption of specific antibodies as part of antibody detection and identification, or prior to crossmatching if the antibody is clinically insignificant. In addition, genes can be engineered to express soluble forms of proteins expressing antigens for antibody inhibition, again as part of antibody detection and identification procedures, or prior to crossmatching.[31-33] For example, concentrated forms of recombinant CR1 (CD35) would be valuable to inhibit clinically insignificant antibodies in the Knops system, thereby eliminating its interference in cross-matching.

Recombinant proteins and transfected cells expressing blood group antigens have been used as immunogens for the production of monoclonal antibodies. This approach has led to the successful production of murine monoclonal antibodies with specificities to blood group antigens not previously made[34,35] (see http://www.nybloodcenter.org). Such antibodies are useful because the supplies of human polyclonal antibodies are diminishing. Molecular manipulations have been used to convert murine IgG anti-Js[b] and anti-Fy[a] to IgM direct agglutinins, which are more practical in the clinical laboratory.[36,37]

REGULATORY COMPLIANCE

In addition to a knowledge of blood groups, their molecular bases, technical aspects of PCR-based assays, and causes of possible discrepancies (be they technical, iatrogenic, or genetic), it is important to be cognizant of issues of regulatory compliance. The laboratory director is responsible for ensuring accuracy of results regardless of whether the test is a laboratory-developed test (LDT; previously known as "homebrew") or a commercial microarray for research use only (RUO). Each facility should have a quality plan that includes test procedures, processes, validation, etc. According to the FDA, DNA testing cannot be used as the sole means of determining the antigen status and a disclaimer statement must accompany reports giving the prediction of blood types. As DNA testing to predict a blood group for the purpose of patient care is not used to identify or diagnose a genetic disease, but is doing a test in a different way (hemagglutination vs. DNA assays) to achieve a similar result, informed consent may not be required. Whether or not informed consent should be obtained from the patient or donor to be tested depends on local laws.

If DNA-based testing is done strictly for patient care, it is exempt from Institutional Review Board (IRB) approval. However, if testing is performed for a research purpose, or is to be published, even as an abstract, then IRB approval is required. The type of research dictates whether the review is expedited or requires full board approval. Influencing factors include whether the sample is linked or unlinked, whether it exists or is collected specifically for the testing, and whether or not the human subject is at risk from the procedure.

SUMMARY

Numerous studies have analyzed blood samples from people with known antigen profiles and identified the molecular bases associated with many antigens.[2] The available wealth of serologically defined variants has contributed to the rapid rate with which the genetic diversity of blood group genes has been revealed. Initially, molecular information associated with each variant was obtained from only a small number of samples and applied to DNA analyses with the assumption that the molecular analyses would correlate with RBC antigen typing. While this is true in the majority of cases, like hemagglutination, PCR-based assays have limitations. Many molecular events result in the DNA-predicted type and RBC type being apparently discrepant (some are listed in Table 7-3). Furthermore, analyses of the null phenotypes have demonstrated that multiple, diverse genetic events can give rise to the same phenotype. Nonetheless, molecular analyses have the advantage that genomic DNA is readily available from peripheral blood leukocytes, buccal epithelial cells, and even cells in urine,

---

Review Questions

1. True or false? The process of changing DNA to RNA is called translation.
2. True or false? A single nucleotide change can give rise to a null blood group phenotype.
3. True or false? A blood group can be predicted by testing DNA extracted from WBCs.
4. A single nucleotide change can cause which of the following:
   a. no change in the codon for an amino acid
   b. a stop codon
   c. a change from one amino acid to another
   d. all of the above
5. A PCR-based assay:
   a. has limitations
   b. gives a prediction of a blood group

   c. amplifies a specific sequence of DNA
   d. all of the above
6. For antigen prediction in the neonatal setting, the most common source of fetal DNA is:
   a. amniocytes
   b. fetal RBCs
   c. cord blood
   d. endothelial cells
7. Antigen prediction by DNA analysis is:
   a. indicated only for patient testing and is not applicable for donor testing
   b. used to determine weakly expressed antigens
   c. used to predict antigens when licensed FDA antisera are not available
   d. b and c

(continued)

REVIEW QUESTIONS (continued)

8. In the transfusion setting, DNA analysis is a valuable adjunct to hemagglutination testing for all of the following circumstances except:
   a. for patients with a negative DAT and no history of transfusion
   b. for patients who require chronic RBC transfusions
   c. for predicting antigens to determine what. alloantibodies a patient can produce
   d. for patients with a positive DAT and a warm autoantibody

9. Which of the following statements is true about antigen testing in a recently multiply-transfused patient?
   a. Antigen typing by routine hemagglutination methods gives accurate results.
   b. The transfused donor RBCs can be easily distinguished from the patient's own RBCs.
   c. DNA analysis is an effective tool for antigen prediction.
   d. Antigen typing is not required to manage these patients.

and it is remarkably stable. The primary disadvantages are that the type determined on DNA may not reflect the RBC phenotype and certain assays can give false results. The prediction of blood group antigens from testing DNA has tremendous potential in transfusion medicine and has already taken a firm foothold. DNA-based assays provide a valuable adjunct to the classic hemagglutination assays. The high-throughput nature of microarrays provides a vehicle by which to increase inventories of antigen-negative donor RBC products and, in this aspect, change the way we practice transfusion medicine.

ACKNOWLEDGMENT

We thank Robert Ratner for help in preparing the manuscript and figures.

REFERENCES

1. Mullis KB, Faloona FA. Specific synthesis of DNA in vitro via a polymerase-catalyzed chain reaction. *Methods Enzymol*. 1987; 155: 335–350.
2. Reid ME, Lomas-Francis C. *Blood Group Antigen Facts-Book*. 2nd ed. San Diego: Academic Press; 2004.
3. Lögdberg L, Reid ME, Lamont RE, et al. Human blood group genes 2004: chromosomal locations and cloning strategies. *Transfus Med Rev*. 2005; 19: 45–57.
4. Daniels G, Castilho L, Flegel WA, et al. International Society of Blood Transfusion Committee on Terminology for Red Cell Surface Antigens: Macao report. *Vox Sang*. 2009; 96(2): 153–156.
5. Cuzin M. DNA chips: a new tool for genetic analysis. *Transfus Clin Biol*. 2001; 8: 291–296.
6. Petrik J. Microarray technology: the future of blood testing? *Vox Sang*. 2001; 80: 1–11.
7. Bennett PR, Le Van Kim C, Colin Y, et al. Prenatal determination of fetal RhD type by DNA amplification. *N Engl J Med*. 1993; 329: 607–610.
8. Nelson M, Eagle C, Langshaw M, et al. Genotyping fetal DNA by non-invasive means: extraction from maternal plasma. *Vox Sang*. 2001; 80: 112–116.
9. Lo YMD. Fetal DNA in maternal plasma: application to non-invasive blood group genotyping of the fetus. *Transfus Clin Biol*. 2001; 8: 306–310.
10. Avent ND, Finning KM, Martin PG, et al. Prenatal determination of fetal blood group status. *Vox Sang*. 2000; 78: 155–162.
11. Lo YMD, Hjelm NM, Fidler C, et al. Prenatal diagnosis of fetal RhD status by molecular analysis of maternal plasma. *N Engl J Med*. 1998; 339: 1734–1738.
12. Faas BH, Beuling EA, Christiaens GC, et al. Detection of fetal RHD-specific sequences in maternal plasma. *Lancet*. 1998; 352: 1196.
13. Bischoff FZ, Nguyen DD, Marquez-Do D, et al. Noninvasive determination of fetal RhD status using fetal DNA in maternal serum and PCR. *J Soc Gynecol Investig*. 1999; 6: 64–69.
14. Avent ND, Reid ME. The Rh blood group system: a review. *Blood*. 2000; 95: 375–387.
15. Reid ME, Rios M, Powell VI, et al. DNA from blood samples can be used to genotype patients who have recently received a transfusion. *Transfusion*. 2000; 40: 48–53.
16. Rios M, Hue-Roye K, Lee AH, et al. DNA analysis for the Dombrock polymorphism. *Transfusion*. 2001; 41: 1143–1146.
17. Wu G-G, Jin Z-H, Deng Z-H, et al. Polymerase chain reaction with sequence-specific primers-based genotyping of the human Dombrock blood group *DO1* and *DO2* alleles and the *DO* gene frequencies in Chinese blood donors. *Vox Sang*. 2001; 81: 49–51.
18. Reid ME. Complexities of the Dombrock blood group system revealed. *Transfusion*. 2005; 45(suppl): 92S–99S.
19. Moulds JM, Zimmerman PA, Doumbo OK, et al. Molecular identification of Knops blood group polymorphisms found in long homologous region D of complement receptor 1. *Blood*. 2001; 97: 2879–2885.
20. Hashmi G, Shariff T, Zhang Y, et al. Determination of 24 minor red blood cell antigens for more than 2000 blood donors by high-throughput DNA analysis. *Transfusion*. 2007; 47: 736–747.
21. Westhoff CM. The structure and function of the Rh antigen complex. *Semin Hematol*. 2007; 44: 42–50.

22. Flegel WA, Khull SR, Wagner FF. Primary anti-D immunization by weak D type 2 RBCs. *Transfusion*. 2000; 40: 428–434.

23. Reid ME, Yazdanbakhsh K. Molecular insights into blood groups and implications for blood transfusions. *Curr Opin Hematol*. 1998; 5: 93–102.

24. Cartron JP, Bailly P, Le Van Kim C, et al. Insights into the structure and function of membrane polypeptides carrying blood group antigens. *Vox Sang*. 1998; 74(suppl 2): 29–64.

25. Reid ME. Molecular basis for blood groups and function of carrier proteins. In: Silberstein LE, ed. *Molecular and Functional Aspects of Blood Group Antigens*. Arlington, VA: American Association of Blood Banks; 1995: 75–125.

26. Tournamille C, Colin Y, Cartron JP, et al. Disruption of a GATA motif in the *Duffy* gene promoter abolishes erythroid gene expression in Duffy-negative individuals. *Nat Genet*. 1995; 10: 224–228.

27. Singleton BK, Green CA, Avent ND, et al. The presence of an *RHD* pseudogene containing a 37 base pair duplication and a nonsense mutation in Africans with the Rh D-negative blood group phenotype. *Blood*. 2000; 95: 12–18.

28. Storry JR, Reid ME, Fetics S, et al. Mutations in *GYPB* exon 5 drive the S−s−U+^{var} phenotype in persons of African descent: implications for transfusion. *Transfusion*. 2003; 43: 1738–1747.

29. Yazdanbakhsh K, Øyen R, Yu Q, et al. High level, stable expression of blood group antigens in a heterologous system. *Am J Hematol*. 2000; 63: 114–124.

30. Ridgwell K, Dixey J, Parsons SF, et al. Screening human sera for anti-Lu antibodies using soluble recombinant Lu antigens [abstract]. *Transfus Med*. 2001; 11(suppl 1): P25.

31. Moulds JM, Brai M, Cohen J, et al. Reference typing report for complement receptor 1 (CR1). *Exp Clin Immunogenet*. 1998; 15: 291–294.

32. Daniels GL, Green CA, Powell RM, et al. Hemagglutination inhibition of Cromer blood group antibodies with soluble recombinant decay-accelerating factor. *Transfusion*. 1998; 38: 332–336.

33. Lee S, Lin M, Mele A, et al. Proteolytic processing of big endothelin-3 by the Kell blood group protein. *Blood*. 1999; 94: 1440–1450.

34. Chu T-HT, Yazdanbakhsh K, Øyen R, et al. Production and characterization of anti-Kell monoclonal antibodies using transfected cells as the immunogen. *Br J Haematol*. 1999; 106: 817–823.

35. Chu T-HT, Halverson GR, Yazdanbakhsh K, et al. A DNA-based immunization protocol to produce monoclonal antibodies to blood group antigens. *Br J Haematol*. 2001; 113: 32–36.

36. Huang TJ, Reid ME, Halverson GR, et al. Production of recombinant murine–human chimeric IgM and IgG anti-Js^b for use in the clinical laboratory. *Transfusion*. 2003; 43: 758–764.

37. Halverson G, Chaudhuri A, Huang T, et al. Immunization of transgenic mice for production of MoAbs directed at polymorphic blood group antigens. *Transfusion*. 2001; 41: 1393–1396.

PRETRANSFUSION TESTING

MARGARET STOE

OBJECTIVES

After completion of this chapter, the reader will be able to:

1. Describe the patient identification process when collecting a patient sample for type and screen.
2. Describe an acceptable sample for pretransfusion testing.
3. Define the AABB standards for pretransfusion testing.
4. Select ABO/Rh-compatible blood for transfusion.
5. Describe the criteria for performing an immediate-spin crossmatch, an indirect antiglobulin test crossmatch, and an electronic crossmatch.
6. Describe the labeling requirements for blood for transfusion.
7. Describe type and screen and crossmatch requirements for infants younger than 4 months of age.
8. Explain the purpose of a maximum surgical blood order schedule.
9. Describe a massive transfusion protocol.
10. Describe an emergency transfusion protocol.
11. Describe the process of issuing blood for transfusion.

KEY WORDS

Abbreviated crossmatch
Antiglobulin crossmatch
Clinically significant antibody
Compatibility testing
Crossmatch
Immediate-spin (IS) crossmatch

Indirect antiglobulin test (IAT)
Major crossmatch
Massive transfusion
Maximum surgical blood order schedule (MSBOS)
Minor crossmatch
Type-specific blood

During the early 19th century, direct transfusion was performed without any serologic testing. It was not until after Landsteiner described the ABO system in the early 1900s that a scientific approach to blood transfusion was appreciated. In 1908, Ottenberg, applying Landsteiner's discovery, reported the importance of blood grouping and crossmatching before a transfusion. The *crossmatch* included the testing of recipient serum against donor red blood cells (RBCs) (*major crossmatch*) and the testing of recipient RBCs against donor plasma (*minor crossmatch*). Because tests were performed at room temperature on glass slides, IgM or "complete" antibodies could be detected. After the Rh antigen was described in 1939, the need to recognize the IgG or "incomplete antibodies" was appreciated. Reports of antibodies detected at various temperatures with a potentiating medium led to the belief that a test for antibody detection and identification should be designed to detect and identify all agglutinins. The importance of albumin as an enhancement medium, a 37°C incubation, and testing phases that included an antiglobulin technique developed in the mid-1940s. By the late 1960s, antibody screens that included saline, albumin, and antiglobulin phases were well established, and the performance of a minor crossmatch and an antibody screen with multiple phases continued to be the standard testing protocol. Technological advances flourished. The growing acceptance of low–ionic-strength salines (LISSs), enzymes, microplates, polyethylene glycol (PEG), and gel tests greatly improved the accuracy and efficiency of antibody detection, but the performance of a minor crossmatch and multiphased antibody and a major crossmatch screen persisted. By the late 1970s, the need to identify all antibodies was challenged, and some important questions were raised:

- What is the significance of performing a minor crossmatch?
- Should antibody screens focus on the detection of only "clinically significant" antibodies?
- Is it necessary to perform an *antiglobulin crossmatch* when the antibody screen failed to detect unexpected antibodies?

The need to perform a minor crossmatch was settled by the late 1960s, when the *Standards* of the American Association of Blood Banks (currently AABB) stated that the minor crossmatch was unnecessary. The need to be cost-effective led to a focus on test processes that detected clinically significant antibodies or those antibodies capable of immediate or delayed destruction of RBCs. The need to perform an antiglobulin crossmatch when the antibody screen fails to detect unexpected antibodies is still debated. What has not changed is the significance of the crossmatch in detection of ABO incompatibility and so the *immediate-spin (IS) crossmatch* gained in popularity. In 1994 the Food and Drug Administration (FDA) approved the first alternative to serologic crossmatch, permitting blood establishments to use a computer or electronic crossmatch.

As this chapter progresses, it is important to keep several things in mind:

- Safety, cost-effective strategies, and an aging workforce have advanced the developments of automated systems for pretransfusion testing.
- Multiple test methodologies are available, and each has advantages and disadvantages.
- A single test methodology cannot guarantee the detection of all antibodies, and the transfusion of a crossmatch-compatible unit cannot guarantee a transfusion without adverse reaction.
- Blood banks and transfusion services are highly regulated. A combination of the *AABB Standards for Blood Banks and Transfusion Services, the Code of Federal Regulations*, and reagent manufacturers' instructions provides guidelines and minimum requirements for testing. An individual institution's standard operating procedures describe how the selection and performance of testing are accomplished. The reader is referred to Chapter 19 of this book for additional information about the role of regulatory agencies in blood bank and transfusion services.

PRETRANSFUSION TESTING

In current blood banking, the crossmatch is only one element of what is referred to as pretransfusion testing, also referred to as *compatibility testing*. Box 8-1 provides a summary of the elements of pretransfusion

BOX 8-1	
Elements of Pretransfusion Testing	
ABO forward testing	Recipient red blood cells with anti-A and anti-B
Rh testing	Recipient red blood cells with anti-D and an Rh control, if needed
ABO reverse testing	Recipient serum (plasma) with A_1 cells and B cells
Antibody screen	Recipient serum (plasma) with screening cells
Crossmatch	Recipient serum with donor red blood cells

testing. A pretransfusion testing protocol includes all of the following:

- A request to perform testing and prepare components
- Receipt of an acceptable blood sample
- Performance of an ABO blood group, Rh type, and a test for unexpected antibodies (antibody screen)
- Review of previous records for blood type and unexpected antibodies
- Selection of crossmatch procedure
- Selection of blood for transfusion
- Performance of a crossmatch

The Requisition

All laboratory testing is generated from a physician's or other authorized health professional's request to perform testing or provide blood components. The *AABB standards* require that the request for blood components and records accompanying the recipient sample contain sufficient information for positive and unique identification of the recipient. This includes two independent identifiers and the date of the sample collection.[1]

Request Forms

In addition to the information described in the preceding section, it is not uncommon to find request forms that provide additional information about the patient/recipient:

- Patient's age or date of birth is useful in determining the extent of testing that will be performed. For example, infants younger than 4 months of age may have abbreviated testing.

- Tests ordered should be marked so that the volume of sample required and the collection container can be assessed. The collection container refers to the blood collection tube.
- "STAT" (at once), "ASAP" (as soon as possible), or "routine" are some of the designations or terms used to define the priority of testing.
- Patient location can also help determine testing priority: for example, a location of ER (emergency room) or OR (operating room) implies urgency.

Patient Identity

Wristbands or a similar form of identification must be worn by patients/recipients of transfusions. A trained and competent phlebotomist, after positively identifying the potential transfusion recipient, should collect a blood sample in a stoppered tube. Positive patient identification can be accomplished by requesting the patient to identify him or herself and comparing this information (1) to the patient's identification band and (2) to the request form. If the patient cannot speak, a parent, guardian, family member, or direct care provider can provide the information needed. If errors in identity are detected, a sample for pretransfusion testing should not be collected until corrections are done satisfactorily. Only after positive identification is established, should the sample be collected. Each sample collected is labeled before leaving the patient's side. The label should be affixed to the container and contain two unique identifiers, for example, patient's last and first name, identification number or birth date, and date of collection. The labeled tube is again compared for accuracy to the information on the requisition and the patient identification band. The identity of the phlebotomist must also be documented.

In an emergency environment, the patient identification may be abbreviated. An individual facility must have a written protocol for establishing patient name and identification number in an emergency. Some facilities may establish a unique patient identification number and may designate patients as John/Jane Doe or Unknown Male/Female.

The Patient Sample

Venous blood usually is collected in a volume sufficient to perform requested testing. The collection container used should be approved for blood bank use and consistent with the manufacturer's recommendations for the test methodology used in the laboratory, for example, a serum collection tube or a tube containing an anticoagulant such as heparin or ethylenediaminetetraacetic acid (EDTA). Plasma, particularly heparinized plasma, has the disadvantage of delayed fibrin formation, resulting in clot formation and enmeshment of RBCs during the 37°C incubation. The blood sample submitted for pretransfusion testing:

- should be as free from hemolysis as possible because hemolysis detected in testing may be indicative of an antibody known to cause hemolysis of antigen-positive cells in the antibody screen or the crossmatch. Antibodies known to produce hemolysis include antibodies in the ABO, P, Lewis, Kidd, or Vel blood group systems.
- should not be contaminated with intravenous infusion fluid. This complication can be avoided by collecting the sample below the infusion site or by using an alternate collection site. If blood must be collected from an intravenous line, the first 5 to 10 mL of blood removed should be discarded before obtaining the blood for testing.
- should not be collected in tubes that contain clot activators or silicone coating or other tubes not approved for blood bank use.

Frequency of Specimen Collection

Pretransfusion samples should reflect the current antibody status of a patient. Samples used for pretransfusion testing should be collected within 3 days (day of collection is day 0) of the scheduled transfusion if:

- the patient/recipient has been transfused within the preceding 3 months with blood or components containing RBCs, or
- the patient/recipient has been pregnant within the preceding 3 months, or
- the history is uncertain or unavailable.[2]

Recent transfusion and pregnancy are opportunities for sensitization to occur. Additional sample collection from infants younger than 4 months of age is not required after the initial infant ABO/Rh and antibody screen is performed.

Sample Retention

Samples should be tested as soon as possible after collection. Samples used in pretransfusion testing are stored at 1°C to 6°C for a minimum of 7 days after transfusion. To accomplish this requirement, samples are usually stored for 7 to 10 days. Some transfusion services have adopted preadmission type and screen programs for some patients where the sample is collected up to 1 month in advance of surgery.

Storage requirements for these samples should reflect an extended storage date.

Previous Record Review

For each sample received for pretransfusion testing, the records of testing for ABO/Rh are reviewed and compared with the ABO/Rh results observed on the current sample tested. Any discrepancy should be resolved before a unit is released for transfusion. A review of patient records for unexpected antibodies is also documented. If the patient's records indicate a previously detected antibody, blood negative for the antigen to which the antibody was directed should be provided. This aids in avoiding an anamnestic response and possible delayed hemolytic sequelae.

TYPE AND SCREEN

Methodologies and Antigen/Antibody Reaction Gradings

There are several test methodologies, including gel technologies, microplates, and tube testing, which are used to perform ABO/Rh and antibody screening tests. Regardless of the method selected, the goal is to detect antigen and antibody interaction. The visible sign of antigen and antibody interaction is dependent on the methodology used. In gel technology, a grading of 0 represents a button of cells at the bottom or tip of the microtube, a grading of 4+ represents a cell "clump" at the top of the gel surface, and 1+, 2+, and 3+ reaction gradings are determined by the dispersion of cells throughout gel in the microtube. Microplates employ solid-phase technology where antigen and antibody react and adhere to sides of wells, which is indicative of a positive test; no adherence or cell buttons in the center of the well indicate a negative test; the strength of reactivity is based on the dispersion of cells throughout the well. For tube testing, agglutination reactions are graded based on the size of a cell button dislodged from the bottom of a test tube. One example of a strength-of-reaction grading scheme is 4+, 3+, 2+, 1+, +/−, and 0^3 (see Table 8-1 and Fig. 8-1). Individual facilities may elaborate further on grading the strength of agglutination.

TABLE 8-1	Interpretations of Agglutination Reactions
Strength of Reaction	**Appearance**
4+	A single agglutinate, no free cells
3+	Strong reaction, many large agglutinates
2+	Large agglutinates with many smaller clumps, no free cell
1+	Many small agglutinates and a background of free cells
+/−	Few agglutinates and weak agglutinates microscopically
0	An even cell suspension, no agglutinates detected

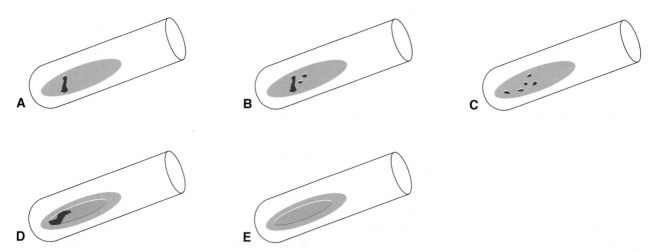

FIGURE 8-1   Agglutination reactions. A: A 4+ reaction. One large clump, clear background. B: A 3+ reaction. One or two large clumps and several small clumps, clear background. C: A 2+ reaction. Several small clumps, clear background. D: A 1+ reaction. Many small clumps, cloudy background. E: Negative. No clumps, red cells stream freely.

The ABO Blood Group

Determining a patient's ABO is the most important test performed in a blood bank or transfusion service. A recipient's ABO grouping includes an antigen (forward) grouping and an antibody (reverse) grouping. The test tube technique is frequently used and is the method used for explanation here. The forward grouping is performed by placing one drop of commercially prepared anti-A and anti-B into a labeled test tube and adding one drop of a 4% to 6% saline suspension of patient's RBCs. The mixture is centrifuged, gently resuspended, and observed for clumping, indicating the presence of the A or B antigen, or both, or no clumping indicating the absence of A or B antigen on the patient's RBCs. Reactions are observed and recorded. The reverse typing is performed by mixing the patient's serum/plasma with A_1 or B RBCs. The serum/plasma and cell mixture is then centrifuged, resuspended, and observed for hemolysis or agglutination indicating the presence of anti-A or anti-B, or both. Reactions are observed and recorded. To prevent misinterpretation of ABO/Rh from occurring, some facilities establish a minimum grading of 2+ before an ABO/Rh can be interpreted. The pattern of reactivity in the forward and reverse typing determines the interpretation of the ABO group. Discrepancies between the forward and reverse group or between the current ABO and historical records must be resolved before issuing group-specific blood. If discrepancies cannot be resolved, group O blood must be used.

The Rh Type

The Rh type is a test for presence of the D antigen on RBCs and is performed by mixing a 4% to 6% saline suspension of RBCs with a commercially prepared anti-D reagent. The mixture is centrifuged, resuspended, observed for agglutination, and observations are documented. Before interpreting a patient as AB Rh(D) positive, a commercial Rh control serum or 6% albumin control should be included in testing and should be negative. This is necessary when a negative control is not present in the forward grouping (group AB). A control is necessary to ensure that spontaneous agglutination that may yield a false-positive result is not present. The control tube must be negative to interpret the Rh(D) typing. A test for weak D antigen is not routinely required in patient testing.

Antibody Detection (Antibody Screen)

As previously mentioned, various technologies are available for performing tests for unexpected antibodies (Table 8-2). The method chosen should have the sensitivity and specificity to

- detect most clinically significant antibodies
- fail to detect unwanted reactions
- allow for timely completion of testing

TABLE 8-2	Phases of the Indirect Antiglobulin Test	
Phase	**Incubation**	**Purpose**
RT immediate spin	None	Detects ABO incompatibility and strongly reactive cold antibodies.
RT	15 min	Detects cold antibodies. Seldom performed because these are clinically insignificant antibodies.
37°C	Time varies depending on enhancement medium used	Allows IgG antibodies, particularly Rh antibodies, or complement to bind to red cells. Sometimes agglutination may be observed directly after this incubation.
Wash	No incubation time; washing should be uninterrupted	Removes unbound proteins.
Antiglobulin	No incubation	Detects IgG or complement bound to red cells.
Check cells	No incubation	Agglutination proves antiglobulin serum was added, washing was adequate, and antiglobulin serum has anti-IgG reactivity.

Screening Cells

Each screening cell represents an individual donor antigenic profile. The combination of the screening cells used must contain antigenic expressions of D, C, c, E, e, Kell, k, Le^a, Le^b, Jk^a, Jk^b, Fy^a and Fy^b, P1, M, N, S, and s.[4] Some facilities require the reagent manufacturer to supply red cells that are homozygous (double dose) for clinically significant antibodies. For example, a red cell that is Jk(a+b−) is desirable because antibodies to Jk^a can show dosage. Dosage is demonstrated when antibody reactivity is observed on cells that have a double-dose expression of antigen (homozygous), and reactivity is weakened or not observed on cells that contain a single dose of antigen (heterozygous). For example, reactivity is observed on red cells that are Jk(a+b−) (homozygous), but no reactivity is observed on red cells that are Jk(a+b+) (heterozygous). The same is common when anti-M is suspected. Reactivity may be observed with M+N− cells, but is weakened or not detected with M+N+ cells.

Test Performance

An antibody screen is performed by testing recipient serum/plasma with screening cells. Commercially prepared, two- or three-cell screens are available. The individual screening cells should not be pooled. Testing must include a 37°C incubation preceding an antiglobulin test. Performing an IS phase and a 15-minute room temperature phase is optional because agglutination found in these phases tends to involve antibodies of no clinical significance.[5] The reading for agglutination after the 37°C incubation is also optional, although there is some risk associated with the possibility of not detecting clinically significant antibodies in the Rh system with the omission of this reading.[6] As with the ABO test, the grading of agglutination is very useful in antibody screens and antibody identification studies. When varying grades of agglutination are observed in the antibody screen, the technologist should consider the possibility of the presence of more than one antibody. When unexpected antibodies are detected, an antibody identification panel is usually performed.

Blood Selection Guidelines

ABO/Rh

The ABO and Rh must be performed if group- and type-specific blood is to be used for transfusion. If there is no sample or the sample is not acceptable, or there is nonagreement of current results with historical results, the transfusing facility must issue group O blood for transfusion. The Rh type should be performed so that a recipient can receive Rh-specific blood. When the Rh cannot be interpreted, Rh(D)-negative blood should be used. Table 8-3 summarizes ABO and Rh selection for whole blood, RBCs, and plasma.

Additional Attributes in Blood Selection

When a blood bank is notified that a potential transfusion recipient has distinct transfusion requirements, this information must be readily available so that donor units selected are appropriate. Some examples follow:

- Recipients of lung transplants are at an increased risk for development of cytomegalovirus (CMV) infection and require CMV-negative or CMV-"safe" (leukocyte-reduced) RBCs.
- Patients undergoing bone marrow transplantation require irradiation to prevent graft-versus-host disease.
- Patients who experience febrile transfusion reactions may benefit from leukoreduced blood.

TABLE 8-3   Blood Component ABO and Rh Compatibility

Patient's ABO Group	Compatible with		Plasma
	Whole Blood	Red Blood Cells	
O	O	O	O, A, B, AB
A	A	A, O	A, AB
B	B	B, O	B, AB
AB	AB	AB, A, B, O	AB

An Rh positive patient may receive Rh positive or Rh negative components.

An Rh negative patient should only received Rh negative components except in unusual circumstances.

Autologous, Directed, and Allogeneic Units

Although group/*type-specific blood* is usually preferred, patient's requests for units from directed donors—individuals designated by the recipient or the recipient's family—may result in the selection of blood that is not group/type specific. For the selection of blood for transfusion, it is important to understand classification of donors. Autologous blood describes blood that a patient donates for his or her own surgery. Individual transfusion facilities may choose to abbreviate routine crossmatch protocols for autologous units. Directed donation is blood collected from individuals designated by the patient as acceptable donors. Directed donations from immediate family members require irradiation before issue. Allogeneic blood is that which comes from the general donor population. When selecting units, the order of transfusion should be: first, autologous units, if available; second, ABO/Rh-compatible directed donor units, if available; and third, allogeneic units.

THE CROSSMATCH

A crossmatch is the final test to determine the compatibility of recipient serum/plasma with donor RBCs. Frequently, the method selected for crossmatch is the same as the method used in the antibody screen. Although saline, IS, albumin, LISS, and the like are valid methods for pretransfusion testing, data collected between January 1994 and January 1995 indicated that 51% of the responders routinely use the IS crossmatch, and 48% routinely use an *indirect antiglobulin test (IAT)* method.[7] For this reason, our discussion is limited to two serologic methods: the IS and IAT methodologies, and one nonserologic method: the "computer" crossmatch. When a serologic crossmatch is performed, the donor blood used for testing in the crossmatch must be taken from an integrally attached segment of the donor unit.[1]

The Immediate-spin Crossmatch

The IS crossmatch detects most ABO incompatibility and may be performed if the antibody screen is nonreactive and there is no history of unexpected antibody. An IS crossmatch is performed by making a 2% to 3% suspension of donor RBCs and mixing with a patient's serum/plasma. After a brief centrifugation, the cell button is gently dislodged and inspected for the presence or absence of agglutination or hemolysis.

Interpretation

The absence of agglutination or hemolysis is a nonreactive test and the unit is considered acceptable for transfusion (compatible). The presence of agglutination or hemolysis at any phase of testing is considered positive and the unit is not considered acceptable for transfusion (incompatible). If the IS crossmatch is reactive, consider the following:

- The unit selected may be ABO incompatible.
- The patient's serum may be exhibiting rouleaux. If the antibody screen does not have an IS phase, the rouleaux may be undetected.
- The patient may have autoantibodies or alloantibodies that were not detected in the antibody screen.
- The test tube may have been contaminated.

The Indirect Antiglobulin Test Crossmatch

Patients who have clinically significant antibodies either by current testing or by history must have a crossmatch performed that includes a 37°C incubation phase and the antiglobulin test. An IAT crossmatch may also be performed for patients who do not demonstrate clinically significant antibodies. An IAT crossmatch consists of testing donor cells and patient serum with an enhancement medium such as albumin or LISS at a 37°C incubation and includes the addition of an antiglobulin phase.

The 37°C incubation time depends on the choice of enhancement solution. The antiglobulin reagent used may be monospecific (IgG) or polyspecific (IgG and C3d). Historically, when it was considered necessary to investigate reasons for reactivity at all testing phases, the IS and a 15-minute room temperature incubation were part of an IAT crossmatch. Studies have reported that compatibility tests performed at 37°C in a LISS solution are as sensitive for the detection of ABO incompatibility as the IS crossmatch and could therefore be eliminated in the IAT crossmatch.[5] As with antibody screen tests, reading for reactivity after 37°C incubation, although frequently performed, is not required.

Additional Considerations for Patients with Antibodies

Patients with identified antibodies, either by current testing or by history, usually require additional testing of the donor unit. When a patient demonstrates a *clinically significant antibody*, the units selected should be tested with commercially prepared antiserum and typed as antigen negative for the offending antibody. For example, a patient has an antibody identified as anti-Kell. A sample of blood from a donor segment, and positive and negative controls are obtained and tested with commercially prepared anti-Kell following the manufacturer's instructions. If the donor cells are Kell negative, and the unit is IAT crossmatch compatible, the unit is considered acceptable for transfusion. Antigen typing of the donor unit may be done before or after the IAT crossmatch.

Interpretation of Crossmatches

Absence of hemolysis or agglutination at all phases of testing may be interpreted as nonreactive, or compatible, and units are considered acceptable for transfusion. Hemolysis or agglutination detected at any phase of testing is interpreted as positive and the unit is not considered acceptable for transfusion, or incompatible.

When an IAT crossmatch is positive, consider the following:

- The unit selected may be ABO incompatible.
- The unit may have a positive direct antiglobulin test.
- The unit may not have been antigen typed or the unit may be designated incorrectly.
- The patient may be developing an additional antibody.
- The patient may have an antibody to a low-incidence antigen that was not present on the screening cells.
- The test system could be contaminated.

Box 8-2 summarizes the potential causes of incompatible crossmatches. The major crossmatch has limitations as listed in Box 8-3.

SPECIAL CONSIDERATIONS FOR INFANTS YOUNGER THAN 4 MONTHS OF AGE

Infants younger than 4 months of age have unique test requirements. After an initial pretransfusion sample is obtained, the necessity of additional sample collections depends on the results of the antibody screen and the selection of blood for transfusion.

ABO/Rh

Determining the ABO group and Rh type is required. The ABO group is determined by testing a sample of infant's RBCs with anti-A and anti-B. The expression of A and B antigens may be weaker in this age group, so that testing with anti-A,B can also be performed and will discriminate a group O from a nongroup O. Because naturally occurring anti-A and anti-B are not

usually demonstrated until approximately 6 months of age, a reverse type is not performed. Repeat testing of ABO/Rh during a single hospital admission is not required.

BOX 8-2

Possible Causes of Incompatible Crossmatches

ANTIBODY SCREEN NEGATIVE

- Alloantibody in recipient to low-incidence antigen on donor red blood cells
- Positive direct antiglobulin test on donor red blood cells
- ABO error—recipient or donor red blood cell
- Contaminant in the test system
- Polyagglutinable donor red blood cells

ANTIBODY SCREEN POSITIVE

- Alloantibody directed toward antigen on donor red blood cells
- Contaminant in the test system

ANTIBODY SCREEN POSITIVE, AUTOCONTROL POSITIVE

- Alloantibody present in recipient who has been transfused
- Autoantibody and alloantibody present in recipient's serum (presence of underlying alloantibody is a major concern when autoantibody is present)
- Rouleaux present
- Reaction with or an antibody to substance in enhancement medium

---

BOX 8-3

Limitations of the Major Crossmatch

- Antibodies exhibiting dosage may not be detected.
- Antibodies reactive only at room temperature may not be detected. (This is of no concern because such antibodies are considered clinically insignificant.)
- Not all ABO grouping errors in the potential recipient or donor can be detected.
- Not all Rh grouping errors in the potential recipient or donor can be detected.
- The normal survival of transfused red blood cells is not ensured.
- There is no assurance that the recipient will not experience an adverse reaction.
- Not all clinically significant antibodies may be detected.

Antibody Screen

An initial antibody screen is usually performed on an infant sample. The maternal sample may be used because antibodies detected at this age are passively acquired from the mother and the difficulty in obtaining an adequate sample volume from an infant of this age is frequently a problem.

Interpretation of Infant's Antibody Screen Results

If the antibody screen is negative, a crossmatch and additional testing are usually not necessary when group O RBCs are selected for transfusion. When other than group O RBCs are selected for transfusion, an initial crossmatch that includes an antiglobulin phase is required.

If the antibody screen is positive, antibody identification studies are performed by testing either the mother's or infant's serum. If clinically significant antibodies are identified, the selection of antigen-negative units or units compatible by antiglobulin crossmatch is required until the passively acquired antibody is no longer demonstrated.

Crossmatch

When selecting a group-specific unit for crossmatch, it is important to crossmatch with RBCs that have a strong antigenic expression. For example, A_1 RBCs have more A antigen sites than a unit that does not type as A_1. If a group A unit is selected for crossmatch, the unit must be tested with anti-A_1 lectin according to the manufacturer's directions. If the unit is positive with anti-A_1 lectin, it is designated as A_1 and is crossmatched. Alternatively, a crossmatch with infant serum and reagent A_1 cells can be performed in lieu of a crossmatch with a donor unit. In either situation, if the initial crossmatch is nonreactive, the infant may receive group-specific blood, and subsequent testing and crossmatching is not required. If the crossmatch is positive, group O blood must be used for transfusion.

The Electronic "Computer" Crossmatch

The computer crossmatch is the verification of ABO compatibility by computer comparison of donor unit information and patient ABO group and Rh type.[8] This nonserologic crossmatch may be performed when only the detection of ABO incompatibility is required, provided the following criteria are met.

The Computer

- The computer must be validated on-site. This establishes the validity of the system as it is used by the customer.
- The computer must contain logic to prevent the release of ABO-incompatible donor units.
- The computer must contain the donor unit information. This includes the donor number, the name of the component, the ABO group and Rh type of the unit, and the ABO confirmation tests performed on the unit.
- The computer must contain the recipient ABO group and Rh type.
- There must be a method to verify the correct entry of data. This is usually accomplished through interpretation tables, truth tables, warning devices, manual overrides, and the like.

The Recipient

There must be two determinations of the recipient's ABO group, and one determination must be performed on a current sample. The other ABO group determination may be made either by retesting the same sample and comparing the results obtained with previous records, or by obtaining a second current sample.

Ideally, the ABO grouping is performed by two different individuals. The performance of a computer crossmatch is enhanced by the use of barcode readers for both patient sample identity and for donor unit information. Although keyboard entry is permitted, the preference is to use a barcode reader.

BLOOD REQUESTS FOR SURGERY

Facilities usually establish protocols to expedite surgery requests for blood. Type and screen refers to a request for an ABO, Rh, and an antibody screen. Boral and Henry proposed the use of a type and screen when blood use is unlikely but blood should be available on demand if needed. Data indicated that the type and screen was 99.99% effective in preventing transfusion of incompatible blood.[9] When there are no clinically significant antibodies detected in a two-cell screen method, the frequency of an incompatible antiglobulin crossmatch ranges from 0.06% to 0.08%.[10] A type and cross in addition to the testing performed in a type and screen includes a request for a specified number of units. Frequently, blood is crossmatched for surgical procedures that rarely use blood. Data collected in a study of pretransfusion testing of surgical patients resulted in the development of a *maximum surgical blood order schedule (MSBOS)* that can be used in conjunction with a type and screen.[11]

An MSBOS is a list of an institution's surgical procedures and the corresponding blood usually available for a particular surgery. An MSBOS represents a maximum blood order, not a minimum blood requirement. Transfusion services that use an MSBOS review the surgical schedule and compare the presurgical blood requests to the MSBOS. Blood requests that exceed the MSBOS are reduced to the MSBOS recommendation; however, a physician may request a larger number of units to be crossmatched if a patient has special needs. Using an MSBOS allows a transfusion service to review the ratio of crossmatches performed to transfusion given (C/T ratio). This ratio is usually an indication of the appropriateness of blood-ordering practices. Blood inventory is managed by use of a type-and-screen protocol and the MSBOS because crossmatches are performed only on surgical cases that have a predictable blood use.

EXCEPTIONAL PROTOCOLS

Blood banks and transfusion services may encounter clinical situations that require a departure or deviation from standard operating procedures. Policies should include protocols that address exceptions from routine. In addition, it is prudent to have a process to document and track events that promulgate a departure from routine operations. The following sections describe examples protocols that are exceptional.

Massive Transfusion

When the total blood volume of an individual has been replaced with donor blood within 24 hours, a *massive transfusion* event has occurred. Because the patient's circulation contains primarily donor blood, the purpose of the crossmatch is somewhat diminished. Frequently during these instances, an *abbreviated crossmatch* may be performed at the discretion of the director of the transfusion service.[12] For the purposes of this discussion, an abbreviated crossmatch reduces the amount of testing that is normally performed. For example, an IS or computer crossmatch is performed when the transfusion recipient qualifies for an antiglobulin crossmatch. Within 24 hours of the massive transfusion event, the recipient's crossmatch status should be reevaluated.

Emergency Requests for Blood

When an urgent blood request is received, the documented need for blood and the life-threatening urgency of the situation outweigh the delay that may occur in the course of pretransfusion testing. The procedure for providing blood in emergency situations should be as uncomplicated as possible.

- The requesting physician must document that the clinical situation was of sufficient urgency to require release of blood without completion of pretransfusion testing.
- Blood issued in emergency situations is usually group O, Rh(D) negative. If an ABO group and Rh type has been determined without relying on previous records, group- and type-specific blood can be given.
- Units must be labeled in a conspicuous way so that it is clear that pretransfusion testing was incomplete at time of issue.

Pretransfusion testing is completed as soon as possible. In the event the patient does not survive the emergency event, sufficient testing should be completed to establish that the transfusion did not contribute to the patient's death.

Autoimmune Hemolytic Anemia

The presence of autoantibody can cause special problems in pretransfusion testing. It is essential that the need for transfusion be well established. It may be necessary to use autoabsorbed serum for pretransfusion testing. If cold autoantibody is present, alternative pretransfusion testing may be indicated. The specificity of the autoantibody is not crucial, if clinically significant alloantibodies have been excluded. Transfused donor RBCs that are no more agglutinated in pretransfusion testing than the potential recipient's autocontrol should survive as long as the individual's own cells.

Transfusion strategies may include infusing a small volume of donor RBCs with close monitoring of the patient, using a blood warmer when cold autoantibodies is the culprit, and using leukocyte-reduced blood to minimize possible adverse reaction.

ISSUING BLOOD

Issuing blood for transfusion is frequently the final opportunity to verify the acceptability of the donor unit before leaving the blood bank. The blood and container are visually inspected immediately before issue for normal appearance. If the unit is visually unacceptable, for example, hemolysis is detected in the donor unit or segments, it is not issued for transfusion. In addition, the individual issuing the blood must verify that the unit has not expired and that the crossmatch label is secured to the unit. The recipient crossmatch label should contain the following information:

- The facility name
- The intended recipient's two independent identifiers
- The donor unit number
- The interpretation of the compatibility test performed

The unit review for acceptability should be documented. After this information has been verified, and is acceptable, the unit may be issued.

SUMMARY

The goal of pretransfusion testing is to provide blood for transfusion that is beneficial to the recipient (Box 8-4). Critical to achieving this goal is accurate patient identification from sample collection to final transfusion. A spectrum of testing is currently available. An understanding of various test methodologies and limitations of testing clarifies the decisions in providing blood that is efficacious to the recipient. The variety in pretransfusion testing protocols permits an individual facility to institute policies and procedures suitable for its environment.

BOX 8-4

Critical Steps in Pretransfusion Testing

Request Type and Screen.
Is Sample Acceptable?
(Yes)
Perform ABO/Rh Screen:
  Is ABO/Rh Valid?
  (Yes)
  Continue Testing.
  (No)
  Problem Solve.
Does ABO/Rh Match History?
  (Yes)
  Document/Review.
  (No)
  Problem Solve.
Is Screen Negative?
  (Yes)
  Document Results/File Sample.
  (No)
  Problem Solve.
Is Blood Requested?
  (Yes)
  Perform Crossmatch.
  Is Crossmatch Compatible?
    (Yes)
    Issue Blood.
    (No)
    Problem Solve.
  (No)
  File Sample.
(No)
Request New Sample.

Review Questions

1. A blood sample is received for type and screen, but the sample is labeled with the patient's last and first names only. What additional information is necessary for the sample to be acceptable for use?
   a. nothing else is required, the label is acceptable
   b. a patient identification number or second patient identifier
   c. physician's name
   d. patient location

2. A crossmatch label should include:
   a. the crossmatch interpretation
   b. the donor unit number
   c. the name and identification of the recipient
   d. all of the above

3. A review of previous records indicates a patient is group O. The current sample testing indicates the patient is group A. Blood is needed urgently. What red blood cells should be selected for transfusion?
   a. group AB
   b. group B
   c. group O
   d. group A

4. The criteria required for a "computer" crossmatch include:
   a. two individuals comparing previous and past records
   b. the optional use of a computer
   c. two concurrent determinations of the recipient's ABO group, one of which is done on a current sample
   d. the use of a computer validated by the manufacturer

(continued)

REVIEW QUESTIONS (continued)

5. A patient has an anti-E. What crossmatch should be performed?
   a. a "computer" crossmatch
   b. an immediate-spin crossmatch
   c. a crossmatch is not required
   d. a crossmatch that includes an incubation phase and testing with an antihuman globulin reagent.

6. For the patient in Question 5, what additional testing should be performed on the donor unit?
   a. additional testing is not required
   b. antigen type the donor unit for E
   c. antigen type the donor unit for c and E
   d. use donor plasma and perform a minor crossmatch

7. Pretransfusion testing requirements for infants younger than 4 months of age include:
   a. an ABO/Rh and antibody screen on the mother
   b. an ABO/Rh and antibody screen on the infant
   c. a forward and reverse grouping on the infant sample
   d. testing is not required if group O red blood cells are selected for transfusion

8. Allogeneic blood is synonymous with:
   a. autologous blood
   b. directed donor blood
   c. homologous blood
   d. nonvolunteer donor blood

9. A maximum surgical blood order schedule (MSBOS) refers to:
   a. the quantity of blood required for a specific surgical procedure
   b. the required testing before a surgical procedure
   c. a crossmatch-to-transfusion (C/T) ratio
   d. a maximum blood order, not a minimum blood requirement for a specific surgical procedure

10. The final check for unit acceptability for transfusion is performed:
   a. before the unit is labeled
   b. just before issuing the unit
   c. at the time a unit is selected for crossmatch
   d. when the unit is labeled after pretransfusion testing

REFERENCES

1. Klein HG, ed. *Standards for Blood Banks and Transfusion Services*. 25th ed. Bethesda, MD: American Association of Blood Banks; 2008.
2. Vengelen-Tyler V, ed. *Technical Manual of the American Association of Blood Banks*. 12th ed. Bethesda, MD: American Association of Blood Banks; 1996.
3. Walker RH, ed. *Technical Manual*. 10th ed. Arlington, VA: American Association of Blood Banks; 1990.
4. U.S. Department of Health and Human Services, Food and Drug Administration. *The Code of Federal Regulations, 21CFR 660.3–660.36*, current edition. Washington, DC: U.S. Government Printing Office; 1996.
5. Trudeau LR, Judd WJ, Butch SH, et al. Is a room-temperature crossmatch necessary for the detection of ABO errors? *Transfusion*. 1983;23:237.
6. Judd WJ, Steiner EA, Oberman HA, et al. Can the reading for serological reactivity following 37°C incubation be omitted? *Transfusion*. 1992;32:304.
7. Maffei LM. *Current State of the Art: The Survey Pretransfusion Testing: AABB Technical Workshop on Pre-Transfusion Testing: Routine To Complex*. Bethesda, MD: American Association of Blood Banks; 1996.
8. Butch SH, Judd WJ, Steiner EA, et al. Electronic verification of donor–recipient compatibility: the computer crossmatch. *Transfusion*. 1994;34:105.
9. Boral LJ, Henry JB. The type and screen: a safe alternative and supplement in selected surgical procedures. *Transfusion*. 1977;17:163.
10. Mintz PD, Haines AL, Sullivan MF. Incompatible crossmatch following nonreactive antibody detection test: frequency and cause. *Transfusion*. 1982;22:107.
11. Friedman BA. An analysis of surgical blood use in United States hospitals with application to the maximum surgical blood order schedule. *Transfusion*. 1979;19:268.
12. Oberman HA, Barnes BA, Friedman BA. The risk of abbreviating the major crossmatch in urgent or massive transfusion. *Transfusion*. 1978;18:137.

THE ABO BLOOD GROUP SYSTEM

EVA D. QUINLEY

OBJECTIVES

After completion of this chapter, the reader will be able to:

1. Discuss the discovery of the ABO blood group system and its importance to modern blood transfusion practice.
2. Describe the inheritance of the red blood cell and soluble A, B, and H antigens, including the importance of the following genes: *A, B, H,* and *Se.*
3. Describe the following reagents, their source, and usefulness in detecting antigens within the ABO blood group system: anti-A, anti-B, anti-A,B, anti-H, *Dolichos biflorus,* and *Ulex europaeus.*
4. Discuss the importance of the subgroups of A and B in transfusion medicine and how they are distinguished.
5. Define ABO discrepancy, and describe the following different causes, testing patterns of each cause, and method of resolution.

KEY WORDS

ABO discrepancy	Isoagglutinins
Acquired B	Naturally occurring
Amorphic	Non–red cell stimulated
Anti-A$_1$	Reverse grouping
Bombay	Secretor
Cis-AB	Subgroups
Dolichos biflorus	Type I precursor chain
Forward grouping	Type II chain
Glycosyltransferase	*Ulex europaeus*

The ABO blood group system (BGS) is the most important human BGS in transfusion practice and was the first to be discovered. The ABO system was first described by Karl Landsteiner in 1900 and was reported in 1901.[1] Landsteiner drew blood from coworkers in his laboratory, separated cells and plasma, and mixed the cells and plasma from the various people on glass tiles. He was able to identify three different patterns of reactivity, which he termed A, B, and C. These were later reclassified as groups A, B, and O, respectively. Von Decastello and Sturli discovered group AB (the rarest of the common ABO types) and reported this blood type in 1902.[2] Routine blood grouping tests were developed from the work of these blood bank pioneers. A, B, O, and AB represent the four major groups in the ABO system. A listing of antigens and antibodies present in these four major ABO groups is given in Table 9-1. Subgrouping within the system is discussed in a later section.

The ABO BGS is the most important in transfusion medicine as almost all normal, healthy people older than 3 months of age have **naturally occurring** antibodies to the ABO antigens that they lack. These antibodies were first called naturally occurring because

TABLE 9-1	Antigens and Antibodies in Various ABO Groups	
Blood Group	**Antigens on Red Cells**	**Antibodies in Plasma**
A	A antigen	Anti-B
B	B antigen	Anti-A
O	Neither A nor B antigen	Anti-A and anti-B
AB	Both A and B antigens	Neither anti-A nor anti-B

TABLE 9-2 Representative Typing Reactions of Common ABO Blood Groups

Blood Group	Forward Grouping Reaction with		Reverse Grouping Reaction with	
	Anti-A	Anti-B	A Cells	B Cells
A	+	0	0	+
B	0	+	+	0
O	0	0	+	+
AB	+	+	0	0

they were thought to arise without antigenic stimulation. It is now known that this is not the case, and they are believed to be stimulated by antigens in nature that are ABO like. These "naturally occurring" antibodies are almost always present and are mostly of the immunoglobulin M (IgM) class. They are capable of agglutinating saline or low–protein-suspended red blood cells (RBCs) without enhancement and may readily activate the complement cascade. This means that a potentially life-threatening situation may exist during the first attempted transfusion of a recipient if appropriate precautions are not taken to provide the correct ABO blood group for transfusion.

In its simplest form, the ABO system can be demonstrated by simple room temperature mixing of RBCs and plasma or serum. The reagents that are used in the laboratory for routine ABO grouping may simply consist of serum from group B people (containing anti-A), serum from group A people (containing anti-B), and cells from known group A and B people. Alternatively, reagents produced by monoclonal technology may be used for ABO typing. Table 9-2 provides a representative example of grouping reactions for the common ABO groups.

INHERITANCE

It was originally believed that the ABO antigens were inherited directly, along with the ability to produce the antibodies to the ABO antigens not produced. It was believed that no antigenic stimulus was necessary to produce the antibody. This theory was soon discarded after it was shown that the naturally occurring antibodies were actually caused by stimulation with antigenically similar substances present in our environment. Experiments with chickens that develop similar, naturally occurring *isoagglutinins* proved this. Isoagglutinins are antibodies that react with some members of the same species. When the chickens were grown in an experimental "germ-free" environment, they failed to develop the naturally occurring isoagglutinins. Further work showed that the isoagglutinins of humans were developed in a similar way. This is why it generally takes 3 to 6 months for newborns to develop sufficient levels of these isoagglutinins to be readily classified. The term "naturally occurring" is most appropriately replaced with the term *non–red cell stimulated* (NRCS) when referring to these antibodies.

The ABO blood group genes code not for the antigens directly, which are carbohydrate in nature, but for the production of *glycosyltransferases*. Glycosyltransferases are enzymes that facilitate the transfer of carbohydrate (sugar) molecules onto carbohydrate precursor molecules. The transferase associated with each blood group is specific for a particular immunodominant sugar. The immunodominant sugar molecule completes the antigenic determinant when combined with the precursor substance. A listing of the specific transferase, along with the immunodominant sugar for each common ABO antigen, is given in Table 9-3.

The *ABO* genes seem to follow simple Mendelian genetic laws and are inherited in a codominant fashion because both *A* and *B* alleles are expressed when present. The *O* gene is an *amorphic* or silent gene in that it appears to have no gene product or to produce a nondetectable product. No specific transferase has been associated with the *O* gene. The *ABO* locus is found on the long arm of chromosome 9. The *A* and *B* genes may be found alternatively at these loci, one on each of the pair of chromosomes in any combination (Fig. 9-1). Variants of *A* and *B* rarely may be found but are simple replacements for the more common gene and are inherited similarly to the more common forms of the *A* and *B* genes. Yamamoto et al. have completed extensive work identifying the molecular genetic basis of the ABO system.[3]

The frequency of blood types in various populations differs depending on their genetic makeup. Table 9-4 gives the approximate frequencies of the ABO blood groups in select population groups in the United States. White people are predominantly group O (44%) and

TABLE 9-3 Transferases and Immunodominant Sugars of the ABO Blood Group System

Gene	Glycosyltransferase	Immunodominant Sugar
H	L-fucosyltransferase	L-fucose
A	N-acetylgalactosaminyl-transferase	N-acetylgalactosamine
B	D-galactosyltransferase	D-galactose

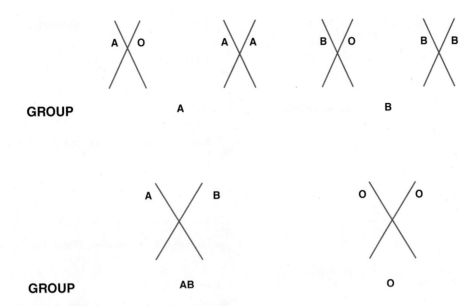

GROUP   A   B

GROUP   AB   O

FIGURE 9-1 Common ABO groups and their inheritance.

TABLE 9-4	Approximate Frequencies of ABO Groups in Various Populations			
Blood Group	White People (%)	African Americans (%)	Native Americans (%)	Asians (%)
O	44	49	79	41
A	42	27	16	28
B	10	20	4	26
AB	4	4	<1	5

group A (42%), with only 10% being group B and only 4% group AB. Group O is slightly more common in African American people (49%), whereas group A is much less frequent (27%), and group B is much more frequent (20%) than in the white population. Group O accounts for 79% of the Native American population in the United States, with only 16% being group A and only 4% group B. Group AB is extremely rare in the Native American population; less than 1% of the Native American population carries the *A* and *B* genes. Asian people have approximately the same frequency of group O as white people (41%), with group A (28%) and group B (26%) being almost identical in frequency. Group AB in Asians is slightly more common (5%) than in white people.

BOMBAY PHENOTYPE

The understanding of the inheritance of the A, B, and O antigens was not complete until the discovery of a rare individual who lacked the A and B antigens on the surface of the RBCs (apparent group O) but had antibodies in the plasma which reacted not only with A and B red cells but also with group O red cells. This rare group was first discovered in **Bombay**, India, in 1952 and is referred to as H deficient or the Bombay phenotype. Through study of the genetic makeup of these people compared with "normal" group O people, a proposed theory of inheritance was developed that explains the existence of the Bombay phenotype and the amorphic nature of the O gene.

The *H* gene is present, in single or double dose, in almost all people and is apparently necessary for the development of the A and B antigens. The silent allele, *h*, is extremely rare and fails to produce the L-fucosyltransferase necessary to convert the ABO precursor substance to the H substance (H antigen). The H antigen serves as a precursor for the A and B transferases. The *H* gene, which is dominant to its amorphic allele *h*, results in the production of a glycosyltransferase that facilitates placement of L-fucose onto an appropriate precursor substance. This H substance (or H antigen) serves as the precursor substance for the A and B transferases. Because the A and B transferases are very specific, failure to produce the H substance results in an inability of the A and B transferases to function normally. Therefore, it is possible for a person with the Bombay phenotype genetically to transmit functional *A* and *B* genes to his or her progeny, although that person is unable to produce the A and B antigens. A proposed diagrammatic representation of the inheritance of the *ABO* and *Hh* genes is shown in Figure 9-2.

Because the Bombay phenotype fails to produce the H antigen, it produces an NRCS anti-H in the serum. When routine ABO grouping is attempted, the people appear to group as a group O. However,

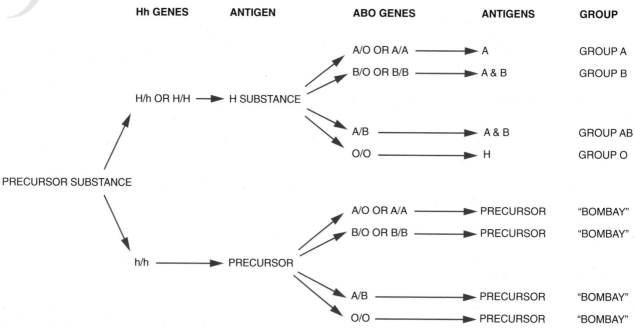

FIGURE 9-2   Inheritance of ABO blood group.

the anti-H present in their sera causes them to react with all normal group O cells. This antibody is primarily IgM in nature and is reactive over a wide thermal range. Thus, the only safe blood donor for an individual possessing anti-H is a donor with the Bombay phenotype. To prove that the individual lacks the H antigen, his or her RBCs may be typed with a product of the plant *Ulex europaeus* (anti-H lectin) or with sera containing anti-H activity from which all anti-A, anti-B, and anti-A,B activity has been adsorbed.

The plant lectin provides a much simpler and more readily available source of anti-H-like activity. This extract of *U. europaeus*, when properly diluted, may be used to determine the presence or absence of the H antigen on the surface of RBCs. Table 9-5 shows the reactions of a Bombay phenotype in routine pretransfusion testing.

Inheritance of the Bombay Phenotype (O_h or ABH_{null})

Normal people inherit a pair of *H* genes at a locus separate from the *ABO* locus. The classic Bombay pheno-

type would be expected to arise most frequently in the children resulting from consanguineous marriages. Consanguineous marriages are marriages between people of close blood relationship, usually closer than third cousins. The Bombay phenotype results from the inheritance of an *h* gene from both parents at the *H* locus, leaving the person unable to produce the H glycosyltransferase and therefore unable to produce H antigen. Regardless of the *A, B, or O* genes inherited by this individual at the *ABO* locus, no A, B, or H antigen is formed. This person appears to be group on in testing, but lacking the H antigen, produces anti-H in his or her serum. These people, therefore, are sometimes termed O_h or ABH_{null}. As will be seen in the study of other BGSs, the understanding of the inheritance of the null phenotype (if present) is crucial to the understanding of the inheritance of a BGS. Figure 9-3 gives a pedigree of a family demonstrating the inheritance of *ABO* and *H/h* genes resulting in a Bombay phenotype.

As shown in this representative pedigree, progeny of Bombay people acquire normal *ABO* genes from their "abnormal" parents. Thus, genes inherited at the *H* locus in no way affect the genetic

TABLE 9-5 Reactions of Bombay Phenotype in Routine Pretransfusion Testing					
Reaction with anti-A	Reaction with anti-B	Reaction with anti-A,B	Reaction with A_1 cells	Reaction with B Cells	Reaction with O Cells
0	0	0	4−	4+	4+

No H demonstrated on subject's red blood cells when subsequently tested with anti-H lectin.

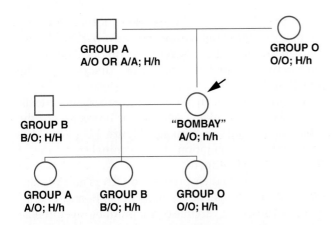

FIGURE 9-3   Inheritance of *ABO* and *Hh* genes in a family exhibiting the Bombay phenotype.

transmission of the A and B transferases. This has been demonstrated by scientific studies revealing the presence of the appropriate A and B transferases in the blood of Bombay phenotype people.

The true O_h individual lacks both the *H* and *Se* alleles. Rare individuals do exist who lack *H* but possess at least one *Se* allele. These individuals can have H, A, and B substance in their secretions while their red cells have no A, B, or H sugars. This phenotype is referred to as para-Bombay.

Cis-AB

Rare examples of apparent unequal crossing-over of genetic information have been documented in the ABO system. Documentation of such events usually occurs with cases of disputed paternity. The most common documented example of apparent unequal crossing-over occurs when a person carries both the *A* and *B*

genes on the same chromosome. This rare occurrence is termed a ***cis-AB*** and results in the ability to genetically transmit both *A* and *B* genes to progeny. An example of this situation is illustrated in Figure 9-4. It has now been documented that at least a portion of those cases of apparent unequal crossing-over are due to gene mutation. Yamamoto et al. have shown that in two cases they studied, the genetic transmission was not due to crossing-over but to a gene mutation resulting from two nucleotide substitutions, one identical to that documented to result in the A_2 allele and the other found at the fourth position of the four amino acids that discriminate A_1 and B transferases.[4]

ANTIGEN DEVELOPMENT

The A and B antigens begin to develop as early as the fifth week of fetal life, but they increase slowly in concentration: less than 50% of the adult antigen sites are present at birth. This may result in an inability to differentiate adequately *subgroups* on newborn cells. Adult levels of A and B antigens usually are not reached until approximately 2 to 4 years of age.

The *O* gene is an amorphic gene and does not result in any conversion of H substance. Therefore, group O has the highest concentration of H antigen. Refer to Box 9-1 for a listing of the common ABO blood groups in order of the concentration of H antigen on their surface.

A and B antigens are formed by a complex interrelationship between the *H/h* genes and the *ABO* genes. As previously noted, the *H*, *A*, and *B* genes do not result directly in the production of H, A, or B antigens, but in the inheritance of the ability to produce specific

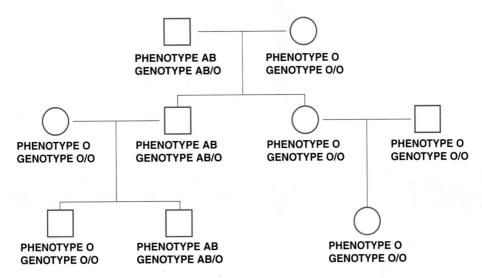

FIGURE 9-4   Inheritance of *ABO* genes in a family exhibiting *cis-AB*.

glycosyltransferases that facilitate placement of terminal sugars onto a precursor substance. The *A* gene codes for the production of *N*-acetylgalactosaminyl-transferase, which facilitates transfer of *N*-acetylgalactosamine onto the H antigen. The *B* gene codes for the production of D-galactosyltransferase, which facilitates transfer of D-galactose onto the H antigen.

The ABH antigens were the first blood group antigens to be so well characterized because similar substances are found in body secretions (see section "Secretor Status"). The glycoprotein precursor of the ABH antigens present in secretions is referred to as a ***type I precursor chain*** because it was the first to be biochemically characterized. The glycolipid precursor chain found on the surface of RBCs is referred to as a ***type II chain***. This glycoprotein versus glycolipid nature of the precursor chain is easy to remember if one remembers that the RBC membrane is a "lipid sandwich." Otherwise, the difference between these precursor chains is slight and does not significantly change the antigenic nature of the A, B, and H antigens made from the different precursors. The difference between type I and type II precursors lies in the attachment of the terminal galactose to the *N*-acetylglucosamine. In type I precursors, the attachment is a $\beta1 \rightarrow 3$ linkage, and in type II precursors, the attachment is a $\beta1 \rightarrow 4$ linkage. Figure 9-5 gives a diagrammatic representation of the terminal structures of the A, B, and H antigens.

In addition to their presence on RBCs and in soluble form in various body fluids, the A, B, and H antigens are present in variable concentrations on epithelial cells, lymphocytes, platelets, and organs such as the kidney. This means that the ABO group of the patient plays an important role in transplantation practice.

ANTIBODIES OF THE ABO SYSTEM

As stated previously, the antibodies of the ABO system arise shortly after birth on exposure to environmental agents for which antigenic makeup is similar to the A and B antigens found on human RBCs. The concentration (or titer) of these antibodies varies widely. The NRCS antibodies of the ABO system are primarily IgM in nature, although some quantity of IgG and IgA may also be present. These antibodies follow the general traits of IgM antibodies (i.e., they react best at room

ANTIGEN   TERMINAL STRUCTURE

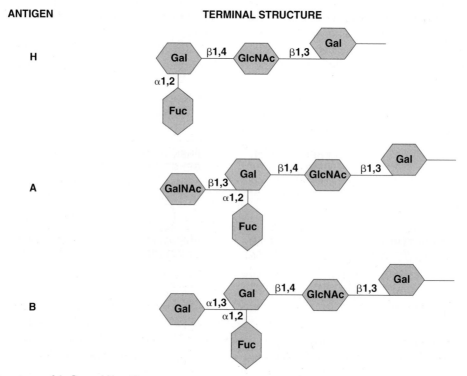

FIGURE 9-5   Structure of A, B, and H antigens.

temperature or below, are capable of activating complement, and are saline agglutinins). The IgM and IgA versions of the ABO antibodies do not cross the placental barrier. However, IgG versions cross the placenta and may cause hemolytic disease of the newborn.

The immune form of the ABO antibodies results from the exposure to incompatible RBCs or other sources of ABO antigens. It is more common for immune forms to be IgG, resulting in an increased risk of transplacental transfer of ABO antibodies during pregnancy. Further, the immune forms of the ABO antibodies are not readily inhibitable by soluble A and B antigens. This indicates that the antibody that arises due to RBC sensitization is able to detect the subtle difference between type I and type II precursor chains that produce the A and B antigens.

Unlike most other examples of IgG antibody, which have an optimum temperature of reactivity at 37°C, these IgG ABO antibodies agglutinate RBCs readily at room temperature. Both the NRCS and immune forms of these antibodies readily activate complement, and do so best at 37°C. Occasionally, the ABH antibodies may cause hemolysis at room temperature when serum samples are used for testing. Hemolysis should be considered a positive result, and caution should be observed when using hemolyzed specimens for ABO grouping. Lack of ability to detect complement activation when using plasma acquired through the use of anticoagulants that bind calcium (thereby inhibiting complement activation) may lead to less-than-satisfactory results in ABO grouping. The preferred sample for grouping is a nonanticoagulated specimen or one anticoagulated with heparin.

Anti-A

Anti-A arises in the sera of group B people on exposure to environmental agents similar to the A antigen and will agglutinate the RBCs of all group A and AB people. Most of this anti-A is IgM, although small amounts of IgG and IgA may be present. Therefore, anti-A is able to agglutinate RBCs suspended in saline and activate complement with ease. It may cause rapid intravascular destruction of RBCs carrying the A antigen. Anti-A can be functionally split into two components: *anti-A$_1$*, which reacts with A$_1$ cells but not with A$_2$ cells, and anti-A$_{common}$, which reacts with both A$_1$ and A$_2$ cells. A$_1$ and A$_2$ are the two most common subgroups of A, representing approximately 80% and 20%, respectively, of the total number of group A people. Other subgroups are very rare and are discussed later in this chapter.

Although functionally separable, this anti-A$_1$ also can be shown to be removed with A$_2$ cells on exhaustive adsorption. This may be explained by a slight

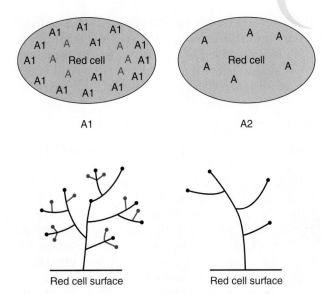

FIGURE 9-6   Quantitative difference between an A$_1$ red blood cell and an A$_2$ red blood cell.

difference in the A$_{common}$ antigen on the surface of the RBCs of the A$_2$ person. It has been proposed that this apparent difference in the antigen between the RBCs of A$_1$ and A$_2$ people lies in the relative amount of branching that occurs in the precursor structures for the ABH antigens. The A$_1$ antigen is more branched and therefore reacts differently with anti-A than the lesser-branched A$_2$ antigen. This also explains why newborns, who will ultimately express the A$_1$ phenotype, may initially type as A$_2$. Thus, the antibody known as anti-A$_{common}$ may actually be a form of anti-A that reacts differently because of the steric hindrance caused by the superbranched A$_1$ antigen. Figure 9-6 gives a diagrammatic representation of this relationship.

Anti-A$_1$

Anti-A from a group B person, when mixed with A$_2$ cells, can cause adsorption of a component of anti-A called anti-A$_{common}$, leaving a component with apparent anti-A$_1$ activity. This reagent is called anti-A$_1$ (adsorbed) and can be used to distinguish between A$_1$ and A$_2$ cells. A reagent made from the plant *Dolichos biflorus* (lectin), when properly diluted, can easily differentiate between A$_1$ and A$_2$ cells and is the preferred reagent for distinguishing A$_1$ and A$_2$ cells.

Anti-B

The serum from group A people contains an antibody that agglutinates essentially all group B and group AB RBCs. Anti-B, like anti-A, appears most frequently without RBC stimulation as IgM, which may have a small component of IgG and IgA. Immune forms of this antibody react similarly to immune forms of anti-A.

This antibody readily agglutinates cells suspended in saline, activates complement, and may rapidly destroy incompatible RBCs by intravascular hemolysis. Weak subgroups of B may react variably with anti-B and are discussed later in this chapter.

Anti-A,B

Anti-A,B is found in the sera of all group O people along with some component of anti-A and anti-B. Anti-A,B is not simply a mixture of anti-A and anti-B, as can be demonstrated by differential adsorption with either A or B cells. Either of these cells is capable of completely adsorbing all anti-A or anti-B activity. Further, when elution studies are performed, anti-B-like activity can be demonstrated by the antibody reacting with the A cells, and anti-A-like activity can be demonstrated by the antibody eluted from B cells. The antibody is not only capable of reacting with either A or B cells, but usually has a higher titer and avidity than NRCS anti-A or anti-B.

This is why anti-A,B may be used to confirm group O donors, in the testing of newborn blood samples, and as an aid in identification of weak subgroups of A and B. The IgG form of anti-A,B is more likely to occur in the sera of group O people who have been sensitized by the A or B antigen. Therefore, group O mothers are more likely to have the IgG anti-A,B in their sera when carrying a group A or B fetus. The fetus will be more likely to suffer from hemolytic disease of the newborn from the IgG form of anti-A,B in conjunction with IgG anti-A or anti-B or from anti-A,B alone. This should always be considered when eluates from newborn samples are tested for apparent ABO incompatibility. The antibody on the surface of the newborn's RBCs is most likely anti-A,B and should be reported as such.

Anti-H

Anti-H may be found as a weak, cold-reacting antibody in the sera of group A_1 and be A_1B people. It is also found as a strong, NRCS antibody in the sera of people expressing the Bombay phenotype (Oh). The H antigen present in A_1 and A_1B people is in the lowest concentration of all the ABO types. This may result in a failure of these people to recognize the H antigen as "self" and to make an antibody to H. This is the explanation for the weak anti-H that is sometimes present in the sera of A_1 and A_1B people.

A reagent with anti-H-like activity can be prepared from the plant *U. europaeus*. When properly diluted, this lectin can differentiate among cells with varying concentrations of H antigen and may used for testing for **secretor** status. When tested with either anti-H or the *U. europaeus* lectin, the RBCs of the Bombay phenotype are negative.

Forward Grouping

Forward grouping refers to the testing of RBCs to determine the presence of A or B antigens on the surface. Other common terms used to describe forward grouping include front typing, cell typing, cell grouping, and forward typing. Forward grouping is accomplished by testing a sample of RBCs with known anti-A and anti-B. Anti-A,B may be used for typing all group O blood donors. As discussed previously, anti-A,B is a reagent that is best used to help detect weak subgroups of A and B. Routine use of anti-A,B for the testing of patient populations is not recommended unless ABO discrepancies occur. The detection of a weak subgroup of A or B simply leads to confusion and usually does not alter the choice of donor blood for the patient.

Testing is classically performed at room temperature by either manual or automated techniques. Slide typing, the mixture of cells and testing serum on a slide or glass tile, may be performed by mixing a drop of the appropriate antiserum with a drop of a 20% to 30% suspension of RBCs in their own serum or an equivalent number of RBCs attached to a wooden mixing stick. The cells are mixed well with the antiserum and rocked for several minutes while observing for agglutination. Agglutination appears as a clumping of RBCs and may be visualized macroscopically.

Tube typing is another classic method of performing ABO grouping. Tube typing is performed by adding one drop of a 2% to 5% saline suspension of RBCs to a 10×75-mm or 12×75-mm tube containing one drop of appropriate antiserum followed by centrifugation with sufficient force to develop a loose cell button. All manufacturer's directions must be followed exactly. The cells are resuspended using an optical aid while observing macroscopically for agglutination. Refer to Table 9-2, which gives the results of forward grouping for the common ABO blood groups.

Microplate and Gel Testing

Microplate testing has been adopted by many larger blood centers for donor typing. It is performed in 96-well microtiter plates. Small quantities of diluted antiserum along with small quantities of RBCs combine with ease of testing of large volumes to make this technique useful in these larger blood centers. Further information on microplate testing may be found in the American Association of Blood Banks' *Technical Manual*.

Many blood banks have gone to alternative methods of testing, including gel and solid-phase techniques. In gel testing, reagents are suspended in a gel medium in columns on cards. Red cells are added to the columns and reactions occur in the gel if the appropriate antigen is present. A buffered gel column is used for *reverse grouping* using plasma or serum. As with all testing techniques, manufacturer's instructions must be adhered to during performance of the testing. Automated testing utilizing these methodologies is becoming more and more prevalent, particularly in donor centers.

Reverse Grouping

Reverse grouping refers to the testing of a serum to determine the presence or absence of anti-A or anti-B. Other common names for this testing include serum grouping, confirmation grouping, and back typing. Reverse grouping is routinely accomplished by reacting the serum to be tested with a suspension of known A_1 cells and known B cells. A_1 cells are used in reverse grouping because they have the greatest quantity of A antigen on their surface. The testing is performed at room temperature and consists of mixing two drops of the serum to be tested with a drop of the known cell suspension (2% to 5% suspension of reagent cells). As stated previously, almost all normal, healthy people older than 3 months have detectable ABO antibodies in their serum to the ABH antigens that they lack. Table 9-2 gives common reactions found in reverse grouping of the four major blood groups. Detection and proper identification of these antibodies are essential if proper ABO typing is to be performed. In all cases, the reverse grouping must match the forward grouping. If these tests do not agree, a cell–serum group discrepancy exists. See section "Discrepancies in ABO Grouping" for a discussion of various causes of cell–serum group discrepancies and how they may be resolved.

Molecular Testing

In recent years, molecular testing has become more prevalent. This is discussed in detail in Chapter 7.

ABH SYSTEM IN DISEASE

Many disease states may lead to an alteration in the ABH antigens on the RBC surface or the antibody found in a subject's serum. Sometimes, the changes are real, as in the progressive decrease in antigen strength in some patients suffering from leukemia. The loss of antigen in this case seems to correlate with the severity of the disease.

Other diseases, such as carcinoma of the stomach, may result in an apparent reduction in antigenic strength. Patients suffering from carcinoma of the stomach may produce excess blood group–specific soluble substances (BGSS), which may partially or completely neutralize the reagent antisera used for ABO testing. In this case, the loss of antigenic strength is only apparent, and sufficient washing of the subject's RBCs before testing to remove all BGSS results in proper typing.

Other diseases may affect the level of antibody present in the patient's serum. Diseases that are caused by, or may lead to, alterations in the immune system should be suspected when the patient fails to react properly in the reverse grouping. Examples of diseases that may alter the level of antibody to ABO antigens include diseases resulting in hypogammaglobulinemia, such as chronic lymphocytic leukemia and non-Hodgkin lymphoma.

SECRETOR STATUS

As stated previously in this chapter, the presence of ABH antigens in the secretions of some people allowed for the relatively straightforward biochemical characterization of the ABH antigens. Although inherited separately, the gene that controls the presence of the ABH antigens in these secretions is called *Se*. *Se* is dominant over its allele *se*. The presence of *Se*, in single (*Sese*) or double (*SeSe*) dose, results in the presence of the H antigen in secretions. Box 9-2 lists the fluids that may contain ABH-soluble substances. Approximately 78% of random adults in the United Sates have the secretor gene and are said to be secretors. The remainder (22%) inherit a double dose of the *se* gene (*sese*) and are said to be nonsecretors. Although important to the ABO system, the secretor status is even more important to the discussion of the Lewis system. Table 9-6 gives the concentrations of various ABH antigens in saliva of secretors and nonsecretors.

The secretor gene controls only the presence or absence of the H substance (i.e., the L-fucosyltransferase)

BOX 9-2

Fluids Containing ABH-soluble Substances

- Saliva
- Urine
- Tears
- Bile
- Amniotic fluid
- Milk
- Exudative fluids
- Digestive fluids

Table 9-6   ABH Antigens in Saliva

	ABO Group	Concentration of Antigens in the Saliva		
		A	B	H
Secretors	O	Absent	Absent	Present
Secretors	A	Present	Absent	Present (small amounts)
Secretors	B	Absent	Present	Present (small amounts)
Secretors	AB	Present	Present	Present (small amounts)
Nonsecretors	A, B, O, AB	Absent	Absent	Absent

in body secretions. It does not affect the presence of the H substance on erythrocytes.

The presence of the A and B transferases on erythrocytes is not controlled by the secretor gene. If a person is a secretor and independently inherits the A or B transferase, these transferases result in an altering of the H substance in secretions and on the surface of the erythrocytes, resulting in ABH antigens in the secretions as well. The conversion of H substance is incomplete because it is on the RBC surface. Some residual H antigen remains in the secretions regardless of the presence of the A or B transferases.

Test procedures for detection of the presence of A, B, and H antigens in secretions are found in the Procedural Appendices to this chapter.

Presence of the H substance on the surface of RBCs is controlled by another hypothetical gene combination (Zz) inherited at a locus different from ABO, $Sese$, and Hh. Failure to inherit at least one Z gene is extremely rare.

SUBGROUPS OF A

Within a decade of the discovery of the ABO system, the first subgroup of A was discovered. Subgroups of A are phenotypes that differ quantitatively or qualitatively from the A antigen carried on the RBCs and found in the saliva of secretors. A_1 and A_2, the two major subgroups of A, constitute 99% or more of group A people tested. They both react strongly with reagent anti-A when routine testing protocols are followed. Most blood group A people are now classified as A_1 (80%), whereas approximately 20% of group A people are classified as A_2. The frequency of A_2 versus A_1 differs somewhat depending on the race (gene pool) of the population. Reagent anti-A is apparently a mixture of two antibodies. The anti-A or anti-A_{common} reacts with A_1 and A_2 cells, and anti-A_1 reacts with A_1 cells but not A_2 cells in simple testing. These two antibodies can be separated functionally by adsorption with A_2 cells.

The antigen of these two common subgroups of A appears to be qualitatively and quantitatively different. Qualitative differences are known to exist because 1% to 8% of A_2 people and 22% to 35% of A_2B people produce a readily identifiable anti-A_1 in their serum. Therefore, there are subtle qualitative differences between A_1 and A_2 antigens because the immune systems of these people fail to recognize the A_1 antigen as self, and these people make an antibody that reacts preferentially with A_1 cells and does not react with self. Anti-A_1 is usually nonreactive at body temperature and therefore is considered clinically insignificant. The differences in the transferases have been demonstrated by Yamamoto et al. However, it should be noted that an example of anti-A_1 reactive at 37°C is clinically significant and should be handled with utmost care. The antibody is predominantly IgM and may lead to in vivo RBC destruction.

Quantitative differences in the antigen of these subgroups are more readily identified. It is clear that A_2 cells carry approximately 25% as many A antigen sites as A_1 cells. Further study of A_2 people has also demonstrated a quantitative difference (reduction) in the amount of N-acetylgalactosaminyltransferase. Thus, it is not surprising that A_2 people have more residual H antigen on the surface of their RBCs than do A_1 people.

A plant lectin prepared from *D. biflorus* serves as the preferred reagent for differentiating A_1 and A_2 cells. The plant product, when properly diluted, may be used to separate these two subgroups. The reagent agglutinates A_1 cells and A_1B cells but not A_2 and A_2B cells.

Subgroups of A weaker than A_2 are rare and usually are not of great importance in clinical populations. However, weak subgroups occurring in donor populations may cause major problems when they are not properly identified. A failure to properly classify a weak subgroup of A may lead the donor to be classified as a group O and to be used to transfuse a group O patient. For this reason, although it is not usually recommended that anti-A,B be used for patient testing, it is mandatory that all group O donors be tested

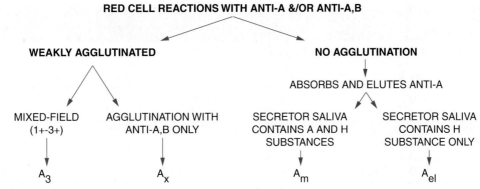

FIGURE 9-7   Investigation of A subgroups.

with anti-A,B to confirm that they are not actually weak subgroups of A.

The reason for this special caution is that all group O people have in their serum anti-A,B, which is the most potent antibody capable of reacting with the weaker subgroups of A. Failure to detect a weak subgroup of A or B in a patient population usually causes few if any problems. If the people fail to demonstrate a cell–serum group discrepancy, they would be transfused with RBCs as if to disregard the presence of the weak A or B antigen. The weaker examples of the A or B antigen also are unlikely to lead to significant hemolysis if transfused with incompatible plasma because the plasma will be diluted with existing patient blood volume (e.g., a weak subgroup of A transfused with group O plasma).

RBCs of the A_{int}, A_3, A_x, A_m, or A_{el} subgroups are rarely seen in transfusion practice. Classification of the subgroups of A depends on several different testing procedures. Correct classification of the subgroups of A depends on patterns of reactivity with anti-A, A_1 lectin, anti-A,B, and H lectin, as well as the presence or absence of anti-A_1 in the subject's serum and the presence of A or H antigens in the saliva of secretors. Box 9-3 lists the

---

BOX 9-3

Methods of Classification of the Subgroups of A

- Agglutination pattern with anti-A and anti-A_1
- Agglutination pattern with anti-A,B
- Agglutination pattern with *Ulex europaeus* (H lectin)
- Presence or absence of anti-A_1 in the patient's serum, resulting in ABO discrepancy
- Presence or absence of A and H substances in the saliva of secretors

---

procedures used in the classification of the subgroups of A, and Figure 9-7 demonstrates a flow chart that may be used systematically to classify these subgroups. Table 9-7 gives the reactions expected with suggested testing.

SUBGROUPS OF B

The subgroups of B are even more infrequent than the weaker subgroups of A. They are initially identified by variability of reaction with anti-B and anti-A,B. The subgroups B_3, B_x, B_m, and B_{el} are classified similarly to their counterparts in the classification of the A subgroups. See Table 9-7 for representative reactions of these weak subgroups of B.

DISCREPANCIES IN ABO GROUPING

The importance of ABO blood grouping is underscored by the fact that all ABO blood grouping, with the exception of newborns, consists of both a cell grouping and a serum grouping. In most cases, the interpretation of these two tests supports a common conclusion, and the ABO group is confirmed. In some instances, cell grouping and serum grouping tests result in different interpretations of the ABO type of the patient. In these cases, a cell–serum group discrepancy exists. All discrepancies between cell and serum grouping must be resolved before a definitive type can be assigned to the patient. Discrepancies can be grouped according to their probable causes to facilitate resolution of the discrepancy. Common causes of discrepancy are discussed in the following sections.

Technical Errors

Technical errors leading to *ABO discrepancy* are common in student laboratories and may occur more

TABLE 9-7   Results of Testing that May Be Used for Subgrouping of A and B

| Type | Reaction of Subject Red Blood Cells with | | | | NRSC Antibodies | | Antigen in Secretions | Presence of A/B Transferases |
	Anti-A	Anti-B	Anti-A,B	Anti-H	Common	Other		
A₁	4+	0	4+	0	Anti-B		A, H	A
A₂	3 to 4+	0	3 to 4+	2 to 3+	Anti-B	Anti-A₁	A, H	A
A₃	2 + mf	0	2 + mf	3+	Anti-B	Anti-A₁	A, H	Weak A
Aₓ	Weak/0	0	1 to 2+	4+	Anti-B	Anti-A₁	H	Very weak A
A_end	Weak mf	0	Weak mf	4+	Anti-B	Anti-A₁	H	No A
Aₘ	0	0	0	4+	Anti-B		A, H	Weak A
A_el	0	0	0	4+	Anti-B	Possible anti-A₁	H	No A
B	0	4+	4+	2+	Anti-A		B, H	B
B₃	0	2 + mf	2 + mf	3+	Anti-A		B, H	Weak B
Bₓ	0	Weak/0	Weak/1+	3+	Anti-A	Weak Anti-B	H	No B
Bₘ	0	0	0	3 to 4+	Anti-A		B, H	Weak B
B_el	0	0	0	3 to 4+	Anti-A	May be weak anti-B	H	No B

NRCS, non–red cell stimulated.

frequently than they should in the clinical laboratory. The best defense against technical errors is a well-written and meticulously followed testing protocol and attention to detail. Common errors that may lead to ABO discrepancies are listed in Box 9-4. The best way to prevent these errors is to follow the testing procedure exactly, and the first step in resolving a discrepancy is to repeat the testing procedure to ensure it was followed.

Weak or Missing Antibodies

The most frequent ABO discrepancy is due to weak or missing antibodies. ABH antibodies have been traditionally reported as being in highest titer during adolescence and gradually weakening with age. It has been demonstrated repeatedly that reduction in titer of ABH antibodies does not come necessarily with age but with poor health and nutritional status. The very young and the very sick or debilitated may demonstrate such a low titer of ABH antibodies that routine testing may not detect them (Box 9-5). Other patients may show a depression of the normal levels

BOX 9-4

Errors that May Cause ABO Discrepancies

Clerical errors
- Improper identification of patient sample/testing
- Improper recording of reactions

Technical errors
- Failure to follow manufacturer's directions
- Contaminated or expired reagents
- Improper concentration of subject red blood cells
- Failure to add reagents/sample or improper amounts
- Improper centrifugation
- Warming of test

of ABH antibodies due to disease or iatrogenic causes.

This discrepancy may best be resolved by optimizing the reverse grouping reaction. Although routine serum grouping is performed at room

Patients Who May Express ABO Discrepancy Due to Weak or Missing Isoagglutinins

- Neonatal patients
- Elderly patients
- Patients with hypogammaglobulinemia
- Immunosuppressed patients (drug/disease)
- Bone marrow transplant patients

temperature, the antibodies that are detected in this procedure react best at reduced temperatures. Therefore, enhancement will occur if the testing is performed at 18°C or 4°C. However, care must be taken that other cold-reacting antibodies are not mistaken for ABH antibodies. When incubating the reverse grouping at reduced temperature, an autocontrol and group O screening cells should be included to rule out autoantibodies or alloantibodies, causing the expected pattern of agglutination. If the autocontrol and the screening cells are negative and the expected reaction occurs after incubation for 15 to 60 minutes, the discrepancy is resolved and may be attributed to weakened antibodies. An appropriate note should be included in the person's record. Table 9-8 shows an example of a discrepancy due to weak or missing isoagglutinins and the proper resolution of the discrepancy. Most discrepancies in this category may be resolved with testing under enhanced conditions. However, rare people may lack detectable ABH antibodies in their serum for a variety of reasons.

Weak or Absent Antigens

Causes of discrepancies under this classification may include the presence of subgroups of A or B and weakening of antigenic strength in leukemia, as previously mentioned. If apparent weakening of the antigen is suspected, attempts to prove the presence of the antigen with adsorption and elution may be worthwhile. Refer to the Procedural Appendices at the end of this chapter for instructions on the demonstration of weak antigens by adsorption and elution. The depression is rarely complete, and it should be possible properly to group the patient.

Unexpected Cold-reactive Autoantibodies

Panagglutination is the ability of a particular serum to agglutinate all or almost all cells in a particular population. A good example of a panagglutinin is a person whose serum contains a strong auto anti-I. This antibody agglutinates all but approximately 0.01% of the adult population because the I antigen is strongly expressed in almost all adults. Patients with cold-reactive autoantibodies such as autoanti-I may demonstrate ABO discrepancies. Patients with high titers (>126) of cold agglutinins may have cells that autoagglutinate at room temperature. The cooler the testing temperature, the greater the likelihood that a patient with cold autoagglutinins will have an ABO discrepancy. High-titered cold autoagglutinins also may interfere with reverse grouping if the reagent cells have the appropriate antigens on their surface. Refer to Table 9-9 for an example of ABO discrepancy due to cold-reactive autoantibodies.

The resolution of discrepancies due to cold-reactive autoantibodies may be difficult without first obtaining a new specimen. Two problems exist. As the person's sample is allowed to cool after drawing, the cells become sensitized or coated with IgM antibody. This antibody may cause autoagglutination and not only interfere with blood bank testing, but may cause the RBCs to clump together, interfering with the counting and sizing necessary for automated hematologic testing. Prewarming the specimen tube and keeping it at 37°C prevents the autoantibody from attaching to the person's RBCs in vitro. The patient's cells should be washed with 37°C saline three or more times before being used for testing to remove any previously

TABLE 9-8	Example of ABO Discrepancy Due to Weak or Missing Isoagglutinins							
	Forward Grouping Reaction of Subject RBCs with			Reverse Grouping of Subject Serum with Reagent RBCs				
	Anti-A	Anti-B	Anti-A,B	A₁ Cells	A₂ Cells	B Cells	O Cells	Auto
RT testing	4+	0	NT	0	NT	0	0	0
18/4 C^a testing	4+	0	NT	0	NT	2+	0	0

^{a}Repeat testing of subject sample at reduced temperature will enhance reaction. O cells and autotesting must be included and show no agglutination.
RBCs, red blood cells; RT, room temperature; NT, not tested.

TABLE 9-9   Example of ABO Discrepancy Due to Unexpected Cold-reactive Autoantibody

	Forward Grouping Reaction of Subject Red Blood Cells with			Reverse Grouping Reaction of Subject Serum with				
	Anti-A	Anti-B	Anti-A,B	A_1 Cells	A_2 Cells	B Cells	O Cells	Auto
RT testing	4+	2+	NT	2+	2+	4+	2+	2+
After adsorption[a]	4+	0	NT	0	0	2 to 4+	0	0

[a]Serum either autoadsorbed or adsorbed with rabbit red blood cell stroma before retesting. Subject's sample redrawn and kept at 37°C. Cells washed five times with warm saline prior to being tested.
RT, room temperature; NT, not tested.

attached warm-reactive antibodies. Reverse grouping of patients with strong cold autoantibodies may be difficult to perform. The sample may be allowed to clot and then stored at refrigeration temperatures to allow autoagglutination to occur.

Alternatively, the person's serum may be autoadsorbed or adsorbed with commercially prepared rabbit RBC stroma to remove all cold-reactive autoantibody before reverse grouping is performed. Ensuring that all reagents have come to room temperature after removal from the refrigerator can sometimes prevent this problem.

Unexpected Cold-reactive Antibodies

Unexpected cold-reactive antibodies may lead to ABO cell–serum discrepancies by causing unexpected reactions in the reverse grouping of subjects. These antibodies may be related to the ABO BGS, such as anti-A_1 in the serum of a group A_2 individual, or they may be completely unrelated to the ABO BGS. It must always be remembered that the reagent A_1 and B cells used for reverse grouping have not only A_1 and B antigen, but many other antigens. Antibodies that react at reduced temperatures (usually the IgM class) may sometimes be

present in the subject's serum and may react with the appropriate antigen on the reagent RBCs. The antibody screen performed using O reagent cells usually allows proper identification of these antibodies as being "atypical" as opposed to the typical antibody (ABO isoagglutinins) found in most subjects. Chapter 10 discusses the detection and identification of atypical antibodies. Once the specificity of the atypical antibody has been determined, examples of A_1 and B cells that lack the antigen to this atypical antibody may be selected and the discrepancy resolved. Table 9-10 gives an example of ABO discrepancy due to unexpected cold-reactive antibodies.

Rouleaux

Abnormal levels of proteins, plasma expanders such as Dextran, and Wharton jelly (coating cord tissue of the fetus) can cause RBCs to stick together in a manner that may resemble agglutination. This false agglutination, or rouleaux, may result in an ABO discrepancy. The most common cause of this type of discrepancy is due to elevated protein levels, as might be seen in multiple myeloma, Waldenstrom macroglobulinemia, and other plasma cell dyscrasias. Increased levels of protein may

TABLE 9-10   Example of ABO Discrepancy Due to Unexpected Cold-reactive Antibody

	Forward Grouping Reaction of Subject Red Blood Cells with			Reverse Grouping Reaction of Subject Serum with				
	Anti-A	Anti-B	Anti-A,B	A_1 Cells	A_2 Cells	B Cells	O Cells	Auto
Example 1: RT testing[a]	4+	0	NT	2+	2+	4+	2+	0
Example 2: RT testing[b]	4+	0	NT	2+	0	4+	0	0

[a]Subject shows evidence of atypical antibody. Antibody identification should be performed.
[b]Subject has probable anti-A_1. Subject's cells should be tested with A_1 lectin, and subject's serum should be tested against a panel of at least three different A_1 and A_2 cells. Subject cells should be negative with lectin and should react only with the A_1 cells on the panel.
RT, room temperature; NT, not tested.

TABLE 9-11   Example of ABO Discrepancy Due to Rouleaux

	Forward Grouping Reaction of Subject Red Blood Cells with			Reverse Grouping Reaction of Subject Serum with				
	Anti-A	Anti-B	Anti-A,B	A_1 Cells	A_2 Cells	B Cells	O Cells	Auto
RT testing saline tube	4+	2+	NT	2+	2+	4+	2+	2+
Replacement testing[a]	4+	0	NT	0	0	4+	0	0

[a]Subject demonstrates loose 2+ reactions that when examined under the microscope appear as "stacks of coins." Saline tube replacement can be used to disperse the rouleaux and yield results indicated. In this procedure, the testing is performed as usual, but before resuspending the cell button, all sera are removed with a piper and gently replaced with two drops of saline. The test is then examined for agglutination.
NT, not tested; RT, room temperature.

interfere in cell grouping, serum grouping, or both. Interference in cell grouping tests may be overcome by multiple washing of the cells to be tested so that all nonattached protein is removed. Interference with serum grouping is more difficult to deal with and may be overcome by the saline tube replacement technique. See Table 9-11 for an example of this type of discrepancy.

Miscellaneous

Miscellaneous causes of ABO discrepancy include interferences caused by alterations in normal subject blood samples such as increased BGSS, *acquired B* phenomenon, antibodies to low-incidence antigens present in reagent antisera, and polyagglutination. Problems related to increases in BGSS due to carcinoma of the stomach and pancreas were noted previously. Adequate washing of a person's RBCs before testing alleviates this cause of ABO discrepancy.

Acquired B phenomenon may result from intestinal obstruction, carcinoma of the colon or rectum, or any disorder of the gastrointestinal tract that may lead to obstruction or slowing of intestinal movement, sufficient to allow passage of intestinal bacteria through the intestinal wall and into the bloodstream. Acquired B may result from alteration of A antigen in group A people by bacterial enzymes or by adsorption of a B-like antigen from bacteria, such as may occur in group A or group O patients. In the latter case, bacterial polysaccharide from *Proteus vulgaris* and *Escherichia coli* O_{86} may be adsorbed onto the cell surface and result in alteration of group A to apparent group AB and group O to group B. The result is a person who carries the antibody to an apparent antigen he or she carries on the RBCs but fails to agglutinate his or her own cells. Proof of the nature of the acquired antigen may lie in the testing of secretors for the presence of the antigen in secretions.

Occasionally, a human or animal source reagent serum, although exhaustively tested by the manufacturer, will demonstrate an antibody to a private antigen (one carried by the RBCs of only a few people). When used to group the RBCs of those people carrying the private antigen, the serum reacts positive. This may lead the technologist to believe that he or she is witnessing the reaction of the antibody named in the reagent (e.g., anti-A) with the A antigen on the surface of the cells, rather than the actual interaction of a private antigen. This discrepancy may be resolved by testing the patient with more than one manufacturer's reagent antiserum. The likelihood of two manufacturers' sera containing the same antibody to a private antigen is extremely remote.

Polyagglutination is the spontaneous agglutination of RBCs by all or almost all normal human sera. There are several causes of polyagglutination. The first type to be discovered was due to T activation. Bird showed that a plant lectin made from the peanut, *Arachis hypogaea*, was able to detect an antigen on the surface of the RBCs of rare people who seemed to develop an antigen labeled T on the surface of their RBCs.[5] Further work led to the discovery that a number of lectins could be used to differentiate polyagglutinable cells (Table 9-12). People may sometimes suffer from T activation without pathologic causes, whereas in others the change seems to indicate some potentially serious latent disease. T activation occurs when a portion of the normal RBC membrane is cleaved enzymatically to expose a previously unexposed antigen. This may occur in vivo or in vitro. Once it is exposed, the T antigen is free to react with the IgM anti-T that is normally present in the serum of most normal adults. People who have in vivo T activation do not usually demonstrate anti-T in their serum and thus have a negative autocontrol. T activation in vivo is a transient condition caused by exposure to bacterial enzymes. Once the cause of the exposure is eliminated, the cell will no longer be activated. Organisms noted as a cause of T activation include *E. coli*

TABLE 9-12	Reactions of Polyagglutinable Cells with Various Lectins			
	T	Tn	Tk	Cad
ABO-compatible adult human serum	+	+	+	+
Arachis hypogaea	+	0	+	0
Salvia sclarea	0	+	0	0
Salvia horminum	0	+	0	+
Glycine soja	+	+	0	+
Dolichos biflorus	0	+	0	+

and *Vibrio cholerae* as well as other bacteria and viruses.

Testing with cord serum may allow proper typing of the subject because newborns have not formed the anti-T antibody, anti-A, or anti-B in the cord serum (in appropriate samples) therefore may detect the A or B antigen on the surface of T-activated RBCs without anti-T interfering. In addition, testing the person with a panel of lectins useful in identification of suspected polyagglutination may be helpful.

A similar situation results in the exposure of a different antigen, Tk. Tk activation results from similar causes and reacts in a similar manner to T activation. Also, like T activation, Tk activation is transient.

Another type of polyagglutination is a result of unknown causes and may occur much less frequently. This polyagglutination is permanent and results in Tn activation. It has not been simulated in vitro. However, Tn is destroyed by enzyme, and thus enzyme-treated cells may be used for further testing. Tn activation results in cells that react in a mixed-field pattern and fail to react with the lectin from *A. hypogaea*. Bird and Wingham showed that when properly diluted, a lectin from the plant *Salvia sclarea* had specificity for Tn.[6]

Finally, there are several forms of inherited polyagglutination. The first is that resulting from the presence of the antigen Cad. The Cad antigen (Sd[a]) is present in variable amounts in most people. Some people express an extremely large amount of Cad antigen and react with the sera of most normal people, which contain a small amount of Cad autoantibody.

Hereditary erythroblastic multinuclearity with a positive acidified serum test is a form of chronic dyserythropoietic anemia. It results in increased susceptibility to agglutination and complement destruction by the small amount of cold agglutinins found in most normal sera.

SUMMARY

Although the ABO BGS may seem complex, the level of knowledge required for routine testing is fundamental. The student of immunohematology should be aware of the complex interaction of genes and rare causes of discrepancies that may lead to problems in grouping patients. However, the fundamental principles of ABO grouping are simple and straightforward. Once committed to memory, these simple principles, along with following proper protocols for testing, will suffice in most instances. If the world of immunohematology were a book, then the ABO system would be only the first chapter. Although the study of many other BGSs follows, no other system is more important to the routine practice of blood banking.

Review Questions

1. The H antigen is found in highest concentration on what type of red blood cell?
   a. group A
   b. group B
   c. group AB
   d. group O

2. The lectin used for detection of the H antigen is called:
   a. *Arachis hypogaea*
   b. *Dolichos biflorus*
   c. *Ulex europaeus*
   d. *Salvia sclarea*

(continued)

REVIEW QUESTIONS (continued)

3. Common sources of ABO discrepancies due to technical error include all the following except:
   a. clerical mix-ups
   b. contaminated reagents
   c. warming of the test
   d. patients with agammaglobulinemia

4. An individual must inherit which of the following to be classified as a group AB?
   a. the *A* gene
   b. the *B* gene
   c. the *H* gene
   d. answers a and b
   e. answers a, b, and c.

5. The immunodominant sugar associated with the A antigen is:
   a. L-fucose
   b. *N*-acetylgalactosamine
   c. D-galactose
   d. D-glucose

6. The gene that controls the presence or absence of the H substance in body secretions is the:
   a. *H* gene
   b. *Se* gene
   c. *h* gene
   d. *B* gene

7. Group A_2 constitutes approximately what percentage of group A individuals?
   a. 2%
   b. 20%
   c. 40%
   d. 60%
   e. 80%

8. Approximately what percentage of A_2 individuals have evidence of anti-A_1 in the sera?
   a. none
   b. 1% to 8%
   c. 13% to 18%
   d. 50% or more

9. The antibody normally found in the serum of group B individuals is:
   a. anti-A
   b. anti-B
   c. anti-H
   d. anti-A,B

10. Approximately what percentage of adult levels of A and B antigen are present at birth?
    a. 10%
    b. 25%
    c. 50%
    d. 100%

11. Fetal development of ABO antigens begins in the:
    a. first week of fetal life
    b. second week of fetal life
    c. sixth week of fetal life
    d. second trimester

12. ABO grouping discrepancies may occur due to which of the following causes?
    a. rouleaux
    b. clerical error
    c. atypical antibody
    d. all of the above

REFERENCES

1. Issitt PD. *Applied Blood Group Serology.* 3rd ed. Miami: Montgomery Scientific; 1985.
2. Mollison PL, Englefreit CP, Contreras M. *Blood Transfusion in Clinical Medicine.* 8th ed. Oxford: Blackwell Scientific Publications; 1988.
3. Yamamoto F, Clausen H, White T, et al. Molecular genetic basis of the histo-blood group ABO system. *Nature.* 1990; 345: 229–233.
4. Yamamoto F, McNeill PD, Kominato Y, et al. Molecular genetic analysis of the ABO blood group system: 2, *cis*-AB alleles. *Vox Sang.* 1993; 64: 120–123.
5. Bird GWG. Anti-T in peanuts. *Vox Sang.* 1964; 9: 748.
6. Bird GWG, Wingham J. Haemagglutinins from *Salvia.* *Vox Sang.* 1974; 26: 163.

PROCEDURAL APPENDIX I

ROUTINE ABO GROUPING

Slide Testing

Principle

Anti-A, anti-B, and anti-A,B are prepared from the sera of appropriate people who lack other atypical antibodies. These reagents are used to test for the presence of the A and B antigens on the surface of erythrocytes. The test is routinely performed at room temperature and must not be heated. The manufacturer's directions always must be meticulously followed. Some manufacturers specify the use of whole blood, whereas others specify differing concentrations of RBCs in saline or in autologous serum or plasma.

1. Place one drop of each reagent to be tested (anti-A, anti-B, and, when appropriate, anti-A,B) on a clean glass slide or tile allowing approximately a 20 × 40 mm area for each test. A wax pencil or other method may be used to ensure that the reagents do not become inappropriately mixed together.
2. To each drop of reagent from step 1, add one drop of a well-mixed suspension of RBCs (in saline, autologous serum, or plasma and in a concentration recommended by the reagent manufacturer).
3. Mix the reagents and RBC suspensions thoroughly using a clean wooden applicator stick while spreading the mixture over an area approximately 20 × 40 mm.
4. Gently tilt the slide back and forth for 2 minutes while observing for agglutination. Read and record the results.

Interpretation

Agglutination in the presence of specific reagents indicates the presence of the appropriate antigen on the RBC surface. Lack of agglutination indicates a lack of the appropriate antigen and thus a negative result.

Tube Testing

Tube testing may be used for forward and reverse grouping of RBCs. The manufacturer's directions must be followed at all times.

Forward Grouping

1. Place one drop of the appropriate reagent (anti-A, anti-B, or anti-A,B) in a clean and appropriately labeled 10 × 75-mm or 12 × 75-mm glass test tube.
2. Add one drop of a 2% to 5% suspension of RBCs to be tested (in saline, serum, or plasma) to each tube. Alternatively, an equivalent number of RBCs may be transferred from a whole-blood sample with a wooden applicator stick.
3. Mix the reagent and RBCs, and centrifuge at 100g for 15 to 20 seconds.
4. Gently resuspend the RBC buttons while observing for agglutination and record results.

Interpretation

Agglutination with appropriate reagents indicates the presence of that antigen on the surface of the RBCs tested.

Reverse Grouping

Reverse grouping is performed to confirm the presence of expected naturally occurring antibodies in the serum or plasma. Reagent RBCs demonstrating the strongest antigenic makeup for A and B are used (A_1 and B cells).

1. Place two drops of the serum or plasma to be tested in each of two appropriately labeled tubes (A_1 cells and B cells).
2. Place one drop of reagent A_1 cells in the tube marked "A_1 cells" and one drop of reagent B cells in the tube marked "B cells."
3. Mix thoroughly and centrifuge at 1000g for 15 to 20 seconds.
4. Gently resuspend the RBCs while observing for agglutination, and record results.

Interpretation

Agglutination with the appropriate reagent RBC suspension demonstrates the presence of the appropriate antibody in the serum or plasma tested.

PROCEDURAL APPENDIX II

SECRETOR STUDY

ABH Antigens in Secretion

Principle

Approximately 78% of people (those who inherit at least one *Se* gene) are capable of secreting H substance in their body secretions. If they also inherit *A* or *B* genes, the transferases in their secretions will result in the conversion of this H substance to A or B antigen. The presence of H, A, or B antigens in secretions may be demonstrated by testing the saliva of an individual with agglutination inhibition testing. The saliva is collected, heat inactivated, and used to attempt to neutralize weak reacting antiserum. Neutralization of this antiserum by soluble ABH substances results in complete inhibition of agglutination, resulting from the mixing of the antisera with appropriate RBCs.

Collection of Saliva

1. Collect approximately 10 mL of saliva and place it in an appropriately labeled test tube. To encourage salivation, the subject may be given a small amount of paraffin to chew.
2. Place the test tube in a boiling water bath for 10 minutes to inactivate innate salivary enzyme activity, which may interfere with subsequent testing.
3. Centrifuge the heat-inactivated saliva for 10 minutes at high speed, and remove the clear supernatant. Save the supernatant for further testing.
4. If the test is not to be completed immediately, refrigerate until testing is completed later that day. Alternatively, the sample may be stored frozen until needed.

Dilution of Antisera to be Tested

1. Prepare doubling dilutions of the antisera to be tested.
2. Combine one drop of the diluted antiserum with one drop of a 2% to 5% suspension of appropriate RBCs (A cells when testing for A substance, B cells when testing for B substance, and O cells when testing for H substance).
3. Centrifuge at $1,000g$ for 15 to 20 seconds.
4. Gently resuspend and observe for agglutination. Select for further testing the dilution that gives a 2+ agglutination.

Testing of Neutralized Saliva

1. Add one drop of the appropriately diluted antiserum (see step 4) to an appropriately labeled tube. Repeat for each soluble antigen that you wish to test. A saline control tube also should be used.
2. Add one drop of saliva to each tube from step 1. Allow the tubes to incubate at room temperature for at least 10 minutes.
3. Add one drop of a 2% to 5% saline suspension of appropriate indicator cells to each tube, mix, and incubate for 60 minutes at room temperature.
4. Centrifuge at $1,000g$ for 15 to 20 seconds.
5. Gently resuspend the cells, observe for agglutination, and record the results.

Interpretation

See Table 9-8 for aid in interpretation of saliva testing.

ABSORPTION AND ELUTION TESTS FOR WEAK ANTIGENS

Principle

Erythrocytes having weak A or B antigens may not be directly agglutinated by anti-A, anti-B, or anti-A,B in routine forward grouping tests. However, the presence of A or B antigens on the erythrocyte surface can be proven by the adsorption and subsequent elution of one or more of these antibodies.

1. Wash 1 mL of the RBCs to be tested at least three times with a large volume of saline. Remove the supernatant from the last wash, and save for a control.
2. Add an equal volume (1 mL) of appropriate reagent (anti-A, anti-B, or anti-A,B).
3. Mix the RBCs and antiserum, and incubate for 1 hour at 4°C.
4. Centrifuge the mixture for 10 minutes at 1,000g to ensure that the RBCs and antiserum are well separated.
5. Remove the antiserum and discard. Wash the RBCs at least five times with large volumes of saline (at least 10 × RBC volume). Save an aliquot of the final wash, and label as a control.
6. Add an equal volume of saline or 6% albumin to the washed, packed RBCs and mix well.
7. Elute the adsorbed antibody (if any) by placing the tube in a 56°C water bath for 10 minutes.
8. Mix the sample several times during the elution procedure.
9. Centrifuge the eluate at 1,000g for 10 minutes to pack the RBCs and separate the saline or 6% albumin containing any eluted antibody. Remove the supernatant, and discard the RBCs and RBC stroma. The supernatant (eluate) will be cherry red because of the amount of RBC hemolysis that has occurred.
10. Test the eluate and final wash (control) from step 5 with at least three examples of group O, group A, and group B RBCs by placing two drops of the eluate or control in an appropriately labeled tube, along with one drop of a 2% to 5% saline suspension of the RBCs to be tested.
11. Test the eluate and control at 4°C, 37°C, and in the AHG phase.

Interpretation

The final wash (control) sample should show no agglutination at any phase of testing, indicating that no antibody remained in the supernatant of the final wash. Agglutination of group A cells would indicate that there is a weakened form of the A antigen on the surface of the RBCs tested. Agglutination of group B cells would indicate that there is a weakened form of the B antigen on the surface of the RBCs tested. It is important that no reactivity be demonstrated against group O cells. Reactivity with O cells would indicate the presence of an atypical antibody that would not support the determination of a weak subgroup of A or B.

THE Rh BLOOD GROUP SYSTEM

CONNIE WESTHOFF

OBJECTIVES

After completion of this chapter, the reader will be able to:

1. Describe the Rh system antigens, including:
   a. The alleles inherited at each locus.
   b. The causes of weak D and partial D expression.
   c. Variations in C and e antigen expression.
   d. Compound antigens.
   e. How to determine an individual's most probable genotype.
2. Discuss causes of the Rh$_{null}$ phenotype.
3. Describe Rh system antibody reactivity and characteristics.
4. Discuss the administration of Rh immune globulin.
5. Describe the reagents used in Rh typing and the appropriate controls.
6. List causes of discrepancies in Rh typing.

KEY WORDS

Compound antigen	Rh haplotype
Deleted or partially deleted phenotype	Rh immune globulin
	Rh negative
Fisher and Race	Rh positive
G antigen	Rh$_{null}$
ISBI	Weak D
Partial D	Wiener terminology

The Rh blood group system is one of the most polymorphic and antigenic blood group systems. It is second only to ABO in importance in blood transfusion and is well known as a primary cause of hemolytic disease of the fetus and newborn (HDFN). The principal antigen is D, and the terms *Rh positive* and *Rh negative* refer to the presence or absence of D antigen. Caucasians of European extraction have the highest incidence of the Rh-negative phenotype (15% to 17%), and Rh-negative type is much less common in Africa (5%) and Australia and is considered a rare blood type not routinely tested for in some parts of Asia (<1%). Other common Rh antigens include the antithetical C and c, and E and e antigens. Patients are not routinely typed for these unless they have developed atypical antibodies or are facing long-term transfusion support for diseases such as myelodysplasia or sickle cell disease (SCD). In addition to the five principal antigens (D, C, c, E, and e), more than 50 other Rh system antigens are known. Because they are not often encountered in the routine blood bank, they will not be covered here in detail. References at the end of the chapter provide further information for interested readers.

GENES

Two genes *RHD* and *RHCE* encode the Rh proteins: one encodes the D antigen and the other encodes CE antigens in various combinations (ce, cE, Ce, or CE)

(Fig. 10-1). The RhD and RhCE proteins encoded by the two genes differ by 32 to 35 amino acids. This contrasts with most blood group system antigens that are encoded by single genes, with alleles that differ by only one or a few amino acids. Most D-negative (Rh-negative) phenotypes are the result of complete deletion of the *RHD* gene. The large number of amino acid differences between RhD and RhCE proteins explains why RhD is so antigenic when encountered by the immune system of someone who is Rh negative and has only RhCE.

The *RHCE* gene encodes C and c antigens, which differ by four amino acids: Cys16Trp (cysteine at residue 16 replaced by tryptophan) encoded by exon 1, and Ile60Leu, Ser68Asn, and Ser103Pro encoded in exon 2. E and e differ by one amino acid, Pro226Ala encoded in exon 5 (Fig. 10-1).

NOMENCLATURE

The Rh system was discovered in the 1940s, and several terminologies developed over the years. These reflected differences in thinking regarding the inheritance of the antigens. *Fisher and Race* believed that the Rh system consisted of three closely linked genes or alleles: D at one locus, C or c at the second, and E or e at the third, as reflected in the DCE terminology (Table 10-1). This terminology is used most often in written discussions of the Rh system antigens. The *Wiener terminology* was based on the belief that the Rh antigens were the products of a single gene coding for an "agglutinogen" composed of multiple "blood factors." The names given to each of the five major Rh antigens were Rh0, rh′, rh″, hr′, and hr″, but the original Wiener terminology is obsolete. A modified

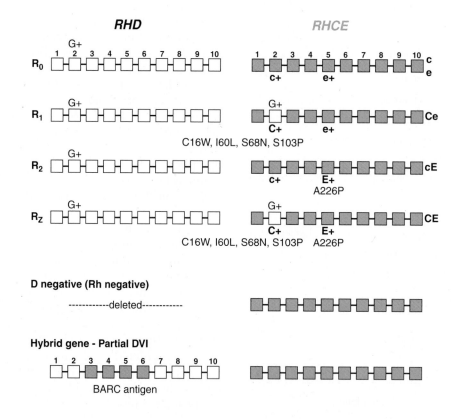

FIGURE 10-1 RH genes. Diagram of the *RHD* and *RHCE* genes indicating the changes associated with the common antigen polymorphisms, the haplotypes (R_0, etc.), and an example of a hybrid gene encoding partial DVI. The 10 coding exons of the *RHD* gene are shown as *white boxes* and the 10 exons of *RHCE* are shown as *red boxes*. The amino acid changes associated with the common antigens are indicated by single-letter designations and the position in the protein. For example, an E+ RBC phenotype results when alanine (A) at amino acid position 226 is changed to proline (P), which is encoded in exon 5 of RHCE. The c+ versus C+ phenotype is associated with changes also encoded by *RHD* (*white box*). The shared exon 2 of *RHD* and *RHCE* explains the expression of G antigen (G+) on RhCe and RhD proteins. Most Rh negatives (D negatives) are due to deletion of the *RHD* gene. Example of one of the gene rearrangements between *RHD* and *RHCE* that results in a partial D phenotype, as well as a new Rh antigen, BARC.

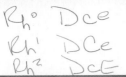

TABLE 10-1 Rh Nomenclature and Incidence of Common Haplotypes

Fisher-Race Haplotype	Modified Wiener Haplotype	Incidence (%) Caucasian	African Black	Asian
Rh positive				
Dce	R_1	42	17	70
DcE	R_2	14	11	21
Dce	R_0	4	44	3
DCE	R_z	<0.01	<0.01	1
Rh negative				
ce	r	37	26	3
Ce	r'	2	2	2
cE	r"	1	<0.01	<0.01
CE	r^y	<0.01	<0.01	<0.01

version (Table 10-1) is useful in spoken language to convey the **Rh haplotype**. Uppercase R is used to describe haplotypes that produce D antigen, and lowercase r (or little r) is used when D is absent. The C or c and E or e Rh antigens carried with D are represented by 1 for Ce (R_1), 2 for cE (R_2), 0 for ce (R_0), and z for CE (R_z) (Table 10-1). The symbols prime (′) and double prime (″) are used with r to designate the CcEe antigens; for example, "prime" is used for Ce (r′), "double prime" for cE (r″), and "y" for CE (r^y). The R versus r terminology allows one to convey the common Rh antigens present on one chromosome in a single term (a phenotype). Dashes are used to represent missing antigens of the rare deletion (or CE-depleted) phenotypes; for example, D– – (referred to as D dash, dash) lacks C/c and E/e antigens.

International Society of Blood Transfusion (ISBT) terminology assigns each antigen a number. For example, D is Rh1, C is Rh2, E is Rh3, c is Rh4, and e is Rh5, and so on. The presence or absence of each antigen on the red blood cell (RBC) is noted by the designation Rh:1 for the presence of D and Rh:−1 for the absence of D, and so forth. An RBC that is nonreactive for D, C, and E, but positive for c and e would be designated as Rh:−1, −2, −3, 4, 5. ISBT terminology is difficult for oral communication, but it is precise for manuscript and computer usage, although it has not gained widespread use.

Recent Rh terminology distinguishes between the antigens, genes, and proteins. The antigens are referred to by the letter designations, D, C, c, E, and e. The RH genes are designated by capital letters, with or without italics, and include erythroid *RHD*, *RHCE*, and *RHAG*. The alleles are designated by the gene followed by an asterisk (*); for example, alleles of the *RHCE* gene are designated *RHCE*ce*, *RHCE*Ce*, *RHCE*cE*, and so on, according to which antigens they encode. The proteins are indicated as RhD, RhCE, or according to the specific antigens they carry, Rhce, RhCe, RhcE, or RhCE.

Most Probable Genotype

Typing RBCs for the five major Rh antigens yields the RBC phenotype. The probable genotype coding for the phenotype can be deduced from gene frequency estimates. This is useful when a person is multiply transfused or when typing a father to determine the probability that a fetus may suffer from hemolytic disease when the mother has an Rh antibody. The prevalence of Rh haplotypes by ethnic group is shown in Table 10-1. Knowledge of ethnicity is important when determining the most probable genotype. As an example, if the RBCs phenotype D+C−c+E−e+ and the patient is European American, the most probable genotype would be Dce/ce (R_0r); however, if the patient is African American, Dce/Dce (R_0R_0) would be more likely because the occurrence of the R_0 haplotype is higher (44%) than that of the r haplotype (26%) in African Americans. More accurate determination of the RH genotype, specifically *RHD* zygosity, is of significance when the mother has anti-D. Serologic testing of the father's RBCs cannot determine whether they are from a homozygote (D/D) or heterozygote (D/d), as anti-D seldom shows any difference in reactivity between RBCs with a single or double dose of D antigen. *RHD* zygosity can be determined by DNA molecular testing by assaying for the presence of an *RHD* gene deletion or an inactive *RHD*, and testing is available in some specialized blood bank molecular reference laboratories.

D ANTIGEN

D antigen is very antigenic and before the routine use of **Rh immune globulin**, anti-D was the most frequently encountered unexpected and clinically significant antibody seen in pretransfusion testing. As indicated above, it represents the presence (D+) or absence (D−) of an entire RBC protein rather than a single amino acid difference (i.e., K/k, Jka/b, etc.) and is composed of many antigenic epitopes. Approximately 2% of individuals of European extraction, and even more with African ethnicity, have changes in the *RHD* gene. These encode changes in the protein, which often cause variations in the expression of D antigen and include weak D, D_{el}, and partial D phenotypes.

Weak D

Some RBCs exhibit a weaker than normal form of the D antigen, giving weaker than expected reactivity with anti-D on initial spin testing or requiring the antiglobulin phase for detection. (Formerly known as Du, that terminology is no longer recognized and should not be used.) **Weak D** antigen expression is primarily found in persons with a single *RHD* that has a mutation encoding an amino acid change. Many different *RHD* changes encode weak D. To date, these are designated types 1 through 57, but the number of different mutations found continues to grow. Importantly, types 1, 2, and 3 are more common and make up 90% of the weak D cases found in Europeans. The number of D antigen sites in RBCs with weak D varies, depending on the severity of the effect of the mutation on the level of protein expression. RBCs with very reduced D antigen numbers, such as weak D type 2, can be missed with some commercial anti-D reagents or with some test methods. This can result in D-typing discrepancies, that is, the patient could be D+ or D− at different institutions or at the same institution after changing reagent manufacturer or typing method. Investigation of D-typing discrepancies is discussed below. Some RBCs with extremely low levels of D antigen are not detected by any routine typing method or reagents. These are revealed only with adsorption–elution studies with anti-D and are designated D_{el} for elution or by molecular *RHD* genotyping. D_{el} are more often found in Asian ethnic

groups. Lastly, position effects can also influence D antigen expression. This occurs when a Ce allele is found in *trans* to *RHD* and the amount of D antigen in the membrane is reduced. Samples that exhibit this phenomenon have an R_1r' (DCe/Ce), R_0r' (Dce/Ce), or R_2r' (DcE/Ce) haplotype.

Testing for Weak D

Testing the RBCs for weak D is not required for patients, unless typing the RBCs of an infant to determine if an Rh-negative mother is a candidate for Rh immune globulin. Weak D testing is also sometimes performed on the Rh-negative mother before the delivery of the infant if the facility uses microscopic reading of the weak D test, or a rosetting test with anti-D, to detect large D+ fetal–maternal bleed after delivery. Testing for weak D in an apparent D-negative patient needing large-volume or long-term transfusion could conserve the use of D− blood supplies.

Testing for weak D is required by the *AABB Standards for Blood Banks and Transfusion Services* for donor units, and the unit must be labeled "Rh positive" if the test is positive. For AABB-accredited hospitals, the D type of units labeled "Rh negative" must be confirmed from an integrally attached segment before transfusion, but testing for weak D is not required. Discrepancies must be reported to the collecting facility and resolved before issue of blood for transfusion. As mentioned above, serologic methods do not detect some rare RBCs with very low to undetectable levels of D antigen. Blood with very weak D antigen is not as antigenic as blood with normal levels of D antigen, but donor units transfused to a patient who presents with anti-D after receiving Rh-negative blood (anti-G must be ruled out) should be reported to the donor facility so as to investigate the *RHD* status by adsorption–elution or RH genotyping.

Partial D

RBCs with **partial D** are primarily due to inheritance of hybrid genes in which portions of *RHD* are replaced by the corresponding portions of *RHCE* (Fig. 10-1). This results in loss of some D epitopes. The RBCs type as D positive, but individuals make anti-D following transfusion or pregnancy. Note, the new hybrid protein resulting from regions of RhD joined to RhCE can generate antigens; for example, DVI RBCs carry the Rh antigen called BARC (Rh52).

Clinical Significance of Weak D and Partial D

The majority of patients with weak D RBCs are unlikely to make anti-D and can receive D-positive blood. Rare weak D types (11, 15, and 21) have made anti-D, suggesting that they have altered D epitopes.

Patients with partial D RBCs are at risk for production of anti-D, and females should receive D-negative blood and be considered candidates for Rh immune globulin. Unfortunately, serologic reagents cannot distinguish some variant D antigens or differentiate weak D from partial D. RH genotyping is required.

C AND c ANTIGENS

C and c are encoded by alleles or alternative forms of the *RHCE* gene (Fig. 10-1). The C and c antigens are codominant, and if both are present, one on each chromosome, both are expressed on the RBC. The C antigen has an approximate frequency of 68% in the white population, and 80% express the c antigen. The frequency of C antigen is higher in Eastern Asia, but much lower in African Blacks. Both antigens are less immunogenic than D antigen.

Altered C and c Antigens

Other alleles inherited at the RHCE locus encode antigens that are of low frequency. C^W (Rh8) and C^X (Rh9) antigens are due to single amino acid changes most often encoded by *RHCE*Ce* and associated with an R_1 haplotype. C^W is more often seen than C^X and has an incidence of approximately 1% in the American population. The incidence of C^W explains why anti-C^W is not a rare antibody found in transfused patients in a routine blood bank. C^W and C^X are variations of the RhCe protein, and although the RBCs type as C+, some patients make antibodies with anti-C (or −Ce) specificities following transfusion. Another important example of expression of variant C antigen occurs primarily in African Blacks and hence in patients with SCD. This altered C is encoded by a hybrid *RHD-CE-D* gene and is associated with a haplotype designated (C)ce^S or r$'^S$. This haplotype encodes an altered C antigen, designated as (C) because the RBCs react more weakly than normal with most polyclonal anti-C (but are strongly reactive with commercial monoclonal anti-C reagents), and also encodes altered e antigen, designated e^S. Hence, the RBCs type as C+ and e+, but patients make anti-C, anti-e, and/or anti-Ce. These multiple and complex Rh antibody specificities are often called anti-hr^B. The RBCs of patients homozygous for (C)ce^S, or even heterozygous for (C)ce^S with a second altered Rh haplotype on the other chromosome, type as hr^B−.

E AND e ANTIGENS

E and e are encoded by alleles of the *RHCE* gene (Fig. 10-1). The E and e antigens are codominant, and in all populations e is more frequent than E.

Approximately 30% of the white population express E and 98% have the e antigen. E is a more effective immunogen than e.

Altered E and e Antigens

Altered or variant forms of the E antigen, designated EI through EIV, are rare, and their discussion is beyond the scope of this chapter. Expression of the e antigen is easily altered by other changes in the Rh proteins. For example, as many as 30% of blacks express the Rh antigens V and VS, which result from a Leu245Val amino acid change in the protein that is located close to the e antigen, Ala226. This 245Val change causes a conformation change in the protein and weakens and alters the expression of e antigen on RBCs that are V/VS positive. Although the RBCs type as e+, the patients can make allo anti-e directed to conventional e because their e antigen is altered. Expression of e antigen can be influenced by many other genetic changes in *RHCE* genes common in individuals of African ancestry. Again, although the RBCs type as e+, patients make alloantibodies with e-like specificities following transfusion. The antibodies, designated anti-hr^S, −hr^B, −RH18, and −RH34, have complex specificities and are difficult to identify serologically. The antibodies can be clinically significant, and rare blood is sometimes needed from the American Rare Donor Program (ARDP). Importantly, because of the multiple and different RH genetic backgrounds, the antibodies produced are not all serologically compatible with donors designated as hr^B− and hr^S− by serologic testing. Molecular genotyping is now being used to find compatible blood for transfusion, and molecular matching is an important tool for transfusion support in these patients.

Deleted or Partially Deleted Phenotypes

In rare cases, people may inherit inactivated, or partially inactive, *RHCE* genes that do not encode E or e and may or may not encode some level of expression of C or c. These are called *deleted or partially deleted phenotypes* and are found primarily in Caucasians whose parents may be consanguineous or distant cousins. The D antigen is present, usually in increased amounts, and the deletion types that have been described include Dc−, DC^W−, and D−−. People homozygous for these haplotypes lack high-prevalence Rh system antigens. When they are exposed to conventional RBCs during transfusion or pregnancy, they form antibodies usually characterized as anti-Rh17 (Hr$_0$). The presence of these antibodies causes the serum of the individual to agglutinate all RBCs except those of

D–– homozygotes or Rh$_{null}$, making transfusion very difficult. People who have formed antibodies to conventional RhCE proteins are counseled to donate autologous blood for themselves and to have it frozen to provide for transfusion requirements. These antibodies have been responsible for severe, and sometimes fatal, HDFN.

THE G ANTIGEN

The *G antigen* is a product of exon 2 of *RHD* or exon 2 of *RHCE*Ce*, as these are identical and encode the same amino acids (Fig. 10-1). Therefore, RBCs that are *either* D positive or C positive are also G positive. In antibody identification studies, anti-G appears to be anti-D plus anti-C on routine antibody identification because of the presence of G antigen on both D+ and C+ RBCs. Anti-G versus anti-D+C can be discriminated by adsorption and elution studies, but this is not usually necessary in the pretransfusion setting, as patients with anti-G must receive D– and C– blood. However, for obstetric patients, further testing is important because Rh immune globulin prophylaxis is indicated if the mother does not have anti-D.

COMPOUND ANTIGENS

Compound antigens in the Rh system are direct to the shared epitopes of C or c and E or e antigens on the same protein. These are ce (f), Ce (rh$_i$), cE (Rh27), and CE (Rh22) (see Table 10-2). The f antigen is encoded by the Rhce protein, rhi by RhCe, and so on . Cells of the genotype Ce/DcE would express the compound antigens Ce (rh$_i$) and cE (Rh27). These cells would not express f even though they carry the c and e antigens because c and e are not encoded on the same protein. In the routine laboratory, antibodies to compound antigens are encountered less frequently than single-specificity Rh antibodies and may be components of sera with multiple antibody specificities.

TABLE 10-2	Compound Antigens and the Haplotypes that Produce them
Compound Antigens	**Haplotypes**
Ce (rh$_i$)	DCe (R$_1$) and Ce (r')
cE (Rh27)	DcE (R$_2$) and cE (r'')
ce (f)	Dce (R$_0$) and ce (r)
CE (Rh22)	DCE (Rz) and CE (r^y)

Rh$_{null}$

Rh$_{null}$ red cells carry no Rh system antigens. This is very rare, and no D, C, c, E, or e antigen is detectable when typing the RBCs. The cells also lack Rh29, often called "total Rh." Two genetic pathways can lead to an Rh$_{null}$ phenotype: Rh-negative person (lacking *RHD*) who also has an inactive *RHCE* gene, referred to as an Rh$_{null}$ amorph, or, more often, inheritance of inactive *RHAG* gene, referred to as an Rh$_{null}$ regulator. RhAG protein is required for expression and trafficking of RhCE and RhD to the RBC membrane; so, although the Rh blood group proteins are made in the Rh$_{null}$ regulator individuals, they cannot reach the membrane due to mutation in RhAG. Rh$_{null}$ individuals who have been transfused or who are pregnant may form, among other Rh system antibodies, anti-Rh29. The serum of the people who form these antibodies agglutinates cells from all people except another Rh$_{null}$. Owing to the paucity of Rh$_{null}$ blood, it is recommended that people who have this rare blood type donate autologous blood and have it frozen for transfusion needs.

Rh ANTIBODIES

Rh system antibodies are principally RBC stimulated. Immunization occurs when the individual receives RBCs carrying Rh antigens not present on his or her own cells, either through a transfusion, pregnancy, or needle-sharing. Most Rh antibodies are of the immunoglobulin G (IgG) class, usually the IgG1 or IgG3 subclass. IgG antibodies may occur in mixtures with a minor component of immunoglobulin M (IgM). The antibodies usually appear between 6 weeks and 6 months after exposure to the Rh antigen. The Rh system antibodies do not agglutinate saline-suspended RBCs carrying the corresponding antigen unless they have a major IgM component, but the presence of the antibodies can be demonstrated by the indirect antiglobulin technique. IgG Rh system antibodies react best at 37°C and are enhanced when enzyme-treated RBCs are tested. The antibodies do not bind complement except in rare instances, probably because the Rh antigens are too far apart on the RBC membrane to allow two antibodies to bind close enough to initiate the classic complement cascade through activation of C1q. If a transfusion recipient receives blood carrying an Rh antigen to which he or she has an antibody, the removal of the cells will be extravascular owing to the lack of complement activation. Transfusion reactions may be immediate or delayed.

D is the most immunogenic of the common Rh antigens, followed in decreasing order of immunogenicity by c, E, C, and e. Estimates vary from 30% to 85% as to the number of D– persons who will make anti-D following exposure to D+ RBCs and clearly the RBC dose and immune status of the patient are important variables. Nevertheless, it is generally accepted that D+ RBCs should only be given to D− patients in an emergency, when there is a D− blood shortage, or in massive transfusion. Rh-negative girls and women of childbearing age should always receive D− blood and blood products, but if that is not possible, the use of Rh immune globulin to prevent anti-D must be considered.

When Rh system antibodies are encountered in the routine blood bank laboratory, it is important to be aware of the Rh antibodies that often occur together. For example, sera containing anti-D often contain anti-G as well. R_1R_1 people who make anti-c have probably been exposed to E antigen as well and may also have low-level anti-E.

Rh IMMUNE GLOBULIN

The cause of HDFN was discovered when it was realized that the mother was reacting to a paternal antigen inherited on the RBCs of the fetus. These women often had healthy first babies, but subsequent pregnancies often resulted in severe anemia in the fetus or stillbirth and spontaneous abortion. Because fetal RBCs enter the maternal circulation in small amounts during pregnancy and in larger amounts during childbirth, the first pregnancy with an Rh-positive fetus may sensitize the mother to anti-D. Anti-D is predominantly IgG1 and IgG3 and will cross the placenta and attach to the D antigen, which is well developed on fetal RBCs. Thus, in any subsequent Rh-positive pregnancy, the maternal anti-D crosses the placenta, resulting in the destruction of the fetal RBCs. The observation that ABO incompatibility between a mother and the fetus had a partial protective effect against production of maternal antibodies led to the development of Rh immune globulin. The protective effect suggested that maternal, naturally occurring anti-A or anti-B bound to the incompatible fetal A-positive or B-positive RBCs, preventing production of anti-D. By the 1960s, a mere 20 years after the discovery of RhD incompatibility, HDFN due to anti-D could be effectively prevented if the mother received an injection of passive antibody. The incidence of HDFN due to anti-D has decreased dramatically in the Western world owing to treatment with Rh immune globulin. Rh immune globulin is a solution containing human IgG anti-D. In the United States, it is administered to Rh-negative women during the 28th week of pregnancy (antepartum dose) and again after the delivery of an Rh-positive infant (postpartum dose) or at the time of an induced or spontaneous abortion. When testing the mother after delivery for the presence of anti-D, the antenatal Rh immune globulin may still be weakly demonstrable when the serum is tested against D-positive RBCs. It is important to recognize this possibility and to not exclude the woman from receiving postpartum Rh immune globulin. Rh immune globulin must be administered in each pregnancy if the fetus is Rh positive to prevent maternal sensitization and formation of anti-D. Unfortunately, many women in poor or developing countries do not have access to Rh immune globulin prevention, and HDFN due to anti-D is still seen in some parts of the world.

Other Rh antibodies may also cause severe HDFN. Rh immune globulin prevents only anti-D, not the formation of other Rh antibodies such as anti-C, anti-c, anti-E, and anti-e. Women should be screened early in each pregnancy for Rh antibodies as well as other IgG blood group antibodies like anti-Kell, which may cause HDFN.

Rh MOLECULAR TESTING

Serologic reagents detect the principal antigens, D, C, e, E, and e, but there are many other Rh antigens, including altered or variant antigens, which are not uncommon in African Black and Hispanic groups. No commercial serologic reagents are available to detect these. DNA-based genotyping has the potential to modernize selection of compatible blood for patients with complex Rh antibodies.

Rh SEROLOGIC REAGENTS

Reagents used to detect the D antigen in the slide, tube, microplate, automated, and gel tests often have different formulations and performance characteristics. Each manufacturer's anti-D reagents may contain different antibody clones, potentiators, additives, or diluents, and reagents that contain the same antibody clone can also vary, for example, in antibody dilution or the preservative present. Hence, instructions for testing may differ and must be consulted and carefully followed for accurate testing.

High-protein polyclonal reagents prepared from pools of human sera and containing high concentrations of protein (20% to 24%) were originally used for Rh typing. These reagents are potent and reliable, but were associated with false-positive reactions when the test RBCs are coated with immunoglobulin. A control consisting of the diluent used by the manufacturer to prepare the reagent must be tested in parallel for valid results.

Many polyclonal anti-D have been replaced with monoclonal reagents, and in the United States, most Food and Drug Administration (FDA)–licensed anti-D contain a mixture of monoclonal IgM and monoclonal or polyclonal IgG. The IgM anti-D component causes direct agglutination of positive RBCs at immediate spin, and the IgG anti-D is reactive in the antiglobulin phase of testing, making the reagent suitable for weak D testing. Spontaneous agglutination causing a false-positive result is much less frequent than seen with high-protein reagents, but controls performed as described by the reagent manufacturer are still required. Proper controls for false positives are usually a negative test result, performed concurrently, for example, the absence of agglutination of the RBCs with anti-A or -B. If a separate control test must be done (AB sample), 6% albumin is an appropriate control.

Chemically modified IgG antisera have been treated with a sulfhydryl compound that weakens the disulfide bonds at the hinge region of the IgG molecule. This allows greater distance between the two antigen-binding sites in the hypervariable regions of the antigen-binding (Fab) portions of the molecule, converting the IgG anti-D to a direct agglutinin.

Reagents are also commercially available for determining the presence of C, c, E, and e antigens on RBCs. Most of these are monoclonal blends intended for direct testing only and are not appropriate for anti-human globulin (AHG) phase of testing. Follow manufacturer's instructions. Appropriate negative controls for false-positive typing, as discussed above for anti-D, also apply.

Slide Testing

A glass slide containing a drop of 40% to 50% serum or plasma suspension of RBCs and a drop of anti-D is mixed and placed on a heated Rh view box that is tilted continuously for 2 minutes to observe for agglutination. To achieve rapid warming of the materials on the slide to 37°C, the Rh viewing box is kept at a temperature between 40°C and 50°C. Slide testing is rarely performed owing to the imprecise nature of the test method and risk of biohazard exposure.

Tube Testing

Tube testing is performed in either 10 × 75-mm or 12 × 75-mm test tubes. The washed RBCs to be tested are suspended in saline at approximately 2% to 5% cell suspension. One drop of the cell suspension is added to the test tube containing one drop of antiserum and centrifuged. The mixture is resuspended and observed for agglutination. Tube testing is relatively easy to read and, for some reagents, can be continued to the indirect antiglobulin phase of testing, depending on the specific manufacturers' instructions.

Automated and Microplate Testing

Automated testing (e.g., Olympus PK) or microplate testing has been adopted by larger blood centers for donor typing. The antiserum used must state that it is formulated for automation or microplate Rh testing and may require that the blood be collected in a specific anticoagulant. Always consult and follow manufacturers' instructions.

Gel Testing

Rh typing may also be done using a gel technique. The antiserum is distributed throughout the gel particles. Antigen-positive RBCs react with the antisera, and the agglutinins are trapped and cannot pass through the gel when centrifuged. This method has the advantage that the gel card can be saved for later review of the results.

Technical Considerations for Rh Typing

False-positive Results

False-positive results can result from the following:

- Cold autoagglutinins. Washing the cells, sometimes multiple times, with warm saline and retyping should correct the problem.
- Warm autoagglutinins. Washing the cells multiple times and retesting or using IgM reagents may be required. Treatment of the cells to remove IgG can also be done.
- Positive direct antiglobulin test (DAT). Indirect antiglobulin testing for weak D will not be valid on RBCs coated with IgG with a positive DAT. Treatment of the cells to remove IgG can also be done.
- Using a posttransfusion sample, including D typing in patients who are D− and have received large amounts of D+ blood during massive or emergency transfusion. Always obtain an accurate transfusion history for valid typing.
- Use of the wrong antiserum. Careful reading of labels on each reagent vial is required. Antiserum labels must not be obscured, and those with unreadable labels should be discarded.

- Reagent contaminated with a low-incidence antibody. Testing with another manufacturer's reagent or with a known antibody from a patient or donor aids in clarification.
- Contaminated reagents. Reagent vials can become contaminated with bacteria, proteins, or other reagents owing to sloppy technique. Workers must be careful not to touch the dropper tip or remove the droppers from multiple vials simultaneously.
- Polyagglutinable cells. These cells will be agglutinated by any reagent that contains human serum. Using a monoclonal reagent should correct the problem.

False-negative Reactions

False-negative reactions may result from the following:

- Failure to add antiserum. Adding the antiserum before the addition of the RBCs aids the worker in seeing whether reagent is present.
- Blocking of antigen sites. In severe HDFN, the RBCs may be so heavily coated with antibody that no antigen sites remain for antisera to bind. The correct Rh type may be obtained if the cells are first heat eluted to remove some of the blocking antibody.
- Incorrect cell suspension. Too heavy or too light a cell suspension can cause false-negative results. If the button after centrifugation is larger or smaller than usual, the test should be repeated.
- Incorrect antiserum-to-cell ratio. Deviation from the manufacturer's instructions can result in using inappropriate amounts of particular antisera. Two drops are often *not* better than one, and the manufacturer's instructions must always be followed.
- Overly vigorous resuspension after centrifugation. Shaking too hard results in dispersal of weak agglutination. Careful resuspension is essential.
- Failure of the antiserum to react with a weak or variant antigen. A specific antibody may not react with weak forms of an antigen or with variant antigens. Using an antiserum from another manufacturer or a known donor or patient antibody may aid investigation. Absorption and elution of the antibody may also be necessary to demonstrate the presence of the antigen.
- Reagent deterioration. Prolonged or incorrect storage of reagents may result in the destruction of the antibody in the reagent. Antiserum should not be used after the expiration date.

- Antiserum in which the predominant antibody is directed against a compound antigen. This can be a problem with anti-C antiserum if the antibodies are actually anti-Ce (anti-rh$_i$). These reagents may not react well with cells of haplotypes other than DCe (R$_1$) and Ce (r'), that is, cells from an R$_z$ (DCE) or CE (r^y).
- Use of wrong antiserum.

Rh TYPING DISCREPANCIES

A patient or donor RBC sample that was previously found to be positive but is now determined to be negative, or vice versa, should always be investigated to rule out identification, clerical, or recording errors. A new sample should be obtained and tested. If the discrepancy is between current testing and historical records, it may be due to the method used, phase of testing (direct or IAT), type of reagent (polyclonal vs. monoclonal), or manufacturer. Different reagents often contain different antibody clones that may show variable reactions with RBCs with weak or partial Rh antigens. Knowledge of the ethnicity of the donor or patient can be helpful when investigating a typing discrepancy because some partial and weak phenotypes are more common in a specific ethnic group. Typing with several reagents from different manufacturers may be helpful.

Reagents licensed by the FDA for D typing have been selected to be nonreactive with partial DVI RBCs in the direct test. This is because girls and women of childbearing age with DVI RBCs are at risk for production of anti-D associated with fatal HDFN and are better treated as D negative for transfusion and as candidates for Rh immune globulin. DVI RBCs will test positive for weak D, which is required for donor testing. Therefore, patients with partial DVI are considered D negative for transfusion but appropriately classified as D-positive donors.

SUMMARY

The Rh system is one of the most important systems in transfusion medicine. It is second only to ABO in transfusion importance. Antibodies or combinations of antibodies often result in individuals who are exposed to antigens that they do not possess. Advances in testing have allowed us to learn much about the complexities of the system, and our ability to test and understand variants has increased. Although once a major cause of HDFN, anti-D does not pose as high a risk today, thanks to the use of Rh immune globulin.

Review Questions

1. The term "Rh positive" refers to the presence of which of the following:
   a. D
   b. E
   c. C
   d. none of the above

2. The use of R to denote the presence of "D" in Rh nomenclature is an example of which terminology?
   a. Fisher–Race
   b. Wiener
   c. ISBT
   d. none of the above

3. True or false? Weak D can result from few D-antigen sites on the red cell or from the presence of Ce allele in *trans* position to D.

4. True or false? For AABB-accredited hospitals, the D type of units labeled Rh negative must be confirmed from an integrally attached segment before transfusion, but testing for weak D is not required.

5. True or false? The E and e alleles are codominant.

6. Anti-G will agglutinate which of the following:
   a. D-positive red cells
   b. C-positive red cells
   c. E-positive red cells
   d. both a and b
   e. both a and c

7. Which of the following is true regarding Rh_{null} individuals?
   a. their cells lack Rh29
   b. their cells lack DCE but have c and e
   c. they can form a weak but harmless antibody
   d. all of the above

8. True or false? The Rh antibodies do not bind complement except in rare instances.

9. Which of the following is the most antigenic?
   a. D
   b. C
   c. c
   d. E
   e. e

10. HDFN has been dramatically reduced by giving Rh-negative women doses of _____.

Please indicate if the following can result in a false positive (P), a false negative (N), or both depending upon the circumstances (B)

11. Contaminated reagent
12. Polyagglutinable red cells
13. Blocking of antigen sites
14. Use of wrong antiserum
15. Reagent deterioration

ADDITIONAL READINGS

Daniels G. *Human Blood Groups*. 2nd ed. Cambridge, MA: Blackwell Science; 2002.

Reid ME, Lomas-Francis C. *The Blood Group Antigen Facts Book*. 2nd ed. San Diego, CA: Academic Press; 2004.

Westhoff CM. Molecular testing for transfusion medicine. *Curr Opin Hematol*. 2006; 13: 471–475.

Westhoff CM. The structure and function of the Rh antigen complex. *Semin Hematol*. 2007; 44:42–50.

PROCEDURAL APPENDIX

RAPID TUBE TYPING FOR D ANTIGEN

This procedure is intended to be a general guide for testing. Follow instructions of the manufacturer.

1. Label two 10×75-mm or 12×75-mm test tubes. Label one tube "D" and the other tube "cont."
2. Wash the RBCs to be tested in normal saline.
3. Prepare a 2% to 5% suspension of the washed cells in fresh normal saline.
4. Add one drop of anti-D to the tube labeled "D."
5. Add one drop of 6% albumin to the tube labeled "cont."
6. Centrifuge for 30 seconds at $1,000g$ (3,200 rpm in a serofuge or immunofuge).
7. Gently resuspend the cell button, watching for agglutination as resuspension occurs. Be sure to fully resuspend the entire cell button before deciding that no agglutination has taken place. The Rh control tube must show no agglutination. If there is agglutination in the Rh control tube, the test is invalid and another antiserum must be used.
8. Record the agglutination reaction as 4+, 3+, 2+, 1+, w+, or negative.

WEAK D TESTING

1. If the reaction is less than 2+, incubate the test and the control at 37°C for 15 to 60 minutes.
2. After incubation, wash the cells in each tube with normal saline.
3. Fill the tube with saline, mixing well. Be sure to completely resuspend the cell button in the saline.
4. Centrifuge for 1 minute at $1,000g$.
5. Decant the saline completely.
6. Repeat steps 3 through 5 for a total of three to four washes.
7. Add two drops of antiglobulin serum, and mix well.
8. Centrifuge for 15 seconds at $1,000g$.
9. Resuspend gently and observe for agglutination. The control tube must show no agglutination to validate the test.
10. Record the results.

OTHER BLOOD GROUP SYSTEMS

TERRY DOWNS

OBJECTIVES

After completion of this chapter, the reader will be able to:

1. Name the major antigens of each blood group system and list the frequencies of the observed phenotypes.

2. Describe carrier molecule structure and possible function for selected blood group systems.

3. Discuss biochemistry and genetics of selected blood group systems.

4. Discuss the characteristics of antibodies associated with each blood group system including:

   a. Serologic characteristics

   b. Clinical significance

   c. Special reagents and techniques useful in identification of the antibody

5. Describe disease conditions associated with selected blood group systems.

KEY WORDS

Blood group system	High-incidence antigens
Carrier molecules	High titer, low avidity
Donath-Landsteiner test	Low-incidence antigens
Dosage effect	Secretor status
Glycolipids	Sialoglycoprotein
Glycoproteins	Silent allele

*O*f the more than 600 antigens that have been described, 302 antigens have been classified by the International Society for Blood Transfusion (ISBT) Committee on Terminology for the red cell surface antigens. The antigens are sorted into blood group systems, collections, and series of independent antigens. There are currently 30 blood group systems recognized as shown in Table 11-1.[1] Table 11-2 lists the gene product of the major blood group alleles. The blood group systems are numbered as ISBT 001 through ISBT 030. They are listed in numerical order in this chapter with the exception of the two groups of antigens. The P blood group system, the Globoside blood group system, and the Globoside collection are discussed together. The I blood group system is discussed with the Ii blood collection. The ABO, H, Rh, and LW blood group systems are presented in other chapters.

The importance of blood groups, antigens, and antibodies relates to the characteristics that determine clinical significance for transfusion purposes and hemolytic disease of the fetus and newborn (HDFN). An understanding of antigens through structure, function, and genetic background is helpful in both transfusion medicine and the study of disease. As molecular techniques have evolved, immunohematologists have a greater understanding of the genetics of the antigens in general.

CLASSIFICATION AND NOMENCLATURE

A *blood group system* is defined by the ISBT as "when one or more antigens are controlled at a single gene locus or by two or more very closely linked

TABLE 11-1 **ISBT Table of Blood Group Systems**

No.	System Name	System Symbol	Gene Name(s)	Chromosome
001	ABO	ABO	ABO	9
002	MNS	MNS	GYPA, GYPB, GYPE	4
003	P	P1	Unknown	22
004	Rh	RH	RHD, RHCE	1
005	Lutheran	LU	LU	19
006	Kell	KEL	KEL	7
007	Lewis	LE	FUT3	19
008	Duffy	FY	DARC	1
009	Kidd	JK	SLC14A1	18
010	Diego	DI	SLC4A1	17
011	Yt	YT	ACHE	7
012	Xg	XG	XG, MIC2	X
013	Scianna	SC	ERMAP	1
014	Dombrock	DO	ART4	12
015	Colton	CO	AQP1	7
016	Landsteiner—Weiner	LW	ICAM4	19
017	Chido/Rogers	CH/RG	C4A, C4B	6
018	H	H	FUT1	19
019	Kx	XK	XK	X
020	Gerbich	GE	GYPC	2
021	Cromer	CROM	CD55	1
022	Knops	KN	CR1	1
023	Indian	IN	CD44	11
024	Ok	OK	BSG	19
025	Raph	RAPH	CD151	11
026	John Milton Hagen	JMH	SEMA7A	15
027	I	I	IGNT	6
028	Globoside	GLOB	B3GALT3	3
029	Gill	GIL	AQP3	9
030	Rh-associated glycoprotein	RHAG	RHAG	6

TABLE 11-2   Blood Group Systems: Gene Product with Carrier Molecule and Function

Name	Gene Product	Structure	N-terminus Orientation	Function
MNS	Glycophorin A Glycophorin B	Type 1 SGP	Exofacial	Carrier of sialic acid Complement regulation
P	Glycosyltransferase	Carbohydrate		Unknown
Lutheran	Lutheran glycoprotein	Single-pass	Exofacial	Adhesion/receptor
Kell	Kell glycoprotein	Single-pass	Exofacial	Unknown
Lewis	Glycosyltransferase			Unknown
Duffy	Fy glycoprotein	Multipass-7	Exofacial	Chemokine receptor
Kidd	Urea transporter	Multipass-10	Cytoplasmic	Urea transporter
Diego	Band 3	Multipass-14	Cytoplasmic	Anion transporter Membrane anchor
Yt	Acetylcholinesterase	GPI linkage	NA	Acetylcholinesterase
Xg	Xgᵃ glycoprotein	Single-pass	Exofacial	Adhesion
Scianna	ERMAP protein	IgSF single-pass		Adhesion/receptor
Dombrock	Do glycoprotein	GPI linkage	NA	ADP-ribosyltransferase
Colton	CHIP-1	Multipass-6	Cytoplasmic	Water transport
LW	LW glycoprotein	Single-pass	Exofacial	Adhesion
Chido/ Rogers	Complement component 4 (C4)			Complement regulation
Kx	Kx glycoprotein	Multipass-10	Cytoplasmic	Transport
Gerbich	Glycophorin C Glycophorin D	Single-pass	Exofacial	Carrier of sialic acid Complement regulation
Cromer	CD55 (DAF)	GPI-linkage	NA	Complement regulation
Knops	CD35 (CR1)	Single-pass	Exofacial	Complement regulation
Indian	CD44	Single-pass	Exofacial	Adhesion
Ok	CD147	Single-pass	Exofacial	Adhesion
Raph				
JMH	SEMA7A			Adhesion/receptor
I				
Globoside	B3GALNT1	Carbohydrate		Unknown
Gil	Aquaporin	Multipass		Water/glycerol channel
RHAG		Type 3—12 span		Unknown

TABLE 11-3   Antigen and Phenotype Designations

Numerical Terminology	Alternative Terminology	Antigen Present on Red Cell
LU:−1,2	Lu(a−b+)	Lu^b
FY: 1,2	FY(a+b+)	Fy^a and Fy^b
GE: 2,3,4,−5,−6,−7,−8,−9	GE: 2, 3, 4 Wb− Ls(a−) An(a−) Dh(a−)	Ge2, Ge3, Ge4
GE:−2,−3,−4	GEIS−	Null
GE:−2,−3, 4	Leach phenotype	Ge4
GE:−2, 3, 4	Gerbich phenotype	Ge3, Ge4
	Yus phenotype	
I:1	I adult	I
I:−1	i adult or cord	i
MNS: 1,2,−3,4	M+N+S−s+	M, N, s

homologous genes with little or no observable recombination between them."[1] The number of antigens in each system varies from 1 (P, H, Kx, Ok, Raph, I, Globoside, Gill) to 49 (Rh). *Collections* describe groups of antigens that have phenotypic, biochemical, or genetic relationships, but there are not enough data to demonstrate their independence from other systems. Examples of blood group collections are Glob, Cost, Er, and Vel. The series of independent antigens are divided into the 700 series of *low incidence* (<1%) and the 901 series of high incidence (>90%). The ISBT maintains a list of obsolete numbers and as the antigens are classified, numbers are retired. Several terminologies have been used over the years to describe the different blood group systems and the various antigens. Sometimes the antigens were named after the individual who made the corresponding antibody. Other times numbers or letters were used, some with a superscript. An ISBT committee was founded in 1980 to devise the numerical terminology for red cell antigens. The committee meets regularly to review new information on antigens and categorize them appropriately. Table 11-3 displays blood group systems by ISBT number, common name, gene name, and chromosome location.

CARRIER MOLECULE TYPE

Red blood cell (RBC) antigens are carbohydrate or protein structures carried on three types of molecules— *glycoproteins, glycolipids,* and proteins. Most of the antigens are carried on glycoproteins and have a specificity determined by the attached oligosaccharide sequence or the amino acid sequence. Carbohydrate antigens include ABO, Lewis, H, I, and P in which the antigen is depicted by the immunodominant carbohydrate and its linkage carried on a glycoprotein or a glycolipid. The polymorphisms arise from glycosyltransferase genes that change the substrate or inactivate it. Protein antigens are located on different types of *carrier molecules* that can be single-pass or multipass through the red cell membrane or have a glycosylphosphatidylinositol (GPI) linkage to the membrane. The single-pass carriers can be oriented with the N-terminus outside (type 1) or inside (type 2) the membrane. Multipass carriers (type 3) typically are oriented with both the N- and C-termini inside the membrane. The exception is the glycoprotein carrying the Duffy antigens in which the N-terminus is extracellular. These molecules generally are glycosylated by *N*- and/or *O*-glycans on one of the extracellular loops. These glycans help to form the glycocalyx or a negatively charged area that prevents spontaneous aggregation of circulating red cells. Other antigens are located on proteins that are adsorbed from plasma onto the red cell such as Lewis and Chido/Rogers.[2]

CARRIER MOLECULE FUNCTION

Molecular techniques have increased our knowledge of the structures of carrier molecules, but the function of carrier molecules has become an intense field of research. The type of carrier molecule may correlate with its function, and information is sometimes deduced from the function of similar molecules found on other tissues. *Null phenotypes* arising from an absent

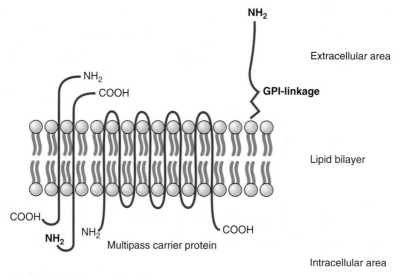

FIGURE 11-1   **Red cell membrane components and antigen carrier protein structures.**

carrier molecule may provide information if a disease condition is present in the individual. However, many null conditions exist with no detriment to the individual.

Multipass membrane proteins tend to have transport functions because they form a transmembranous channel, allowing molecules in or out of the cell. For example, the Gil antigen is a glycerol and water channel. Single-pass carrier proteins appear to have adhesion and receptor functions. The Duffy antigen acts as a receptor for types of cytokines. Several carrier types contain extracellular domains of an immunoglobulin superfamily (IgSF) that function as adhesion and receptors. IgSF glycoproteins contain repeating extracellular domains with sequence homology to immunoglobulin variable (V) or constant (C1 or C2) domains. Antigens carried on molecules with a GPI linkage to the red cell surface often are involved in enzymatic activities. Some carriers, such as the Gerbich glycoprotein, have C-terminal domains that attach to the membrane skeleton and assist with red cell structure. Table 11-2 lists the blood group systems described in this chapter with the type of carrier molecule and possible functions, if known. Figure 11-1 displays some common features of carrier molecules.

PHENOTYPES

The antigen is the structure on the red cell membrane that can complex with a specific antibody. A phenotype describes the antigens that are present on red cells based on the results of serologic tests on those red cells. There are several typical ways to designate phenotype using either the ISBT numerical terminology or the alternative terminology. See Table 11-3 for some examples.

MNS BLOOD GROUP SYSTEM (ISBT 002)

The MNS system was the second human blood group system to be discovered. Landsteiner and Levine reported the M and N antigens in 1927. In 1947, Walsh and Montgomery described the S antigen. The s antigen was found in 1951 by Levine et al. and U in 1953 by Weiner et al.[3]

Biochemistry and Genetics

The system is made up of over 40 antigens carried on two *sialoglycoprotein* (SGP) molecules or hybrid molecules of SGP produced by the *GYPA* and the *GYPB* genes. Also known as glycophorins, they are rich in sialic acid and extend from the external environment of the cell through the membrane and into the cytoplasm. The polypeptide backbone of the structure is N- and O-glycosidically linked oligosaccharides referred as N- and O-glycans. The N-glycans are larger than the O-glycans, but the O-glycans carry most of the sialic acid. It is thought that the sialic acid also plays a role in the serologic expression of the M and N antigens.

The *GYPA* gene produces glycophorin A while *GYPB* produces glycophorin B. A third gene *GYPE*, next to *GYPB*, participates in gene rearrangements, but does not appear to encode a membrane component.

Most of the antigens in the system reside on one of these glycophorins. Other antigens occur because of crossing-over between the genes for GPA and GPB, which results in hybrid glycophorins. Deletions can also occur which result in GPA- or GPB-deficient states. The *GYPA*, *GYPB*, and *GYPE* genes are in close proximity on the long arm of chromosome 4. Although *GYPE* may not encode a membrane component, it is believed to play a role in variant alleles.

Antigens of the MNS System

The most important antigens that affect transfusion are M, N, S, s, and U. The M and N antigens are carried on glycophorin A, while S, s, and U are on glycophorin B. There is a strong association of the M antigen with S and the N antigen with s. The incidence of MNS blood group system antigens are displayed in Table 11-4 along with the affected glycophorins in antigen expression.

TABLE 11-4 MNS Blood Group System Antigens

ISBT Antigen Number	Alternative Terminology	Relative Incidence Whites	Blacks	Antithetical Antigen	Glycophorin or Hybrid
MNS1	M	78	74	N	GPA
MNS2	N	72	75	M	GPA
MNS3	S	57	30	s	GPB
MNS4	s	88	93	S	GPB
MNS5	U	High	99.7		GPB
MNS6	He	<1	3	"N"	Hybrid
MNS7	Miᵃ	<1			Hybrid
MNS8	Mᶜ	Low			Hybrid
MNS9	Vw	Low		HUT, ENEH	Hybrid
MNS10	Mur	Low			Hybrid
MNS11	Mᵍ	Rare			Hybrid
MNS12	Vr	Low			GPA
MNS13	Mᵉ	0.5	Low		
MNS14	Mtᵃ	0.25	Low		GPA
MNS15	Stᵃ	Low			Hybrid
MNS16	Riᵃ	Low			GPA
MNS17	Clᵃ	Low			
MNS18	Nyᵃ	Low			GPA
MNS19	Hut	Low		Vw, ENEH	Hybrid
MNS20	Hil	Low			Hybrid
MNS21	Mᵛ	0.6	Low		GPB
MNS22	Far	Low			
MNS23	Sᴰ	Low			GPB

(continued)

TABLE 11-4   MNS Blood Group System Antigens (continued)

ISBT Antigen Number	Alternative Terminology	Relative Incidence Whites	Relative Incidence Blacks	Antithetical Antigen	Glycophorin or Hybrid
MNS24	Mit	0.12	Low		GPB
MNS25	Dantu	Rare	Low		Hybrid
MNS26	Hop	Low			Hybrid
MNS27	Nob	Low		EnªKT	Hybrid
MNS28	Enª	>99.9			
MNS29	EnªKT	>99.9		Nob	Hybrid
MNS30	"N"	>99.9		He	GPB
MNS31	Or	Low			GPA
MNS32	DANE	0.4 in Danes			Hybrid
MNS33	TSEN	Low			Hybrid
MNS34	MINY	Low			Hybrid
MNS35	MUT	Low			Hybrid
MNS36	SAT	0.01 in Japanese			Hybrid
MNS37	ERIK	Low			GPA
MNS38	Osª	Low			GPA
MNS39	ENEP	High		HAG	GPA
MNS40	ENEH	High		Vw, Hut	Hybrid
MNS41	HAG	Low		ENEP	GPA
MNS42	ENAV	High		MARS	GPA
MNS43	MARS	Low		ENAV	GPA
MNS44	ENDA	High			Hybrid
MNS45	ENEV	High			GPA
MNS46	MNTD	Low			GPA

Glycophorin A

The MN glycoprotein is a single-pass protein that consists of 131 amino acids separated into three regions. Of these amino acids, 70 extend into the extracellular environment and are glycosylated, 26 are contained in the lipid bilayer, and the remaining 35 amino acids are intracellular. There are about 800,000 copies of GPA per red cell. The expression of antigen occurs on the outer or N-terminal extending into the extracellular environment. The amino acid sequence for the M and N antigens has position changes at 1 and 5 of the molecule. See Table 11-5 for a display of the changes.

Sixteen high- and low-incidence antigens that result from single-point mutations causing amino acid substitutions are found on GPA. The Vr antigen arises from a point mutation that changes serine at position 47 to tyrosine. The Mtª antigen arises from a point mutation that codes threonine at position 58 to isoleucine.[4]

TABLE 11-5   Amino Acid Position Changes for the M and N Antigens

	Amino Acid Sequence Positions 1–5	
GPA (M antigen)	Ser-Ser-Thr-Thr-Gly	Ser-Thr-Thr are
GPA (N antigen)	Leu-Ser-Thr-Thr-Glu	O-glycosylated

Ser, serine; Thr, threonine; Gly, glycine; Leu, leucine; Glu, glutamic acid.

Ny^a is another low-frequency antigen that substitutes aspartic acid at position 27 for glutamic acid. The Os^a antigen arises by a proline to serine substitution at position 54.[5] The other low-incidence antigens associated with single nucleotide mutations are Vw/Hut, Ri^a, Or, ERIK, HAG, MARS, and a recent addition to the MNS system, MNTD. *High-incidence antigens* associated with single-nucleotide mutations are ENEP, ENEH, ENAV, and as recent addition to the system, ENEV.

Glycophorin B

The Ss glycoprotein is also a single-pass protein consisting of 72 amino acids. There are approximately 200,000 copies of GPB per red cell. An amino acid substitution at position 29 changes methionine for S to threonine for s. The first 26 N-terminal amino acids on GPB are identical to the GPA that carries the N antigen. Because of the similarity, an N-like or "N" antigen is found on most cells.

There are also low-incidence antigens present on GPB, arising from single-nucleotide mutations causing amino acid substitutions. A proline to arginine substitution at position 39 causes production of the S^D antigen. The M^V antigen is demonstrated by a change from threonine to serine at position 3. The Mit antigen is demonstrated when histidine substitutes arginine at position 35.[6]

Glycophorin Deficiencies

Inheritance of genes with deleted exons can result in absence of either GPA or GPB or both. Two inherited *GYPA* genes with a deletion of exons 2 through 7 result in a lack of GPA. These cells are described as En(a$^-$), but the term reflects several amino acid segments of GPA such as En^{a}TS (trypsin sensitive), En^{a}FS (ficin sensitive), or En^{a}FR (ficin resistant). Normal levels of GPB are carried on these cells. Examples of anti-En^a react with a portion of GPA that is not associated with the M or N antigens. These cells have reduced levels of sialic acid; however, the deficiency does not appear to affect red cell survival.[7,8] Anti-Wr^b is frequently found in the sera of En(a$^-$) individuals.

Deletion of *GYPB* and *GYPE* gives rise to GPB deficiency. Thus, these individuals have the S$-$s$-$U$-$ phenotype.[9] A deletion of *GYPA*, *GYPB*, and *GYPE* results in the M^{k}M^k genotype. These individuals have neither GPA nor GPB, resulting in a lack of all MNS antigens.

Hybrid Glycophorins

As mentioned previously, the MNSs genes *GYPA* and *GYPB* are in close proximity on the chromosome. Modifications arise from unequal crossover or gene conversion. The gene products are described as hybrid

molecules with many variations in the structure. They may carry the N-terminal (amino) of GPA and the C-terminal of GPB or vice versa. Others may carry an insertion of a part of GPA into GPB or an insertion of a part of GPB into GPA. The term *GYP(A-B)* describes the genetic basis of the structure with an N-terminal of GPA and a C-terminal of GPB. Hybrid genes that exist through insertion of one GP into another may be labeled as *GYP(A-B-A)* or *GYP(B-A-B)*. In the former, a piece of GPB crosses and replaces a piece of GPA. The corresponding section of GPA crosses over to GPB to create the haplotype. The resulting glycophorins contain pieces of GPA and GPB. In addition to encoding novel antigens, the expression of the more common MNS system antigens may be affected if the encoding sequence is close to the crossover site. The variants are named with a GP, followed by the name of the variant (e.g., GP.Hil). The system is complex and describes many unusual antigens. Historically, these antigens were previously thought to be low incidence and separate within the MNS system. Many of them were categorized into the Miltenberger subsystem based on reactivity with selected antisera. As molecular techniques have evolved, the Miltenberger subsytem no longer adequately describes the antigens. It is mentioned because of the historical nature of the information and the discussion of it in the literature. Some of the antigens will be described in the following text.

Hybrid Glycophorin Molecules and the Low-incidence Antigens

The three glycophorin GP(A-B) varients that arise from the gene *GP(A-B)* are GP.Hil, GP.JL, and GP.TK. The antigens Hil, MINY, and TSEN are produced from these configurations. *GP(A-B-A)* hybrids include GP.Vw, GP.Hut, GP.Nob, GP.Joh, and GP.Dane. Antigens carried on these glycophorins are Mi^a, Vw, Hut, and MUT. GP(B-A-B) hybrids include GP.Mur, GP.Hop, GP.Bun, and GP.HF. The associated antigens with these glycophorins are Mi^a, Mur, MUT, Hil, and MINY.[10]

Antibodies in the MNS System

Anti-M

Anti-M tends to be a cold-reactive antibody and can be found in the sera of individuals who have never received a transfusion nor have been pregnant. It usually reacts at room temperature or below and may have both an IgM and IgG component. Most examples do not bind complement and it is not a cause of HDFN. Examples of anti-M that do not react at 37°C should be ignored. This is best accomplished by not performing pretransfusion antibody screens and crossmatches at room temperature. For those facilities that perform an immediate spin crossmatch, a prudent policy would be to perform indirect antiglobulin test (IAT) crossmatches as the next step when the immediate spin crossmatch is positive (assuming ABO is compatible). The IAT crossmatches are rarely positive when anti-M is involved unless the antibody is particularly potent. Anti-M may demonstrate a *dosage effect* when tested against cells with "double"-dose *(MM)* versus single-dose *(MN)* cells. Anti-M does not react with cells treated with ficin and papain. Anti-M can be enhanced by testing in an environment designed to lower the pH to 6.5.

Anti-N

Anti-N is uncommon and like anti-M is a naturally occurring IgM agglutinin. As with anti-M, anti-N will not react with cells treated with enzymes and exhibits a dosage effect. Anti-N does not activate complement. The more common anti-N is made by the individual whose red cells type as M+N−, but carry either S or s. Although their cells type as N−, they carry "N" on GPB and the anti-N is really an autoantibody. The second type of anti-N is one made by individuals whose cells type as M+N−S−s−. These cells lack "N" and their serum will react with donor cells that type as M+N− and either S+s− or S−s+. The anti-N made by individuals with "N"− red cells is usually more significant than those made by individuals with "N"+ cells. The individuals whose red cells type as S−s− are rare, so this type of antibody is not common. Another form of anti-N is seen in dialysis patients when the residual formaldehyde in the dialyzer membranes alters the N or "N" antigens of the patient. This specificity of anti-N is not considered clinically significant.

Anti-S and Anti-s

These antibodies are not as common as anti-M and anti-N and they are usually red cell stimulated through transfusion or pregnancy. The majority are IgG reactive at 37°C and IAT. Enzyme treatment of test cells shows variable reactivity and some examples of anti-S may demonstrate a dosage effect. Both antibodies are clinically significant and cause HDFN. There are some rare examples of IgM anti-S.

Anti-U

Anti-U is a rare antibody that can be produced by individuals whose red cells type S−s−U−. It is usually seen in the African American population and is considered clinically significant. It has been associated with HDFN and hemolytic transfusion reaction (HTR). The antibody may be difficult to identify in that most panel cells would test positive, but should be considered when an antibody is positive for the majority of panel cells in a patient of African American descent.

Anti-En^a

Anti-En^a antibodies are directed at several different amino acid sequences on GPA. These are IgG in nature reactive at 37°C and IAT. They are considered clinically significant and capable of causing HDFN.

P BLOOD GROUP SYSTEM (ISBT 003), GLOBOSIDE BLOOD GROUP SYSTEM (ISBT 028), AND GLOBOSIDE BLOOD GROUP COLLECTION

The two blood group systems and collection are discussed together because of the interrelationships between the antigens. There are three different genetic loci that are responsible for the different phenotypes.

History

Animal experiments conducted by Landsteiner and Levine in 1927 led to the discovery of an antigen called P. The researchers injected human red cells into rabbits and tested the resulting rabbit antibody against human red cells, which they called anti-P. The null phenotype, or p, was reported in 1951 describing an antibody called anti-P.[11] The antigen first described by Landsteiner and Levine was changed to P$_1$. In 1959, a new antigen was reported and called P^k.[12] The LKE (Luke) antigen was described in 1965 and associated with the P system.[13] An antibody called anti-p was later reported in 1972.[14] Four antigens were thus described with a relationship to the P system: P$_1$, P, P^k, and LKE.

As the molecular bases have been discovered, the antigens have been reassigned. The P$_1$ antigen is the single antigen in the P blood group system, while the P antigen is the single antigen in the Globoside blood group system. The P^k and LKE antigens are in the Globoside blood group collection until further information can assign them a system.

Phenotypes of the P and Globoside Blood Group System/Collection

Three antigens (P$_1$, P, and P^k) give rise to five phenotypes listed in Table 11-6. The presence of all three antigens results in the P$_1$ phenotype, which has a frequency of 79% in whites and 94% in blacks. The absence of the P$_1$ antigen results in the P$_2$ phenotype with a frequency of 21% in whites and only 6% in blacks. Of note, Cambodians and Vietnamese individuals have red cells

TABLE 11-6   P/GLOB Blood System and GLOB Blood Collection Antigens and Antibodies

Phenotype	Antigens Present	Antigens Absent	Antibody
P_1	P_1, P, and P^k	None	None
P_2	P and P^k	P_1	Anti-P_1
p	None	P, P_1, and P^k	Anti-P, P_1, and P^k
P_1^k	P_1, P^k	p	Anti-P
P_2^k	P^k	P_1 and P	Anti-P

of the P_2 phenotype with an 80% frequency. The amount of P_1 antigen can vary from person to person.

The p phenotype could be referred to as the null phenotype of both the P and GLOB systems and is rare. These individuals do not carry the P_1, P, and P^k antigens. Anti-P, anti-P_1, and anti-P^k occur as naturally occurring antibodies.

Individuals with the rare P_1^k phenotype have red cells that express the P_1 and P^k antigens. Their cells lack the high-frequency P antigen and they have anti-P in the serum. Another rare phenotype, P_2^k red cells express P^k antigen only. Anti-P and anti-P_1 are present in the serum.

Biochemistry and Genetics

The antigens of the P and Glob systems and Glob collection are carbohydrate epitopes carried on cell membrane glycosphingolipids (GSLs). P-system anti-gens are synthesized by sequential addition of sugars to precursor chains similar to the synthesis of ABH antigens.

Lactosylceramide (CDH) is the common precursor for the different GSLs which are produced as a result of which sugars are added to CDH. See Figure 11-2 for a schematic diagram of the biosynthetic pathways for production of the antigens. There are two structural families into which the antigens are classified. The Globo family comprises the P^k, P, and LKE antigens. In addition, other oligosaccharide structures are built from the P antigen such as NOR1, NOR2, Globo-H, and Gb_5. The P_1 antigen is part of the Neolacto family, but other structural gly-colipids are Lc_3, nLc_4, SPG, X_2, and Sialosyl-X_2. The oligosaccharide structures of each of these vary by the terminal sugars.

The process starts with the synthesis of the P^k anti-gen when a terminal galactose is added to CDH by the action of P^k synthase ($4-\alpha$-galactosyltransferase). The

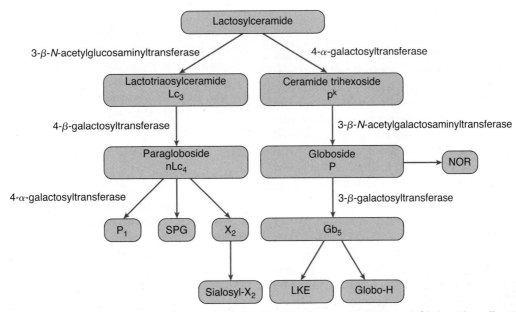

FIGURE 11-2   Biosynthetic pathway for the P and Globoside blood group systems and Globoside collections.

P antigen is formed as a result of P synthase ($3\text{-}\beta\text{-}N$-acetylgalactosaminyltransferase) on the P^k antigen. The polyagglutinable NOR1 phenotype occurs by the addition of a single galactose to P. NOR2 is a disaccharide extension of NOR1.[15] Further action on the P antigen can form Gb5, which is the precursor for structures such as LKE and Globo-H. LKE is the result of a terminal neuraminic acid on Gb5. Globo-H has a fucose added to Gb5.

The P_1 antigen is a member of the Neolacto family or type 2 chain GSLs. A separate pathway starts at CDH to build Lc_3, then paragloboside, and finally P_1. Other structures are also converted from paragloboside such as X_2 and SPG. It is found that the same transferase that adds a terminal galactose to CDH producing the P^k antigen also adds a galactose to paragloboside to form the P_1 antigen.[16] Because of the association, it was thought that there was a genetic association with P_1 and P^k. This hypothesis has been questioned in more recent studies.[17]

The genetic background for P and Globoside is not completely understood at this time. The P antigen is encoded by the *GLOB* gene on chromosome 3. Mutations with this gene can cause either the P_1^k or the P_2^k phenotype when the transferase that makes P from P^k is not produced. The gene encoding the P_1 antigen is not named but is located on chromosome 22. The P^k antigen is encoded by the P^k or $\alpha\text{-}4GAL\text{-}T$ gene on chromosome 22. Mutations occurring in the P^k gene produce the p phenotype. The transferase that converts paragloboside to P_1 also converts lactosylceramide to P^k in a separate pathway.

P Antibodies

Anti-P_1

Anti-P_1 antibodies are often found in P_2 individuals. The antibody can be naturally occurring and reacts as an IgM cold-reacting agglutinin. Anti-P_1 can bind complement. Since it does not usually react above room temperature, it may not be detected in routine pretransfusion testing. The antigen is weakly expressed on cord cells, so the antibody is not associated with HDFN. Rare examples of anti-P_1 have been associated with HTRs. Enzymes enhance reactivity and may cause in vitro hemolysis.

Anti-P

Allo-anti-P can be made by individuals of the P_1^k and P_2^k phenotypes. It is a potent hemolysin and must be considered when selecting blood for transfusion. Since these phenotypes are rare, allo-anti-P is a rare antibody.

Auto-anti-P is associated with an autoimmune hemolytic anemia called paroxysmal cold hemoglobinuria (PCH). Auto-anti-P is sometimes referred to as the Donath-Landsteiner antibody. It is a biphasic antibody that binds to red cells in the reduced temperature of peripheral circulation and activates complement, which leads to severe intravascular hemolysis. The ***Donath-Landsteiner test*** is used to diagnose PCH. The test is performed by preparing three tubes of patient's serum with antigen-positive red cells. One tube is incubated in the cold, a second tube incubated at 37°C, and a third tube incubated first in the cold and then at 37°C. After incubation, the tubes are examined for hemolysis. Because of the biphasic nature of the antibody, only the third tube (incubated in the cold and then at 37°C) shows hemolysis.

Anti-PP_1P^k

This antibody which was once called anti-Tj^a or anti-Jay is found in individuals with the p phenotype. It represents a mixture of anti-P and anti-P_1P^k antibodies. The components are mainly IgG antibodies. Pregnant women with the antibodies experience a higher rate of spontaneous abortions. It is unknown whether the anti-P or the anti-P_1P^k components are involved. Because the P antigens are not well developed on fetuses, the mechanism is not understood. Placental tissue may be involved as it is a rich source of P and P^k antigen and could thus be the target of the antibodies.[18]

Disease Association with P/Globoside

The three antigens (P, P_1, and P^k) act as cellular receptors for uropathogenic *E. coli*. The P^k antigen is a receptor for toxins produced by *S. dysenteriae* and enterohemorrhagic *E. coli*. The P antigen is a receptor for parvo-B19 virus, also known as the agent for fifth disease. Individuals lacking the antigens appear to be naturally resistant to infection from these organisms and viruses.[19]

P_1 Neutralization

As with Lewis, there is commercially available P_1 substance for neutralizing anti-P_1 activity in sample. The test is useful for antibody identification because the anti-P_1 activity is removed, permitting identification of clinically significant antibodies. The substance is incubated with the patient's plasma and tested. A control-substituting saline should be performed in a separate tube.

LUTHERAN BLOOD GROUP SYSTEM (ISBT 005)

History of Lutheran

The Lutheran blood group system was first reported in a patient with lupus who received a series of transfusions and developed a remarkable succession of antibodies.[20] The system is named after the donor of the blood that caused the antibody formation. In 1956, the Lu[b] antigen was described. The first example of blood with the phenotype Lu(a−b−) was noted in 1961. The individual was a noted immunohematologist, Dr. Crawford, who found her own cells to be Lu(a−b−). The Lutheran system gradually expanded when Lu4 was described in 1971. The authors decided at this time to begin numbering the antigens.[21] Lu5, Lu6, Lu7, and Lu8 were then reported in 1972.[22]

The Lutheran system now comprises a set of 19 antigens numbered LU1 to LU21. LU10 and LU15 have been designated obsolete. The most recent antigen, LU21, was reported in 2004.[23]

Lutheran Biochemistry and Genetics

The Lutheran antigens are carried on two type 1 integral membrane glycoproteins present as isomers, the Lu glycoprotein and the epithelial cancer antigen (B-CAM). The Lu glycoprotein is a member of the Ig superfamily and is a receptor for the extracellular matrix protein laminin. Laminin is a major component of basement membranes. The biologic function of the glycoprotein at this time is unclear and individuals of the Lu$_{null}$ phenotype are asymptomatic. However, sickle cells exhibit an increased expression of Lu antigens, which bind increased quantities of laminin and may contribute to vaso-occlusion events in sickle cell patients.[24] The discovery that the location of the laminin-binding site is at the flexible junction of Ig domains 2 and 3 may lead to possible therapies for the disease.[25]

The carrier molecule is a single-pass membrane with five extracellular disulfide-bonded domains. The Lutheran antigens are distributed among the domains. Both forms of the isomer are encoded by the *Lu* gene located on chromosome 19.

Lutheran Antigens

As previously stated, there are 19 antigens associated with the Lutheran system, numbered LU1 through LU21 (LU10 and LU15 are obsolete). There are four pairs of allelic and polymorphic antigens: Lu[a]/Lu[b]/(LU1/LU2), LU6/LU9, LU8/LU14, and Au[a]/Au[b]

TABLE 11-7 Lutheran Blood Group System Phenotypes

Phenotype	Frequency (Most Populations) (%)
Lu(a+b−)	0.2
Lu(a−b+)	92.4
Lu(a+b+)	7.4
Lu(a−b−)	Rare

(LU18/LU19). The remaining antigens are of high incidence. Table 11-7 lists the phenotypes and frequencies for Lu[a] and Lu[b]. Table 11-8 lists the Lutheran antigens with amino acid position and IgSF domain.

Lutheran Null Phenotypes

The Lutheran null phenotype, Lu$_{null}$ or Lu(a−b−) can arise from three circumstances: inheritance of the recessive form, *LuLu*, inheritance of an autosomal suppressor *In(Lu)*, and X-linked. The only true null phenotype is the recessive form in which the Lutheran antigens are not detected by any techniques. The recessive form appears to result from homozygosity for an inactive *LU* gene. These individuals do not produce any Lutheran antigens on their red cells. In three individuals with the characteristics of the Lu$_{null}$ phenotype, each had a Lutheran glycoprotein with a disrupted structure based on nonsense mutations.[26]

The inheritance of an autosomal suppressor gene, *InLu*, is more common compared to the recessive form. The phenotype is associated with reduced red cell surface antigens from several other independent blood group systems, most notably P$_1$ and I. In addition, this phenotype is associated with weakened Lutheran antigens that appear to be missing, but using adsorption and elution techniques, the antigens that are present can be found. The molecular basis for *In(Lu)* has recently been established. The InLu phenotype is most likely caused by inheritance of a loss-of-function mutation on one allele of *EKLF*. EKLF is a transcription factor regulating erythroid differentiation. The inheritance of a single, normal allele and the mutated allele results in reduced levels of EKLF and thus reduced transcription of erythroid genes. Thus, the In(Lu) phenotype results from reduced transcription rather than the action of dominant inhibitor gene.[27]

The X-linked form is very rare and is presumably caused by an X-born inhibitor gene, *XS2*. It is also associated with weakened Lutheran antigen expression, but adsorption and elution studies may indicate the presence of the antigens.

TABLE 11-8   Lutheran Antigens

Name	Incidence	Antithetical Antigen	Amino Acid/Position	IgSF Domain
LU1 (Luᵃ)	Low	LU2 (Luᵇ)	His77	1
LU2 (Luᵇ)	High	LU1 (Luᵃ)	Arg77	1
LU3 (Luᵃᵇ)	High		Unknown	
LU4	High		Arg175	2
LU5	High		Arg109	1
LU6	High	LU9	Ser275	3
LU7	High		Unknown	4
LU8	High	LU14	Met204	2
LU9	Low	LU6	Phe275	3
LU11	High			
LU12	High		Deletion of Arg34 and Leu35	1
LU13	High		Ser447	
Gln 581 transmembrane	5			
LU14	Low	LU8	Lys204	2
LU16	High		Arg227	2
LU17	High		Glu114	1
LU18 (Auᵃ)	80%	LU19 (Auᵇ)	Ala539	5
LU19 (Auᵇ)	50%	LU18 (Auᵃ)	Thr539	5
LU20	High		Thr302	3
LU21	High		Asp94	1

Lutheran Antibodies

Anti-Luᵃ most frequently presents as a cold-reacting agglutinin. It is predominately an IgM antibody, but can have an IgG component. When reacting as an agglutinin, the antibody is noted to react with a mixed field appearance (small clumps in a background of unagglutinated cells). Anti-Luᵇ is also seen as a cold-reacting agglutinin, but more frequently at IAT than anti-Luᵃ. Because the Lutheran antigens are poorly developed at birth, the incidence of HDFN is rare and only of mild form when present. There are reports of mild transfusion reactions to anti-Luᵇ. The individual that is truly Lu(a−b−) may produce anti-Lu3.

KELL BLOOD GROUP SYSTEM (ISBT 006)

History

In 1946, the newly introduced antiglobulin test was used to investigate a case of HDFN that could not be attributed to Rh. As a result, the K antigen was first described in a woman named Mrs. Kelleher and the system was called Kell.[28] The antithetical antigen was later found by Levine et al. in 1949 during the investigation of a mild case of HDFN. This high-incidence antigen was named Cellano and linked to the K antigen.[29] It was not until 1957 that the system began to expand with the discovery of the antithetical antigens, Kp^a and Kp^b as well as K_0 (Kell$_{null}$).[30-32] The antigen Js^a was described in 1958 named after the producer of the antibody, John Sutter. The antithetical antigen, Js^b was found in 1963 in a Memphis female who made the corresponding antibody.[33,34] The Js^a and Js^b antigens were added to the Kell system in 1965. There are two other pairs of antithetical antigens in the system. K11, a high-incidence antigen first reported in 1971 is antithetical to K17 (also called Wk^a), a low-incidence antigen first described in 1974.[35] The Kp^c antigen (initially called Levay in 1946 and considered to be a low-incidence antigen) joined the Kell system in 1979.[36-38] K14, another antigen of high incidence first described in 1973 has the low-incidence antithetical antigen, K24 found in 1985. The Kell system now includes 24 antigens. The ISBT numbering is not sequential as some antigens are now obsolete.

Biochemistry and Genetics

The Kell antigens are located on a single-pass type II glycoprotein with the N-terminal 47 amino acids in the cytoplasmic region.[39] The transmembrane domain contains 20 amino acids. The large extracellular C-terminal area has 665 amino acids and contains 15 cysteine residues that suggest multiple disulphide bonds and folding of the protein. The structure of the Kell protein suggests a sequence homology with a family of zinc-binding endopeptidases and is an endothelin-3–converting enzyme. Endothelins are involved in the regulation of vascular tone, but absence of the Kell glycoprotein does not result in red cell abnormalities. The K_0 or null phenotype can be caused by several different genetic defects that lead to truncation of the protein and is very rare.[40] The Kell$_{mod}$ phenotype results in weak expression of Kell antigens and is not well understood at this time.

The glycoprotein is covalently linked by a disulfide bond at Cys72 of KELL to Cys347 of the XK glycoprotein. The *XK* gene is located on the short arm of the X chromosome. Point mutations in the gene result in the absence or reduction of the XK protein called the McLeod phenotype. There are several types of mutations that lead to the McLeod phenotype.[41] Regardless of the type of mutation, they all lead to weak expression of Kell antigens and a truncated, lacking, or aberrant Kx glycoprotein.[42]

The *KEL* gene consists of 19 exons and is located on chromosome 7q33.[43,44] The different Kell system antigens are the result of nucleotide mutations causing single amino acid substitutions, the glycoprotein. The *Kell* complex might be expected to produce haplotypes of various combinations of the antithetical antigens. However, this has not been shown to be the case. The production of more than one of the low-incidence antigens in a haplotype has not been found. The hap-

TABLE 11-9	Kell Blood Group System Phenotypes and Frequencies (%)	
Phenotype	Whites	Blacks
K−k+	91	98
K+k+	8.8	2
K+k−	0.2	Rare
Kp(a−b+)	97.7	100
Kp(a+b+)	2.3	Rare
Kp(a+b−)	Rare	0
Js(a−b+)	100	80
Js(a+b+)	Rare	19
Js(a+b−)	0	1

lotype that makes K always makes Kp^b, Js^b, and K11 and never makes Kp^a, Kp^c, Js^a, or Wk^a. Consequently, the haplotype that makes Kp^a always makes k, Js^b, and K11, but never K, Js^a, or Wk^a.[3] It is not clear why this occurs, but has been suggested that the low-incidence antigens representing a single mutation are rare as it is and a double mutation to express two low-incidence antigens would be extremely rare.

The Kell System Antigens

Kell is a complex system containing 24 antigens described to date. There are five sets of alleles expressing high- and low-frequency antigens as well as at least 14 other independent antigens. Table 11-9 lists the common Kell system phenotypes and frequencies. Kell antigens show variation in different populations. The K antigen occurs in 9% of whites but only 2% of blacks. The Kp^a antigen has a frequency of 2% in whites but is rare in blacks. The Kp^c antigen may be found in about 0.2% of Japanese and is rare in other groups. The Js^a antigen can occur in up to 20% of blacks but rarely in whites. The Ul^a antigen is a low-incidence antigen, but is noted in 2.6% of Finns and 0.46% of Japanese. The rest of the antigens are either of high incidence or low incidence. The Ku antigen represents the "total Kell" antigen and individuals that lack Ku are considered to be K null.

The molecular basis for the antigens has been determined.[40] Table 11-10 lists the ISBT and common nomenclatures, frequencies, and amino acid substitutions for the Kell system antigens. Some of the mutations cause changes in the carrier molecule. The amino acid substitution for the KEL1 antigen disrupts an *N*-glycosylation site resulting in four instead of five

TABLE 11-10 Kell Blood Group System Antigens and Amino Acid Substitutions

ISBT	Antigen	Other Names	Incidence	Amino Acid Substitution	Comments
KEL1	K	Kell/Kelleher	Low	Methionine at 193	Antithetical to k
KEL2	k	Cellano	High	Threonine at 193	Antithetical to K
KEL3	Kp^a	Penney	Low	Tryptophan at 281	Antithetical to Kp^b and Kp^c
KEL4	Kp^b	Rautenberg	High	Arginine at 281	Antithetical to Kp^a and Kp^c
KEL5	Ku	Peltz/K$_o$	High		Missing on K$_0$
KEL6	Js^a	Sutter	Low	Proline at 597	Antithetical to Js^b
KEL7	Js^b	Matthews	High	Leucine at 597	Antithetical to Js^a
KEL10	Ul^a	Karhula	Low	Glutamic acid → Valine at 494	
KEL11		Côté	High	Valine at 302	Antithetical to K17
KEL12		Bockman	High	Histidine → Arginine at 548	
KEL13		SGRO	High	Leucine → Proline at 329	
KEL14		Santini	High	Arginine at 180	Antithetical to K24
KEL16	k-like		High		
KEL17	Wk^a	Weeks	Low	Alanine at 302	Antithetical to K11
KEL18		Marshall	High	Arginine → Tryptophan or Glutamine at 130	
KEL19		Sublett	High	Arginine → Glutamine at 492	
KEL20	Km	MacLeod	High		Missing on K$_0$
KEL21	Kp^c	Levay	Low	Glutamine at 281	Antithetical to Kp^a and Kp^b
KEL22	NI	Ikar	High	Alanine → Valine at 322	
KEL23		Centauro	Low	Glutamine → Arginine at 382	
KEL24	Cls	Callais	Low	Proline at 180	Antithetical to K14
KEL25	VLAN		Low	Arginine → Glutamine at 248	
KEL26	TOU		High	Arginine → Glutamine at 406	
KEL27	RAZ		High	Glutamic acid → Lysine at 249	

N-linked oligosaccharides. The proline at 597 for Js^a may cause structural changes by introducing kinks.

The K$_0$ or Kell$_{null}$ phenotype lacks the entire Kell glycoprotein and thus all Kell antigens, but the red cells express larger amounts of the Kx antigen, an antigen in the Kx blood group. The red cell morphology in individuals with the K$_0$ phenotype is normal.

There are conditions where Kell antigens are expressed weakly due to inherited or acquired and transient conditions. When the XK glycoprotein is absent, the condition is known as the McLeod phenotype. The phenotype is characterized by absence of the Kx antigen, weakened expression of Kell system antigens, acanthocytes, and has an X-linked inheritance. In addition, individuals have elevated levels of serum creatine phosphokinase. There are other symptoms associated with the McLeod phenotype that are variable, such as muscular myopathy and neuropathy usually occurring later in life. It is possible that the type of mutation causing the phenotype may be responsible for the degree of myopathy and neuropathy. The Kell antigens may be so weak that adsorption–elution studies are necessary to demonstrate their presence.

Chronic Granulomatous Disease

Chronic granulomatous disease (CGD) is an inherited disorder characterized by a predisposition to severe bacterial and fungal infections. The ability of polymorphonuclear leukocytes to phagocytize certain microorganisms is impaired due to a granulocytic enzyme defect.[45] Some individuals with CGD also have the McLeod phenotype. Other X-linked inherited disorders are retinitis pigmentosa (RP) and Duchenne-type muscular dystrophy (DMD). The genes responsible for the various disorders appear to be located very close to each other on the X chromosome. In at least one patient, a minor Xp21 deletion caused all the disorders to manifest.[46] Partial deletions of the X chromosome may be responsible for the type of disorder.

Other findings are associated with weakened Kell antigens. The effect of Kp^a in a *cis* position results in weakened high-incidence Kell antigens. Although the Gerbich blood system is independent of the Kell system, some Gerbich (Ge:$-2,-3$) and Leach (Ge:$-2,-3,-4$) phenotypes have weakened Kell antigen expression (see Table 11-11). It is speculated that the product of exon 3 of GYPC somehow alters the availability of antigens on the Kell glycoprotein. A K$_{mod}$ phenotype has been described that also results in weakened high-incidence Kell antigens. Different point mutations causing amino acid substitutions and possibly altering the glycoprotein configuration could inhibit transport of Kell proteins to the cell surface.[47]

Kell System Antibodies

After ABO and Rh, the K antigen is the most immunogenic blood group antigen causing both hemolytic disease of the newborn and immediate and delayed HTRs. The antibody is usually IgG and predominantly IgG1. Patients with antibodies to the Kell blood group system should receive antigen-negative blood.

The antibody reacts best at the antiglobulin phase, but there are examples of direct agglutinating antibodies.

There are reports of "naturally occurring" anti-K1 as a result of microbial infections. In one case of mycobacterium infection, the antibody showed agglutination with K:1 red cells at room temperature, but not at the antiglobulin phase. Testing the sample with 2-mercaptoethanol showed the antibody to be IgM. These "naturally occurring" antibodies were no longer detectable when the infections cleared.[48–50] There are other reports of naturally occurring anti-K1 in the serum of individuals who had not had red cell stimulation. These antibodies reacted at 4°C and 22°C, but were negative at 37°C and IAT.[51,52]

Anti-K does appear to be less severe in cases of HDFN than anti-D. The K antigen appears on fetal red cells earlier than Rh proteins. Consequently, the anti-K facilitates phagocytosis at an earlier stage before the cells produce hemoglobin. The anemia may be severe because anti-K causes a suppression of erythropoiesis rather than the immune destruction that occurs with anti-D.[53]

Anti-k is usually reported as an alloantibody, although it is not a common antibody since most individuals are k+. As with anti-K, anti-k has been found as a direct agglutinating antibody, though it tends to be IgG in nature. The antibody has been implicated in both severe and mild forms of HDFN and HTR.

Antibodies to Kp^a, Kp^b, Kp^c, Js^a, and Js^b are also encountered and in these cases, race should be considered when identifying the antibodies. The Kp^a antigen is only found in whites and Kp^c is only found in Asians. Both Kp^a and Kp^c are low-incidence antigens, so the majority of individuals will be Kp(a$-$b$+$c$-$). The Js^a antigen is more common in blacks than the Kp^a antigen is in whites or Kp^c in Asians.

Immunized individuals who lack Kell antigens make an antibody called anti-Ku (K for Kell and u for universal). In addition, their serum may contain antibodies to other high-incidence Kell antigens.

LEWIS BLOOD GROUP SYSTEM (ISBT 007)

History

The Lewis blood group was discovered in 1946 and named after one of the two original donors in whom anti-Le^a was identified.[54] Le^b was described in 1948.[55]

Lewis Antigens

There are six antigens assigned to the Lewis system. The two main antigens are Le^a and Le^b, which lead to phenotypes Le(a+b$-$), Le(a$-$b+), Le(a$-$b$-$), and

TABLE 11-11	Gerbich Antigens		
Phenotype Name	Historical Name	Frequency	Antibody
Ge:2,3,4	Gerbich positive	>99.9%	NA
Ge:-2,3,4	Yus type	<0.1%	Anti-Ge2
Ge:-2,-3,4	Ge type	<0.1%	Anti-Ge2 or Ge3
Ge:-2, -3,-4	Leach type (null)	Very rare	Anti-Ge2, $-$Ge3, or $-$Ge4

TABLE 11-12	Lewis Blood Group Frequencies (%)		
Phenotype	White	Black	Asians
Le(a+b−)	22	23	0.2
Le(a−b+)	72	55	73
Le(a−b−)	6	22	10
Le(a+b+)	Rare	Rare	10–40

Le(a+b+). The frequency of distribution is listed in Table 11-12. The Le(a+b+) phenotype is very rare, but can be seen in young children and some individuals of Asian descent. The expression of the antigens is a result of two separate, independent genes (*Le* and *Se*) and is discussed further in the chapter. In a nonsecretor, the *Le* gene produces an enzyme that fucosylates a type 1 chain to make the Le^a antigen. An individual with the *Le* gene, who is a secretor, produces an enzyme that fucosylates a type 1 H chain to make the Le^b antigen.

The Le^{ab} antigen is another antigen of the Lewis system. It originally was referred to as Le^x, but was reassigned to its current name by ISBT in 1998. The antigen is on all red cells that are Le(a+b−) and Le(a−b+) and 90% of cord cells. Even though cord samples type as Le(a−b−), they demonstrate reactivity if they have the *Le* gene. It is thought that the binding site for Le^{ab} is at the α1→4 binding site between GlcNAc and fucose.

Another antigen in the system is Le^{bH}. It was originally thought to be Le^b, but named Le^{bH} in 1959 and allocated an ISBT number in 1998. It is present on group O and A$_2$ Le(b+) red cells.

The last two antigens of the Lewis system are ALe^b and BLe^b. The first, ALe^b is found on all A$_1$ Le(b+) and A$_1$B Le(b+) individuals. The second, BLe^b is found on all B Le(b+) and A$_1$B Le(b+) red cells. That is to say that these are group A$_1$, B, or A$_1$B individuals having *FUT2* (*Se*) and *FUT3* (*Le*) genes. The molecular basis for these antigens is the same as for Le^b with the addition of the blood group determinations.

Antigen Development

Lewis antigens are not well developed at birth and most infants will type as Le(a−b−). If more sensitive techniques are used, infant samples may test as Le(a+).[56] Several studies have indicated a lower amount of the *Se* gene–specified transferase and a higher amount of the *Le* gene–specified transferase in infants who have both the *Se* and *Le* genes. Thus, the Le^a specificity is added to type 1 chains before the *Se* gene acts to make the type 1 H chains leading to the development of the Le^b antigen. As time continues, the *Se* gene–specified transferase increases, and by about 1 year of age, the type 1 H chains

are starting to be produced. At this time, the phenotype Le(a+b+) may be common until 2 to 3 years of age when the levels approach adult levels and the Lewis phenotype will be clear.[3]

Biochemistry and Genetics

The antigens of the Lewis system are not synthesized on red cells, but are absorbed from the plasma. The Lewis antigens are derived from a type 1 oligosaccharide chain. The terminal disaccharide unit carries the carbohydrate residues that determine the Lewis properties. Lewis antigens are found in both plasma and secretions such as saliva. The Lewis antigens are carried on type 1 oligosaccharide chains bound through D-glucose to sphingolipids in plasma producing a GSL. But in the saliva, the antigens are carried on the same oligosaccharides but are bound through N-acetyl-D-galactosamine to proteins, producing a glycoprotein.[57] The Lewis substances on type 1 chains in plasma and in secretions are identical, but the carrier molecule is different. It is the GSL that is inserted on the red cell membrane and thus is of plasma origin.

The biosynthesis of Lewis antigens results from interactions of two independent genes at different loci: *Se (FUT2)* and *Le (FUT3)*. *FUT2* enables the A, B, and H antigens to be secreted by coding for the production of the enzyme, α1-2 fucosyltransferase. This enzyme is responsible for adding an α-1 → 2 fucose to the subterminal galactose residue on type 1 chains, forming type 1 H chains in secretions. The inheritance of at least one *FUT2 (SeSe or Sese)* gene permits expression of soluble ABH antigens in secretions. If two recessive alleles (*sese*) are inherited, the A, B, and H antigens are not secreted. Several types of nonsense mutations cause a stop codon that truncates the enzymatically active domain of the fucosyltransferase, resulting in nonsecretion. *FUT3* is responsible for the presence of Lewis antigens. The product of *FUT3* is an α-1 → 4 fucosyltransferase that adds fucose to the subterminal N-acetylglucosamine residue. The term *le* denotes the absence of the *Le (FUT3)* gene. The inheritance of these two genes (*FUT2* and *FUT3*) determines the Lewis antigen expression. Table 11-13 lists the effect of gene interactions on Lewis antigen expression.

The Le^a antigen is characterized by α-1 → 4 fucose attachment to the subterminal N-acetylglucosamine residue. The Le^b antigen is determined by the same α-1 → 4 fucose attachment to the subterminal N-acetylglucosamine (like the Le^a antigen) with the addition of the H determinant, the α-1 → 2 fucose attached to the terminal galactose residue. Thus, the combination of Lewis and *secretor status* determines whether Le^a or Le^b is expressed on the red cells and whether Le^a or both Le^a and Le^b are expressed in the

TABLE 11-13	Effect of Gene Interactions on Lewis Antigen Expression		
Genes Present	Lewis Phenotype	Antigen in Plasma/ Secretions	Lewis Antigen on Red Cells
Le sese	Le(a+b−)	Le^a	Le^a
Le Se	Le(a−b+)	Le^b	Le^a, Le^b
lele sese	Le(a−b−)	None	None
lele Se	Le(a−b−)	None	None

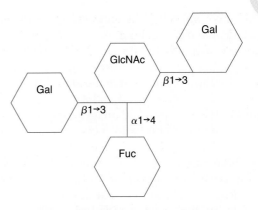

Le^a structure (*sese* gene with *Le* gene)

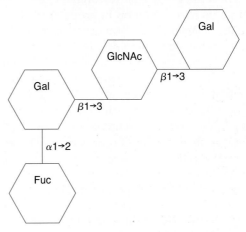

H type 1 chain (*Se* gene)

plasma and secretions. Since the Lewis antigens are assembled in the plasma, if an *Le* gene is present, some type of Lewis antigen will be present in the secretions and plasma regardless of the secretor status. So although the secretor status determines if A, B, or H antigens are present in secretions and plasma, it also determines which Lewis antigen is present. When the recessive *sese* gene is present with *Le*, Le^a is expressed on the red cells and is present in the plasma and secretions. When *Se(FUT2)* is present with *Le*, Le^b is expressed on the red cells and Le^a and Le^b are present in the plasma and secretions. See Figure 11-3 for a depiction of the structures.

Individuals who have the *lele* genotype do not produce Le^a or Le^b antigens regardless of the other genes present. The red cells have a phenotype of Le(a−b−) and there are no Lewis antigens in the plasma or secretions. There are several types of nucleotide changes in the *FUT3* gene that code for amino acid changes, causing an inactivation of the fucosyltransferase.

A weak secretor gene (*Se^w*) has also been described that leads to the Le(a+b+) phenotype in some individuals of Asian descent.[58] The nucleotide mutation leads to an amino acid change of isoleucine to phenylalanine at position 129 in the fucosyltransferase. This causes a reduction of activity in the enzyme, leading to partial secretion and thus both Le^a and Le^b antigen absorption on the red cell.

Group A$_1$ and B individuals can have further modifications because of the ABO glycosyltransferases that form ALe^b, BLe^b, type 1 A, and type 1 B antigens.

Lewis Antibodies

Anti-Le^a

Anti-Le^a is a common antibody that can be naturally occurring or immune stimulated. Individuals who have the Le(a−b+) phenotype secrete Le^a antigen in their plasma and have a small amount on their red cells and thus do not usually make anti-Le^a. It occurs

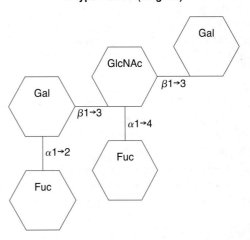

FIGURE 11-3 Lewis structures—Le^a, H type 1 chain, and Le^b structure (*Se* gene with *Le* gene).

almost exclusively in individuals whose red cells type as Le(a−b−). Anti-Le^a is often found with anti-Le^b.

There have been a few examples of anti-Le^a made by persons with the Le(a−b+) phenotype. In one, the patient had a squamous cell carcinoma of the esophagus. Although the saliva contained Le^a, Le^b, and H substances, the Le^b antigen content of his red cells was half that of control cells. The antibody was described as being an autoantibody because it did not react with the patient's own cells, but it was inhibited by his own saliva. It is thought that the disease process was responsible for the development of the antibody.[59] Other examples have been described and it was determined that none of the examples had an IgG component.[60]

There are other observations concerning anti-Le^a in Le(a−b−) individuals that have not been fully explained. Some researchers have described that secretor status affects the ability of individuals to make anti-Le^a. Miller et al. noticed that anti-Le^a is usually made by individuals with the *lele* and *Se* gene combination.[61] Several groups of researchers have noted that anti-Le^a is more common in group A, B, and AB individuals. When anti-Le^a is made by group O individuals, it often occurs with anti-Le^b.[61,62]

Most examples of anti-Le^a are clinically insignificant because they react best at room temperature and do not bind to Le(a+) red cells at 37°C. The antibody is usually IgM in nature, although examples of anti-Le^a have been found that have an IgG component. The IgM form of the antibody can bind complement. The use of enzyme-treated cells enhances reactivity and hemolysis is sometimes noted. Soluble Le^a antigen can be used to neutralize the antibody to permit detection of other clinically significant antibodies.

Anti-Le^a is not associated with HDFN for two reasons. The antibody is often IgM and does not cross the placenta and also because the antigen is not present on fetal cells. There have been some examples of IgG anti-Le^a that crossed the placenta, but HDFN did not occur presumably because of the low levels of Le^a antigen on fetal red cells.[63] There have been some reports of anti-Le^a causing in vivo destruction of transfused red cells.[64-66]

Anti-Le^b

Anti-Le^b is also a common antibody occurring with weak reactivity in the sera of individuals with the Le(a−b−) phenotype, who have made a potent anti-Le^a. It also occurs on its own in people who are *lele* and *sese* genetically. It is thought that those individuals who are *lele* and *Se* genetically already make a type 1 H chain and this is similar enough to Le^b so that the antibody is generally not made. The antibody is also made by individuals with the Le(a+b−) phenotype because they do not have Le^b substance in their plasma or saliva.

There are two forms of anti-Le^b described. Anti-Le^{bH} reacts with Le(b+) cells that are group O and A$_2$, but not group A$_1$ or B cells. It can be neutralized by saliva that contains H or H and Le^b. Anti-Le^{bL} reacts with Le(a−b+) red cells regardless of the ABO type and is inhibited by saliva that contains H and Le^b, but not by saliva that contains H only.

Anti-Le^b is typically an IgM, room temperature–reacting agglutinin that also can bind complement. The use of enzyme-treated cells enhances reactivity and the antibody can be neutralized with soluble Le^b substance.

Other Lewis System Antibodies

Anti-Le^{ab} is a fairly common antibody frequently found with anti-Le^a and/or anti-Le^b. It occurs mainly in individuals who are secretors and blood groups A$_1$, B, or A$_1$B. Anti-Le^{bH} is predominately a room temperature–agglutinating IgM antibody that can cause complement binding. Anti-ALe^b acts as single specificity that cannot be separated from anti-A and anti-Le^b. The same holds true for BLe^b.

Lewis Antigens and Antibodies in Pregnancy

Lewis antigens are much weaker in pregnancy, and some females of the Le(a−b+) phenotype may lose Le^b altogether during pregnancy. In pregnancy, the ratio of lipoprotein to red cell mass increases more than fourfold. More of the available Le^b-active glycolipid is attached to lipoprotein and less is attached to GSLs (which attach to the red cell). These individuals with a transient phenotype of Le(a−b−) may even produce anti-Le^b. The antibody disappears once delivery occurs and the normal Lewis phenotype is restored.

Clinical Significance of Lewis System Antibodies

The antibodies of the Lewis system are rarely involved in either HDFN or HTRs. Although there are reports of anti-Le^a causing an HTR or anti-Le^b causing in vivo destruction of Le(b+) red cells, the majority are incapable of causing problems. The main reason is that the antibodies are unable to complex with red cells at 37°C. Since the antibodies are usually IgM, they do not cross the placenta. In addition, the Lewis antigens are poorly developed at birth, so that even if an IgG antibody did cross the placenta, it is not likely to cause harm.

In those individuals in whom the antibody appears to be able to cause destruction of antigen-positive red cells, it is usually not necessary to look for antigen-negative blood. Routine compatibility testing at 37°C followed by IAT should suffice to find compatible blood. People with a history of Lewis antibodies that are currently not showing reactivity can even have an immediate spin or computer crossmatch performed.

Phenotype	Genotype: Whites	Genotype: Blacks	Whites	Blacks
Fy(a+b−)	FY*A/FY*A	FY*A/FY*A or FY*A/FY*Fy	20	9
Fy(a+b+)	FY*A/FY*B	FY*A/FY*B	47	1
Fy(a−b+)	FY*B/FY*B	FY*B/FY*B or FY*B/FY*Fy	33	22
Fy(a−b−)	FY*amorph	FY*Fy/FY*Fy	Very rare	68

TABLE 11-14 Duffy Blood Group Genotypes and Phenotype Frequencies (%)

DUFFY BLOOD GROUP SYSTEM (ISBT 008)

History

The Duffy blood group was first described in 1950 by Cutbush et al.[67] in a multiply transfused hemophiliac who made the corresponding antibody to the antigen that was called Fy[a]. The system was named after the patient, Mr. Duffy, using the last two letters in his name for the abbreviation. At the time, an antithetical antigen was predicted and named Fy[b].[68] In 1951, Ikin et al. described anti-Fy[b] in the serum of Mrs. Hahn following the birth of her third child.[69] In 1955, Sanger reported the phenotype Fy(a−b−) in American blacks in which a third allele that is silent was also part of the system.[70] A new allele, Fy[x], was described in 1965 by Chown that appeared to produce an antigen that reacted weakly with selected anti-Fy[b] sera.[71] In 1971, the antigen Fy3 was reported when the corresponding antibody was found in a white Australian woman who had been transfused and was pregnant. The antibody reacted with all Fy(a+b−), Fy(a+b+), and Fy(a−b+) red cells but not with Fy(a−b−).[72] The antigens Fy4 and Fy5 were reported in 1973.[73,74] Fy6 was added to the system in 1987.[75]

Biochemistry and Genetics

The Duffy system is made up of six antigens that reside on an acidic glycoprotein encoded by the *DARC* gene located on chromosome 1. The glycoprotein spans the membrane seven times with the N-terminus in the extracellular region and the C-terminus intracellular. The carrier molecule, also known as the Duffy antigen receptor for chemokines (DARC) functions as a cytokine/*Plasmodium vivax* receptor. It binds a variety of proinflammatory cytokines playing a role in recruitment of leukocytes to sites of inflammation. The Duffy glycoprotein is also a receptor for the malaria parasite, *P. vivax*.

The two main alleles *FY*A* and *FY*B* encode the principle antigens, Fy[a] and Fy[b], which are antithetical and codominant. The glycoprotein is the same except

for a single amino acid substitution from glycine for the Fy[a] antigen to aspartic acid for Fy[b]. A third allele, *FY*Fy*, encodes no antigen on the red cells that results in the phenotype Fy(a−b−). The fourth allele, *FY*X*, is responsible for a weakened form of Fy[b] expression. Table 11-14 lists the frequency of the phenotypes of the Fy[a] and Fy[b] antigens.

The null phenotype Fy(a−b−) is rare in Caucasians, but common in blacks. For many years, it was thought that the null phenotype was the result of an inheritance of two Fy genes that encoded no production of Fy[a] or Fy[b]. But Blacks whose red cells test Fy(a−b−) have genes that are identical to Fy[b] in the region that encodes production of the Fy[b] antigen; yet the antigen is not expressed on their red cells. However, the antigen is expressed normally on their tissue cells. It is now known that most blacks carry an *FYB* allele with a single nucleotide substitution (T to C at −46). This mutation impairs the promoter activity in red cells by disrupting a binding site for the GATA1 erythroid transcription factor.[76] So although they do not carry the Duffy glycoprotein on their red cells, it is found on their tissues. Although these individuals may make anti-Fy[a], they do not make anti-Fy[b].

Another very rare form of the null phenotype is caused by nonsense mutations in the coding sequence of either *FY*A* or *FY*B*. The mutated genes have premature stop codons that cause the Duffy glycoproteins to truncate and they are not present on the cell surface nor are they on the tissues.[77] These individuals can make anti-Fy[b] as well as anti-Fy3.

The Fy[x] phenotype (*FY*X*) arises from an arginine to cystine substitution at position 89 in the first cytoplasmic loop, which leads to protein instability and weak expression of the Fy[b] antigen.[78]

The High-incidence Antigens: Fy3, Fy4, Fy5, and Fy6 and their Antibodies

The Fy3 antigen is present on all red cells except those of the Fy(a−b−) phenotype. Although initially, it appeared that this might compound antibody to Fy[a] and Fy[b], it was unusual in that the antigen was resistant to enzymes unlike other Duffy antigens that are sensitive. The occurrence of the antigen nears 100% in Caucasians and Asians, but is only 32% in blacks.

The Fy4 antigen is a high-incidence antigen produced by the majority of the population. In individuals with the Fy(a−b−) phenotype, blacks carry the Fy4 antigen, but whites with the rare Fy(a−b−) phenotype do not carry it. The antigen is not destroyed by enzymes. The Fy5 antigen is another high-incidence antigen that is not found only on Rh$_{null}$ cells. The Fy6 antigen is present on all cells except those of the Fy(a−b−) phenotype, but it is destroyed by enzymes.

Duffy Antigens and Malaria

The Duffy glycoprotein is a receptor for *P. vivax*, one of the parasites responsible for malaria infection. Studies have shown that the merozoites are able to bind to Fy(a−b−) red cells, but are unable to invade the cells. This Fy allele would be advantageous in areas where *P. vivax* is endemic. Although the red cells lack chemokine receptors when the Duffy glycoprotein is missing, the built-in resistance to malaria infection would be helpful. Additionally, the tissues would still carry the glycoprotein and could possibly function as needed.

Duffy Antibodies

Anti-Fy^a is a relatively common antibody, while anti-Fy^b is less common. They are IgG antibodies, reacting at IAT. They rarely cause complement binding. Duffy antibodies are associated with mild to severe HTRs and HDFN. The Fy^a and Fy^b antigens are sensitive to ficin and papain. The antigens are expressed on cord cells.

Anti-Fy3 is very rare. It mimics a combination anti-Fy^a and anti-Fy^b in that it reacts with both Fy(a+b−) and Fy(a−b+) cells, but Fy3 is resistant to ficin/papain. Anti-Fy3 from whites reacts strongly with cord cells that are Fy positive, but anti-Fy3 from blacks reacts weakly or not at all.[79] Mild HDFN has been attributed to anti-Fy3.[80]

Anti-Fy5 reacts with Fy(a+) or Fy(b+) and white Fy(a−b−) red cells, but not black Fy(a−b−) red cells. It was originally thought to be anti-Fy3 when first reported, but further investigation revealed that it did not react with Rh$_{null}$ cells.

KIDD BLOOD GROUP SYSTEM (ISBT 009)

The Kidd blood group system is a relatively straightforward system with only three antigens. The antibody to Jk^a was first described in 1951 in the serum of Mrs. Kidd, whose infant suffered from HDFN.[81] The first example of the antibody to Jk^b was reported in 1953.[82] The phenotype Jk(a−b−) was later described in 1959 when a patient had a transfusion reaction after four units of blood.[83]

Biochemistry and Genetics

The Kidd antigens are located on a multipass glycoprotein that spans the membrane 10 times. Both the C- and N-termini are contained in cytoplasm. The glycoprotein is involved in urea transport in the red cell.[84] It transports urea into and out of red cells as they pass through the high urea concentration in the renal medulla. A urea transport deficiency exists in Jk(a−b−) individuals.[85] They do not suffer a clinical syndrome, but they are unable to concentrate their urine.

The expression of Kidd antigens is controlled by the *HUT 11* gene with three alleles, *Jk^a*, *Jk^b*, and the **silent allele** *Jk*. The polymorphism of the two antigens is caused by a single nucleotide mutation that has aspartic acid for Jk^a and asparagine for Jk^b at residue 280 on the fourth extracellular loop. The Jk(a−b−) phenotype has several mutations found in various ethnic groups. The Kidd gene has been assigned to chromosome 18.[86]

Kidd Antigens

Two antigens, Jk^a and Jk^b, are responsible for the common phenotypes. The phenotypes and their frequencies are listed in Table 11-15. The red cells of Jk(a−b−) individuals are unique in their resistance toward lysis in 2 M urea.[87]

Kidd Antibodies

Kidd antibodies are stimulated by pregnancy and blood transfusion, although they are not particularly immunogenic. Anti-Jk^a is often found with other specificities, but anti-Jk^b is usually found with other

TABLE 11-15	Kidd Blood Group Phenotypes and Frequencies		
	Frequency (%)		
Phenotype	Whites	Blacks	Asians
Jk(a+b−)	26.3	51.1	23.2
Jk(a−b+)	23.4	8.1	26.8
Jk(a+b+)	50.3	40.8	49.1
Jk(a−b−)	Rare	Rare	0.9 (Polynesian)

antibodies. They are often weakly reacting IgG antibodies showing dosage. Reactivity is enhanced with enzymes. They bind complement and may be more readily detectable if polyspecific antiglobulin reagent is used instead of anti-IgG reagent. Some examples have been known to be agglutinating. Kidd antibodies are notorious for weakening over time and even becoming undetectable. When pretransfusion testing is performed, the antibody may not be found.

Despite this, they cause severe delayed HTRs. Patients needing transfusions should receive antigen-negative blood. Anti-Jk[a], anti-Jk[b], and anti-Jk3 have been implicated in HDN, but it is usually mild even though they are IgG, bind complement, and the antigens are well developed on fetal cells.

DIEGO BLOOD GROUP SYSTEM (ISBT 010)

The Diego blood group was first described in 1955 in a case of HDFN and named after Mrs. Diego, the person who made the antibody to the low-incidence antigen Di[a]. The antithetical antigen Di[b] was described in 1967. In 1953, a low-incidence antigen named Wr[a] was found, but the association with the Diego blood system was not apparent. The Diego system has implications in population genetics because the Di[a] antigen is found in people of Mongolian descent.

Biochemistry and Genetics

The *SLC4A* gene, located on chromosome 17, contains 20 exons. The Diego protein is a transmembrane glycoprotein spanning the membrane 14 times. The protein accounts for 25% of total red cell protein. Only GPA rivals this in abundance. The Diego antigens are carried on the erythroid band 3 protein (anion exchange 1 or AE1).[88] The long N-terminus is in the cytoplasmic region and functions as an anchor point for the membrane skeleton through interaction with peripheral membrane proteins. It also serves as a binding site for hemoglobin and glycolytic enzymes. The C-terminus is cytoplasmic and binds carbonic anhydrase II (CAII).[89] One of the major functions of blood is to transport respiratory gases (oxygen to the tissues and carbon dioxide to the lungs). Carbon dioxide is hydrated to bicarbonate by CAII. Band 3 acts as ion exchanger that permits bicarbonate ions to cross the membrane in exchange for chloride ions. Band 3 deficiency results in membrane surface area loss and the generation of spherocytic red cells. The genetic background to the polymorphisms is a single-nucleotide change in the band 3 gene that gives rise to an amino

TABLE 11-16   Di[a]/Di[b] Phenotype Frequencies

Phenotypes	Caucasians/Blacks	Asians/South American Indians
Di(a−b+)	>99.9%	64−90%
Di(a+b+)	Rare	10−36%
Di(a+b−)	Very rare	Rare

acid substitution. In addition, for at least the Wr[b] antigen, an interaction of the band 3 protein and GPA is required for expression.

Di[a] and Di[b]

There are 21 antigens associated with the system. The first antigens described were the low-incidence antigen, Di[a] and the antithetical high-incidence antigen, Di[b]. The Di[a] antigen is very rare except in Chinese, Japanese, and native peoples of North and South America where it can approach 54% frequency. The Di[a] and Di[b] antigens are located on the seventh extracellular loop of band 3. The single amino acid substitution changes from leucine for Di[a] at position 854 to proline for Di[b]. Table 11-16 displays the frequencies of Di[a] and Di[b] antigens.

Wr[a] and Wr[b]

A new antibody responsible for a fatal case of HDFN was first described by Holman in 1953.[90] The low-incidence antigen, Wr[a], was named after the antibody maker, Mrs. Wright. Further examples of anti-Wr[a] causing severe transfusion reactions appeared shortly after. The high-incidence antibody defining Wr[b] was discovered in 1971 in the serum of a woman who was positive for the low-incidence Wr[a] antigen.[91] Her antibody was provisionally called anti-Wr[b]. The antigens were poorly understood for many years. In 1988, the antigens were proven to be antithetical to each other.[92] Early serologic studies initially showed an association with GPA, the glycoprotein that carries the MNS system antigens. Wr[b] expression is dependent on the presence of GPA. En(a−) cells, which lack GPA, type as Wr(a−b−). Other GPA variants are also associated with the lack of expression of Wr[b]. Later, two individuals with the phenotype En(a+) Wr(a+b−) were identified casting doubt on the association with the MNS system. It now appears that the Wr[b] antigenic structure is formed by both GPA and band 3 protein sequences.

Low-incidence Diego Blood Group Antigens

As of 1995, there were 37 low-incidence antigens listed in the ISBT 700 series of antigens not assigned to a

TABLE 11-17	Low-incidence Diego Antigens 5–21		
ISBT Number	Antigen	Amino Acid Substitution	Year Assigned to Diego
DI5	Wdᵃ	Val557Met	1996
DI6	Rbᵃ	Pro548Leu	1996
DI7	WARR	Thr552Ile	1996
DI8	ELO	Arg432Trp	1998
DI9	Wu	Gly565Ala	1998
DI10	Bpᵃ	Asn569Lys	1998
DI11	Moᵃ	Arg656His	1998
DI12	Hgᵃ	Arg656Cys	1998
DI13	Vgᵃ	Tyr555His	1998
DI14	Swᵃ	Arg646Gln or Arg646Trp	1998
DI15	BOW	Pro561Ser	1998
DI16	NFLD	Glu429Asp and Pro561Ala	1998
DI17	Jnᵃ	Pro566Ser	1998
DI18	KREP	Pro566Ala	1998
DI19	Trᵃ	Lys551Asn	Provisional
DI20	Frᵃ	Glu480Lys	2000
DI21	SW1	Arg646Trp	2000

particular blood group system. Researchers suspected that more antigens could be linked to the Diego blood group system because of the size and amount of band 3 proteins on red cells. They began looking at various antigens in the 700 series to see if there was a connection. Seventeen antigens (Table 11-17) have now been assigned to the Diego system. The location of the antigens on the molecule has been determined. There are seven loops in the extracellular area of the band 3 protein. ELO is located on loop 1 and Frᵃ is on loop 2.[93] Eleven antigens are located on loop 3 with six more antigens on loop 4. Diᵃ and Diᵇ are on the seventh loop. It is thought that the closeness of the antigens on the loops may account for some of the characteristics of the antigens and antibodies that define them.

Diego Antibodies

Nineteen of the 21 Diego antigens are of low incidence. The likelihood of being transfused with a unit positive for one of the antigens is rare and the antibodies are rarely encountered. With the exception of ELO, they have not been implicated with HDFN. The first report of anti-ELO causing HDFN occurred in 1992 with a second report in 1993 when the same patient had another baby.[94,95] It has been noted that some individuals have antibodies to several low-incidence antigens. BOW and NFLD each arise from amino acid substitutions at position 561.[96] The substitution for Jnᵃ and KREP is found at position 556. The assignment of so many low-frequency antigens to the band 3 protein helps explain some observations among reference laboratory workers. In addition, some of the specificities are Rh– and GPA related, further indicating the relationship between band 3, GPA, and the Rh proteins.

In routine pretransfusion testing, the antigens are not likely to be carried on the screening cells. In addition, if immediate spin or computer crossmatches are performed, the individual with an antibody to one of the low-incidence antigens will generally not be detected. Some of the antibodies are naturally occurring and are of no clinical significance for transfusion.

Anti-Diᵃ and anti-Wrᵃ have caused severe and fatal HDFN and have been involved in immediate and delayed transfusion reactions. Anti-Diᵃ is rare in most populations, but ethnicity should be considered during an investigation of an antibody to a low-incidence antigen. In contrast, anti-Wrᵃ is commonly found as an apparent, naturally occurring agglutinin or as an immune IgG antibody with other antibodies to low-incidence antigens and associated with autoimmune hemolytic anemia. In the IgG form, anti-Wrᵃ is associated with HDFN and HTR.

Antibodies to the high-incidence Diᵇ antigen cause problems in locating compatible blood because of the rarity of the negative phenotype. The antibody has caused mild HND, moderate immediate and delayed transfusion reactions. Not much is known about anti-Wrᵇ as few individuals have been described with the antibody, but it is suggested that it could cause accelerated destruction of antigen-positive red cells.

Yt BLOOD GROUP SYSTEM (ISBT 011)

The Yt blood group system has historically been referred to as the Cartwright system. It was first described in 1956 when anti-Ytᵃ was first described.[97] It consists of two antithetical antigens, Ytᵃ and Ytᵇ. The carrier molecule for the antigens is an enzyme, GPI-linked glycoprotein called acetylcholinesterase (AChE).[98] Although AChE has enzymatic functions in neurotransmission, the function of AChE on red cells is unknown.

The genetic locus for Yt is on chromosome 7. A single nucleotide mutation causes an amino acid change from histidine for Ytᵃ to asparagine for Ytᵇ at position 353.[99] The mutation does not have any effect on the

TABLE 11-18	Yt System Phenotype Frequencies
Phenotype	**Frequency (%)**
Yt(a+b−)	91.9
Yt(a+b+)	7.8
Yt(a−b+)	0.3
Yt(a−b−)	Transient—extremely rare

overall structure of AChE nor on its functions in nervous tissues.[100]

The Yt[a] antigen is a high-frequency antigen found in 99.8% of populations. Yt[b] is infrequent, except in Israeli Jew, Israeli Arabs, and Israeli Druse where the incidence can be as high as 26%. A transient null phenotype has been described in a patient that developed a probable antibody to AChE. The loss of AChE coincided with the loss of Yt[a] antigen. As AChE levels returned to normal, the antigen was ditected.[101] The phenotypes and their frequencies are listed in Table 11-18.

GPI-linked Molecules and PHN

AChE is an example of a carrier molecule for blood group antigens that is linked to the red cell membrane by a glycosyl phosphatidylinositol (GPI) anchor. The acquired hematopoietic stem cell disorder paroxysmal nocturnal hemoglobinuria (PNH) results from the absence or deficiency in expression of GPI-linked proteins. All red cell antigens that are carried on a GPI-linked carrier molecule will not be expressed in PNH.[102]

Even though the Yt(a−b+) phenotype is relatively low, many examples of anti-Yt[a] have been described. Yt[b] appears to be a poor immunogen and is rarely seen except in individuals who make other blood group antibodies. Both antibodies are the result of transfusion or pregnancy and are not known to be naturally occurring. They are generally not implicated in transfusion reaction or HDFN. In fact, there are several reports of women with anti-Yt[a] bearing a Yt(a+) child and no indication of HDFN. The same holds true for a woman with anti-Yt[b] bearing a Yt(b+) child. Some patients with anti-Yt[a] have received transfusions of Yt(a+) blood with no ill effects while others showed evidence of decreased red cell survival.

The antigens are sensitive to ficin, papain, and DTT. The antibodies are IgG, reacting optimally at IAT. Some Yt[a] antibodies may cause complement binding, but anti-Yt[b] does not. Consequently, the clinical significance of Yt antibodies has been the subject of research. Various studies have been conducted to try to examine the significance of transfusing incompatible blood by using ^{51}Cr survival studies, monocyte monolayer assay (MMA), and even transfusion of antigen-positive red cells.

Xg BLOOD GROUP SYSTEM (ISBT 012)

The Xg blood group system consists of two antigens—Xg[a] and CD99. This is the only blood group whose genetic locus is assigned to the X chromosome. The Xg[a] antibody was first described in 1961 in a male who had received many transfusions.[103] An antithetical antigen to Xg[a] has not been found; thus the phenotypes are Xg(a+) and Xg(a−). In females, the Xg[a] and CD99 antigens escape X-chromosome inactivation, also known as the Lionization effect. The carrier molecules for both Xg[a] and CD99 are single-pass glycoproteins with an exofacial N-terminus. The function of the Xg[a] molecule is unknown but CD99 functions as an adhesion molecule. The gene encoding the antigen is *PBDX* located on the X chromosome.[104]

Xg[a]

Because the *Xg* locus is on the X chromosome, females can be *Xg[a]Xg[a]*, *XgXg*, or *Xg[a]Xg*. Males can be *Xg[a]Y* or *XgY*. The genotypes *Xg[a]Xg[a]*, *Xg[a]X*, and *Xg[a]Y* all result in the Xg(a+) phenotype. *XgXg* females and *XgY* males have the Xg(a−) phenotype. Because the *XG* genetic locus is on the X chromosome, the phenotype frequencies are different. The prevalence of Xg[a] is 66% in males and 89% in females.

Anti-Xg[a] is an uncommon antibody, is IgG in origin, and detectable by IAT. It is usually red cell stimulated but some are naturally occurring. Anti-Xg[a] rarely occurs with other alloantibodies. It is not associated with HTRs or HDFN. The antigen is sensitive to ficin and papain, but resistant to DTT.

CD99

CD99 is the other antigen of the system. It became part of the Xg system because the two genes, *MIC2* and *XG* are adjacent and homologous to each other. The frequency of the antigen is >99%. Two CD99 individuals have been reported with the antibody. The antibody is IgG reacting at IAT. It is sensitive to ficin and papain, but resistant to DTT. There are not enough data to determine whether it is associated with HTR or HDFN.

SCIANNA BLOOD GROUP SYSTEM (ISBT 013)

The first Scianna antibody was reported in 1962 and called anti-Sm.[105] An antibody defining a new antigen Bu-a was reported in 1963.[106] At the time of publication, neither group was aware of the findings of the other so there was no exchange of materials. In 1964, the possible relationship of the two antigens was described.[107] By 1974, the relationships were established and the system was named after the original antibody maker.

Scianna Antigens

There are five antigens recognized to be part of the Scianna system. Sc1 and Sc3 are high-incidence antigens, while Sc2 is a low-incidence antigen. Sc3 is expressed on all RBCs except those of the rare Sc1- and Sc2-negative phenotype. The antigens are expressed on the ERMAP protein (erythroblast membrane–associated protein).[108] The function of ERMAP is not clear at this time. Another low-frequency antigen, Sc4 or Rd, is expressed by a variant ERMAP protein. The high-prevalence antigen, Sc5 or STAR, occurs because of an amino acid change in the extracellular portion of ERMAP.[109]

Scianna Antibodies

The phenotype frequency in Caucasians of the Sc:1, −2 phenotype is 99.7% so anti-Sc1 is rarely seen. The antibodies are rare and are not associated with HTR or HDFN, but anti-Sc2 has caused a positive DAT.

DOMBROCK BLOOD GROUP SYSTEM (ISBT 014)

The first example of a Dombrock antigen was found in 1965 when anti-Do^a was found in an individual, Mrs. Dombrock, who had been multiply transfused.[110] In 1973, anti-Do^b was described and Do^b was noted to be the antithetical antigen to Do^a.[111] These two antigens comprised the Dombrock system for many years. Three high-prevalence antigens have been assigned to the Dombrock system: Gy^a, Hy, and Jo^a.[112]

The carrier molecule is a GPI-linked, single-pass molecule with an unknown function at this time. The sequence of the protein suggests that it transfers adenosine diphosphate (ADP) ribose to various protein receptors, but it is not known if this is active on red cells.[113] In fact, individuals with the absence of the glycoprotein, characterized by the Gy(a−) phenotype

TABLE 11-19 Dombrock System Phenotype Frequencies

Phenotype	Do^a	Do^b	Gy^a	Hy	Jo^a	Whites (%)	Blacks (%)
Do(a+b−)	+	−	+	+	+	18	11
Do(a+b+)	+	+	+	+	+	49	44
Do(a−b+)	−	+	+	+	+	33	45
Gy(a−)	−	−	−	−	−	Rare	0
Hy−		−	+^{w}	+^{w}	−	−	0	Rare
Jo(a−)	+^{w}	+/−^{w}	+	+^{w}	−	0	Rare

are not clinically affected. Like other GPI-linked antigens, Dombrock antigens are not expressed on PNH III cells (see Yt Blood Group System). *ART4*, the gene that encodes the Dombrock glycoprotein is found on chromosome 12.

Dombrock Antigens

The frequencies of the phenotypes of Dombrock antigens are listed in Table 11-19. *Do^a* and *Do^b* are codominant alleles that differ in three nucleotide positions that encode Do^a and Do^b, respectively. Do^a has aspartic acid at position 265 while Do^b has asparagines. The high-prevalence Hy antigen has glycine at position 108 and is associated with the Do(a−b+) phenotype. Another high-frequency antigen is Jo^a which has threonine at position 117. There is a null phenotype in the system called Gy(a−) or Do$_{null}$. There are several different mutations that cause the null phenotype. The antigens are resistant to enzymes and sensitive to DTT.

Dombrock Antibodies

Antibodies to Dombrock antigens are not common and often present with other antibodies. They appear to be clinically significant, but only mild HDN with a positive DAT has been reported.

COLTON BLOOD GROUP SYSTEM (ISBT 015)

An antibody to a high-frequency antigen was reported in 1967 and called anti-Co^a.[114] Anti-Co^b was reported in 1970, and the Co(a−b−) phenotype was described in 1974.[115,116] The Colton antigens are carried on a multipass membrane glycoprotein, aquaporin 1 (AQP1) responsible for water homeostasis and urine concentration.[117] The gene, *AQP1*, is located on chromosome 7. The Colton polymorphism is determined by an amino acid substitution at position 45 of the protein. Alanine is present when the Co^a antigen is expressed and valine is present when Co^b is expressed.

Co^a is the high-frequency antigen present in 98% of the population, while Co^b is the antithetical antigen present in 8% of the population. A third antigen Co3 is always present when Co^a and/or Co^b are expressed. Co3 is not present on Co(a−b−) red cells. These red cells also lack or have low amounts of aquaporin 1; however, there does not seem to be a medical condition associated with it.

Colton Antibodies

Antibodies to Colton antigens have caused both mild to moderate HTRs and mild to severe (rare) hemolytic disease of the newborn. Anti-Co3 is only seen in the null phenotype. The antibodies are IgG in nature and some have been shown to bind complement. The antigens are resistant to the effect of enzymes and chemicals.

CHIDO/ROGERS BLOOD GROUP SYSTEM (ISBT 017)

The Chido/Rogers system is a little different from most blood group systems. For instance, the antigens are located on the fourth component of complement (C4) instead of a red cell structure. Before the antigens were associated with C4, they were considered to be like other antigens because they were detected on red cells with blood grouping reagents and thus were adopted as a system. The first antigen, Ch, was reported in 1967 when the antibody was responsible for crossmatching difficulties.[118] The Rg^a antigen was later described in 1976 when an antibody was reacting with 97% of individuals in the British population.[119]

Chido/Rogers Antigens

The system has nine antigens, which are found on red cells and in plasma. There are six high-frequency Ch antigens (Ch1 through Ch6) and two high-frequency Rg antigens (Rg1 and Rg2). The ninth antigen, WH, is a hybrid antigen and is associated with the Ch:6, Rg:1, −2 phenotype.

Chido/Rogers Biochemistry and Genetics

The antigens are located on the C4d fragment of the fourth component of complement (C4) and adsorbed onto the red cell membrane. The two components to C4, C4A and C4B, are identical in their amino acid sequences, but C4A binds to protein while C4B binds to carbohydrate. The Chido antigen is found on C4B, while the Rogers antigen is on C4A.[120] The C4 molecule is a glycoprotein composed of three disulfide-linked polypeptide chains, α, β, and γ. The mechanism for the antigens to become bound to the red cells occurs in the course of the classical pathway of complement activation. C4 becomes activated by one of two mechanisms and binds to the red cell as C4b. The C4b undergoes proteolytic degradation to split into two fragments, C4c and C4d. C4d, which contains the antigens, remains attached to the red cell membrane.[121]

The antigens are inherited by two closely linked genes, *C4A* and *C4B*, which both encode the isotypes. The genes are located on chromosome 6.

Ch/Rg Antibodies

The antibodies are usually IgG in nature and react best at IAT induced by blood transfusion in Chido or Rogers individuals. They usually react weakly and if titration studies are performed, have a high titer with continued weak reactivity. In addition, the reactions are not reproducible, causing difficult identification. These antibodies are rarely significant and are not implicated in HTR or HDFN.

Kx BLOOD GROUP SYSTEM (ISBT 019)

Biochemistry and Genetics

The Kx antigen is carried on the XK protein encoded by the *XK* gene located on the short arm of the X chromosome. The glycoprotein spans the membrane 10 times with both the N- and C-terminal domains in the cytoplasm. It has structural characteristics of a membrane transport protein. The XK protein is linked to the Kell glycoprotein by a single disulfide bond. Absence of the protein is associated with abnormal red cell morphology and late-onset forms of nerve and muscle abnormalities also known as the McLeod syndrome. There is a decrease of Kell antigen expression in individuals missing the Kx antigen.

GERBICH BLOOD GROUP SYSTEM (ISBT 020)

The Gerbich blood group system was first reported in 1960 and named after the original person who made the antibody, Mrs. Gerbich.[122] A year later, another anti-Ge was reported in an individual named

Mrs. Yus. The serum of Mrs. Yus was compatible with the red cells of Mrs. Gerbich, but the serum of Mrs. Gerbich was incompatible with the red cells of Mrs. Yus. Later a third type called Leach was introduced to the confusion.[3]

Biochemistry and Genetics

The Gerbich blood group system antigens are carried on the single-pass membrane proteins glycophorin C (GPC), glycophorin D (GPD), or both. A single gene on chromosome 2, *GYPC*, produces the highly glycosylated glycophorins.[123] The two glycophorins are identical except that GPD lacks the 21 amino acids at the terminal sequence of GPC. Both glycophorins play a role in maintaining red cell integrity by an interaction with protein 4.1 in the cytoplasm. Three high-incidence antigens are associated with the Gerbich system—Ge2, Ge3, and Ge4. GPC carries Ge3 and Ge4 while GPD carries Ge2 and Ge3. The five low-incidence antigens are Ge5 (Wb), Ge6 (Ls[a]), Ge7 (Ana[a]), Ge8 (Dh[a]), and GEIS. The lack of one or more of the high-incidence antigens results in three types of Gerbich-negative phenotypes. The Leach phenotype results from absence of Ge2, Ge3, and Ge4 and is the null phenotype (Ge:−2, −3, −4). The Gerbich phenotype lacks Ge2 and Ge3 (Ge:−2, −3, 4), while the Yus phenotype lacks Ge2 (Ge:−2, 3, 4).[124] Table 11-20 displays the four phenotypes and the associated antibodies.

Antibodies

Correspondingly, the antibodies produced by Ge-negative individuals can be of three types: anti-Ge2, anti-Ge3, or anti-Ge4. All three antigens are destroyed by trypsin; in addition, Ge2 and Ge4 are destroyed by papain. Ge3 is resistant to papain and can be used to distinguish anti-Ge2 from anti-Ge3 (assuming the very rare Ge:−2, −3, −4 phenotype is excluded). Gerbich antibodies may be immune in origin or can occur without red cell stimulation.

TABLE 11-20 Lutheran Blood Group System Phenotypes

Phenotype	% Occurrence
Lu(a+b−)	0.2
Lu(a−b+)	92.4
Lu(a+b+)	7.4
Lu(a−b−)	Rare

They are not considered clinically significant, but anti-Ge3 has been associated with HDFN manifesting 2 to 4 weeks after birth.

CROMER BLOOD GROUP SYSTEM (ISBT 021)

Biochemistry and Genetics

Fifteen antigens comprise the Cromer blood group system carried on the glycoprotein called decay accelerating factor or DAF or CD55.[125] The glycoprotein is linked to the red cell membrane via GPI linkage. The antigens are a product of the gene, *DAF*, found on chromosome 1.[126] Complement regulation is one function of the protein in that it helps to protect red cells from lysis by autologous complement by inhibition of C3-convertases. Twelve of the antigens are of high incidence and the remaining three of low incidence. Table 11-21 shows the incidence of the various antigens. The polymorphisms are the result of single nucleotide substitutions except

TABLE 11-21 Cromer System Antigens

Name	ISBT Name
	High frequency >99.9%
Cr[a]	CROM1
Tc[a]	CROM2
Dr[a]	CROM5
Es[a]	CROM6
IFC	CROM7
WES[b]	CROM9
UMC	CROM10
GUTI	CROM11
SERF	CROM12
ZENA	CROM13
CROV	CROM14
CRAM	CROM15
	Low frequency <0.01%
Tc[b] (6% in blacks)	CROM3
Tc[c]	CROM4
WES[a]	CROM8

for the multiple epitope IFC antigen. Red cells lacking the IFC antigen (CROM7) are of the INAB phenotype. Two different single-point mutations result in a truncation of the protein, which cannot attach to the red cell membrane and the majority of the DAF protein is lacking.

Cromer system antibodies are rare. The clinical significance is variable with some showing decreased survival in transfusion. An example of anti-Tc^a causing an HTR has been reported in the literature. Cromer system antibodies have not been shown to cause hemolytic disease of the newborn possibly because placental tissue is rich in DAF, which may absorb the antibody. The antibody can be inhibited by plasma and urine from antigen-positive individuals and platelet concentrates.

KNOPS BLOOD GROUP SYSTEM (ISBT 022)

Biochemistry and Genetics

Knops system antigens are located on CR1, the primary complement receptor on red cells.[127] The carrier molecule is a single-pass membrane glycoprotein. The high-incidence antigens are Kn^a, McC^a, Sl^a, Yk^a, and Sl3. The low-incidence antigens are Kn^b, McC^b, and Vil. There is variable frequency with the antigens between black and white individuals.

Antibodies

Knops system antibodies historically were described as *"high titer, low avidity"* due to their weak reactions even at high titer. The antibodies are IgG and do not bind complement. They do not seem to be a cause of HTRs or HDFN.

INDIAN BLOOD GROUP SYSTEM (ISBT 023)

The Indian antigens are located on CD44 and encoded by the gene, *CD44*, on chromosome 11. The carrier molecule is a single-pass membrane glycoprotein with a disulfide-bonded N-terminal domain that acts as a cellular adhesion molecule. Two allelic antigens are In^a and In^b. The In^a antigen is low frequency in Caucasian, Asians, and blacks at 0.1%, but Indians have a 4% incidence and Arabs up to 11.8%. The antithetical antigen is In^b with a 99% incidence in Caucasians and 96% in Indians. Two missense mutations in the CD44 gene have been reported to encode two antigens-INFI (IN3) and INJA (IN4).[128] They are both high incidence.

Antibodies to Indian antigens are IgG in nature. They are associated with decreased red cell survival and positive DAT, but not HDFN.

Ok BLOOD GROUP SYSTEM (ISBT 024)

The Ok blood group system was established in 1999, although the antigen was first described in 1979 when Morel and Hamilton found the antibody in the serum of a Japanese woman who had been transfused but not pregnant.[129] The Ok antigen is carried on a single-pass type 1 membrane glycoprotein (CD147) with two IgSF (immunoglobulin superfamily) domains. CD147 is encoded by a gene on chromosome 19. The high-incidence antigen Ok^a nears 100% distribution. Absence of Ok(a) arises from an amino acid change from glutamic acid to lysine at position 92 on the first IgSF domain. The rare instances of the Ok(a)-negative phenotype are most frequently seen in individuals of Japanese descent, but there are two reports in individuals, one each of Iranian and Hispanic descent.[130]

The alloantibody is an IgG antibody reactive at IAT. It is not known to cause complement binding and is not associated with HDFN. The antibody does appear to be clinically significant with indications of reduced RBC survival.

RAPH BLOOD GROUP SYSTEM (ISBT 025)

The Raph blood group system comprises a single antigen, MER2. It is carried on CD151, a glycoprotein, a member of the Tetraspanin family that is encoded by a gene on chromosome 11. Tetraspanins are proteins with four transmembrane segments. Both the N- and C-termini lie on the intracellular side of the membrane. Of the two extracellular loops, one of the domains is longer than the other. It is thought to function as an adhesion molecule. The antigen is common; about 92% of Caucasian individuals express the antigen and it shows some variability in strength, particularly decreased expression over time.[131] Of MER2-negative individuals, there are at least two mutations described. One type is associated with a truncation of the protein that prevents extracellular expression of the domains. These individuals are CD151 deficient and have renal failure and other disorders associated with the deficiency. The other is a single amino acid change from arginine to cysteine at position 171 and is not associated with renal failure. The extracellular domains are expressed and the substitution does not appear to affect the role of the protein.

Although anti-MER2 has not been considered to be clinically significant, a recent report of clinical significance has appeared in the literature in individuals with the single amino acid substitution.[132]

JMH BLOOD GROUP SYSTEM (ISBT 026)

The JMH (John Milton Hagen) antigen is carried on Semaphorin 7A or CD108, a glycoprotein bound to the red cell membrane by GPI linkage. *SEMA7A*, the gene that encodes Semaphorin 7A is located on chromosome 15. Although Semaphorin 7A has functional aspects on other cells and tissues, its function on red cells is unknown. There are four variants to the JMH antigen resulting from single amino acid substitutions in the semaphorin domain of the molecule.[133] The JMH antigen is absent on PNH III red cells, indicating a possible role of other complement proteins.

The antibody has not been demonstrated to be of clinical significance, although there may be decreased survival in the variant types. It is an IgG antibody, principally, IgG4 reacting at IAT. It is not associated with HDFN.

I BLOOD GROUP SYSTEM (ISBT 027) AND Ii BLOOD GROUP COLLECTION

History of the I System/Ii Collection

The I antigen was first described in 1956 when Wiener et al. found a panagglutinating autoantibody from a patient with CHD (cold hemagglutinin disease).[134] The antibody was called anti-I and the antigen it detects, I. Of 22,000 donor samples, 5 were negative for I and labeled as I negative or i. Anti-i was reported in 1960.[135]

Biochemistry and Genetics

The I blood group system was established in 2002 and is composed of a single antigen-I encoded by the gene *IGnT* on chromosome 6.[136] The i antigen remains in the Ii collection because it is not a product of the *IGnT* gene. Like, ABO, Lewis, and P, the Ii antigens are carbohydrate structures. Synthesis of the antigen occurs by the addition of sugar residues to a common precursor substance in a branched formation. The I antigen is present on the interior structures of the oligosaccharides that form the A, B, and H antigens. That is, the antigens are carried on the same glycoprotein and glycolipid chains that carry A, B, and H antigens, but are closer to the red cell membrane. However, the nature of the antigens on

the red cells is not purely linear and some folding occurs, bringing the different antigenic determinants close to each other. I and i antigens are based on type 2, βGal1-4GlcNAc, chains. The i antigen is produced from a sequential action of β-3-N-acetylglucosaminyltransferase and β-4-galactosyltransferase. The I antigen is a branched form of the i antigen. The enzyme that causes the branching is β-6-N-acetylglucosaminyltransferase that attaches a GlcNAc $\beta1\rightarrow6$ linkage from Gal to create a branch. See Figure 11-4.

Development of I and i Antigens

The expression of the antigen occurs as a reciprocal relationship in that fetal and infant red cells express little I antigen while adult red cells express little i antigen. As development occurs, the branching of the antigen converts i to I. The process is usually complete by the age of 18 months. The amount of I antigen on red cells is variable. The adult i phenotype is uncommon.

Antibodies in the Ii System

Anti-I is present in the sera of most individuals if tests are carried out at 4°C. It may not always be detectable because of absorption of the antibody. Rarely, clinically insignificant auto-anti-I will react at temperatures above room temperature. This is usually when complement binding occurs at room temperature and is carried over to the IAT reading using polyspecific reagent. Anti-i is rarely encountered. It is usually a cold-reactive IgM antibody. Auto-anti-I can also be a cause of cold agglutinin syndrome.

Compound antibodies sometimes occur because of the folding of the chains bringing the A, B, H, I, P, and Le^b antigens and an antibody to parts of several determinants. The most common is anti-HI. This cold-reacting agglutinin reacts with cells expressing H and I antigens, namely Group O and A$_2$ adults.

Reagents and Testing Methods

The ideal method for handling cold reactive, benign autoantibodies is to not detect them in the first place. Room temperature readings should be avoided. It may be helpful to perform IAT readings with anti-IgG only and not use polyspecific reagent that may pick up complement components.

Anti-I can interfere with antibody identification testing if the reactions carry over to 37°C readings. Trying to distinguish anti-HI from anti-I can confuse the picture. To identify cold agglutinins, a panel of selected cells can be run at room temperature and 4°C. The panel can include group O adult red cells, group O cord cells,

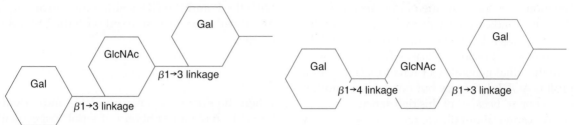

Type 1 oligosaccharide chain

Type 2 oligosaccharide chain

Type 1 and type 2 oligosaccharide chains with linkage positions

Type 2 chain with $\beta1{\rightarrow}6$ linkage showing branches

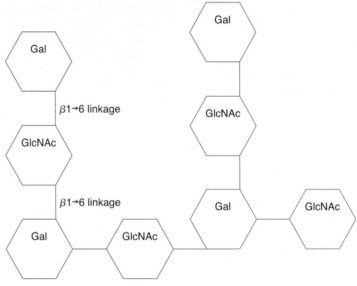

FIGURE 11-4   I and i antigen structures built on type 2 oligosaccharide chain. Gal, galactose; GlcNAc, *N*-acetylglucosamine.

group A_1 or B adult cells, and group A_1 or B cord cells. The group O cells will contain a lot of H antigen, while the A_1 or B cells will not. The group O cord cells will not contain a lot of I antigen, but the A_1 or B cells will.

Although there are ways to obtain soluble I substance from saliva or other secretions, it is not very reliable. A commercial preparation of rabbit erythrocyte stroma (rich in I antigen) is available for adsorption of the antibody. Always consult the manufacturer's instructions as other specificities may be adsorbed as well.

Prewarmed techniques are sometimes advised to eliminate reactivity due to cold agglutinins. Although procedures exist for prewarmed testing, it is generally not advisable as clinically significant antibodies can be removed in the process.[137]

Autoadsorptions can be performed to remove autoantibody, but care must be taken to ensure that recent transfusions have not occurred or alloantibody can be removed in the process.

I and Disease

The adult i phenotype in Japanese is associated with congenital cataracts. The association does not seem to be as pronounced in whites. Molecular changes in the IGnT gene have been reported that are associated with the adult i phenotype. It has been reported that a defect in the I locus may lead directly to the development of congenital cataracts.[138]

GIL BLOOD GROUP SYSTEM (ISBT 029)

The Gill antigen is of high incidence carried on aquaporin 3 (AQP3), coded by *AQP3*, on chromosome 9. AQP3 is a water channel molecule that facilitates the transport of glycerol. Because of the association of AQP1 with the Colton blood group system, researchers looked for a linkage with AQP3 and found the Gill antigen. The monomer spans the membrane six times with both the amino and carboxy termini located intracellularly.[139] The antigen is resistant to enzymes and DTT. The GIL-negative phenotype arises from a homozygous mutation that generates a premature stop codon. The result is AQP3 deficiency but no disease condition has been reported because of this deficiency.

Little is known about the characteristics of GIL antibody. It is an IgG antibody with optimal reactivity at IAT. There is some indication of the potential for destruction of transfused red cells, but the antibody is so rare that further studies are indicated.

RH-ASSOCIATED GLYCOPROTEIN (ISBT 30)

RHAG is a multipass membrane protein that exists as part of the Rh immune complex. In the absence of the RHAG protein, neither RHD nor RHCE proteins will be expressed.

BLOOD GROUP COLLECTIONS

The ISBT defines a blood group collection as two or more antigens that are related serologically, biochemically, or genetically, but which do not fit the criteria required for system status. Table 11-22 shows a list of the current antigens that fall into this category. The Globoside collection is discussed with the P and the Globoside blood group systems. The Ii collection is discussed with the I blood group system.

Cost

When the serum of three unrelated individuals was found to have an antibody of similar specificity, the Cs^a antigen was found. It was named after two of the patients in which the antibody was found, Mrs. Co. and Mrs. St.[140] The antithetical antigen was reported in 1987 when the antibody was described.[141] In 1988, the collection was established and named "Cost." The incidence of Cs^a is >98% in most populations, but 96% in blacks. The Cs^b antigen has a prevalence of about 34% in all populations. Both antigens are resistant to enzyme treatment and there is a variable effect with DTT. The antibodies are IgG, reacting best at IAT, and do not bind complement. Anti-Cs^a is not associated with transfusion reactions or HDFN. Only one example of anti-Cs^b has been reported.

Er

A new high-frequency antibody reported in 1982 and called anti-Er^a was found in three unrelated individuals.[142] In 1988, the antithetical antigen was described and called Er^b. At the time, a *silent allele* was postulated that would present as a null phenotype.[143] In 2003, there was another report of an antibody to an E-related antigen in an individual with the phenotype, Er(a−b−).[144] There appears to be apparent heterogeneity with anti-Er^a in that not all examples of anti-Er^a react with Er(a+) red cells. The antibodies are IgG and react at IAT. They do not cause complement binding and are not associated with HTR. Anti-Er^a can cause a positive DAT, but clinical HDFN has not been reported.

Vel

Anti-Vel was first described in 1952 and named after the antibody maker. The antigen has a frequency of about 0.02% in all populations except Norwegians and Swedes, where the incidence is about 0.07%. The strength of the Vel antigen can be variable, making identification difficult. The antigen is resistant to enzymes and DTT treatment. The antibody is found as an IgM-agglutinating antibody and IgG reacting at IAT. The IgM form can present as a complement-binding hemolysin. Anti-Vel is a clinically significant antibody and Vel-negative blood should be used for transfusion in patients with the antibody. Since Vel is weakly expressed on cord cells and it is often of IgM form, it generally does not cause HDFN.

TABLE 11-22   Collections of Antigens

Collection			Antigen		
ISBT Number	Name	Symbol	ISBT Number	Symbol	Frequency (%)
205	Cost	COST	205001	Cs^a	95
			205002	Cs^b	34
207	Ii	I	207002	I	Low (presumed)
208	Er	ER	208001	Er^a	>99
			208002	Er^b	<1
			208002	Er3	>99
209		GLOB	209002	p^k	>99
			209003	LKE	98
210			210001	Le^c	1
			210002	Le^d	6
211	Vel	VEL	211001	Vel	>99
			211002	ABTI	>99

Another antigen, ABTI, has recently been associated with Vel. It was first reported in 1996 named after the three people in one family who made the antibody. Little is known outside of these cases, but the antibody is IgG reacting optimally at IAT. There are no data on clinical significance for HTR or HDFN. ABTI-negative red cells have a weakened expression of Vel.

The Vel antigen was originally located in the 901 series of high-incidence antigens, but has now been placed in the blood group collections when the association with ABTI was established.

SERIES OF LOW- AND HIGH-INCIDENCE ANTIGENS

There are a number of both high- and low-incidence antigens that are not associated with a blood group system. The ISBT Working Party on Terminology has categorized these as belonging to either the 700 (low incidence) series of antigens (Table 11-23) or the 901 (high incidence) series (Table 11-24).

Low-incidence Antigens

There are currently 18 antigens in the 700 series of *low-incidence antigens*. These antigens occur in less than 1% of the population, do not have a known allele, and have no association with a blood group collection or system. Most of the antibodies described from these antigens are only found when a case of HDFN is being investigated. The antigens are usually not present on screening cells and are thus not detected in pretransfusion testing. The antibodies thus far that have reports of HDFN are Batty, Biles, Reid, Livesay, Rasmussen, JVF, Katagiri, JONES, HJK, HOFM, and REIT. Of those, only Katagiri and REIT have reported severe HDFN. Some of the antibodies are found in autoimmune hemolytic anemia (AIHA).

High-incidence Antigens

There are nine antigens in 901 series of high-incidence antigens. They are characterized as having an incidence of >90%, do not have a known allele, and have no association with a blood group collection or system. Thus, VEL and ABTI were moved to a collection when they became associated with each other.

Lan and Anti-Lan

The Lan antigen occurs in all but about 1 in 20,000 people. The Lan-negative phenotype is inherited in a recessive manner. Despite the fact it is so rare, there

TABLE 11-23   700 Series of Low-incidence Antigens

ISBT Number	Name	Symbol
700002	Batty	By
700003	Christianson	Chr^a
700005	Biles	Bi
700006	Box	Bx^a
700017	Torkildsen	To^a
700018	Peters	Pt^a
700019	Reid	Re^a
700021	Jensen	Je^a
700028	Livesay	Li^a
700039	Milne	
700040	Rasmussen	RASM
700043	Oldeide	Ol^a
700044		JFV
700045	Katagiri	Kg
700047	Jones	JONES
700049		HJK
700050		HOFM
700052		SARA
700054		REIT

TABLE 11-24   901 Series of High-incidence Antigens

ISBT Number	Name	Symbol	Year Reported
901002	Langereis	Lan	1961
901003	August	At^a	1967
901005		Jr^a	1970
901008		Emm	1987
901009	Anton	AnWj	1982
901012	Sid	Sd^a	1967
901013	Duclos		1978
901014		PEL	1980/1996
901016		MAM	1993

are several examples of anti-Lan in the literature. The antibody has an immune origin, is IgG in nature, and optimally reactive at IAT. Anti-Lan has been implicated in an immediate HTR, but has not caused severe HDFN, although the DAT may be positive. Individuals with anti-Lan should receive blood negative for the Lan antigen.

Sd^a

The Sd^a antigen is one of the more unusual ones. The antigen is also widely distributed in secretions, excretions, and tissues. Urine contains the largest amounts. The antigen is famous for its mixed field appearance when tested with anti-Sd^a. The strength of the antigen on red cells varies widely with individuals that have Cad(+) red cells, having marked reaction with anti-Sd^a. There is a marked depression of antigen expression during pregnancy and women who are positive for the Sd^a antigen will appear to be Sd(a−) at full term. In spite of this, the level of Sd^a in urine remains at the normal levels. The antigen is not well developed at birth, and infant cells will often test Sd(a−). Again, if the infant has inherited the *Sda* gene, the urine will contain the soluble substance.

Many examples of anti-Sd^a are non–red cell stimulated. The antibody is usually IgM, reacting better at room temperature. If it is found at IAT, it may be a carryover from room temperature testing. Since most antigen screening cells do not contain the Sd^a antigen, most cases of anti-Sd^a are not found. That is fortunate because the antibody is benign. It is not known to cause HDFN either.

Other High-incidence Antigens

The antigen called At^a was reported in 1967 when the antibody was discovered in the serum of Mrs. August who had never been transfused, but whose third baby's cells gave a weak, positive, direct antiglobulin reaction.[145] The individual and her brother both had At(a−) red cells. The At(a−) phenotype has only been found in blacks, but it is not common. The antigen is present on cord cells and resistant to enzymes and DTT. Anti-At^a has been reported and it appears that pregnancy seems to stimulate the antibody because many of the antibody makers have been pregnant but never transfused. The antibody class is IgG reacting at IAT. It does not appear to bind complement or cause HDFN. Two reports have identified the potential for an HTR.

The Jr^a antigen was reported in 1970 when seven examples were described. Approximately half of the known Jr(a−) individuals are of Japanese origin. It appears to be a recessively inherited condition. The antigen is resistant to enzymes and DTT. Survival studies have indicated that there is shortened survival when Jr(a+) red cells are transfused to a patient with anti-Jr^a. The antibody can be IgM or the more common IgG. A positive DAT, but not clinical HDFN has been described.

The antigen called Emm was described in 1987 when the antibody was found in the serum of four individuals, three of whom had never been transfused.[146] It is thought that the antigen is carried on a phosphatidylinositol-linked protein because anti-Emm is not reactive with PNH III red cells (which lack PI-linked proteins). The antigen is resistant to enzymes and DTT treatment. The antibody has been found to be both IgG and IgM and exhibits some complement binding.

Another antigen, originally called Anton, but now named AnWj is carried on a CD44 glycoprotein. There is altered expression (weak) of the antigen when an individual has the InLu phenotype. The antigen shows resistance to enzyme treatment and a variable reaction to DTT. The antibody is IgG and rarely binds complement. It does not appear to cause HDFN, but there has been one severe case of HTR.[147]

The Duclos antigen was reported in 1978 after the first and only producer of the antibody. The antigen is not found on Rh$_{null}$ U−, Rh$_{mod}$ U−, red cells and those of the original antibody maker. There are little data available on the significance of the antibody.

The antigen PEL was described in 1996 when the antibody was found in the serum of two PEL-negative French-Canadians.[148] The antigen is resistant to enzymes and DTT treatment. The antibody is presumed to be IgG, but little is known of the significance.

The MAM antigen, first reported in 1993 and assigned to the 901 series in 1999 is resistant to enzymes and DTT. The antibody is IgG reacting well at IAT. There appears to be a potential for HTR and HDFN.

SUMMARY

The study of antigens (and their corresponding antibodies) continues to be an intense field of research, particularly since molecular testing methods have been developed. Our understanding of the biochemistry and genetics is ever increasing, while at the same time opening up more questions. Further awareness of the functions of carrier molecules may lead to further insight into disease states. The study of antibodies will always be an important aspect in the field of blood banking because of the desire to provide the best possible blood component for a patient.

Review Questions

1. Antigens carried on molecules with a GPI linkage to the red cell surface are often involved in which of the following functions?
   a. cytokine receptor
   b. glycerol and water transport
   c. enzymatic activities
   d. adhesion function

2. Which of the following is a carbohydrate antigen?
   a. Jk^a
   b. Le^b
   c. AnWj
   d. GIL

3. Which of the following multipass carrier molecule has the unusual exofacial N-terminus orientation?
   a. Fy glycoprotein
   b. CHIP-1
   c. Kx glycoprotein
   d. Do glycoprotein

4. Select the correct numerical terminology to describe an individual with the Leach phenotype.
   a. GE:−2, −3, −4
   b. GE:−2, −3, 4
   c. GE:−2, 3, 4
   d. GE:2, 3, 4

5. Anti-U may be found in individuals with which of the following phenotype?
   a. M−N−S−s+
   b. M+N−S−s+
   c. S−s−
   d. S+s−

6. Which of the following antigens are destroyed by ficin?
   a. M
   b. Jk^b
   c. Le^a
   d. Do^a

7. Which one of the following characteristics is common for anti-Lu^a?
   a. warm reacting
   b. mixed field appearance
   c. IgG only
   d. hemolysis at 37°C

8. Inheritance of which of the following genes determines Lewis antigen expression?
   a. *FUT1*
   b. *FUT2*
   c. *FUT2/FUT3*
   d. *FUT3*

9. Blacks whose red cells type as Fy(a−b−) may have which of the following antigen(s) on their tissue cells?
   a. Fy^a
   b. Fy^b
   c. Fy^a and Fy^b
   d. Fy^c

10. Which of the following blood system antibodies are notorious for weakening over time?
    a. Rh
    b. Duffy
    c. Diego
    d. Kidd

11. The expression of Wr^b is dependent on the presence of which of the following?
    a. AE1
    b. GPA
    c. GPB
    d. GPC

12. Individuals with PNH will not express which of the following antigens?
    a. MNS
    b. Duffy
    c. Yt
    d. Ok

13. Which of the following antigens are carried on a component of complement?
    a. Kx
    b. Lutheran
    c. Chido/Rogers
    d. Gil

14. Which of the following antigens is linked to the Kell glycoprotein by a single disulfide bond?
    a. JMH
    b. Kx
    c. Gerbich
    d. Dombrock

15. Red cells that type as Ok(a−) are typically found in which of the following populations?
    a. Blacks
    b. Whites
    c. Norwegian
    d. Japanese

REFERENCES

1. Daniels G, Flegel A, Fletcher A, et al. International Society of Blood Transfusion Committee on Terminology for Red Cell Surface Antigens: Cape Town report. *Vox Sang.* 2007; 92:250–253.

2. Reid ME, Mohandas N. Red blood cell blood group antigens: structure and function. *Semin Hematol.* 2004; 41(2):93–117.

3. Issitt PD, Anstee DJ. *Applied Blood Group Serology.* 4th ed. Durham, NC: Montgomery Scientific Publications; 1998.

4. Storry J, Coghlan G, Poole J, et al. The MNS blood group antigens, Vr (MNS12) and Mta (MNS14), each arise from an amino acid substitution on glycophorin A. *Vox Sang*. 2000; 78:52–56.

5. Daniels G, Bruce L, Mawby WJ, et al. The low-frequency MNS blood group antigens Nyᵃ and Osᵃ are associated with GPA amino acid substitutions. *Transfusion*. 2000; 40:555–559.

6. Storry J, Reid M, Maclennan S, et al. The low-incidence MNS antigens Mᵛ, sᴰ, and Mit arise from single amino acid substitutions on GPB. *Transfusion*. 2001; 41:269–275.

7. Gahmberg CG, Myllyla G, Leikola J, et al. Absence of the major sialoglycoprotein in the membrane of human En(a–) erythrocytes and increased glycosylation of band 3. *J Biol Chem*. 1976; 251(19):6108–6116.

8. Tanner MJ, Anstee DJ. The membrane change in En(a−) human erythrocytes. *Biochem J*. 1976; 153:271–277.

9. Huang CH, Johe K, Moulds JJ, et al. Delta glycophorin (glycophorin B) gene deletion in two individuals homozygous for the S–s–U– blood group phenotype. *Blood*. 1987; 70:1830–1835.

10. Storry JR, Poole J, Condon J, et al. Identification of a novel hybrid glycophorin gene encoding GP.HOP. *Transfusion*. 2000; 40:560–565.

11. Levine P, Bobbitt OB, Waller RK, et al. Isoimmunization by a new blood factor in tumor cells. *Proc Soc Exp Biol Med*. 1951; 77(3):403–405.

12. Matson GA, Swanson J, Noades J, et al. A "New" Antigen and antibody belonging to the P blood group system. *Am J Hum Genet*. 1959; 11(1):26–34.

13. Tippett P, Sanger R, Race RR, et al. An agglutinin associated with the P and the ABO blood group systems. *Vox Sang*. 1965; 10:269–280.

14. Engelfriet CP, Beckers D, Borne AE von dem, et al. Haemolysins probably recognizing the antigen p. *Vox Sang*. 1972; 23(3):176–181.

15. Duk M, Singh S, Reinhold VN, et al. Structures of unique globoside elongation products present in erythrocytes with a rare NOR phenotype. *Glycobiology*. 2007; 17(3):304–312.

16. Iwamura K, Furukawa K, Uchikawa M, et al. The blood group P1 synthase gene is identical to the Gb3/CD77 synthase gene. *J Biol Chem*. 2003; 278(45):44429–44438.

17. Tilley L, Green C, Daniels G. Sequence variation in 5′ untranslated region of the human *A4GALT* gene is associated with, but does not define, the P1 blood-group polymorphisms. *Vox Sang*. 2009; 90:198–203.

18. Lindstrom K, Von Dem Bourne AE, Breimer ME, et al. Glycosphingolipid expression in spontaneously aborted fetuses and placenta from blood group p women. Evidence for placenta being the primary target for anti-Tja-antibodies. *Glycoconj J*. 1992; 9(6):325–329.

19. Moulds JM, Moulds JJ. Blood group associations with parasites, bacteria and viruses. *Transfus Med Rev*. 2000; 14(4):302–311.

20. Callender S, Race RR, Paykoc ZV. Hypersensitivity to transfused blood. *Br Med J*. 1945; 2:83–84.

21. Bove JR, Allen FH Jr, Chiewsilp P, et al. Anti-Lu4: a new antibody related to the Lutheran blood group system. *Vox Sang*. 1971; 21(4):302–310.

22. Marsh WL. Anti-Lu5, anti-Lu6, and anti-Lu7. Three antibodies defining high frequency antigens related to the Lutheran blood group system. *Transfusion*. 1972; 12(1):27–34.

23. Crew VK, Poole J, Banks J, et al. LU21: a new high-frequency antigen in the Lutheran blood group system. *Vox Sang*. 2004; 87:109–113.

24. Cartron JP, Colin Y. Structural and functional diversity of blood group antigens. *Transfus Clin Biol*. 2001; 8:163–169.

25. Mankelow TJ, Burton N, Stefansdottir FO, et al. The Laminin 511/521-binding site on the Lutheran blood group glycoprotein is located at the flexible junction of Ig domains 2 and 3. *Blood*. 2007; 110:3398–3406.

26. Crew VK, Mallinson G, Green C, et al. Different inactivating mutations in the LU genes of three individuals with the Lutheran-null phenotype. *Transfusion*. 2007; 47:492–498.

27. Singleton BK, Burton NM, Green C, et al. Mutations in EKLF.KLF1 form the molecular basis of the rare blood group In(Lu) phenotype. *Blood*. 2008; 112:2081–2088.

28. Coombs RR, Mourant AE, Race RR. In-vivo isosensitisation of red cells in babies with hemolytic disease of the newborn. *Lancet*. 1946; 247:264–266.

29. Levine P, Backer M, Wigod M, et al. A new human hereditary blood property (Cellano) present in 99.8% of all bloods. *Science*. 1949; 109:464–466.

30. Allen FH Jr, Lewis SJ. Kpᵃ (Penney), a new antigen in the Kell blood group system. *Vox Sang*. 1957; 2(2):81–87.

31. Allen FH Jr, Lewis SJ, Fudenberg H. Studies of anti-Kpᵇ, a new antibody in the Kell blood group system. *Vox Sang*. 1958; 3(1):1–13.

32. Chown B, Lewis M, Kaita K. A 'new' Kell blood-group phenotype. *Nature*. 1957; 180:711.

33. Walker RH, Argall CI, Steane EA, et al. Anti-Jsᵇ, the expected antithetical antibody of the Sutter blood group system. *Nature*. 1963; 197:295–296.

34. Walker RH, Argall CI, Steane EA, et al. Jsᵇ of the Sutter blood group system. *Transfusion*. 1963; 3:94–99.

35. Strange JJ, Kenworthy RJ, Webb AJ, et al. Wkᵃ (Weeks), a new antigen in the Kell blood group system. *Vox Sang*. 1974; 27(1):81–86.

36. Callender S, Race RR, Paykoc ZV. Hypersensitivity to transfused blood. *Br Med J*. 1945; 2:83–84.

37. Yamaguchi H, Okubo Y, Seno T, et al. A "new" allele, Kpᶜ, at the Kell complex locus. *Vox Sang*. 1979; 36(1):29–30.

38. Gavin J, Daniels GL, Yamaguchi H, et al. The red cell antigen once called Levay is the antigen Kpᶜ of the Kell system. *Vox Sang*. 1979; 36(1):31–33.

39. Lee S, Zambas ED, Marsh WL, et al. Molecular cloning and primary structure of Kell blood group protein. *Proc Natl Acad Sci USA*. 1991; 88:6353–6357.

40. Lee S. Molecular basis of Kell blood group phenotypes. *Vox Sang*. 1997; 73:1–11.

41. Russo DC, Lee S, Reid M, et al. Point mutations causing the McLeod phenotype. *Transfusion*. 2002; 42:287–293

42. Lee S, Zambas ED, Marsh WL, et al. The human Kell blood group gene maps to chromosome 7q33 and its expression is restricted to erythroid cells. *Blood*. 1993; 81:2804–2809.

43. Lee S, Zambas E, Green ED, et al. Organization of the gene encoding the human Kell blood group protein. *Blood*. 1995; 85:1364–1370.

44. Walker R, Danek A, Uttner I, et al. McLeod phenotype without the McLeod syndrome. *Transfusion*. 2007; 47: 299–305.

45. Hitzig WH, Seger RA. Chronic granulomatous disease, a heterogeneous syndrome. *Hum Genet*. 1983; 64: 207–215.

46. Francke U, Ochs HD, de Martinville B, et al. Minor Xp21 chromosome deletion in a male associated with expression of Duchenne muscular dystrophy, chronic granulomatous disease, retinitis pigmentosa and McLeod syndrome. *Am J Hum Genet*. 1985; 37:250–267.

47. Lee S, Russo DC, Reid ME, et al. Mutations that diminish expression of Kell surface protein and lead to the K_{mod} RBC phenotype. *Transfusion*. 2003; 43:1121–1125.

48. Marsh WL, Nichols ME, Oyen R, et al. Naturally occurring anti-Kell stimulated by *E. coli* enterocolitis in a 20-day-old child. *Transfusion*. 1978; 18(2):149–154.

49. Kanel GC, Davis I, Bowman JE. "Naturally occurring" anti-K1: possible association with mycobacterium infection. *Transfusion*. 1978; 18(4):472–473.

50. Judd WJ, Walter WJ, Steiner EA. Clinical and laboratory findings on two patients with naturally occurring anti-Kell agglutinins. *Transfusion*. 1981; 21(2):184–188.

51. Morgan P, Bossom E. "Naturally occurring" anti-Kell (K1): two examples. *Transfusion*. 1963; 3:397–398.

52. Mukumoto Y, Konishi H, Ito K, et al. An example of naturally occurring anti-Kell (K1) in a Japanese male. *Vox Sang*. 1978; 35(4):275–276.

53. Daniels G, Hadley A, Green C. Causes of fetal anemia in hemolytic disease due to anti-K [Letters to the editor]. *Transfusion*. 2003; 43:115–116.

54. Mourant AE. A "new" human blood group antigen of frequent occurrence. *Nature*. 1946; 158:237–238.

55. Andresen PH. The blood group system L. A new blood group L2, a case of epistasis within the blood groups. *Acta Pathol Microbiol Scand*. 1948; 25:728.

56. Cutbush M, Giblett ER, Mollison PL. Demonstration of the phenotype Le(a+b+) in infants and in adults. *Br J Haematol*. 1956; 2(2):210–220.

57. Watkins WM, Morgan WT. Possible genetical pathways for the biosynthesis of blood group mucopolysaccharides. *Vox Sang*. 1959; 4(2):97–119.

58. Henry S, Mollicone R, Fernandez P, et al. Molecular basis for erythrocyte Le(a+b+) and salivary ABH partial-secretor phenotypes: expression of a FUT2 secretor allele with an A → T mutation at nucleotide 385 correlates with reduced $\alpha(1,2)$fucosyltransferase activity. *Glycoconj J*. 1996; 13(6): 985–993.

59. Judd WJ, Steiner EA, Friedman BA, et al. Anti-Le^a as an autoantibody in the serum of Le(a-b+) individual. *Transfusion*. 1978; 18(4):436–440.

60. Cowles JW, Spitainik SL, Blumberg N. Detection of anti-Le^a in Le(a−b+) individuals by kinetic ELISA. *Vox Sang*. 1986; 50(3):164–168.

61. Miller EB, Rosenfield RE, Vogel P, et al. The Lewis blood factors in American Negroes. *Am J Phys Anthropol*. 1954; 12(3):427–443.

62. Walker RH, Griffin LD, Kashgarian M. The distribution of the ABO blood groups in persons with Lewis antibodies. *Am J Clin Pathol*. 1969; 51(1):3–8.

63. Spitalnik S, Cowles J, Cox MT, et al. Detection of IgG anti-Lewis (a) antibodies in cord sera by kinetic Elisa. *Vox Sang*. 1985; 48(4):235–238.

64. Vries de SI, Smtiskamp HS. Haemolytic transfusion reaction due to an anti-Lewis^a agglutinin. *Br Med J*. 1951; 1:280–281.

65. Matson GA, Coe J, Swanson J. Hemolytic transfusion reaction due to anti-Lea. *Blood*. 1955; 10:1236–1240.

66. Mollison PL, Cutbush M. Use of isotope-labelled red cells to demonstrate incompatibility in vivo. *Lancet*. 1955; 268(6878):1290–1295.

67. Cutbush M, Mollison PL, Parkin D. A new human blood group. *Nature*. 1950; 165:188–189.

68. Cutbush M, Mollison PL. The Duffy blood group system. *Heredity*. 1950; 4(3):383–389.

69. Ikin E, Mourant AE, Pettenkofer HJ, et al. Discovery of the expected haemagglutinin, anti-Fy^b. *Nature*. 1951; 168:1077–1078.

70. Sanger R, Race RR, Jack J. The Duffy blood groups of New York Negroes: the phenotype Fy(a–b–). *Br J Haematol*. 1955; 1(4):370–374.

71. Chown B, Lewis M, Kaita H. The Duffy blood group system in Caucasians: evidence for a new allele. *Am J Hum Genet*. 1965; 17:384–389.

72. Albrey JA, Vincent EE, Hutchinson J, et al. A new antibody, anti-Fy3, in the Duffy blood group system. *Vox Sang*. 1971; 20(1):29–35.

73. Behzad O, Lee CL, Gavin J, et al. A new anti-erythrocyte antibody in the Duffy system: anti-Fy4. *Vox Sang*. 1973; 24(4):337–342.

74. Colledge KI, Pezzulich M, Marsh WL. Anti-Fy5, an antibody disclosing a probable association between the Rhesus and Duffy blood group genes. *Vox Sang*. 1973; 24(3):193–199.

75. Nichols ME, Rubinstein P, Barnwell J, et al. A new human Duffy blood group specificity defined by a murine monoclonal antibody. *J Exp Med*. 1987; 166:776–785.

76. Tournamille C, Colin Y, Cartron JP, et al. Disruption of a GATA motif in the Duffy gene promoter abolishes erythroid gene expression in Duffy-negative individuals. *Nat Genet*. 1995; 10(2):224–228.

77. Rios M, Chaudhuri A, Mallinson G, et al. New genotypes in Fy(a–b–) individuals: nonsense mutations (Trp to stop) in the coding sequence of either *FYA* or *FYB*. *Br J Haematol*. 2000; 108(2):448–454.

78. Olsson M, Smythe JS, Hansson C, et al. The Fy(x) phenotype is associated with a missense mutation in the Fy(b) allele predicting Arg89Cys in the Duffy glycoprotein. *Br J Haematol*. 1998; 103(4):1184–1191.

79. Oberdorfer CE, Kahn B, Moore V, et al. A second example of anti-Fy3 in the Duffy blood group system. *Transfusion*. 1974; 14(6):608–611.

80. Buchanan DI, Sinclair M, Sanger R, et al. An Alberta Cree Indian with a rare Duffy antibody, anti-Fy3. *Vox Sang*. 1976; 30(2):114–121.

81. Allen FH Jr, Diamond LK, Niedziela B. A new blood-group antigen. *Nature*. 1951; 167:482.

82. Plaut G, Ikin EW, Mourant AE, et al. A new blood-group antibody, anti-Jk^b. *Nature*. 1953; 171:431.

83. Pinkerton FJ, Mermod Le, Liles BA, et al. The phenotype Jk(a–b–) in the Kidd blood group system. *Vox Sang*. 1959; 4:155.

84. Olivès B, Mattei MG, Huet M, et al. Kidd blood group and urea transport function of human erythrocytes are carried by the same protein. *J Biol Chem*. 1995; 270(26):15607–15610.

85. Frohlich O, Macey RI, Edwards-Moulds J, et al. Urea transport deficiency in Jk(a–b–) phenotypes. *Am J Physiol*. 1991; 260(4 pt 1):C778–C783.

86. Geitvik GA, Høyheim B, Gedde-Dahl T, et al. The Kidd (JK) blood group locus assigned to chromosome 18 by close linkage to a DNA-RFLP. *Hum Genet*. 1987; 77(3):205–209.

87. Heaton DC, McLoughlin K. Jk(a–b–) red blood cells resist urea lysis. *Transfusion*. 1982; 22(1):70–71.

88. Bruce LJ, Anstee DJ, Spring FA, et al. Band 3 Memphis variant II. Altered stilbene disulfonate bonding and the Diego (Dia) blood group antigen are associated with the human erythrocyte band 3 mutation Pro854→Leu. *J Biol Chem*. 1994; 269(23):16155–16158.

89. Vince J, Reithmeier A. Carbonic anhydrase II binds to the carboxyl terminus of human band 3, the erythrocyte Cl$^-$/HCO$_3^-$ exchanger. *J Biol Chem*. 1998; 273(43):28430–28437.

90. Holman CA. A new rare human blood group antigen (Wr^a). *Lancet*. 1953; 265(6777):119–120.

91. Adams J, Broviac M, Brooks W, et al. An antibody, in the serum of a Wr(a+) individual, reacting with an antigen of very high frequency. *Transfusion*. 1971; 11(5):290–291.

92. Wren MR, Issitt PD. Evidence that Wr^a and Wr^b are antithetical. *Transfusion*. 1988; 28(2):113–118.

93. Zelinski T, Punter F, McManus K, et al. The ELO blood group polymorphism is located in the putative first extracellular loop of human erythrocyte band 3. *Vox Sang*. 1998; 75(1):63–65.

94. Ford DS, Stern DA, Hawksworth DN, et al. Haemolytic disease of the newborn probably due to anti-ELO, an antibody to low frequency red cell antigen. *Vox Sang*. 1992; 62(3):169–172.

95. Better PH, Ford DS, Frascarelli A, et al. Confirmation of anti-ELO as a cause of haemolytic disease of the newborn. *Vox Sang*. 1993; 65(1):70.

96. McManus K, Pongoski J, Coghlan G, et al. Amino acid substitutions in human erythroid protein band 3 account for the low-incidence antigens NFLD and BOW. *Transfusion*. 2000; 40(3):325–329.

97. Eaton BR, Morton JA, Pickles MM, et al. A new antibody, anti-Yt^a, characterizing a blood-group antigen of high incidence. *Br J Haematol*. 1956; 2(4):333–341.

98. Spring FA, Gardner B, Anstee DJ. Evidence that the antigens of the Yt blood group system are located on human erythrocyte acetylcholinesterase. *Blood*. 1992; 80:2136–2141.

99. Bartels CF, Zelinski T, Lockridge O. Mutation at codon 322 in the human acetylcholinesterase (ACHE) gene accounts for YT blood group polymorphism. *Am J Hum Genet*. 1993; 52:928–936.

100. Masson P, Froment MT, Sorenson RC, et al. Mutation His322Asn in human acetylcholinesterase does not alter electrophoretic and catalytic properties of the erythrocyte enzyme. *Blood*. 1994; 83:3003–3005.

101. Rao N, Whitsett CF, Oxendine SM, et al. Human erythrocyte acetylcholinesterase bears the Yta blood group antigen and is reduced or absent in the Yt(a–b–) phenotype. *Blood*. 1993; 81:815–819.

102. Telen MJ. Glycosyl phosphatidylinositol-linked blood group antigens and paroxysmal nocturnal hemoglobinuria. *Transfus Clin Biol*. 1995; 2(4):277–290.

103. Mann JD, Cahan A, Gelb AG, et al. A sex-linked blood group. *Lancet*. 1962; 1(7219):8–10.

104. Ellis NA, Tippett P, Petty A, et al. *PBDX* is the *XG* blood group gene. *Nat Genet*. 1994; 8(3):285–290.

105. Schmidt RP, Griffitts JJ, Northman FF. A new antibody, anti-Sm, reacting with a high incidence antigen. *Transfusion*. 1962; 2:338–340.

106. Anderson C, Hunter J, Zipursky A, et al. An antibody defining a new blood group antigen, Bu^a. *Transfusion*. 1963; 3:30–33.

107. Lewis M, Chown B, Schmidt RP, et al. A possible relationship between the blood group antigens Sm and Bu^a. *Am J Hum Genet*. 1964; 16:254–255.

108. Wagner FF, Poole J, Flegel WA. Scianna antigens including Rd are expressed by ERMAP. *Blood*. 2003; 101(2):752–757.

109. Hue-Roye K, Chaudhuri A, Velliquette RW, et al. STAR: a novel high-prevalence antigen in the Scianna blood group system. *Transfusion*. 2005; 45:245–247.

110. Swanson J, Polesky HF, Tippett P, et al. A "new" blood group antigen, Do^a. *Nature*. 1965; 206:313.

111. Molthan L, Crawford MN, Tippett P. Enlargement of the Dombrock blood groups system: the finding of anti-Do b. *Vox Sang*. 1973; 24(4):382–384.

112. Banks JA, Hemming N, Poole J. Evidence that the Gy^a, Hy and Jo^a antigens belong to the Dombrock blood group system. *Vox Sang*. 1995; 68(3):177–182.

113. Gubin AN, Njoroge JM, Wojda U, et al. Identification of the Dombrock blood group glycoprotein as a polymorphic member of the ADP-ribosyltransferase gene family. *Blood*. 2000; 96:2621–2627.

114. Heisto H, van der Hart M, Madsen G. Three examples of a red cell antibody, anti-Co^a. *Vox Sang*. 1967; 12:18.

115. Giles CM, Darnborough J, Aspinall P, et al. Identification of the first example of anti-Co^b. *Br J Haematol*. 1970; 19:267.

116. Rogers MJ, Stiles PA, Wright J. A new minus-minus phenotype: three Co(a–b–) individuals in one family [abstract]. *Transfusion*. 1974; 14:508.

117. Smith BL, Preston GM, Spring FA, et al. Human red cell aquaporin CHIP. *J Clin Invest*. 1994; 94:1043–1049.

118. Harris JP, Tegoli J, Swanson J, et al. A nebulous antibody responsible for cross-matching difficulties (Chido). *Vox Sang*. 1967; 12(2):140–142.

119. Longster G, Giles CM. A new antibody specificity, anti-Rga, reacting with a red cell and serum antigen. *Vox Sang*. 1976; 30(3):175–180.

120. Yu CY, Belt KT, Giles CM, et al. Structural basis of the polymorphism of human complement components

C4A and C4B: gene size, reactivity and antigenicity. *EMBO J*. 1986; 5(11):2873–2881.

121. Atkinson JP, Chan AC, Karp DR, et al. Origin of the fourth component of complement related Chido and Rogers blood group antigens. *Complement*. 1988; 5(2):65–76.

122. Rosenfield RE, Haber GV, Kissmeyer-Nielsen F, et al. Ge, a very common red-cell antigen. *Br J Haematol*. 1960; 6:344–349.

123. Reid ME, Spring FA. Molecular basis of glycophorin C variants and their associated blood group antigens. *Transfus Med*. 1994; 4(2):139–146.

124. Anstee DJ, Ridgwell K, Tanner MJ, et al. Individuals lacking the Gerbich blood-group antigen have alterations in the human erythrocyte sialoglycoproteins β and γ *Biochem J*. 1984; 221:97–104.

125. Telen MJ, Hall SE, Green AM, et al. Identification of human erythrocyte blood group antigens on decay-accelerating factor (DAF) and erythrocyte phenotype negative for DAF. *J Exp Med*. 1988; 167:1993–1998.

126. Lublin DM, Kompelli S, Storry JR, et al. Molecular basis of Cromer blood group antigens. *Transfusion*. 2000; 40: 208–213.

127. Moulds JM, Nickells MW, Moulds JJ, et al. The C3b/C4b receptor is recognized by the Knops, McCoy, Swain-Langley and York blood group antisera. *J Exp Med*. 1991; 173:1159–1163.

128. Poole J, Tilley L, Warke N, et al. Two missense mutations in the CD44 gene encode two new antigens of the Indian blood group system. *Transfusion*. 2007; 47:1306–1311.

129. Morel PA, Hamilton HB. Oka: an erythrocyte antigen of high frequency. *Vox Sang*. 1979; 36(3):182–185.

130. Crew VK, Thomas R, Gillen B, et al. A novel variant in the Ok blood group system. *Transfus Med*. 2006; 16(suppl 1):41 (poster).

131. Crew VK, Burton N, Kagan A, et al. CD151, the first member of the tetraspanin (TM4) superfamily detected on erythrocytes, is essential for the correct assembly of human basement membranes in kidney and skin. *Blood*. 2004; 104:2217–2223.

132. Crew V, Poole J, Long S, et al. Two MER2-negative individuals with the sample novel *CD151* mutation and evidence for clinical significance of anti-MER2. *Transfusion* [online]. 2008.

133. Seltsam A, Strigens C, Yahalom V, et al. The molecular diversity of Sema7A, the semaphoring that carries the JMH blood group antigens. *Transfusion*. 2007; 47:133–146.

134. Wiener AS, Unger, LJ, Cohen L, et al. Type-specific cold auto-antibodies as a cause of acquired hemolytic anemia and hemolytic transfusion reactions: biologic test with bovine red cells. *Ann Intern Med*. 1956; 44:221.

135. Marsh WL, Jenkins WJ. Anti-i: a new cold antibody. *Nature*. 1960; 188:753.

136. Yu LC, Twu YC, Chang CY, et al. Molecular basis of the adult I phenotype and the gene responsible for the expression of the human blood group I antigen. *Blood*. 2001; 98(13):3840–3845.

137. Leger RM, Garratty G. Weakening or loss of antibody reactivity after prewar technique. *Transfusion*. 2003; 43: 1611–1614.

138. Yu LC, Twu YC, Chou ML, et al. The molecular genetics of the human I locus and molecular background explain the partial association of the adult i phenotype with congenital cataracts. *Blood*. 2003; 101(6):2081–2088.

139. Roudier N, Ripoche P, Gane P, et al. AQP3 deficiency in humans and the molecular basis of a novel blood group system, GIL. *J Biol Chem*. 2002; 277:45854–45859.

140. Giles CM, Juth MC, Wilson TE, et al. Three examples of a new antibody, anti-C8a, which reacts with 98 per cent of red cell samples. *Vox Sang*. 1965; 10(4):405–415.

141. Molthan L, Paradis DJ. Anti-Csb: the finding of the antibody antithetical to anti-Csa. *Med Lab Sci*. 1987; 44(1): 94–96.

142. Daniels GL, Judd WJ, Moore BP, et al. A "new" high frequency antigen Era. *Transfusion*. 1982; 22(3):189–193.

143. Hamilton JR, Beattie KM, Walker RH, et al. Erb, an allele to Era, and evidence for a third allele, Er. *Transfusion*. 1988; 28(3):268–271.

144. Arriaga F, Mueller A, Rodberg K, et al. A new antigen of the Er collection. *Vox Sang*. 2003; 84:137–139.

145. Applewhaite F, Ginsberg V, Gerena J, et al. A very frequent red cell antigen Ata. *Vox Sang*. 1967; 13(5):444–445.

146. Daniels GL, Taliano V, Klein MT, et al. Emm. A red cell antigen of very high frequency. *Transfusion*. 1987; 27(4): 319–321.

147. De Man AJ, van Dijk BA, Daniels GL. An example of anti-AnWj causing haemolytic transfusion reaction. *Vox Sang*. 1992; 63(3):238.

148. Daniels GL, Simard H, Goldman M, et al. PEL, a "new" high-frequency red cell surface antigen. *Vox Sang*. 1996; 70(1):31–33.

ADDITIONAL READINGS

Daniels G. *Human Blood Groups*. Oxford: Blackwell Science; 1995.

Issitt PD, Anstee DJ. *Applied Blood Group Serology*. 4th ed. Durham, NC: Montgomery Scientific Publications; 1998.

Klein HG, Anstee DJ. *Mollison's Blood Transfusion in Clinical Medicine*. 11th ed. Malden, MA Blackwell Publishing; 1997.

Reid ME, Lomas-Francis C. *The Blood Group Antigen Facts Book*. 2nd ed. New York: Elsevier; 2004.

Roback JD, Combs MR, Grossman BJ, et al. *Technical Manual*. 16th ed. Bethesda, MD: AABB; 2008.

Schenkel-Brunner H. *Human Blood Groups*. 2nd ed. New York: SpringerWien; 2000.

HUMAN LEUKOCYTE ANTIGENS

SUSAN HSU

OBJECTIVES

After completion of this chapter, the reader will be able to:

1. Describe the most salient features of the HLA system.
2. Discuss the role of HLA in immune response.
3. Define class I and class II genes.
4. Describe the various methodologies for histocompatibility testing.
5. Discuss the clinical applications of HLA.
6. Discuss HLA association with disease.

KEY WORDS

Adaptive immunity

Alloreactivity

American Society for Histocompatibility and Immunogenetics (ASHI)

Class I genes

Class II genes

Complement-dependent microlymphocytotoxicity

Epitope

Exon

Genomic DNA

HLA

Intron

Linkage disequilibrium

Major histocompatibility complex

MHC restriction

Polymorphism

Private epitope

Public epitope

Refractoriness

*E*very vertebrate species possesses a chromosomal region called the *major histocompatibility complex* (MHC). The best-studied MHC models are the human *HLA* (human leukocyte antigen) and the murine H-2 (histocompatibility antigen 2) systems. The terms MHC and HLA have been used interchangeably in the field. The HLA genes encoding the histocompatibility antigens are classified into *class I genes* (i.e., HLA-A, B, and C) and *class II genes* (HLA-D–related genes, i.e., HLA-DR, DQ, and DP). The class I and class II genes are highly *polymorphic*, and each of these genes has many alleles. The HLA complex represents the most polymorphic genetic system known to date. Although the HLA complex was discovered only a little more than half a century ago,[1] it has become one of the most intensely studied biomedical science. This is due to the central role of MHC in the fields of immune responses, transplantation, and autoimmune diseases. In addition, it also serves as the most informative genetic marker for anthropological and epidemiology studies.

The most important biologic function of MHC genes is their involvement in controlling and modulating the adaptive immune response. The primary role of the *adaptive immunity* is to employ both the cellular and the humoral arms of the immune system to protect the host against a wide range of intracellular and extracellular pathogenic and/or infectious invaders (e.g., viruses and bacteria). To accomplish this, the immune system must discriminate between "self" and "nonself" (i.e., foreign). The HLA class I and class II molecules are intimately involved in regulating the adaptive immune response by presenting a complex composed of self-HLA molecule and the bound nonself peptide for recognition of clonally expressed T-cell receptors (TCR).[2–6] This phenomenon is termed

MHC restriction.[7] After thymic selection, mature T-cell repertoire is biased toward recognition of peptides following the principle of MHC restriction: the CD4+ T lymphocytes recognize peptide antigens together with self-MHC class II molecules, while the CD8+ T lymphocytes recognize peptide antigens in the context of self-MHC class I molecules.[8] This mechanism for generating T lymphocyte–mediated immune responses utilizes self-MHC antigens as the background on which nonself peptide antigens are recognized.[9,10] This is in contrast to immune responses generated when T lymphocytes recognize an allograft, which presents foreign MHC antigens to the immune system. The immune response generated against nonself MHC molecules is termed *alloreactivity*.[10] There are two types of allorecognition pathways. In the direct pathway, the T lymphocytes recognize the protein-derived peptides, which are bound to allogeneic MHC molecules expressed on foreign cells (e.g., allograft). In the indirect pathway, T cells recognize the peptides derived from the allogeneic MHC molecules that are bound and presented by the self-MHC class II molecules. Both types of allorecognition are clinically important phenomena responsible for allograft rejection following organ transplantation, immune response to platelet transfusion, and for graft-versus-host (GVH) disease following bone marrow transplantation.[10]

It is not possible to provide a comprehensive review of the molecular genetic aspects and the immunologic relevance of HLA in clinical medicine in a book chapter. The intention here is to provide a brief overview of the most salient features of HLA, the principle of testing methodologies commonly used in histocompatibility-testing laboratories, and clinical applications of HLA with emphasis on transplantation and platelet transfusion therapy. Readers interested in gaining in-depth knowledge and understanding of the essential functions of HLA in immune responses, transplantation, disease association, and the anthropological/population aspects of HLA may refer to several key reference sources provided for a more detailed and comprehensive discussion.

GENOMIC ORGANIZATION OF THE HLA SYSTEM

The genes that encode the HLA class I and class II molecules are closely linked and are located on the short arm of chromosome 6 (6p21.31). This genetic segment encompasses over 4,100 kilobases (kb) and contains more than 200 genes.[11,12] Within the HLA complex, gene loci are constituently grouped into three regions. See Figure 12-1.

The class I region contains both the classical HLA-A, B, and C genes, the nonclassical HLA-E, F, G, MICA, and MICB genes, as well as the nonfunctional pseudogenes H, J, K, and L genes. The class II region, also known as HLA-D region, contains the classical HLA-DR, DQ, DP, DM, and DO genes; the nonclassical class II genes: transporter associated with antigen processing (TAPs) and large multifunctional protease (LMPs); and the pseudogenes. The class III region does not contain HLA genes; however, it does contain genes encoding the complement components (C2, C4, and factor B), 21-hydroxylase, tumor necrosis factors (TNFs), and the heat-shock protein (HSP), to name a few.[11,12]

The following discussions will be focused primarily on the classical HLA-A, B, and C (class I) genes and the classical HLA-DR, DQ, and DP (class II) genes, while the nonclassical HLA genes will only be discussed wherever it is applicable.

STRUCTURES AND FUNCTIONS OF MHC MOLECULES

HLA Class I Molecules

All the HLA-A, B, and C molecules share very similar biochemical structures. Each consists of two polypeptides with different molecular weight (mol.wt.). The heavy chain (α) has a mol.wt. of approximately 45,000 D, which is anchored to the cell membrane, while the light chain (β) also called β_2-microglobulin (β_2 m) has a mol.wt. of 12,000 D. The β_2 m is mapped on chromosome 15 and is nonvalently bound to the heavy chain.[13] Both the heavy and light chains are folded into globular domains similar to the immunoglobulin domains. See Color Plate C-1.

The heavy chain has five domains: three extracellular domains (i.e., α1, α2, and α3), each of which contains 90 amino acids; the transmembrane (TM) domain that contains 40 amino acids; and the intracellular cytoplasmic tail (CYT) that contains 30 amino acids. The extracellular portion begins with the amino (NH_2) terminus, and the carboxy (COOH) terminus lies within the cytoplasm. The β_2 m folds into a single domain and is noncovalently bound to the α3 domain.[12]

The genes encoding class I and class II molecules have the characteristic structure of eukaryotic genes in which the coding regions (*exons*) are separated from one another by the noncoding regions (*introns*). The exon–intron organization of a class I gene parallels that of a three-dimensional configuration of a class I molecule as demonstrated in Color Plate C-1. The class I heavy-chain protein domains are encoded by eight exons. Exon 1 encodes the leader sequence that

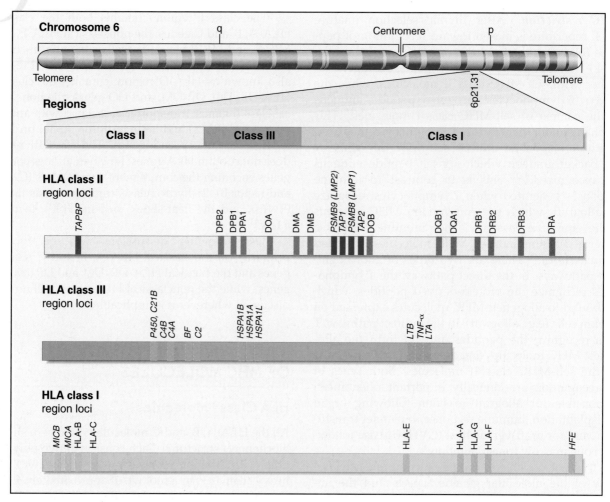

FIGURE 12-1   Location and organization of the HLA complex on chromosome 6. The complex is conventionally divided into three regions: I, II, and III. Each region contains numerous loci (genes), only some of which are shown. Of the class I and II genes, only the expressed genes are depicted. Class III genes are not related to class I and class II genes structurally or functionally. BF, complement factor B; C2, complement component 2; C21B, cytochrome P-450, subfamily XXI; C4A and C4B, complement components 4A and 4B, respectively; HFE, hemochromatosis; HSP, heat-shock protein; LMP, large multifunctional protease; LTA and LTB, lymphotoxins A and B, respectively; MICA and MICB, major-histocompatibility-complex class I chain genes A and B, respectively; P-450, cytochrome P-450; PSMB8 and 9, proteasome $\beta8$ and 9, respectively; TAP1 and TAP2, transporter associated with antigen processing 1 and 2, respectively; TAPBP, TAP-binding protein (tapasin); TNF-α, tumor necrosis factor α; and HSPA1A, HSPA1B, and HSPA1L, heat-shock protein 1A A-type, heat-shock protein 1A B-type, and heat-shock protein 1A-like, respectively. (Reproduced with permission from Klein J. The HLA system: first of two parts. *N Engl J Med.* 2000;343:703.)

is cleaved off and is not incorporated into the matured HLA polypeptide on the cell surface. Exons 2 to 4 encode $\alpha1$, $\alpha2$, and $\alpha3$ domains, respectively. Exon 5 encodes the TM anchor, while exons 6 and 7 encode the CYT. Exon 8 encodes the 3′-untranslated region that is present in all class I genes.[12]

While there are high degrees of interlocus homology, there are specific amino acids to distinguish each class I locus: met-138 and met-189 for HLA-A; arg-239 for HLA-B; val-52, Glu-183, and Glu-268 for HLA-C.[14] The extreme polymorphism detected either at the antigen (by serologic method) or at the allele (by molecular genetic methods) level for any given class I locus is due to the amino acid differences located mostly in the $\alpha1$ and $\alpha2$ domains. These differences are not distributed uniformly throughout the $\alpha1$ and $\alpha2$ domains; instead, they are clustered in seven so-called hypervariable regions that correspond to amino acid residues 9 to 12, 40 to 45, 62 to 83, 94 to 97, 105 to 116, 137 to 163, and 174 to 194.[12] This high degree of protein polymorphism of the class I gene is generated by a variety of mechanisms such as point mutation, deletion, insertion, homologous but unequal crossing-over, recombination, and gene conversion.[12] These hypervariable regions represent the functional regions of the class I molecules. By contrast, $\alpha3$ and β_2 m domains do not exhibit this variability.

Function of Class I Molecules

The function of class I molecules is intimately related to their three-dimensional structures.[15–17] The $\alpha1$ and $\alpha2$ domains generate a platform consisting of eight antiparallel β-pleated sheet and two strands of antiparallel α-helices. A groove is thus created with the characteristic structure of two α-helices overlaying a platform of the β-pleated sheet that serves as the binding site for the processed peptide antigens. The $\alpha3$ domain and the β_2 m together form a pedestal-like structure on top of which sits the peptide-binding groove.[12] Although class I and class II molecules exhibit the same three-dimensional structure, a very subtle change in the α-helical region does result in significant differences in their respective peptide-binding grooves. The class I groove is closed at both ends; therefore, it limits the length of the peptides that it can accommodate. The peptides are usually 8 to 10 amino acids long, and each peptide has two to three key anchoring residues that bind to allele-specific pockets of the class I molecule. By contrast, the class II groove is open at both ends and can accommodate peptides of 10 to 30 amino acids that extend beyond the groove. See Color Plate C-2 . Also, the class II peptides have three or four anchoring residues that bind to the class II allele–specific binding pockets in the groove.[12]

Loading of processed peptides into the binding groove occurs when the new class I and class II molecules are being synthesized. Class I molecules are synthesized in the endoplasmic reticulum (ER). Except in viral infection, peptides bound to class I molecules are self-peptides derived from protein synthesized endogenously in the cytoplasm. The endogenous proteins are degraded by LMP proteasome complex into peptides and transported into the ER facilitated by the ATP-dependent transport proteins. The transport proteins are encoded by the TAP1 and TAP2 genes. Once inside the ER, the peptides are loaded into the groove of the membrane-bound class I molecules. See part A of Color Plate C-3. The peptide–class I complex is then transported to the cell surface and is ready for presentation to the TCRs on CD8+ lymphocytes.[5,6,12]

Each class I molecule binds to particular amino acid side chains of one peptide; therefore, only a few peptides from any protein can bind to a given class I molecule. For example, peptides bound to HLA-A2 molecules share more common structural features than peptides that are bound to HLA-A1 or HLA-B8. The limited number of peptides that can bind to a given class I molecule is compensated both at the individual level and at the population level. Each individual inherits multiple class I (HLA-A, B, and C) molecules that permit the binding of thousands of self-peptides.[9] Since nearly all the polymorphisms that distinguish individual alleles are located in the peptide-binding groove, it provides an effective immune surveillance, besides contributing to the survival of the population. The extreme polymorphisms with different HLA allele frequencies existing in the major or subsets of ethnic population further provide credence that HLA polymorphism and linkage disequilibrium arise through selection pressure during migration and adaptation for species survival.[9,12]

HLA Class II Molecules

The class II molecules that include HLA-DR, DQ, and DP all share similar biochemical structures. Each consists of two noncovalently associated polypeptides, and both chains are anchored on the cell membrane. The heavy chain (α) has a mol.wt. of 33 to 35 kD, while the light chain (β) has a mol.wt. of 26 to 28 kD. Unlike the class I molecule, both the α and β chains of class II molecules are encoded by genes within the class II region. The α- and β-chain genes also have similar exon–intron organization in which exon 1 encodes the leader peptide, while exons 2 and 3 encode the two extracellular domains. In the β-chain genes, exon 4 encodes the TM domain, while exon 5 encodes the CYT. By contrast, in the α-chain genes, both the TM region and the CYT are encoded by exon 4.[12] The exon 5 and exon 6 encode the 3"-untranslated region for α and β chains respectively. The α- and β-chain genes are arranged as matched pairs (i.e., DRα and DRβ, DQα and DQβ, DPα and DPβ), but the number of DRβ genes and pseudogenes may differ, depending on the haplotypes. See Figure 12-2. As proteins, DRα, DQα, and DPα preferentially pair with their respective β-chains, although cross-pairing is also observed.[18]

Each of the class II α and β chain has four domains: the peptide-binding domain ($\alpha2$ and $\beta2$), the TM region, and the CYT (Color Plate C-1). Most of the polymorphisms of class II molecules are located in the exon 2 of DR$\beta1$, DQ$\beta1$, and DP$\beta1$ gene products. This exon encodes the α-helical "walls" and the β-pleated sheet "floor" of the peptide-binding groove formed by the α–β heterodimer (Color Plate C-3). Among the α-chain loci, only DQα and DPα loci show extensive polymorphisms.

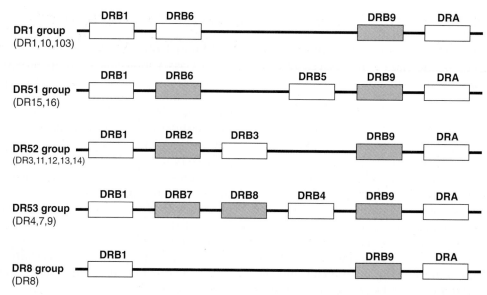

FIGURE 12-2   Expression of DRB genes based on haplotype (shaded bars denote pseudogenes).

Function of Class II Molecules

Class II molecules are also synthesized in the ER. Unlike class I molecules, class II molecules are prevented from binding with processed peptides in the ER; instead, they bind to the so-called invariant chain (Ii). The class II–Ii complexes then travel and intersect with endosomal compartment containing the proteases-degraded exogenous protein peptides (e.g., bacteria).[5] It is in this compartment, with the facilitation of HLA-DM heterodimer that the Ii chain is released, and loading of peptide in the groove can take place. The peptide-laden class II molecules are then transported to the cell surface and presented to the TCR of CD4+ T cells (part B of Color Plate C-3). The key function of CD4+ T cells, stimulated through class II molecules, is to promote production of appropriate antibodies to the offending extracellular antigen.[18–20]

Expression and Tissue Distribution

The class I and class II molecules are codominantly expressed but have different tissue distributions. The class I molecules are found on most nucleated cells but can also be found on anucleated platelets, immature red cells, and reticulocytes. The class II molecules, however, have limited tissue distributions. They are primarily found on antigen-presenting cells (i.e., B cells), endothelial cells, monocytes, macrophages, dendritic cells, Langerhans cells as well as activated T cells.[21,22] The expression of both class I and class II molecules may be upregulated during inflammatory response or can be induced by cytokines, particularly interferon. Their expression may also be downregulated in pathologic condition (e.g., on cancerous cells or various virus-infected cells). The reduced expression or the absence of HLA molecules on the neoplastic or virus-infected cells allows them to escape immune surveillance.[21,22] However, such evasion is countered by natural killer (NK) cells, which mediate killing to detect the decreased expression of class I molecules on tumor or virus-infected cells. This alternative immune defense strategy is termed "missing self."[23] The relationship between NK cell immunoglobulin–like receptors (KIR) and HLA class I molecules in NK cell–mediated cytotoxicity as well as in hematopoietic stem cell transplantation (HSCT) is discussed in detail elsewhere.[24–27]

NOMENCLATURE OF HLA

Currently, there are two nomenclature systems that are used according to the typing techniques employed to identify the gene products. Historically, the various class I gene products were detected through serologic methods, while those in the class II region, also known as the "D" region, were originally defined by cellular techniques.

The conventional HLA nomenclature was first established in 1964 by the HLA Nomenclature Committee under the auspices of the WHO. The nomenclature underwent many revisions between 1965 and 1991. The current rule for naming of the HLA gene products by both serologic and cellular techniques is as follows: HLA followed by a hyphen; capital letters (i.e., A, B, C, DR, DQ, and DP) denoting the individual locus; and a number denoting the antigenic specificity. See Table 12-1. Additionally, the provisional antigenic specificities previously designated with a

TABLE 12-1   WHO Listing of HLA Serologically Defined Specificities

A	B		C	DR	DQ	DP
A1	B5	B50 (21)	Cw1	DR1	DQ1	DPw1
A2	B7	B51 (5)	Cw2	DR103	DQ2	DPw2
A203	B703	B5102	Cw3	DR2	DQ3	DPw3
A210	B8	B5103	Cw4	DR3	DQ4	DPw4
A3	B12	B52 (5)	Cw5	DR4	DQ5 (1)	DPw5
A9	B13	B53	Cw6	DR5	DQ6 (1)	DPw6
A10	B14	B54 (22)	Cw7	DR6	DQ7 (3)	
A11	B15	B55 (22)	Cw8	DR7	DQ8 (3)	
A19	B16	B56 (22)	Cw9 (w3)	DR8	DQ9 (3)	
A23 (9)	B17	B57 (17)	Cw10 (w3)	DR9		
A24 (9)	B18	B58 (17)	Cw15	DR10		
A2403	B21	B59	Cw17	DR11 (5)		
A25 (10)	B22	B60 (40)		DR12 (5)		
A26 (10)	B27	B61 (40)		DR13 (6)		
A28	B2708	B62 (15)		DR14 (6)		
A29 (19)	B35	B63 (15)		DR1403		
A30 (19)	B37	B64 (14)		DR1404		
A31 (19)	B38 (16)	B65 (14)		DR15 (2)		
A32 (19)	B39 (16)	B67		DR16 (2)		
A33 (19)	B3901	B70		DR17 (3)		
A34 (10)	B3902	B71 (70)		DR18 (3)		
A36	B40	B72 (70)				
A43	B4005	B73		DR51		
A66 (10)	B41	B75 (15)				
A68 (28)	B42	B76 (15)		DR52		
A69 (28)	B44 (12)	B77 (15)				
A74 (19)	B45 (12)	B78		DR53		
A80	B46	B81				
	B47	B82				
	B48	Bw4				
	B49 (21)	Bw6				

Reproduced with permission from Rodey GE. *HLA Beyond Tears. Introduction to Human Histocompatibility.* 2nd ed. Houston, Texas: De Novo Inc.; 2000.

TABLE 12-2   Examples of WHO Molecular Nomenclature[a]

Standard Allele	Silent Nucleotide Substitutions	Substitutions in Noncoding Regions
HLA-A*0202	HLA-A*03011	HLA-A*2402101[b]
HLA-A*2406	HLA-A*03012	HLA-A*2402102L[c]
	HLA-A*03013	
HLA-B*0801		HLA-B*5111N[c]
	HLA-B*35091	
HLA-Cw*1801	HLA-B*35092	HLA-DRB4*0103101[b]
		HLA-DRB4*0103102N[c]
HLA-DQA1*0101	HLA-DQA1*0501	
	HLA-DQA1*05011	
HLA-DRB1*0404	HLA-DQA1*05012	
HLA-DRB4*01[d]		

[a]See text for detailed definitions of the nomenclature rules.
[b]This allele is fully expressed.
[c]This allele is expressed at low (L) levels, or is not expressed at all (null or N). The use of L and N is optional.
[d]The two-digit nomenclature is used when sequence information is incomplete.
Reproduced with permission from Rodey GE. *HLA Beyond Tears. Introduction to Human Histocompatibility*. 2nd ed. Houston, Texas: De Novo Inc.; 2000.

letter "w" were dropped with the following three exceptions. To distinguish the HLA-C locus specificities from the complement component, the "w" was permanently retained for the Cw locus. The DP and Dw specificities also retained the "w" to indicate that the original specificities were defined by cellular typing methods. Lastly, Bw4 and Bw6 also retained the "w" to distinguish them as epitopes from other B-locus specificities or alleles.[28]

The second nomenclature system, based on the correlation of nucleotide sequences with the expressed proteins, was first established in 1987 by the HLA Nomenclature Committee. However, revisions were also made between 1989 and 2004 to accommodate the extreme genetic complexity to adopt the sequence-based nomenclature.[29]

The sequence-based HLA nomenclature is illustrated below using HLA-A*240201 and HLA-A*240202L alleles as examples.

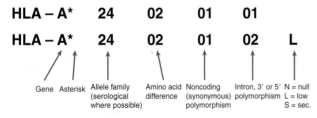

The first four digits are used to distinguish alleles encoding different amino acid sequences. Sequences specifying silent mutation (i.e., identical protein is synthesized) are assigned additional digits, for example, HLA-A*240201. The letter "N" denotes null alleles. Since there is no transcribed or expressed gene product from a null allele, subject possessing a null allele (e.g., HLA-A*0301N) will recognize foreign tissue carrying any normal HLA-A*03 allele as foreign and may mount both cellular or humoral immune responses to such tissues. The letter "L" denotes low expression, while the letter "S" denotes secreted form of an allele. See Table 12-2.

For practical purposes, either four or six digits are used by the typing laboratories for allele assignment. Due to the continued allele expansion, new HLA alleles are identified almost on a weekly basis (Table 12-3). HLA typing laboratories supporting HSCT in particular should update the sequence-based nomenclature list on a quarterly basis.

For more detailed information on both nomenclature systems, their evolution as well as the rationales behind the naming principles for each, readers may refer to the latest HLA Nomenclature Committee Report.[29]

INHERITANCE OF HLA

The HLA gene products are codominantly expressed on the cell surface. The close linkage of class I, class II, and class III genes enables the transmission of the gene

TABLE 12-3	The Complexity of HLA System	
Locus	Number of Serotypes	Number of Alleles
A	25	733
B	54	1,115
C	12	392
DRB1	18	608
DQB1	9	95
DPB1	6	132

Source: IMGT/HLA Database 01/2009.

complex from parent to child "en bloc." The closely linked genes inherited as one unit are termed *haplotype*. Family studies demonstrated that the parental haplotypes are inherited as Mendelian codominant traits. Color Plate C-4 illustrates the segregation patterns of the four parental haplotypes in a family. According to Mendel's law, any two siblings will have a 25% chance of being genotypically identical (i.e., sharing two identical parental haplotypes), 50% chance of being haploidentical (i.e., sharing one parental haplotype), and another 25% chance of being HLA nonidentical (i.e., sharing no identical haplotype). Two parental haplotypes, each inherited from one parent, constitute a "genotype." A child is always haploidentical to each parent and only siblings may have a 25% chance of being genotypically identical to one another. The recombination frequency between HLA-A and HLA-B loci and between HLA-B and HLA-DR loci were each estimated to be about 1%. There is, however, a recombination hot spot between HLA-DR and DP loci. Therefore, two siblings may be genotypically identical for HLA-A, B, C, DR, and DQ loci but may differ for DP alleles.

Linkage Disequilibrium

At the population level, certain combination of alleles (i.e., haplotypes), either within class I or class II genes or between class I and class II genes will occur more frequently than expected by chance. This phenomenon is defined as *linkage disequilibrium*. For example, the gene frequencies for HLA-A1, HLA-B8, and HLA-DR3 in the North American Caucasians are 0.16, 0.10, and 0.14, respectively. If there is no linkage disequilibrium, one would expect the A1, B8, and DR3 haplotype frequency in this population to be 0.02% ($= 0.16 \times 0.1 \times 0.14 \times 100$). The observed haplotype frequency, however, is 5.2%. The difference between the observed and the expected haplotype frequency defined as delta (or D) is 5.18. The linkage disequilibrium of various haplotypes varies vastly in different ethnic populations. Among the speculations to account for this phenomenon, the most plausible one is that these haplotypes may confer survival advantages. They were generated under the selection pressure during the migration and adaptation of the major human populations to their respective continents and subcontinents over the millennia. From the perspective of anthropology and population genetics, haplotype frequencies provide better markers to characterize populations.[30]

CLINICAL HISTOCOMPATIBILITY TESTING

The *American Society for Histocompatibility and Immunogenetics (ASHI)* is the governing organization for clinical and developmental histocompatibility in the United States. ASHI has taken a leadership role in providing guidelines (standards for histocompatibility testing) for the establishment and operation of clinical HLA laboratories in the United States.[31,32] HLA laboratories that provide clinical HLA services in support of solid organ and HSCT transplantation are required to be accredited by ASHI. Although it is not mandatory for laboratories providing HLA services in support of platelet transfusion therapy to be accredited by ASHI, it is advisable to do so because ASHI standards are recognized as the gold standards for histocompatibility testing worldwide. The ASHI procedure manual[33] contains the most current source of technical information related to histocompatibility standards, standard operating procedures (SOPs), and quality assurance programs to name a few, for the operation of clinical HLA laboratories. Readers are encouraged to use it as a reference for detailed information on various testing protocols.

Depending on the scopes of the clinical services and the sizes of the HLA laboratories, a variety of tests may be offered to support solid organ transplantation: HSCT; platelet transfusion; posttransplant monitoring for solid organ and/or for HSCT, clinical research projects. Irrespective of the services provided and the laboratory sizes, the major responsibilities of a clinical HLA laboratory are: HLA typing of recipients and donors either by serologic or molecular genetic (DNA-based) techniques, antibody screening and specificity identification in recipients receiving solid organ transplantation, HSCT and platelets transfusion therapy, and crossmatching (XM) of both solid organ transplant and/or HSCT recipient's serum with lymphocytes of prospective donors. The methods used for XM, antibody screening, and specificity identification can be either serologic or solid phase. Although the classical serology methods are still routinely used by many HLA laboratories, the state-of-the-art techniques for clinical histocompatibility testings are DNA-based and solid phase–based methods for HLA typing and antibody workups, respectively.

Serologic Methodologies

Private, Public Epitopes, and Cross-reactive Groups

Serologic HLA typing reagents were historically derived from alloantisera immunized against HLA antigenic determinants. An antigenic determinant is also called an *epitope*. An epitope is defined as the minimum structure unit with six to seven amino acids that can be perceived as foreign by T- or B-cell receptors. Epitopes that differ among individuals of the same species are called alloepitopes.[32] Since HLA molecules consist of several hypervariable regions, there are multiple alloepitopes residing on the class I molecules, which can elicit immune response following HLA alloimmunization events such as pregnancy, blood transfusion, or tissue transplantation. The serologically defined epitopes can be divided operationally into two types. Antibodies produced against a single HLA gene product (e.g., HLA-A2 or HLA-B44) are referred to as *private epitopes*. Some of the private epitopes identified earlier to specify different HLA antigens were found later by the availability of discriminatory alloantisera to contain two or more mutually exclusive private epitopes. For example, cells carrying HLA-A9 antigen were later found to be either HLA-A23 or HLA-A24. This was due to the fact that alloantisera against the unique private epitope for A23 and 24 were identified subsequently. The epitope specific for A9 thus became known as public or cross-reactive epitope shared by cells carrying HLA-A23 and A24.

Antibodies produced against more than one gene products (e.g., HLA-A2, 28, 9 or HLA-B7, 22, 27) were detected as shared *public epitope* or cross-reactive epitope.[32] There are many public epitopes that reside in the HLA class I molecules. The best-known examples of public epitopes are Bw4 and Bw6. Their differences were due to the amino acid sequence located at positions 77 to 83[34] in the α1 domain: Bw4 has arginine at position 82, while Bw6 has aspartic acid at position 80. The HLA-A locus antigens A23, A24, A25, and A32 also possess Arg-82; therefore, these antigens react positively with anti-HLA Bw4 antisera. The Bw4- and Bw6-specific epitopes are mutually exclusive and all the B-locus antigens can be grouped into antigens either shared by Bw4 or Bw6 public epitopes.

Based on the sharing of public epitopes other than Bw4 and Bw6, the HLA-A and HLA-B locus antigens can be categorized into the following major cross-reactive groups (CREGs): 1 CREG, 2 CREG, 5 CREG, 7 CREG, 8 CREG, and 12 CREG (see Table 12-4). To thoroughly understand the immunogenetic relationships among private epitopes, public epitopes, and CREGs, it is crucial for HLA laboratory personnel to grasp this concept because they have significant clinical implications and relevance in solid organ transplantation as well as platelet transfusion therapy, which will be discussed in relevant sections.

Complement-dependent Microcytotoxicity

The *complement-dependent microlymphocytotoxicity (CDC)* technique has been used as the standard serologic typing method for HLA class I and class II antigens since 1964.[35] The basic and modified CDC assay[36] is shown in Figure 12-3. The tissue source is lymphocytes (i.e., the purified T cells and B cells are used to type class I and class II antigens, respectively). The typing sera are mostly obtained from alloimmunized, multiparous women, and the reagent-grade sera are procured from extensive screening of these sera against a large panel of lymphocytes derived from well HLA-typed subjects. Since the majority of the alloantisera obtained from multiparous women tend to be low titer with broad specificities, monoclonal antibodies raised from immunized mice have also been used since the 1990s as typing reagents.[32] There are frozen class I or II typing trays available from many different HLA vendors. Because the frequencies of HLA antigens vary among major populations (black, Caucasian, and Asia-Pacific islanders), certain HLA antigens are found more prevalent in a particular ethnic population than others; therefore, commercial class I typing trays are specifically configured for typing of black or Asiatic population. Tissue-typing technologists must use the appropriate typing trays or use the ethnic typing tray as supplementary tray when typing black or oriental subjects.

Serologic HLA typing for class I and class II antigens is a well-established procedure. Briefly, 1 μL of well-suspended and purified lymphocytes (T or B cells) is plated into each well containing alloantisera specific for an HLA class I (for class I typing tray) or class II (for class II typing tray) antigen. The cells and antisera are then gently mixed and incubated at room temperature for 30 minutes, followed by the addition of 5 μL of appropriately titered, screened, and freshly frozen rabbit serum (complement source). The tray is then incubated for an additional hour at room temperature.

TABLE 12-4   CREG Frequencies in Some American Ethnic Populations

CREG Frequency[a]	Antigen Inclusions	CREG			
		Asians	Blacks	Latinos	Whites
1C	A1, 3, 11, 23, 24, 29, 30, 31, 36, 80	95.5	97.3	85.9	101.8
2C	A2, 23, 24, 68, 69, B57, 58	105.6	91.1	82.5	85.2
10C	A11, 25, 26, 32, 33, 34, 66, 68, 69, 74	52.5	52.8	65.1	43.9
5C	B18, 35, 46, 49, 50, 51, 52, 53, 57, 58, 62, 63, 71, 72, 75, 76, 77, 78	86.7	88.8	99.8	99.8
7C	B7, 8, 13, 27, 41, 42, 47, 48, 54, 55, 56, 59, 60, 61, 67, 81, 82	81.9	48.8	40.6	76.3
8C	B8, 18, 38, 39, 59, 64, 65, 67	13.5	23.3	26.2	47.4
12C	B13, 37, 41, 44, 45, 47, 49, 50, 60, 61	49.1	42.9	67.9	61.4
4C	A23, 24, 25, 32 ("Aw4"), Bw4 group	59.8 58.6	31.7 71.8	56.5 83.5	29.9 78.1
6C	Bw6 group	143.8	98.9	128.0	114.4

[a]Numbers represent the sum of antigen frequencies within each CREG group. (Reproduced with permission from *HLA Beyond Tears,* by G. E. Rodey, 2000).

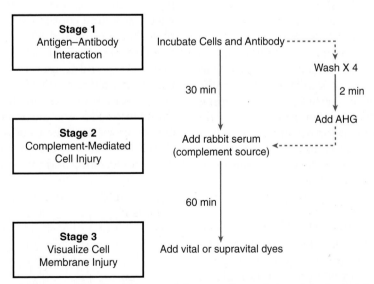

FIGURE 12-3   This figure shows the three basic steps of the complement-dependent microlymphocytotoxicity assay (CDC). The antiglobulin-augmented CDC assay (AHG-CDC) includes extra steps between stages 1 and 2 as noted. (Reproduced with permission from Rodey GE. *HLA Beyond Tears. Introduction to Human Histocompatibility*. 2nd ed. Houston, Texas: De Novo Inc.; 2000.)

When the lymphocytes carrying specific HLA antigens correspond to the alloantisera in the wells, the binding of HLA-specific antibodies to the HLA antigens on the target cells will activate complement, therefore, mediating cell lysis, which in turn will result in cell death. When a vital dye is added to each well (e.g., acridine orange/ethidium bromide), the dead cells will take up the dye denoting a positive result and stain orange/red, while the live cells will stain green denoting a negative result. The scoring of a positive or negative cytotoxic reaction in each well is based on the percentage of cell death read under an inverted phase microscope. Positive reactions indicate that the HLA-specific antisera correspond to the HLA antigens on the target cell surface. Negative reactions indicate that the alloantisera did not correspond to the HLA antigens on the target cells. The scoring system used by HLA laboratories is as follows:

> 1 = 0% to 10% cell death
> 2 = 11% to 20% cell death
> 4 = 21% to 50% cell death
> 6 = 51% to 80% cell death
> 8 = 81% to 100% cell death
> 0 = unreadable due to any reasons

Scores of 1 or 2 indicate negative reactions, a score of 4 indicates weak or doubtful reactions, and scores of 6 or 8 indicate definite positive reactions. In CDC assay, a score of 4 requires a lot of considerations and good judgment depending on whether it is used for HLA typing, antibody screening, or XM. When a false-negative reaction is critical in a crossmatch test, reaction scores of 2 or 4 may be considered positive. When false positive is critical, a reaction score of 4 may be considered negative.[32] However, the best practice in regards to a reaction score of 4 should be clearly spelled out in the laboratory's SOP concerning HLA typing, antibody screening, and XM to avoid making bad judgments or mistakes. Currently, most of the commercial, serologic HLA typing reagents are of high quality; therefore, when good laboratory practices are applied in performing HLA typing, only two HLA antigens (heterozygote) or one HLA antigen (homozygote) per locus are identified.

The Mixed Lymphocyte Culture Test

The mixed lymphocyte culture (MLC) was first introduced in 1964 as an in vitro cellular test to evaluate histocompatibility.[37] The test involves coculturing the sterility-separated lymphocytes from two individuals together. One population of the cells will recognize the different antigenic determinants located in the HLA-D region (i.e., class II region genes DR, DQ, and DP) of the opposite cell population and vice versa. The cell interactions result in lymphoproliferation and DNA synthesis. In order to estimate accurately the proliferative response of one cell population (responder cells) to the other (stimulator cells) in the so-called one-way MLC, one cell population can be treated either with mitomycin C or X-irradiation to prevent cell division but still maintains the ability to stimulate the other cell population.[38] The extent of the lymphoproliferative response of the untreated cell population can be quantitatively measured by pulse labeling of the coculture for 10 to 18 hours with radiolabeled H^3-thymidine. Reciprocal MLC tests are normally performed between two individuals to assess the differences between their class II genes. In the MLC, the responding cells are T cells and the stimulator cells are antigen-presenting cells (e.g., B cells, dendritic cells, macrophages epithelial cells, and Langerhans cells in the skin). The MLC test per se is currently being replaced by DNA-based typing of class II genes. Many laboratories still use this testing methodology for assessing the cellular immunity of patients.

DNA Methodologies

Molecular Genetic Method

Before discussing the various DNA-based HLA typing techniques, a brief review of the biochemical structure and properties of deoxyribonucleic acid (DNA) as well as an introduction of a few molecular genetic terminologies commonly used in DNA-based testing are in order.

DNA is composed of two complementary polynucleotide chains twisted into a double helix. Each nucleotide consists of a deoxyribose sugar(s), a phosphate group, and one of the four bases [Adenine, Thymine (Uracil for RNA), Guanine, and Cytosine]. The A, T, G, and C are the four building blocks commonly referred to as dNTPs that are incorporated into DNA during synthesis (Fig. 12-4). One end of the DNA strand is called 5′ and the other end is called 3′. The sequence of the coding strand is always written in the 5′ to 3′ direction. There are two hydrogen bonds between A–T pairing and three hydrogen bonds between

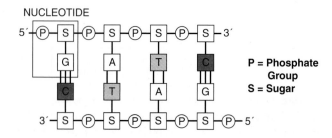

FIGURE 12-4   Biochemical structure/properties of DNA.

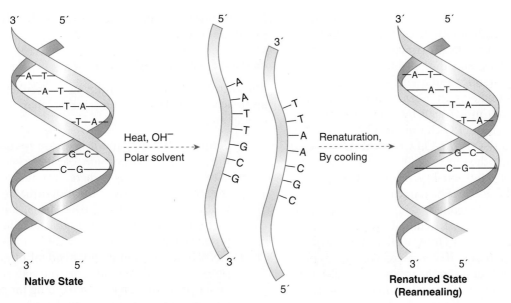

FIGURE 12-5 Denaturation and renaturation of DNA.

G–C pairing; therefore, more energy is required to break the bond of G–C pairing. The length of double-stranded (ds) DNA is measured by base pair (bp) or kb (1 kb = 1,000 bp). The ds DNA can be denatured into two single-stranded DNA by heating, alkali (NaOH), or polar solvent (DMSO and Formamide). Upon cooling (<60°C), the two complementary, single-stranded (ss) DNA will reanneal (renatured) to form ds DNA. The properties of denaturation, renaturation (reannealing), and base pairing of DNA are applied in DNA-based typing methods (Fig. 12-5).

Primers and probes are a short stretch of nucleotides, which are designed to be complementary to the known polymorphic (region) sequences of the genes or alleles to be detected. A *primer* is referred to as a ss synthetic oligonucleotide with 20 to 30 bases in length and provides a free 3'-OH end to which dNTPs are added by Taq polymerase to initiate DNA synthesis of the complementary strand from 5' to 3'. Two ss primers (set or pair) must each flank the opposite strands of the target region to be amplified, for example:

5'-ATGTCACGTTACTCGTAGCATG-3'

←——— 3'-CGTAC-5'

5'-ATGTC-3'——→

3'-TACAGTGCAATGAGCATCGTAC-5'

The forward (5') primer is complementary to the 3' end of the noncoding (antisense) strand, and the reverse (3') primer is complementary to the 3' end of the coding (sense) strand.

A *probe* is a ss synthetic oligonucleotide with 12 to 18 bases in length, and the sequences of the bases are complementary to the polymorphism of an allele or allele group to be detected. An example is depicted in Figure 12-6 to show how a DR1-specific probe is hybridized to its complementary DNA strand after alkali denaturation.

Genomic DNA

The tissue source for DNA-based HLA typing is any nucleated cell. The total amount of DNA extracted from nucleated cells is referred to as *genomic DNA*. The quantity and quality of DNA extracted varies depending on the DNA extraction methods and sample sizes. Currently, a majority of clinical laboratories are using commercial DNA extraction kits available for various sample sources that include whole blood, buccal swab, tissue, hair follicle, or paraffinized tissue

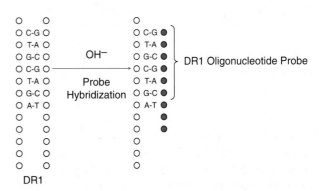

FIGURE 12-6 Hybridization of DR1 probe with complementary DNA sequence.

block. Genomic DNA can either be extracted manually or through automation. There are different models of automatic DNA extraction robotic workstations available to suit the needs and size of each laboratory. The quantity and quality of DNA or RNA can easily be estimated from O.D. readings at 260 nm (A260) and at 280 nm (A280) by a UV spectrophotometer. By definition, 1 O.D. unit at A260 is equal to 50 μg/mL of ds DNA. The O.D. ratio of A260/A280 is used to indicate the purity of DNA because protein is read at A280. High-quality or pure DNA has a ratio between 1.7 to 2.0. For clinical typing, an O.D. ratio $\geq$1.65 is recommended, while a DNA concentration of 10 to 50 ng/μL will satisfy most testing methods. The amount of DNA needed may vary between 10 and 100 μL. If commercial DNA typing reagents are used, one should follow the DNA concentration specified in the product insert. The DNA used for PCR can also be called a template and the gene product obtained after PCR can be referred to as amplicon.[32]

Quality Control of DNA Laboratory

The polymerase chain reaction (PCR) is capable of amplifying large numbers of copies of sequences from minute quantity of DNA template. The ability has not only revolutionized the fundamental approach in biomedical research, but it also created unprecedented problems of cross-contamination of samples and reagents. While high standards and quality performance should be set and applied to all laboratories, cross-contamination that is not due to viruses or infectious agents but due to aerosols (e.g., vortexing, opening, and closing of microcentrifuge tubes); utilizing open-end pipette tips; and/or leaving traces of DNA on work benches, is only unique to PCR process because of the power of PCR amplification. Therefore, it is quintessential that all laboratory personnel are specially trained and follow stringent guidelines in order to operate a creditable DNA-testing laboratory. It is imperative that all staff, as well as the laboratory director, understand the grave consequences created by DNA cross-contamination while performing PCR-related experiments. The steps for establishing a contamination-free DNA laboratory include designing two separate areas (pre-PCR and post-PCR), designating special equipment to those particular areas (pipettes and pipette tips), sample handling, and implementing strict quality control and guidelines to define the competency of the staff. A staff must be trained for all the procedures to prevent cross-contamination in a PCR laboratory before he/she is trained to physically perform the tasks. Excellent guidelines and recommendations to implement a quality assurance program for a DNA-testing laboratory are described in the ASHI procedure manual.[32]

Reason for DNA-based Typing

The primary reasons for utilizing molecular genetic approaches for HLA typing rather than serologic typing are:

- Serologic typing cannot keep up-to-date with the continued expansion of new class I and class II alleles (e.g., there are no serologic reagents to distinguish the individual alleles of DRβ1*0401, 0402, 0403, 0404, 0405, and 0406; therefore, the end result is that all alleles are typed as DR4).
- DNA-based typing is independent of gene expression of HLA molecules on cell surfaces, hence providing an accurate typing for patients with certain hematologic malignancies or patients undergoing chemotherapy.
- The flexibility of using either live or dead nucleated cells as a sample source eliminates restrictions on sample requirement or geographic distance from the point of origin to the typing facility.
- Unlimited sources of DNA typing reagents exist for better quality control and data comparisons.
- HSCT recipients and donors require high-resolution typing for class I and II alleles.
- Family genotyping by serology can differ from genotyping by DNA-based high-resolution typing because there are no serologic reagents available to detect many of the new alleles. See Table 12-5.

DNA-based typing can be carried out at different levels of resolution depending on the typing requirement and time available to perform the test. In general, low-resolution typing is equivalent to serologic antigen typing. These tests are often sufficient for typing pheresis recipients or donors, as well as recipients or prospective donors for solid organ transplant. While low resolution determines allele groups, high-resolution typing determines the nucleotide sequence specific for a particular allele. Allele-level typing is required for recipients and their prospective unrelated donors for HSCT or for disease association studies. There are also limitations with DNA-based typing. The major drawbacks and approaches to circumvent these limitations are discussed in more detail in another section.

DNA-based Typing

DNA typing techniques commonly used in the majority of the HLA laboratories are sequence-specific

TABLE 12-5 Genotyping by Serology Vs. High-resolution Typing

	A	B	DRB1	Methods
PT*	1, 29	8, 44	03XX, 15XX	Serology Class I
Sib1	1, 29	8, 44	03XX, 15XX	Molecular Class II
Sib2	1, 29	8, 44	03XX, 15XX	(Serology Equivalent)
PT	1, 29	8, 44	0301, 1501	Serology Class I
Sib1	1, 29	8, 44	0301, 1502	Molecular High Resolution
Sib2	1, 29	8, 44	0301, 1501	Typing for Class II
PT**	0101, 2901	0801, 4402	0301, 1501 (ac)	Molecular High Resolution
Sib1	0101, 2901	0801, 4403	0301, 1502 (bc)	Typing for Class I & II
Sib2	0101, 2901	0801, 4402	0301, 1501 (ac)	
Father	a 2901	4402	1501	
	b 2901	4403	1502	Genotyping
Mother	c 0101	0801	0301	
	d 0201	5702	1301	

*PT, Sib1, and 2 appear as HLA genotypically identical.
**PT is HLA genotypically identical to Sib2 only.

primer (SSP), sequence-specific oligonucleotide probe (SSOP), and sequence-based typing (SBT) methods. The genetic polymorphic regions that must be included for typing by these methods are exons 2 and 3 for HLA-A, B, and C (class I) genes and exon 2 for HLA-DR, DQ, and DP (class II) genes.

PCR-SSP

The principle of this methodology is designed to identify individual HLA allele (e.g., HLA-A*0201) or group of alleles within a particular antigen group. In order to discriminate polymorphic differences, often with a single nucleotide, SSPs are designed on the basis of the amplification refractory mutation system (ARMS).[39] This entails matching of the 3' end of the primer with the target sequence polymorphism. See Figure 12-7A. A mismatch at the 3' residue of the primer with the target sequence will inhibit PCR amplification. See Figure 12-7B. Internal control of a non-HLA gene must be included to validate the PCR condition for each SSP reaction. Following the PCR process, the products, along with a molecular weight marker are electrophoresed on an agarose gel. At the end of electrophoresis, the presence and/or the absence of the appropriate-size fragments in each lane can be visualized under a UV box. To complete the HLA typing, a panel of SSP primer pairs is required. There are commercial SSP typing trays available to perform either low- or high-resolution HLA class I and class II typing.

PCR-SSOP

The principle of PCR-SSOP technique is based on using a pair of locus-specific primer to amplify the hypervariable regions of a single class I (exons 2 and 3 minimally) or a single class II (exon 2) locus. Following

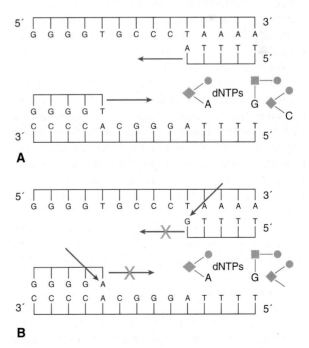

FIGURE 12-7 A: A positive PCR-SSP reaction. B: A negative PCR-SSP reaction.

the PCR process, the gene product is immobilized onto a membrane support. After the membrane-bound DNA is denatured, it can then be probed (i.e., hybridized to a panel of synthetic oligonucleotide probes to identify the alleles present in the amplified DNA sample). This technique was first standardized and introduced to the HLA community worldwide for large-scale typing of class II genes. Many technical refinements have been made, and it includes replacing the radioisotope (^{32}P) for probe labeling by nonisotopic methods, extending the SSOP typing for all class I (HLA-A, B, and C) and class II (DR, DQ, and DP) genes at both low- or high-resolution levels, and developing a variation of the SSOP methodology called reverse SSO (rSSO).[32] In the rSSO assay, instead of the amplified DNA samples, the oligonucleotide probes are individually immobilized onto a membrane support or a strip of the membrane. This variation allows HLA typing for one subject or for a large number of subjects at a time. Recently, the rSSO method was adapted onto the Luminex platform. This technology combines two of the most powerful detection and identification tools, the exquisite binding specificity between biotin and streptavidin, and the versatility of the flow cytometry. Therefore, this technology and principle applied to both DNA-based HLA typing and antibody testing deserve detailed discussion.

Luminex Technology

The Luminex system allows 100 target analyte preparations to be evaluated in a single, multiplexed assay. This is possible because of the unique combination of two different-colored fluorescent tags incorporated into each discrete bead. Thus, every bead population is identifiable by the laser-detection instrument so that a positive reaction is automatically "read" as the proper specificity for that target. The concept is based on a simple permutation model, with increasing proportions of color #1 incorporated into different batches of beads containing color #2 in a similar dosage series. The optical system measures the red and infrared fluorescence to identify the color-coded microspheres and orange fluorescence (at 575 nm) to determine the amount of indicator dye used to indicate a positive assay result. The principle of Luminex-based rSSO typing discussed below uses the LABType method[40] as an example.

LABType SSO Typing Tests

The principle of LABType is that it applies Luminex technology to the rSSO DNA typing method. First, target DNA is amplified by a PCR using HLA locus–specific primers. The PCR product is biotinylated, which allows for later detection using R-phycoerythrin conjugated streptavidin (SAPE). The PCR product is denatured and allowed to rehybridize to complementary DNA probes conjugated to fluorescently coded microbeads. A flow analyzer, the LABScan 100, identifies the fluorescent intensity (FI) of the SAPE indicator on each microsphere. The assignment of the HLA typing is based on the reaction pattern compared to patterns associated with published HLA gene sequences.

Since the amplification of the target DNA by PCR coupled with hybridization and detection all take place in a single reaction mixture, it makes this method suitable for both small- and large-scale testing. LABType generic typing tests provide medium resolution of common alleles in each HLA locus (A, B, C, DR, DQ, or DP). High-definition (HD) assays can resolve common typing ambiguities, for example, caused by Bw4 or Bw6 CREG sequences, and provide high-resolution typing by distinguishing between HLA antigen subtypes (alleles). Each bead-probe set includes negative and positive control beads for subtraction of nonspecific background signals and normalization of raw data to adjust for possible variation in sample quantity and reaction efficiency. Detailed assay protocols, data acquisition from Luminex flow cytometer, and HLA typing analysis are available from the manufacture's product insert.[40]

PCR-SBT

There are limitations in using both PCR-SSP and SSOP for tissue typing because unique polymorphic differences are not always within known hypervariable regions. The gold standard to definitively detect all relevant class I and class II polymorphisms is through DNA sequencing of a particular region of interest. The most common SBT method currently in use by many HLA labs is Sanger's enzymatic dideoxy chain-terminating technique, using PCR products containing the polymorphic regions (to be sequenced) as a template.[32] SBT is a two-step process that is outlined as follows:

1. Prepare the template for subsequent sequencing reactions from genomic DNA. For sequencing of class I genes/alleles, the PCR product must include sequences from at least exons 2 and 3, while for sequencing of class II genes/alleles, the PCR product must include sequences from exon 2. The unincorporated primers and dNTPs affect the subsequent sequencing reactions. The PCR products, therefore, are purified by using spin columns or enzymes (exonuclease 1 and shrimp alkaline phosphatase).

2. The purified PCR products are then used for cycle-sequencing reactions followed by automated sequencing. Sequencing reaction is similar to DNA synthesis (replication). It requires a single-stranded DNA as template, a single primer, DNA polymerase, dNTPs, and a small, but optimal amount of dideoxynucleotides (ddNTPs). The sequencing reactions are performed in a thermocycler. DNA polymerase requires a primer with a free 3'-OH group to initiate DNA replication (synthesis) by incorporating dNTPs into the growing complementary polynucleotide chains. Once a ddNTP is incorporated in place of a dNTP, the replication process immediately stops at the residue occupied by the ddNTP, because ddNTPs lack a free 3'-OH group to form phosphodiester bond with the next dNTP. The incorporation of ddNTP to any growing chain is random. The end product of the cycle-sequencing reaction produces populations of nucleotides of different lengths, each differing from the other by one-nucleotide increments. These different sizes of fragments all begin at a fixed point (primer) and end where a specific ddNTP is incorporated. These fragments are each complementary to the original template (e.g., with N nucleotides) but vary in number of nucleotides in the orders of $n - 1$, $n - 2, n - 3, n - 4$, etc. The principle of sequencing typing relies on the ability to identify and distinguish the different lengths of the newly synthesized fragments. This can be accomplished by using either dye-labeled primer (dye primer chemistry) or dye-labeled ddNTPs (dye terminator chemistry) in the sequencing reactions. The populations of different-length fragments are then resolved by high-resolution gel electrophoresis or capillary electrophoresis connected to an automated DNA sequencer (e.g., ABI Prism models). When automated sequencing is performed, each fluorochrome fluoresces at a different wavelength; the fluorescence emission of each fragment is interrogated by a laser and recorded by a charge-coupled device (CCD) camera. The information collected is analyzed by data management—sequencing software provided by the ABI Company or purchased separately. The software is written to perform sequence alignment and make comparison of sequences from known alleles in the IMGT/HLA database to identify alleles of the template prepared (i.e., sample). It is advisable to perform sequencing on both strands to obtain unequivocal results for heterozygous alleles.

While there are practical limitations (i.e., sequencing ambiguities), SBT does provide the most information compared to the other two methods. The pros and cons of each typing methods and their clinical utilities are listed in Tables 12-6 and 12-7.[41]

Limitations of DNA-based Typing

The major shortcomings associated with DNA-based HLA typing are ambiguous typing, failure to

TABLE 12-6	**Pros and Cons of Various DNA Typing Methods**	
Method	Pros	Cons
SSP	Rapid Low or high resolution Small volume typing STAT tests	Lower throughput Large number of reactions Limited by number of thermocyclers in the lab
SSOP	High throughput Robust High or low resolution Large volume typing Amendable for automation	Slow (membrane based) Batch mode Not for small volume typing (except Luminex-based rSSO)
SBT	Highest resolution Direct identification of new alleles Semi-automation	Lowest throughput More technically demanding Cis-/trans-polymorphism causing sequencing ambiguities Capital equipment costs

TABLE 12-7   HLA Service Categories Vs. Typing Methodologies

		Methodologies			
Categories		Serology	SSP	SSOP	SBT
HSCT	Autologous	X	X	X	
	Related	X	X	X	X
	Unrelated		X	X	X
Solid organ	Living related	X	X	X	
	Cadaveric	X	X		
Transfusion	Patients	X	X	X	
	Donors	X	X	X	
Disease association	Patient	X	X	X	X
Vaccine studies	Participants		X	X	X
Paternity	Parties involved	X	X	X	X

identify new alleles, or allele dropout. Ambiguities stem from the fact that typing reagents are mostly designed to typing polymorphisms located in exons 2 and 3 for class I alleles and in exon 2 for class II alleles. Many individual class I alleles or pairs of heterozygous allele combinations may share identical sequences at the probing exons but differ at other nonprobing exons. For example, HLA-B*0705 and B*0706 share identical sequences at exons 2 and 3, but they differ from each other at exon 5. Since exon 5 is not included in the SSOP- or SBT-typing reagents, SBT-typing result obtained will indicate that the subject could be either 0705 or 0706. Additional testing using high-resolution SSP reagents or another round of group-specific amplification followed by SBT will distinguish B*0705 from B*0706. Another type of ambiguity commonly obtained involves two or more pairs of heterozygous allele combinations after SBT or SSOP typing. Some of the allele combinations may be ambiguous by one typing technique, but may be resolved with another typing method. HLA reagent vendors that provide DNA-based typing kits also provide information for ambiguous combinations. To illustrate, the allele combination of DRB1*1101 and *1501 cannot be distinguished from the combination of *1104 and *1519 by regular SBT typing (see Table 12-8). The polymorphisms occur at codons 71 and 86. At position 71, *1101 and *1104 have the sequence AGG, while *1501 and *1519 have the sequence GCG. At position 86, *1101 and *1519 have the sequence GGT, while *1104 and *1501 have the sequence GTG. A regular SBT

test of either heterozygote combination would give the same typing results, that is, *1101/*1501 could not be distinguished from *1104/*1509.

Invariably, additional testing becomes necessary to resolve the ambiguous typing results. Depending on the laboratory's policies, different methods can be used. For the given example (Table 12-8), one can use high-resolution SSP reagent for DRB1*15 allele group to determine whether the subject is 1501+ or 1519+. If the subject was typed as 1501+, the ambiguous SBT results are then resolved as DRB1*1101 and *1501.

The null alleles present problems to both solid organ and HSCT transplantation. Since recipients and prospective donor candidate in HSCT are always high-resolution typed, subjects carrying null alleles are easily identified. However, it is not required to perform high-resolution typing for solid organ in order to avoid recipient who carries null allele to become alloimmunized; it is advisable to perform additional serology class I typing of recipient who may be homozygous for a rare allele. New alleles with polymorphisms located outside the regions of amplification or with sequence overlapping with primer pair used for amplification will not be detected. In order to overcome these shortcomings, a paper[42] published recently on behalf of ASHI has put forward guidelines concerning DNA-based typing for laboratories to follow. ASHI standards also recommend that laboratory should use two different DNA-based methods for typing patient and donors to prevent allele drop during amplification or other anomalies in the testing process.

TABLE 12-8	Nucleotide Sequences of Two Pairs of HLA-DRB1 Alleles Sharing the Same Nucleotide Polymorphisms in Exon 2															

	Selected Sequence Regions															
Allele	71	72	73	74	75	76	77	78	79	80	81	82	83	84	85	86
1101	AGG	CGG	GCC	GCG	GTG	GAC	ACC	TAC	TGC	AGA	CAC	AAC	TAC	GGG	GTT	GGT
1501	GCG	CGG	GCC	GCG	GTG	GAC	ACC	TAC	TGC	AGA	CAC	AAC	TAC	GGG	GTT	GTG
1104	AGG	CGG	GCC	GCG	GTG	GAC	ACC	TAC	TGC	AGA	CAC	AAC	TAC	GGG	GTT	GTG
1519	GCG	CGG	GCC	GCG	GTG	GAC	ACC	TAC	TGC	AGA	CAC	AAC	TAC	GGG	GTT	GGT

SCREENING AND CHARACTERIZATION OF HLA ANTIBODY

Relevance of Antibody in Solid Organ Transplantation

A deleterious effect of antibody specific for mismatched donor antigens has been amply demonstrated in every type of organs that have been transplanted.[43–46] Antibodies to several antigen systems on the transplanted tissue are all capable of damaging the transplant. Of all the possible antigens expressed on the tissues, HLA and the ABO blood group systems are the two major barriers in tissue transplants. Since a vast majority of organ transplants are ABO compatible, the most important functions of the HLA laboratories supporting solid organ transplantation will include performing HLA typing on patient and donor as well as thoroughly and comprehensively assessing the patient's immune system in terms of defining clinically relevant HLA antibodies.[44] Pretransplant testing of a patient's serum is used to detect and characterize HLA antibody resulting from alloimmunizing events such as pregnancy, transfusion, or prior transplantation. If a thorough and comprehensive characterization of antibody specificities and titers is available on the recipient, this information can be used to predicate crossmatch outcome. Growing evidence indicates that post-Tx monitoring of donor-specific HLA antibodies developed following transplantation serves as useful prognostic indicator to identify high risk for early graft loss or chronic rejection.[47] In order to perform these tests, it is necessary to freeze lymphocytes from cadaveric organ donors. This practice helps the laboratory to resolve any doubt cast on the original crossmatch results and provide live donor lymphocytes for post-Tx crossmatch monitoring.

It is also important that detailed information concerning a patient's previous transplants, histories of transfusion, pregnancy, therapeutic treatment, or medications, etc. are well documented and kept in the patient's file. This information is equally relevant to the detection, characterization, and interpretation of a patient's antibody workup prior to and following transplantation.[44]

Relevance of Antibody in Platelet Transfusion Therapy

HLA class I antigens are expressed not only on the cell surface of most nucleated cells but also on anucleated platelets. In general, patients with thrombocytopenia or patients undergoing chemotherapy that receive repetitive random-donor platelet transfusion may become alloimmunized and immunologically refractory to subsequent platelet transfusion. Although ABO and platelet-specific antigens are also expressed on platelets, most immunologic platelet refractoriness results from antibodies against HLA class I antigens.[48–51] The corrected count increment (CCI) is used clinically to identify refractory patient. The CCI is calculated using the platelet count within an hour after transfusion and the platelet count before transfusion and corrected for the patient's body surface area (BSA) and the number of platelets transfused using the following formula:

$$CCI = \frac{(\text{Post count} - \text{pre count}) \times 10^9/\text{L} \times BSA\ (m^2)}{\text{Platelet transfused} \times 10^{11}}$$

Refractoriness is defined as two, 1-hour post-transfusion CCIs of less than 5 after sequential platelet transfusion.[50,51] Once a multitransfused patient becomes refractory, HLA antibody screening is necessary to ensure that the refractoriness is not due to nonimmune causes. In order to support a refractory patient effectively with HLA-compatible platelets, the most critical information needed is the identification of class I antibody specificities and the patient's HLA phenotyping. If the patient does not respond to HLA-compatible platelets, screening serum for platelet-specific antibody and identifying other nonimmune cases for the refractoriness are necessary.

Techniques for Antibody Testing

Antibody screening tests provide the following information: presence or absence of antibody; percent panel-reactive antibody (PRA) for classes I and II; immunoglobulin isotypes (i.e., IgG vs. IgM); antibody titer and antibody specificities for class I and class II antigens. This information, in turn, is useful to predicate crossmatch outcome for solid organ transplantation and to provide compatible single-donor platelets to refractory thrombocytopenic patients. Currently, most HLA laboratories that support solid organ transplantation, HSCT, or platelet transfusion therapy use commercial reagents for both antibody screening and for the characterization of antibody specificities. Detailed step-by-step protocols to perform the test, data analysis, and interpretation are provided from vendors' product inserts. Therefore, only the principles and comparisons of the advantages and disadvantages of the major techniques will be discussed herewith.

There are two broad types of techniques differentiated by target used: those that use cells as target (i.e., cytotoxicity and flow cytometry) and the other utilizes the solubilized HLA molecules in a sold-phase immunoassay.[44]

Cell-based Techniques

The complement-dependent microcytotoxicity described for serologic HLA typing (Fig. 12-3) is also used for antibody screening and characterization. The difference is that the test serum is plated into the wells that contain panel of HLA-typed frozen cells. Because of the extreme HLA polymorphisms, a panel should include between 60 and 100 racially mixed subjects in order to cover all the HLA antigens. Since there are high-frequency HLA antigens in the population (e.g., HLA-A2) and linkage disequilibrium haplotypes (e.g., HLA-A1, B8 or HLA-A2, B44, etc.), a good panel must not contain too many cells carrying high-frequency antigens or those carrying known linkage disequilibrium haplotypes. The antibody screening trays are prepared separately for class I and class II antigens. Each tray contains positive and negative controls to validate the results obtained. The sensitivity of the microcytotoxicity can be modified by altering the incubation time, washing steps, and the addition of antiglobulin reagent. The most sensitive microcytotoxicity for antibody screening or XM is the AHG-CDC method. It is well established that only the IgG

HLA antibody is of clinical relevance for solid organ transplantation. Since microcytotoxicity detects both IgG and IgM antibodies, it is important to treat test serum with dithiothreitol (DTT) or by heating serum at 63°C for 10 minutes to inactivate IgM.

Using the complement-dependent microcytotoxicity or other methods for antibody screening, the extent of alloimmunization (i.e., breadth) and the antibody specificities can be simultaneously obtained. The percent of PRA is calculated as the number of positive reactions obtained divided by the total number of cells in a panel. This is used to indicate how broad a patient is alloimmunized. The PRA varies depending on the panel compositions and if a constant panel is not used, the PRA is a poor predicator of crossmatch outcome.

The cell-based flow cytometry is an indirect assay that measures the binding of antibody to cells through the use of an antiglobulin labeled with fluorescent marker. The specificity of the antiglobulin reagent (IgG or IgM, etc.) permits the identification of cell-bound antibody. Further characterization of the cells can be achieved by gating on cells defined by physical parameters and staining the cells with labeled monoclonal antibodies specific for cell subsets (e.g., T or B cells).[32,44] The cell-based flow test, which is time-consuming and costly to perform, is now being largely replaced by bead-based flow test.

Solid-phase Immunoassays

These methods utilize the affinity-purified soluble HLA antigens bound to solid-phase matrices. There are three formats of this assay in use depending on the bound matrices.

ELISA Test
Similar to the classical enzyme-linked immunosorbent assay (ELISA), the HLA antigens are bound to individual wells of a microtiter plate. After the addition of test serum to the wells, the presence of HLA antibody is detected by the addition of an enzyme-conjugated substrate, which results in color development in wells containing HLA-specific antibody. The color reactions are read by an ELISA reader. To increase efficiency and to reduce cost, the ELISA assay can be performed in two different stages: the initial screening to determine the presence or absence of HLA antibody in test serum followed by the characterization of antibody specificities of those that tested positive. For the initial screening, the test well may contain either pooled soluble class I or class II antigens that were collected from multiple individuals covering all HLA antigens.

Flow Cytometry
Flow cytometry tests utilize antigens from a single individual bound to 2- to 4-m-diameter polystyrene

beads. Mixtures of up to 30 different bead preparations, each carrying a different phenotype, can be used for the initial antibody screening. Patients that tested positive for antibodies will then undergo additional testing with the use of several different bead mixture preparations each containing 8 to 11 phenotypes to determine the exact antibody specificities.[32]

Luminex Technology
The same technology discussed earlier for DNA-based rSSO typing is also applicable for antibody testing. The example used to illustrate this principle is LABScreen method.[52]

LABScreen Antibody Detection Assay
LABScreen reagents use Luminex microbeads coated with purified class I or class II HLA antigens. Up to 100 different color-coded beads may be combined in one suspension for a single test. Test serum is first incubated with LABScreen beads. Any HLA antibodies present in the test serum will bind to the antigens and then label with R-phycoerythrin (PE)-conjugated goat anti-human IgG. The LABScan 100 flow analyzer detects the fluorescent emission of PE from each bead, allowing almost real-time data acquisition. The reaction pattern of the test serum is compared to the lot-specific worksheet defining the antigen array to assign PRA and HLA specificity.

The mixed bead assay (for antibody screening) uses pooled HLA antigens to detect the presence of antibody to class I, MICA, and/or class II HLA, but does not distinguish between antibody reactions with different antigens in each pool.

The PRA tests (beads coated with extracts from different human lymphoblastoid cell lines) can detect antibodies and their specificities against the HLA antigens included in each panel. For closer scrutiny, the single antigen assay allows confirmation of antibody suggested by a previous PRA test. It eliminates the analytical difficulties common in PRA antigen panels due to multiple phenotypic antigens (from a single cell source) being coated on the same bead. Single antigen products utilize individual recombinant HLA antigens coated on each bead, so there are no "masked" antibody reactions. However, even a single HLA antigen may contain several immunogenic epitopes, so that both specific and cross-reactive antibodies can be detected in this assay. Currently, this is the most sensitive in vitro diagnostic assay available for HLA antibody detection, and it allows a semiquantitative measurement of the antibody reactivity in a specific test specimen, based on the FI of each individual antigen reaction.[53] A negative control serum is used to establish the background value for each bead in a test batch. For

detailed data acquisition and analysis, consult product insert.[52]

In order to anticipate the reactivity of transplant patient's serum to a potential donor's HLA specificities (prior to the identification of such a donor), the HLA laboratory may choose to run a single antigen assay as a type of "virtual crossmatch" test. The theory is that any forbidden allele specificities for that patient represented in the single antigen panel will be identified by a positive reaction with that patient's serum. Any donors in the registry with an HLA typing, including one of these unsuitable alleles, would then be eliminated from consideration as an organ donor for this patient. This preliminary assessment would thus save time and prevent the loss of an organ due to an unexpected positive crossmatch test. The single antigen panel is also especially suited for highly sensitized patients who are refractory to platelet transfusion therapy. It helps to reveal all the class I HLA antigens to which the patient has not been sensitized as yet. This information, in turn, can be used to select compatible but mismatched product.

Crossmatch

XM is performed between the recipient's serum and the donor's purified T and B cells. This is to detect the presence of HLA antibody in the recipient serum reactive against mismatched donor antigens. Since a positive crossmatch is a contraindication for kidney and/or pancreas transplantation, it is standard practice that the XM technique must be equal or more sensitive than the techniques used for antibody testing. AHG-CDC and Flow XM are currently used by most laboratories. For the retransplant recipients, Flow XM is recommended. Several dilutions of the recipient's serum should be included in the final XM test. The laboratory must have established policy jointly with its transplant program concerning all aspects of antibody screening and XM in terms of test frequencies and serum samples used for final XM and so on.

Comparison of Antibody Testing Techniques

The major advantages and disadvantages of the techniques are listed in Table 12-9.[44] In terms of sensitivity the consensus among most HLA laboratories is that both types of flow cytometry techniques (i.e., the conventional and Luminex platform) are comparable to each other. Both techniques are more sensitive than ELISA and ELISA is more sensitive than regular CDC or AHG-CDC.[44,50,53]

TABLE 12-9   Comparison of Antibody Testing Techniques

Types of Techniques	Advantages	Disadvantage
Microcytotoxicity	Less technically demanding Low reagent cost Low equipment cost	Less sensitive than the other methods Interference from non-HLA antibodies present in serum samples Cell viability affecting test results Affected by immunosuppressive treatment (e.g., OKT3) or other medications (hydroxyzine)
Solid-phase immunoassay	High sensitivity Elimination of interferences from non-HLA antibody present in serum Batch testing possible Amenable for automation	More technically demanding, moderate to high reagent cost Expensive instrument (Luminex machine) Interference from immune complex, high level of IgM Ab, or discoloration of serum samples High background from serum reactivity to plastic/beads More quality control needed
Flow cytometry (bead based)	High sensitivity Simultaneous identification of class- and cell-type specific antibodies	Technically demanding High reagent cost Expensive instrument, more quality control needed

CLINICAL APPLICATIONS

Solid Organ Transplantation

In the United States, various types of solid organs can be donated by living related, living unrelated, and deceased donors. Living donors are mostly for kidneys. The United Network for Organ Sharing (UNOS) not only administers deceased donor organ procurement and allocation, it also monitors national policies for solid organ transplantation.[54] UNOS has developed separate allocation policies for different types of solid organs. In order to receive an organ, all patients must be registered and placed on the UNOS waiting list. Each type of solid organ has a different and separate priority list. For example, the UNOS algorithm for allocating deceased donor kidney is locally first and then regionally determined by the patient's waiting time, HLA matching, HLA alloimmunization status, age, and medical urgency of the patient's conditions.[54,66] Similar allocation policies are established for nonrenal solid organs (e.g., liver and heart, etc.). Since these patients have no artificial means (kidney dialysis) to sustain them over a long period of time, the preference is placed primarily on medical urgency and waiting time.[32,54]

As of February 2009, there are more than 100,380 patients on the UNOS waiting list to receive organ donations. There were only 25,625 patients who have received organ transplants between January and November 2008. The lack of deceased kidney donors and the large number of highly sensitized patients on the waiting list present the greatest challenges to kidney transplantation. Over the last 10 to 15 years, innovative approaches and alternative options have been developed. The implementation of desensitization protocols using intravenous immunoglobulin (IVIG), rituximab, and plasmapheresis have either reduced the recipient's donor-specific antibody level to minimum or converted a positive XM to negative to allow the highly sensitized patient group access to kidney transplantation.[55–62] While the desensitization therapy is still in limited practice, and with unanswered questions still remaining, early successful transplant outcomes were encouraging. Continued refinement of the protocols would benefit those patients unlikely to receive a kidney transplant.

The benefits of HLA matching were demonstrated from living family donors. The best outcome for patient is from HLA-identical sibling donors followed by haploidentical family donors.[43,63] Kidney transplants donated from living unrelated donors also demonstrated to be superior than those from deceased donors.[64,65] The favorable outcome may be attributed to shorter ischemic time and the patient's high compliance for medications.[66] Recently, the implementation of living donor exchange program[67–69] also helps to reduce organ shortage in kidney transplants. There are many recipients who may have living related or unrelated volunteer donors available; however, transplantations are not performed because of biologic incompatibility (i.e., ABO blood groups) with their intended donor. For example, donor 1 (blood group A) wants to donate a kidney to her husband (blood group B), but she cannot because they are ABO incompatible. Another pair is excluded for the same reason but in this pair, the donor is blood group B and the recipient is blood group A. By exchanging the donors, two new ABO-compatible pairs are created.[54] There are many logistics to overcome and coordination to be arranged, etc. for the living donor exchange program; such programs, however, have been launched with enthusiasm in many countries, including the United States, Europe, and Asia. As with any new program, it will take time to accumulate outcome data on exchange success rates. The benefits of HLA matching in liver and thoracic organs are uncertain. As discussed earlier, allocation of livers and hearts is based on medical urgency and waiting time.[32,66] However, for sensitized heart transplant recipient, final prospective crossmatch is mandatory.

Hematopoietic Stem Cell Transplantation

HSCT is the therapy of choice for most hematologic malignancies, including all forms of leukemia, lymphoma, and multiple myeloma (nonresponsible to first-line chemotherapeutics), myelodysplastic and myeloproliferative disorders.[70,71] The major clinical complication of HSCT is GVHD, which is caused predominantly by the mismatches of HLA class I and class II alleles between recipient and donor. The overall incidence of acute GVHD (aGVHD) varies between 35% and 80% for all patients receiving an HLA-matched related or unrelated donor stem cells, and aGVHD is the primary cause of death in 10% to 20% of HSCT patients.[70–73] Since 20% to 35% HSCT performed between HLA genotypically identical siblings still experience aGVHD, the additive effects of minor histocompatibility antigens therefore, also contribute to aGVHD.[74,75] Because of these obvious reasons, HLA genotypically identical siblings serve as the best HSCT donors. Unfortunately, more than 65% of the HSCT recipients worldwide do not have HLA-matched family donors. Due to the collaborative efforts of the patients' families, several respected physicians in the fields of HSCT and blood banking, as well as from government funding support, the National Marrow Donor Program (NMDP) was established in 1987.[76,77] Analogous to UNOS, NMDP has taken the leadership role in research, recruiting the largest list of registered donors and cord blood units in the world. NMDP is actively involved in helping donor search using innovative science and technology to identify the best match, supporting patients and their physicians throughout the transplant process.

NMDP maintains relationships with other international NMDP transplant centers and registries.[77]

Since 1992, NMDP has contracted ASHI-accredited HLA laboratories to perform intermediate or high-resolution DNA-based HLA typing for both the registered marrow donors and cord blood units. These contract laboratories are under stringent NMDP quality controls, and the contracts are also periodically undergoing competitive renewal.[78–80] Currently, there are more than 7 million potential marrow donors and 90,000 cord blood units representing all the races and ethnic populations in the United States on the NMDP registry.[80] NMDP facilitates on average more than 350 transplants each month for patients who do not have HLA-matched family donors.[80–82]

Recently, two important advances have been made in the field of allogeneic HSCT: the use of umbilical cord blood (UCB) as an alternative source of stem cell for HSCT and the reduced-intensity conditioning regimen. Since the first successful allogeneic UCB transplant (UCBT) performed in 1988 to treat a child with Fanconi anemia by Gluckman et al.,[83] the development of cord blood bank (CBB) and transplants have been increasing steadily.[83,84] Currently, there are more transplants that are being performed using UCB than peripheral blood stem cells or bone marrow cells for pediatric patients. Originally, the main obstacles to UCBT in adult have been the risks of graft failure and delayed hematologic recovery of neutrophils and platelets.[85] The unfavorable outcomes are primarily due to the disproportions between the body size of adult and the limited number of hematopoietic progenitor cells that can be collected from a UCB. It is clearly demonstrated that UCBT outcome is correlated with cell dose infused.[85] Recent registry studies using UCB grafts contained a median of 2.2 to 2.5 × 10^7 total nucleated cells per kilogram; zero to three HLA mismatches and under a myeloablative conditioning have established UCBT as a safe and feasible alternative to bone marrow transplantation in adults lacking HLA-matched donors.[86–88] One approach to facilitate widespread use of UCB in adult patients is the double-unit transplantation.[89] The minimum criteria used for selecting of the double units are: no more than two HLA disparities and it must contain greater than 3 × 10^7 TNC/kg. Results published from double-unit UCBT[89] under both myeloablative and nonmyeloablative setting indicated that there are slightly higher aGVHD than single-unit transplant, but transplant-related mortality rates remain low and 1-year overall survival ranged from 31% to 79%. Clearly, the double-unit transplant can be extended to almost all adults who do not have HLA-matched family or unrelated donors. The many advantages of utilizing UCB include reducing the risk of GVHD because they are less immunogenic, minimizing stringent HLA matching, and decreasing the waiting time of searching for a donor.[83,84]

Recently, interest in performing antibody testing and XM between HSCT recipient and donor pair has been renewed, particularly for cord blood transplantation. A positive XM between recipient and cord blood unit (or donor) may contribute to graft failure.[90–92] While many HLA laboratories routinely provide antibody testing and XM to their respective HSCT programs, a majority of the HSCT centers do not request these services from their HLA laboratories. Since using CBU when there more than one HLA mismatch with the recipient is routinely practiced for cord blood transplantation, the donor-directed host antibodies become relevant. The limited access to cord blood cells precludes XM. Therefore, performing antibody specificity identification using a single antigen panel, as a type of virtual XM, provides an alternative to predict XM-negative cord blood units or donors for unrelated HSCT.[92]

Reduced-intensity (nonmyeloablative) conditioning regimen have been developed for allograft patients ineligible for myeloablative conditioning because of age (>50 years) or comorbid conditions. This regimen based on the concept of graft-versus-leukemia (GVL) responses, rather than high-dose cytoreductive therapy alone, are the key to preventing disease relapse.[93–96] The primary requirement in developing a reduced-intensity regimen is the need to achieve adequate immunosuppression to permit the development of hematopoietic chimerism, which became feasible with the development of the purine analog family of drugs.[93–96] This treatment option has offered real hope for older patients unlikely to receive this treatment modality.

Platelets Transfusion Therapy

Adverse transfusion reactions attributable to HLA antibodies include platelet refractoriness, febrile transfusion reaction, and transfusion-related acute lung injury (TRALI). When patients are suspected of immune refractoriness, serum screening to determine the presence or absence of HLA class I and platelet-specific antibodies (HPA) is performed. Once the clinical and laboratory diagnosis of immune refractoriness is made, the use of special platelet products is indicated. Two general approaches can be employed to provide compatible single-donor platelets to refractory thrombocytopenic patients. One approach is to crossmatch every prospective donor with the patient's serum and select only crossmatch-negative donors. Platelets from crossmatch-negative donors are generally effective for

low PRA patients, and HLA typing is not required if XM is the only criteria for donor selection.[33] Unfortunately, XM alone is not always practical because many of the alloimmunized patients have HLA antibodies that react with more than 90% of the random population. In many centers that provide single-donor apheresis products, XM is not used as the major donor selection criterion, but is important as a supplemental or alternative procedure.[32] The second approach is to select donors based on HLA types, coupled with knowledge of HLA antibody specificities that the refractory patient has developed. When HLA-matched products are not available, donor selection is based upon selective mismatching; that is, choosing HLA antigen mismatches to which the patient is not yet alloimmunized.[32,50] Therefore, at our blood center, an initially HLA screening–positive refractory patient is automatically placed on single antigen panel for detailed characterization of antibody specificities. We believe that knowledge of the HLA specificity of antibodies in a patient's serum is critical for rational selection of "safe" but mismatched donors. The algorithm used to select compatible platelet products varies according to each institution's transfusion practices. The following briefly summarizes our blood center's practice.

A sample is requested from patients suspected of alloimmune platelet refractoriness for HLA antibody screening and HLA class I typing. While awaiting the results of these tests, the patient can be supported with crossmatch-compatible platelets or HLA matched (if the patient's HLA type is previously known). If the HLA antibody screen is positive and the antibody specificities are identified, the patient is now supported with antigen-negative or crossmatch negative platelets. HLA-typed donors may be recruited to provide antigen-negative platelets. If the HLA screen is negative, an HPA antibody screen and specificity identification are considered. If the HPA screen is positive, the patient is supported with HPA antigen-negative or crossmatch-compatible platelets. If only ABO antibodies are detected, the patient is supported with platelets from ABO-identical or group O donors.[50] Donor selection can also be improved by "HLA matchmaker" developed by Duquesnoy et al.[97] This matching program has been successfully applied to select compatible donors or platelet product for highly sensitized kidney recipient or refractory patients, respectively.[98,99]

Febrile nonhemolytic transfusion reaction (FNHTR) is caused by either an interaction between the recipient's antileukocyte antibodies and the donor's leukocytes contained in the blood components or pyrogenic cytokines produced in the blood components during storage. They are now prevented by transfusing leukocyte-reduced blood component.

TRALI is a rare complication resulting in pulmonary edema, which was first described by Popovsky and Moore.[100] TRALI is caused by antibodies against neutrophil (HNA) and/or HLA class I and class II antigens.[100–105] The implicated antibodies are usually found in the plasma of transfused components; less common antibodies are found in the recipient.[66] Currently, the demonstration of HLA class I or class II or neutrophil-specific antibodies in donor plasma and the presence of the cognate antigen in the recipient is a laboratory evidence for TRALI.[66] TRALI has emerged as the main cause of transfusion-related death in the United States.[103] This elevation most likely relates to improved knowledge and education about the signs/symptoms of this entity.[103,104] Since the AABB standards specify that blood centers need to take steps by November 2008 to reduce the risk of TRALI,[106] many blood centers have already begun HLA antibody screening of their pheresis donors or female blood donors. Many other blood centers are still in the process of identifying the best practice to conduct antibody screening. At present, there is no cost-effective antibody screening technique available for HNA antibodies. Many commercial companies are working toward the development of such a technique.

HLA AND DISEASE ASSOCIATION

Since the first report of a weak HLA association with Hodgkin disease in 1967,[107] a plethora of papers have been published on HLA associations with various disease categories. The list of such diseases includes more than 500 entries.[108,109] Most of the associations are weak or may be fortuitous; more than 50 statistically significant associations, however, have been found. While a wide range of diseases were investigated, diseases demonstrating moderate to strong HLA association appear to share some common features: low incidence in the population; nonmalignant, with strong autoimmune component; and most of the diseases have multifactorial etiologies.[32] There are four diseases (21-hydroxylase deficiency, hemochromatosis, C2, and C4 deficiencies) which are not associated with a particular HLA allele because the genes responsible for disease manifestation happen to locate within the HLA region. Hemochromatosis, a disease in which the body becomes overloaded with iron, is controlled by an autosomal recessive gene mapped approximately 4-MB telomeric to HLA-A locus. Congenital adrenal hyperplasia (CAH) is due to defective alleles of CYP21 genes that encode steroid 21-hydroxylase, an enzyme involved in the biosynthesis of steroids by cortical cells of the adrenal gland.[12] The CYP21 genes and the C2 and C4 genes are all located in class III region.

TABLE 12-10 Some Examples of Significant HLA and Disease Associations

Disease	HLA[1]	Relative Risk[2]
Birdshot retinopathy	A29	200
Ankylosing spondylitis	B27	90
Psoriasis vulgaris	Cw6	35
Subacute thyroiditis	B35	19
Behçet disease	B51	8
Narcolepsy	DR2, DQ6	200
Celiac disease	DR3/5/7, DQ2	30
Goodpasture syndrome	DR2	17
Type I diabetes mellitus	DR3,4, DQ2,8	10
Tuberculoid leprosy	DR2	8
Pernicious anemia	DR5	5
Multiple sclerosis	DR2, DQ6	4
Rheumatoid arthritis	DR4	4
Hashimoto thyroiditis	DR5	3
Severe adrenogenital syndrome	CYP21B variant	—
Hemochromatosis	HFE variant	—

[1] HLA specificities are shown for simplicity, although most of the diseases are associated with specific alleles of the specificities as noted in the text.
[2] Relative risks for adrenogenital syndrome and hemochromatosis are not given because the two diseases are not due to class I or II gene disorders (Reproduced with permission from HLA Beyond Tears by G.E. Rodey, 2000. *Introduction to Human Histocompatibility.* 2nd ed. Houston, Texas: De Novo Inc.; 2000.)

Among the most striking HLA associations (see Table 12-10) that are beneficial to aid clinical diagnosis are HLA-DQB1*0602/DRB1*1501 for narcolepsy, HLA-B27 for ankylosing spondylitis, and HLA-DQB1*02 for celiac disease. Type I diabetes mellitus is strongly associated with DRB1*0301, 0401, 0402, 0405, and DQB1*0201 and 0302. Rheumatoid arthritis (RA) is associated with DRB1*0401, 0404, 0405, and 0408 alleles as well as DRB1*0101 and 1401. All these DR4 alleles encode a similar stretch of amino acids on DRB chain at positions 67 to 74. There are also HLA alleles found that confer protections for type I diabetes mellitus and RA, etc.[109]

Recent new studies also reported strong HLA association with susceptibility to drug hypersensitivity.[110–114] Drug hypersensitivity commonly involves the skin and mucosal surfaces, and in severe cases can lead to hepatitis, renal failure, gastrointestinal bleeding, pneumonitis, bone marrow suppression, blindness, and death.[115] It is estimated that more than 7% of the general population develops some type of drug hypersensitivity.[112] The HLA association observed can be drug specific, such as HLA-B*1502 with carbamazepine-induced Stevens–Johnson syndrome and toxic epidermal necrolysis (SJS/TEN); HLA-B*5701 with abacavir hypersensitivity, and HLA-B*5801 with allopurinol-induced severe cutaneous adverse reactions. The HLA associations can also be ethnicity specific for the association of B*1502, with SJS/TEN only observed in south-east Asians and not in Caucasians.[110-115] This difference can be attributed to the high allele frequency (2.7% to 11.6%) of B*1502 detected in south-east Asians in contrast to no more than 0.1% observed in Caucasian population. It is advocated that screening for these alleles is necessary before prescribing the respective drugs to high-risk patient group.[115]

Many hypotheses have been put forward to explain the association of HLA with disease.[12,116,117] These include presentation of a pathogenic peptide by HLA molecules; thymic selection of T-cell receptor repertoire on HLA molecules with self-peptides; peptide contribution by HLA molecules; interaction of HLA (class II) molecules with superantigens; specific binding and internalization of microorganisms; linkage of HLA locus to a non-HLA disease-associated gene; regulation of T-cell development; and cross-reactive antibody responses. It is beyond the scope of this chapter to discuss these mechanisms. Readers may refer to several publications[12,116-119] on this topic.

SUMMARY

Representing the most polymorphic genetic system known to date, the HLA complex has become one of the most intensely studied biomedical sciences. It has a central role in immune response, transplantation, and autoimmune disease. Advancements in testing technologies have provided accurate tissue typing as well as unequivocal identification of antibody specificities to benefit clinical transplantation. By understanding their role in transplantation, investigators have been able to develop innovative approaches to improve the survival of transplants. Much has been learned and it is certain that more will be learned about this most fascinating genetic system.

Review Questions

1. True or false? The HLA complex is the most polymorphic genetic system known to date.
2. What is the most important biologic function of the MHC genes?
3. Which region does not contain HLA genes but does contain genes that code for complement components?
   a. class I
   b. class II
   c. class III
4. Coding regions of genes are called
   a. exons
   b. introns
   c. polyons
   d. none of the above
5. True or false? The class I and class II molecules are codominantly expressed but have different tissue distributions.
6. True or false? Class I molecules can only be found on nucleated cells.
7. HLA-DR, HLA-DQ, and HLA-DP are which type of molecules?
   a. class I
   b. class II
   c. class III
   d. class IV
8. Closely linked genes are inherited as a block which is known as a:
   a. polytype
   b. haplotype
   c. diplotype
   d. triplotype
9. True or false? A child is haploidentical to each parent and only siblings may have a 25% chance of being genotypically identical to each other.
10. Define linkage disequilibrium.
11. Define epitope.
12. What is the tissue source for DNA-based typing?
13. Why is quality control particularly important in the HLA laboratory?
14. What two blood group systems are the major barriers to transplantation?
15. Most immunologic refractoriness to platelets results from antibodies to:
    a. HLA class I antigens
    b. HLA class II antigens
    c. HLA class III antigens
    d. ABO antigens
16. Name at least two ways to screen for HLA antibodies.
17. True or false? The best outcomes for graft survival are those from HLA-identical sibling donors.
18. What is the major complication of HSCT?
19. The demonstration of HLA class I or class II or neutrophil-specific antibodies in donor plasma and the presence of cognate antigen in the recipient is laboratory evidence for what condition?
20. HLA-B27 is associated with which disease?
    a. narcolepsy
    b. celiac disease
    c. type I diabetes mellitus
    d. ankylosing spondylitis

REFERENCES

1. Dausset J. Iso-leuco-anticorps. Paris, France. *Acta Haematol*. 1958; 20: 156–166.

2. Bjorkman PJ, Saper MA, Samraoui B, et al. The foreign antigen binding site and T cell recognition regions of class I histocompatibility antigens. *Nature*. 1987; 329: 512–518.

3. Kaufman J, & McMichael A. Evolution of the major histocompatibility complex and MHC-like molecules. In: *HLA and MHC Genes, Molecules and Function*. Oxford, UK: BIOS Scientific Publishers; 1996: 1–17.

4. Pamer E, Cresswell P. Mechanisms of MHC class I restricted antigen processing. *Annu Rev Immunol*. 1998; 16: 323–358.

5. Klein J, Sato A. The HLA system. First of two parts. *N Engl J Med*. 2000; 343: 702–709.

6. Rudolph MG, Stanfield RL, Wilson IA. How TCRs bind MHCs, peptides, and coreceptors. *Annu Rev Immunol*. 2006; 24: 419–466.

7. Zinkernagel RM, Doherty PC. Restriction of in vitro T cell-mediated cytotoxicity in lymphocytic choriomeningitis within a syngeneic or semiallogeneic system. *Nature*. 1974; 248: 701–702.

8. Whitelegg A, Barber LD. The structural basis of T cell allorecognition. *Tissue Antigens*. 2004; 63: 101–108.

9. Fleisher T, Rich R, Schroeder H, et al. The major histocompatibility complex. In: *Clinical Immunology Principles and Practice*. 3rd ed. Philadelphia, PA: Elsevier Limited; 2008: 79–90.

10. Dupont B, Ekkehard A, & Marsh S, et al. A new approach. The HLA system: an introduction. In: *The HLA System*. Springer-Verlag; 1990: 1–27.

11. Beck S, Trwsdal J. The human major histocompatibility complex: lessons from the DNA sequence. *Annu Rev Genomics Hum Genet*. 2000; 1: 117–137. Available at: http://www.immuno.path.cam.ac.uk/~immuno/mhc/mhc.html.

12. Marsh SG, Parham P, Barber LD. *The HLA Facts Book*. San Diego, California: Academic Press; 2000.

13. Nakmuro K, Tanigaki N, Pressman D. Multiple common properties of human β_2—microglobulin and the common portion fragment derived from HLA antigen molecules. *Proc Natl Acad Sci USA*. 1973; 70: 2863–2865.

14. Parham P, Lomen CE, Lawlor DA, et al. Nature of polymorphism in HLA-A, B and C molecules. *Proc Natl Acad Sci U S A*. 1988; 85: 4005–4009.

15. Bjorkman PJ, Saper MA, Samraoui B, et al. Structure of the human class I histocompatibility antigen, HLA-A2. *Nature*. 1987; 329: 506–512.

16. Bjorkman PJ, Parham P. Structure, function and diversity of class I major histocompatibility complex molecules. *Annu Rev Biochem*. 1990; 59: 253–288.

17. Browning M & McMichael A. Function of HLA class I restricted T cells. In: *HLA and MHC Genes, Molecules and Function*. Oxford, UK: BIOS Scientific Publishers; 1996: 309–320.

18. Browning M, McMichael A, & Trowsdale J. Molecular genetics of HLA class I and class II regions. In: *HLA and MHC Genes, Molecules and Function*. Oxford, UK: BIOS Scientific Publishers; 1996: 23–36.

19. Cresswell P. Assembly, transport and function of MHC class II molecules. *Annu Rev Immunol*. 1994; 12: 259–293.

20. Van der Merwe PA, Davis SJ. Molecular interactions mediating T cell antigen recognition. *Annu Rev Immunol*. 2003; 21: 659–684.

21. Browning M, McMichael A, Israel A, et al. Regulation of MHC class I gene expression. In: *HLA and MHC Genes, Molecules and Function*. Oxford, UK: BIOS Scientific Publishers; 1996: 139–152.

22. Browning M, McMichael A, & Wassmuth R. HLA/MHC class II gene regulation. In: *HLA and MHC Genes, Molecules and Function*. Oxford, UK: BIOS Scientific Publishers; 1996: 159–178.

23. Ljunggren HG, Karre K. In search of the "missing self": MHC molecules and NK recognition. *Immunol Today*. 1990; 11: 7–10.

24. Jones DC, Young NT. Natural killer receptor repertoires in transplantation. *Eur J Immunogenet*. 2003; 30: 169–176.

25. Lowdell MW. Natural killer cells in hematopoietic stem cell transplantation. *Transfus Med*. 2003; 13: 399–404.

26. Parham P. Immunogenetics of killer-cell immunoglobulin-like receptors. *Tissue Antigens*. 2003; 62: 194–200.

27. Farag SS, Bacigalupo A, Eapen M, et al. The effect of KIR ligand incompatibility on the outcome of unrelated donor transplantation: a report from the Center for International Blood and Marrow Transplant Research, the European Blood and Marrow Transplant Registry and the Dutch Registry. *Biol Blood Marrow Transplant*. 2006; 12: 876–884.

28. Bodmer JG, Marsh GE, Albert ED, et al. Nomenclature for factors of the HLA system, 1991. *Tissue Antigen*. 1992; 39: 161–173.

29. Marsh SGE, Albert ED, Bodmer WF, et al. Nomenclature for factors of the HLA system, 2004. *Tissue Antigen*. 2005; 65: 301–369.

30. Bodmer JG, Kennedy LJ, Lindsay J, et al. Applications of serology and the ethnic distribution of three locus HLA haplotypes. *Br Med Bull*. 1987; 43: 94–121.

31. The American Society for Histocompatibility and Immunogenetics (ASHI). Available at: http://www.ashi-hla.org/about/

32. Rodey GE. *HLA Beyond Tears. Introduction to Human Histocompatibility*. 2nd ed. Houston, Texas: De Novo Inc.; 2000.

33. ASHI Laboratory Manual. 4th ed. 2000 Available at: http://www.ashi-hla.org/publications/lab-manual/

34. Parham P, Lawlor DA, Salter RD, et al. HLA-A, B, C: patterns of polymorphism in peptide-binding proteins. In: Dupong B, ed. *Immunobiology of HLA*. Vol. II. New York: Springer-Verlag; 1989: 10–33.

35. Terasaki PI, McClelland JD. Microdroplet assay of human serum cytotoxins. *Nature*. 1964; 204: 998–1000.

36. Johnson AH, Rossen RD, Butler WT. Detection of alloantibodies using a sensitive antiglobulin microcytotoxicity test: identification of low levels of preformed antibodies in accelerated allograft rejection. *Tissue Antigens*. 1972; 2: 215–226.

37. Bain BM, Vas R, Lowenstein L. The development of large immature mononuclear cells in mixed leukocyte culture. *Blood*. 1964; 23: 108–116.

38. Bach FH, Voynow NK. One-way stimulation in mixed leukocyte cultures. *Science*. 1966; 153: 545–547.

39. Newton CR, Graham A, Heptinstall LE, et al. Analysis of any point mutation in DNA. The amplification refractory mutation system (ARMS). *Nucleic Acids Res*. 1989; 17: 2503–2516.

40. LABType. Product Insert. One Lambda, Inc.; 2008.

41. Hsu SH. *Pros and Cons of Using PCR/SSP or PCR/SSOP or PCR/SBT Methods for Clinical HLA Typing*. Philadelphia, PA: ASHI Regional Educational Workshop; May 2005.

42. Cano P, Klitz W, Mack SJ, et al. Common and well-documented HLA alleles. Report of the ad-hoc committee of the American Society for histocompatibility and immunogenetics. *Hum Immunol*. 2007; 68: 392–417.

43. Terasaki PI, Cho Y, Takemoto S, et al. Twenty-year follow-up on the effect of HLA matching on kidney transplant survival and prediction of future twenty-year survival. *Transplant Proc*. 1996; 28: 1144–1145.

44. Hamilton RG, Rose NR, Sholander JT, et al. Evaluation of the humoral response in transplantation. In: *Manual of Clinical Laboratory Immunology*. 6th ed. Washington DC: ASM Press; 2002: 1153–1163.

45. Terasaki PI, Cai J. Humoral theory of transplantation: further evidence. *Curr Opin Immunol*. 2005; 17: 541–545.

46. Jordan SC, Pescovitz MD. Presensitization: the problem and its management. *Clin J Am Soc Nephrol*. 2006; 1: 421–432.

47. Cai J, Terasaki PI. Post-transplantation antibody monitoring and HLA antibody epitope identification. *Curr Opin Immunol*. 2008; 20: 602–606.

48. Doughty HA, Murphy MF, Metcalfe P, et al. Relative importance of immune and non-immune causes of platelet refractoriness. *Vox Sang*. 1994; 66: 200–205.

49. International Forum. Detection of platelet reactive antibodies in patients who are refractory to platelet transfusions, and the selection of compatible donors. *Vox Sang*. 2003; 84: 73–88.

50. Nance S, Hsu S, Vassallo R, et al. Review: platelet matching for alloimmunized patients—room for improvement. *Immunohematology*. 2004; 20: 80–88.

51. Seftel MD, Growe GH, Petraszko T, et al. Universal prestorage leukoreduction in Canada decreases platelet alloimmunization and refractoriness. *Blood*. 2004; 103: 33–39.

52. LABScreen. Product Insert. One Lambda, Inc.; 2006.

53. Pei R, Lee JH, Shih NJ, et al. Single human leukocyte antigen flow cytometry beads for accurate identification of human leukocyte antigen antibody specificities. *Transplantation*. 2003; 75: 43–49.

54. United Network for Organ Sharing (UNOS). Available at: http://www.unos.org/.

55. Tyan DB, Li VA, Czer L, et al. Intravenous immunoglobulin suppression of HLA alloantibody in highly sensitized transplant candidates and transplantation with a histoincompatible organ. *Transplantation*. 1994; 57: 553–562.

56. Montgomery RA, Zachary AA, Racusen LC, et al. Plasmapheresis and intravenous immune globulin provides effective rescue therapy for refractory humoral rejection and allows kidneys to be successfully transplanted into cross-match-positive recipients. *Transplantation*. 2000; 70: 887–895.

57. Gloor JM, DeGoey SR, Pineda AA, et al. Overcoming a positive cross-match in living-donor kidney transplantation. *Am J Transplant*. 2003; 3: 1017–1023.

58. Jordan SC, Vo A, Bunnapradist S, et al. Intravenous immune globulin treatment inhibits crossmatch positivity and allows for successful transplantation of incompatible organs in living donor and cadaver recipients. *Transplantation*. 2003; 76: 631–636.

59. Becker YT, Becker BN, Pirsch JD, et al. Rituximab as treatment for refractory kidney transplant rejection. *Am J Transplant*. 2004; 4: 996–1001.

60. Montgomery RA, Zachary AA. Transplanting patients with a positive donor-specific crossmatch: a single center's perspective. *Pediatr Transplant*. 2004; 8: 535–542.

61. Vo AA, Toyoda M, Peng A, et al. Effect of induction therapy protocols on transplant outcomes in crossmatch positive renal allograft recipients desensitized with IVIG. *Am J Transplant*. 2006; 6: 2384–2390.

62. Haas M, Montgomery RA, Segev DL, et al. Subclinical acute antibody mediated rejection in positive crossmatch renal allografts. *Am J Transplant*. 2007; 7: 576–585.

63. Terasaki PI, ed. *History of HLA: Ten Recollections*. Los Angeles: UCLA Tissue Typing Laboratory Press; 1990.

64. Terasaki PI, Cecka JM, Gjertson DW, et al. High survival rates of kidney transplants from spousal and living unrelated donors. *N Engl J Med*. 1995; 333: 333–336.

65. Stegall MD, Larson TS, Prieto M, et al. Living-donor kidney transplantation at Mayo Clinic-Rochester. *Clin Transpl*. 2002; 11: 155–161.

66. Choo SY. The HLA system: genetics, immunology, clinical testing, and clinical implications. *Yonsei Med J*. 2007; 48: 11–23.

67. Montgomery RA. ABO incompatible transplantation: to B or not to B? *Am J Transplant*. 2004; 4: 1011–1012.

68. Crew RJ, Ratner LE. Overcoming immunologic incompatibility: transplanting the difficult to transplant patient. *Semin Dial*. 2005; 18: 474–481.

69. Magee CC. Transplantation across previously incompatible immunological barriers. *Transplant Int*. 2006; 19: 87–97.

70. Rowley S, Friedman TM, Korngold R. Hematopoietic stem cell transplantation for malignant disease. In: *Clinical Immunology Principles and Practice*. 3rd ed. Philadelphia, PA: Elsevier Limited; 2008: 1223–1236.

71. Stem Cell Trialists Collaborative Group. Allogeneic peripheral blood stem-cell compared with bone marrow transplantation in the management of hematologic malignancies: an individual patient data meta-analysis of nine randomized trials. *J Clin Oncol*. 2005; 23: 5074–5087.

72. Petersdorf EW, Mickelson EM, Anasetti C, et al. Effect of HLA mismatches on the outcome of hematopoietic transplants. *Curr Opin Immunol*. 1999; 11: 521–526.

73. Petersdorf EW, Malkki M. Genetics of risk factors for graft-versus-host disease. *Semin Hematol*. 2006; 43: 11–23.

74. Wilke M, Goulmy E. Minor histocompatibility antigens. In: *Manual of Clinical Laboratory Immunology*. 6th ed. Washington, DC: ASM Press; 2002: 1201–1208.

75. Dickinson AM, Charron D. Non-HLA immunogenetics in hematopoietic stem cell transplantation. *Curr Opin Immunol*. 2005; 17: 517–525.

76. Karanes C, Confer D, Walker T, et al. Unrelated donor stem cell transplantation: the role of the National Marrow Donor Program. *Oncology (Williston Park)*. 2003; 17: 1036–1038, 1043–1044, 1164–1167.

77. McCullough J, Perkins HA, Hansen J. The National Marrow Donor Program with emphasis on the early years. *Transfusion*. 2006; 46: 1248–1255.

78. Hurley CK, Fernandez Vina M, Setterholm M. Maximizing optimal hematopoietic stem cell donor selection from registries of unrelated adult volunteers. *Tissue Antigens*. 2003; 61: 415–424.

79. Hurley CK, Baxter Lowe LA, Logan B, et al. National Marrow Donor Program HLA-matching guidelines for unrelated marrow transplants. *Biol Blood Marrow Transplant*. 2003; 9: 610–615.

80. The National Marrow Donor Program (NMDP). Available at: http://www.marrow.org.

81. Flomenberg N, Baxter-Lowe LA, Confer D, et al. Impact of HLA class I and class II high-resolution matching on outcomes of unrelated donor bone marrow transplantation: HLA-C mismatching is associated with a strong adverse effect on transplantation outcome. *Blood*. 2004; 104: 1923–1930.

82. Petersdorf EW, Malkki M. Human leukocyte antigen matching in unrelated donor hematopoietic cell transplantation. *Semin Hematol*. 2005; 42: 76–84.

83. Gluckman E, Broxmeyer HE, Auerbach AD, et al. Hematopoietic reconstitution in a patient with Fanconi's anemia by means of umbilical cord blood from an HLA-identical sibling. *N Engl J Med*. 1989; 321: 1174–1178.

84. Bradley MB, Cairo MS. Cord blood immunology and stem cell transplantation. *Hum Immunol*. 2005; 66: 431–446.

85. Schoemans H, Theunissen K, Maertens J, et al. Adult umbilical cord blood transplantation: a comprehensive review. *Bone Marrow Transplant*. 2006; 38: 83–93.

86. Laughlin MJ, Eapen M, Rubinstein P, et al. Outcomes after transplantation of cord blood or bone marrow from unrelated donors in adults with leukemia. *N Engl J Med*. 2004; 351: 2265–2275.

87. Rocha V, Labopin M, Sanz G, et al. Transplants of umbilical cord blood or bone marrow from unrelated donors in adults with acute leukemia. *N Engl J Med*. 2004; 351: 2276–2285.

88. Takahashi S, Iseki T, Ooi J, et al. Single-institute comparative analysis of unrelated bone marrow transplantation and cord blood transplantation for adult patients with hematologic malignancies. *Blood*. 2004; 104: 3813–3820.

89. Barker JN, Weisdorf DJ, DeFor TE, et al. Transplantation of 2 partially HLA-matched umbilical cord blood units to enhance engraftment in adults with hematologic malignancy. *Blood*. 2005; 105: 1343–1347.

90. Ottinger H, Rebmann V, Pfeiffer K, et al. Positive serum crossmatch as predictor for graft failure in HLA-mismatched allogeneic blood stem cell transplantation. *Transplantation*. 2002; 73: 1280–1285.

91. Bray R, Rosen-Bronson SA, Haagenson M, et al. The detection of donor-directed, HLA-specific alloantibodies in recipients of unrelated hematopoietic cell transplantation is predictive of graft failure. *ASH Annual Meeting Abstracts*. 2007; 110: 11.

92. Gutman J, McKinney S, Pereira S, et al. Prospective monitoring for alloimmunization in cord blood transplantation: "virtual crossmatch" can be used to demonstrate donor-directed antibodies. *Transplantation*. 2009; 87: 415–418.

93. Mackinnon S, Papdopoulos EB, Carabasi MH, et al. Adoptive immunotherapy evaluating escalating doses of donor leukocytes for relapse of chronic myeloid leukemia after bone marrow transplantation: separation of graft-versus-leukemia responses from graft-versus-host disease. *Blood*. 1995; 86: 1261–1268.

94. McSweeney PA, Niederwieser D, Shizuru JA, et al. Hematopoietic cell transplantation in older patients with hematologic malignancies: replacing high-dose cytotoxic therapy with graft-versus-tumor effect. *Blood*. 2001; 97: 3390–3400.

95. Crawley C, Lalancette M, Szydlo R, et al. Outcomes for reduced-intensity allogeneic transplantation for multiple myeloma: an analysis of prognostic factors from the Chronic Leukemia Working Party of the EMBT. *Blood*. 2005; 105: 4532–4539.

96. Peggs KS, Hunter A, Chopra R, et al. Clinical evidence of a graft-versus-Hodgkin's lymphoma effect after reduced-intensity allogeneic transplantation. *Lancet*. 2005; 365: 1934–1941.

97. Duquesnoy RJ, Witvliet MJ, Doxiadis IIN, et al. HLA matchmaker-based strategy to identify acceptable HLA class I mismatches for highly sensitized kidney transplant candidates. *Transplant Int*. 2004; 7: 31–38.

98. Duquesnoy R. A structurally based approach to determine HLA compatibility at the humoral immune level. *Hum Immunol*. 2006; 67: 847–862.

99. Nambiar A, Duquesnoy R, Adams S, et al. HLA matchmaker-driven analysis of responses to HLA-typed platelet transfusions in alloimmunized thrombocytopenic patients. *Blood*. 2006; 107: 1680–1687.

100. Popovsky MA, Moore SB. Diagnostic and pathogenetic considerations in transfusion-related acute lung injury. *Transfusion*. 1985; 25: 573–577.

101. Silliman CC, Paterson AJ, Dickey WO, et al. The association of biologically active lipids with the development of transfusion-related acute lung injury: a retrospective study. *Transfusion*. 1997; 37: 719–726.

102. Kopko PM, Paglieroni TG, Popovsky MA, et al. TRALI: correlation of antigen–antibody and monocyte activation in donor-recipient pairs. *Transfusion*. 2003; 43: 177–184.

103. Kleinman S, Caulfield T, Chan P, et al. Toward an understanding of transfusion-related acute lung injury: statement of a consensus panel. *Transfusion*. 2004; 44: 1774–1789.

104. Toy P, Popovsky MA, Abraham E, et al. Transfusion-related acute lung injury: definition and review. *Crit Care Med*. 2005; 33: 721–726.

105. Triulzi DJ. Transfusion-related acute lung injury: current concepts for the clinician. *Anesth Analg*. 2009; 108: 770–776.

106. Mintz PD, Lipton KS. *Transfusion-Related Acute Lung Injury. AABB Association Bulletin 05-09*. Bethesda: American Association of Blood Banks; 2005.

107. Amiel JC. Study of the leukocyte phenotypes in Hodgkin's disease. In: Curtoni ES, Mattiuz PL, Tosi RM, eds. *Histocompatibility Testing 1967*. Copenhagen: Munksgaard; 1967: 79.

108. Tiwari JL, Terasaki PI. *HLA and Disease Associations*. New York: NY; Springer-Verlag; 1985; 1–465.

109. Thorsby E. Invited anniversary review: HLA associated diseases. *Hum Immunol*. 1997; 53: 1–11.

110. Chung WH, Hung SI, Hong HS, et al. Medical genetics: a marker for Stevens–Johnson syndrome. *Nature*. 2004; 428: 486.

111. Hung SI, Chung WH, Chen YT. HLA-B genotyping to detect carbamazepine-induced Stevens–Johnson syndrome: implications for personalizing medicine. *Personalized Med*. 2005; 2: 225–237.

112. Gomes ER, Demoly P. Epidemiology of hypersensitivity drug reactions. *Curr Opin Allergy Clin Immunol*. 2005; 5: 309–316.

113. Bagot M, Bocquet H, & Roujeau JC. Clinical heterogeneity of drug hypersensitivity. *Toxicology*. 2006; 209: 123–129.

114. Hung SI, Chung WH, Jee SH, et al. Genetic susceptibility to carbamazepine-induced cutaneous adverse drug reactions. *Pharmacogenet Genomics*. 2006; 16: 297–306.

115. Chung WH, Hung SL, Chen YT. Human leukocyte antigens and drug hypersensitivity. *Curr Opin Allergy Clin Immunol*. 2007; 7: 317–323.

116. Cucca F, Todd JA. HLA susceptibility to type I diabetes: methods and mechanisms. In: *HLA and MHC Genes, Molecules and Function*. Oxford, UK: BIOS Scientific Publishers; 1996: 383–401.

117. Hall FC, Bowness P. HLA and disease: from molecular function to disease association. In: *HLA and MHC Genes, Molecules and Function*. Oxford, UK: BIOS Scientific Publishers; 1996: 353–376.

118. Wicker L, Wekerle H. Autoimmunity. Editorial overview. *Curr Opin Immunol*. 1995; 7: 783.

119. Winchester R. The genetics of autoimmune-mediated rheumatic disease: clinical and biologic implications. *Rheum Dis Clin North Am*. 2004; 30: 213–227.

TRANSFUSION THERAPY AND THE ROLE OF THE MEDICAL DIRECTOR IN BLOOD BANKING

JULIE CRUZ, STEVEN GREGUREK, DANIEL SMITH, AND DAN WAXMAN

OBJECTIVES

After completion of this chapter, the reader will be able to:

1. List indications for transfusion of various blood components.
2. Describe contraindications for transfusion of specific components.
3. Describe therapeutic benefits of transfusion of specific components.
4. Calculate appropriate dose of platelets and cryoprecipitate.
5. Perform calculations to assess response to platelet transfusion.
6. Describe strategies for platelet provision in refractory patients.
7. Discuss differences in pediatric transfusion of components versus adults.
8. Describe alternatives to homologous transfusion.

KEY WORDS

Absolute platelet increment
Acute normovolemic
  hemodilution
Autologous transfusion
Corrected count increment
Cryoprecipitate
DDAVP
Fresh frozen plasma
Granulocyte colony-
  stimulating factor
Granulocytes
Hemophilia A
Hemophilia B
Intraoperative blood salvage
Packed red blood cells
Platelet concentrate
Postoperative blood salvage
Random donor concentrate
Recombinant factor VIIa
Refractoriness
Single-donor apheresis unit
Transfusion trigger
Whole blood

The transfusion service medical director plays a critical role in ensuring appropriate transfusion to patients in need. In addition to overseeing operations of the hospital or blood center blood bank laboratory, the medical director is an ambassador to clinical staff as well as a consultant. One of the most important roles is educating clinicians and assisting them in achieving an evidence-based approach to transfusion. The transfusion service medical director, along with the facility transfusion committee, must properly manage the blood supply by continually monitoring whether transfusions occur within the appropriate guidelines, and provide corrective action when they do not. The medical director is also the person ultimately responsible for ensuring the service is in regulatory compliance. Blood center medical directors ensure the health of donors and may oversee donor testing laboratories in addition to specialized laboratories such as immunohematology and HLA/DNA labs.

Component therapy is the preferred approach for modern transfusion. The frequently quoted cliché "one unit of blood can save three lives" derives from the ability to separate *whole blood* (WB) into red blood cell (RBC), platelet, and plasma components, each providing a potentially lifesaving transfusion. Component therapy allows the clinician to selectively transfuse according to the patient's deficit (oxygen-carrying capacity, thrombocytopenia with bleeding, etc.) without adding unnecessary volume. This is particularly important for patients at risk for transfusion-associated circulatory overload (TACO). In addition, component therapy allows the blood center, transfusion service, and ordering clinician to be good stewards of a precious resource by transfusing only what is needed. The remaining components from the WB donation may then be used to treat other patients in need.

Current recommendations for allogeneic and *autologous transfusion* will be discussed in this chapter, with a focus on appropriate use of blood components. Recommendations pertain to adult transfusion, unless otherwise noted. Neonatal and pediatric transfusion will be discussed separately.

WHOLE BLOOD

Although the emphasis in modern transfusion medicine is on component therapy, military experiences during the war in Iraq warrant discussion of the use of WB. As military personnel return to the private sector, the transfusion service may receive inquiries regarding the use of WB, and even fresh whole blood (FWB) in the settings of mass casualty and massive transfusion due to trauma.

Repine et al. describe the use of WB in military applications, which arises primarily due to logistical situations. In the theater of war, the necessary equipment for thawing and storage of components is usually present in combat support and field hospitals, but lacking in forward surgical units. These surgical units have a limited capacity for storage of packed red cells (generally 20 units), which may be depleted with a single patient. Long logistical lines of support hamper replacement of transfused products. There are profound limitations in both supply and personnel where the need for aggressive resuscitation is greatest. Thus, in 21st century military applications the "walking blood bank" concept is employed. When situations of mass casualty/massive transfusion arise, donors are immediately procured from in-hospital personnel and/or "walking wounded" (otherwise

healthy soldiers). The FDA has not approved FWB for use in the United States, due to safety concerns such as lack of infectious disease testing. In the military application described before, a "pedigreed" population of personnel who have been regularly tested for infections, screened for HIV, and have up-to-date vaccinations is used. Rapid assays for hepatitis B and C, as well as HIV-1/2, are performed on-site, with additional samples sent for "formal" testing. Fresh WB is not indicated for routine use. However, in the setting of mass casualties requiring massive transfusion (e.g., blast injuries from an explosive device), the risk: benefit ratio favors transfusion.[1] A study by Kauvar et al. compared transfusion requirements in massively transfused patients receiving FWB to those of patients receiving component therapy. Mortality did not differ significantly between the two groups, but the blood product requirements of FWB patients were more than twice that of massively transfused patients receiving component therapy. The authors note that FWB transfusion is currently used when appropriate component therapy is unavailable and is a lifesaving intervention for otherwise untreatable hemorrhage and coagulopathy.[2]

RED BLOOD CELLS

Indications

Transfusion of RBCs is indicated when decreased circulatory oxygen-carrying capacity results in inadequate tissue oxygenation. Oxygen delivery to tissues is expressed as the product of cardiac output and arterial oxygen content. Arterial oxygen content, in turn, may be expressed as the product of hemoglobin concentration, percent saturation, and 1.39 mL/g (1 g of hemoglobin binds 1.39 mL of oxygen when fully saturated). Considering this equation, one can see that tissue hypoxia may occur due to (1) decreased cardiac output, (2) decreased hemoglobin saturation (as occurs with obstructive lung disease), and/or (3) decreased concentration of hemoglobin (anemia). Any or all of these may play a role in a particular patient's ability to deliver oxygen to the tissues.[3]

As a patient becomes anemic, adaptive changes occur to compensate. The oxyhemoglobin dissociation curve shifts to the right as 2,3-diphosphoglycerate (2,3-DPG) increases, resulting in more oxygen released to the tissue at a given PO_2. This shift offsets the decrease in oxygen-carrying capacity initially. Cardiac output is increased, and hemodynamic changes such as decreased systemic vascular resistance occur. In addition, microcirculatory changes such as recruitment of additional capillaries and increased capillary flow serve to increase tissue oxygenation. Symptomatic anemia occurs when the decrease in oxygen-carrying capacity (as represented by the concentration of hemoglobin) becomes severe enough to overwhelm these compensatory mechanisms. This may occur rapidly in cases of acute blood loss, or more slowly as chronic anemia develops due to decreased production or increased destruction of RBCs.

In acute blood loss, volume expansion with crystalloid or colloid solutions is the appropriate initial intervention, since the most important determinant of cardiovascular compensation is the circulatory volume status (left ventricular preload). Transfusion of RBCs should not be performed solely to increase circulatory volume. Acute blood loss represents both a loss of circulatory volume and a decrease in hemoglobin concentration due to loss of RBCs. In young, healthy patients acute blood loss of 30% to 40% of total blood volume may occur before volume expansion alone is inadequate to prevent tissue hypoxia, thus necessitating RBC transfusion. In the elderly and those compromised by underlying disease states, the ability to compensate physiologically with volume expansion alone may be overwhelmed at a loss of a much lower percentage of total blood volume.

Appropriate RBC transfusion in patients with chronic anemia presents a greater challenge. There is no single appropriate *"transfusion trigger"* or level of hemoglobin at which all patients should be transfused. Instead, the decision to transfuse must be driven by the clinical picture, considering the contribution of underlying disease states. For example, anemia is not tolerated as well in the presence of cardiovascular disease. In general, treatment of the underlying disorder to correct the RBC deficit is preferred. Mild symptoms of anemia such as fatigue, weakness, dizziness, and reduced exercise tolerance may not require RBC transfusion, unless they are severe enough to interfere with the patient's functional status. Severe symptoms such as increased respiratory rate, shortness of breath at rest, and mental status changes indicate a severe deficit in oxygen-carrying capacity, and these patients require transfusion. Most patients will present somewhere in the middle of these two extremes, where the decision to transfuse is guided by other clinical factors. The benefit of transfusion must be weighed against transfusion-associated risks (TRALI [transfusion-related acute lung injury], alloimmunization, transfusion-transmitted infectious diseases, etc.). A clear assessment of benefit over risk should be present. "Feel-good" transfusions (performed to enhance the patient or physician's "sense of well-being") should be avoided. Transfusion to promote wound healing is also without merit.

In the largest study to examine the effect of transfusing critically ill patients at different thresholds, the Transfusion Requirements in Critical Care (TRICC) trial, restrictive and liberal transfusion strategies were compared to determine whether they produced equivalent results. A total of 838 critically ill, volume-resuscitated patients were randomly assigned to restrictive (transfuse RBCs at hemoglobin of 7.0 g /dL, then transfuse to maintain hemoglobin between 7.0 and 9.0 g/dL) or liberal (transfuse RBCs at hemoglobin of 10.0 g/dL, then transfuse to maintain hemoglobin between 10.0 and 12.0 g/dL) arms of the study. The 30-day mortality in the restrictive group was slightly lower (18.7% vs. 23.3%), but not statistically significant. Average daily hemoglobin concentrations differed significantly in the two groups (8.5 g/dL in the restrictive group vs. 10.7 g/dL in the liberal group), as did average number of RBC units transfused per patient (2.6 units in the restrictive group vs. 5.6 units in the liberal group). This represented a 54% reduction in the number of transfusions when the lower threshold was used. In fact, 33% of patients in the restrictive group were not transfused at all. The authors concluded that a restrictive strategy of RBC transfusion is at least as effective as, and possibly superior to, a liberal transfusion strategy in critically ill patients. They noted the possible exception of a subgroup of patients with acute myocardial infarction and unstable angina.[5]

In a follow-up study, Hebert et al. analyzed the subpopulation of patients from the TRICC trial who were critically ill with known cardiovascular disease and a hemoglobin concentration of <9.0 g/dL within 72 hours of admission to the intensive care unit ($n = 357$). The same restrictive and liberal transfusion approaches described earlier were employed. Again, there were no significant differences in overall mortality rates. Average hemoglobin concentrations and number of RBC units transfused were significantly lower in the restrictive group (8.5 ± 0.62 g/dL vs. 10.3 ± 0.67 g/dL, $p <0.01$; and 2.4 ± 4.1 vs. 5.2 ± 5.0, $p <0.01$, respectively). The restrictive strategy resulted in a reduction of the average number of RBC units transfused by 53%. The restrictive group experienced significantly fewer changes in multiple organ dysfunction from baseline scores (0.2 ± 4.2 vs. 1.3 ± 4.4, $p = 0.02$). In the subgroup of patients with severe ischemic heart disease ($n = 257$), there were no statistically significant differences in survival measure. The restrictive group was noted to have an overall lower, albeit nonsignificant, absolute survival rate when compared to the liberal group. The authors suggested that most hemodynamically stable, critically ill patients could safely tolerate a decreased hemoglobin concentration to 7.0 g/dL before transfusion, and then be maintained at hemoglobin concentrations between

7.0 and 9.0 g/dL. They again noted the possible exception of patients with unstable coronary ischemic syndromes (such as acute myocardial infarction and unstable angina), who may require transfusion at a greater hemoglobin concentration.[6]

The TRICC trial data echoed the recommendations of the American Society of Anesthesiologists Task Force on Blood Component Therapy. The task force cautioned that RBC transfusion should not be performed based on a single hemoglobin "trigger," but should instead be guided by evaluating the patient's risk of developing complications due to inadequate oxygen delivery. They concluded that RBC transfusion is rarely indicated when the hemoglobin concentration is greater than 10 g/dL and is almost always indicated when it is less than 6 g/dL.[4] The decision to transfuse RBCs for hemoglobin concentrations between 6 and 10 g/dL should be guided by the patient's clinical condition and underlying risk of developing complications due to anemic hypoxia.

Since monitoring of blood utilization is required by many regulatory agencies (The Joint Commission, American Association of Blood Banks [AABB], Centers for Medicare and Medicaid), institutions develop a set of transfusion guidelines for appropriate transfusion specific to their facility. Such guidelines are usually produced by the facility's transfusion committee in consultation with clinical staff. They provide transfusing physicians with an institutional "standard of care" regarding blood transfusions, as well as serving as a template for monitoring appropriate blood utilization. The guidelines also set forth an expectation for adequate documentation of transfusion. Such documentation includes a plan for transfusion, evidence to support the transfusion (hemoglobin/hematocrit, signs/symptoms of anemia, risks of transfusion), and posttransfusion evaluation of the result of the transfusion.

Adverse events associated with transfusion of RBCs range from an insignificant nonhemolytic febrile reaction to fatal hemolysis. The transfused volume alone, especially in a patient who is also receiving intravenous fluids or is with renal dysfunction, may result in TACO. Infectious disease risks, including bacterial contamination, the usual viral infections (HIV, HBV, HCV, WNV), and more esoteric infections such as Malaria, Babesiosis, and Chagas disease should be considered. Although testing interdicts the vast majority of potentially infectious units, residual risk is still present. Other effects such as immunomodulation and alloimmunization are also important considerations. Of particular significance is TRALI occurring with red cell transfusion. For a more thorough discussion of adverse events related to transfusion, see Chapter 14.

Dose and Administration

Transfusion of one unit of RBCs is expected to raise the hemoglobin concentration by 1 g/dL and the hematocrit by 3%. Smaller increases may be seen in patients who are actively bleeding or in disease states such as splenomegaly and renal insufficiency. One unit of RBCs has a volume between 200 and 350 mL, and a hematocrit of 55% to 80%. Most of the donor plasma has been removed and replaced with an additive solution to allow extended storage. These additives have proven to be safe for a broad range of patients, including neonates.[7] Although many clinicians habitually order two units of RBCs for any transfusion, giving a single unit and then assessing clinical response prior to ordering a second unit is also appropriate. If a single unit is enough to relieve symptoms of anemia, the second unit and its attendant risks prove unnecessary. This consideration may be particularly important for volume-sensitive patients, such as those with congestive heart failure or renal failure.[8]

Each unit released from the blood bank for a patient should be crossmatch compatible, or in the case of autoantibodies "least incompatible." The term "least incompatible" is a misnomer, as it implies many or all available units have been screened, with those with the weakest incompatibility being selected for transfusion. Such units are, in fact, correctly described as incompatible, but are appropriate for transfusion when necessary. Use of the term serves to increase the comfort level of the blood bank personnel and transfusing physician, rather than truly describing compatibility status.

When clinically significant alloantibodies have been detected, RBC units negative for the corresponding antigen should be dispensed. Some chronically transfused patients, such as those with sickle cell disease (SCD), may benefit from proactively selecting units matching the patient's phenotype in order to prevent alloimmunization. Simple transfusions may be performed for treatment of symptomatic anemia, multiorgan system failure, splenic sequestration, or acute chest syndrome in SCD patients. The STOP I and STOP II trials have demonstrated the benefit of prophylactic exchange transfusions in SCD patients with high risk of stroke. Supplying fully phenotype-matched RBCs to these patients would prevent alloimmunization, but would also require RBC units with phenotypes that are much less prevalent among random donors. A partial phenotype match limited to Rh and Kell is an alternative.[9,10]

Some facilities utilize an "electronic crossmatch" procedure, when appropriate prior test results are present. The unit should be visually inspected for discoloration of the plasma/additive solution due to hemolysis or bacterial contamination, as well as the presence of clots.

A unit of RBCs should generally be administered over 1 to 2 hours. Once begun, transfusion must be complete by 4 hours or the time and date of expiration of the unit, whichever comes first. This is to reduce the risk of bacterial contamination once the unit becomes an "open system." For patients at risk of circulatory overload, a slower rate of 1 mL/kg/hr may be used. Pretransfusion treatment with a loop diuretic may also be considered for these patients to ameliorate the increased circulatory volume caused by the transfusion.[3] For brisk or massive bleeding, administration may be achieved faster, in order to keep pace with circulatory loss. A standard blood filter should be used. Normal saline is the only acceptable solution to maintain intravenous lines through which blood is administered, to rinse the tubing or blood bag, or to reduce the viscosity in a unit with high hematocrit to promote flow. Medications must not be added to blood components. Hypotonic saline, dextrose, or Lactated Ringer's solution are inappropriate. Hypotonic saline and dextrose cause hemolysis, and Lactated Ringer's contains enough calcium to overcome the citrate anticoagulant present in the stored blood and promote clot formation.[11]

Modifications of Red Cell Components

Leukocyte Reduction

Leukocyte reduction (leukoreduction) may be accomplished pre-storage during manufacture of the components or may occur at the bedside with use of a special filter. Both are designed to reduce the number of leukocytes in the component to $<5 \times 10^6$. Leukoreduction reduces the risk of HLA alloimmunization, transfusion-transmitted infection with cytomegalovirus (CMV), and febrile nonhemolytic transfusion reactions. This last effect is more effective with prestorage leukoreduced components, as not only is the transfusion of intact leukocytes prevented, but accumulation of inflammatory cytokines released by leukocytes into the storage bag is prevented.

Washing

Washed RBCs are indicated to prevent severe recurrent allergic reactions not responsive to premedication with antihistamines and steroids. They may also be used for IgA-deficient patients when RBCs from a deficient donor are unavailable. Patients may also have other plasma protein hypersensitivities requiring washing. Washing may be employed for

patients at risk of hypokalemia (intrauterine transfusion, neonates), but usually can be avoided by administering units that are as fresh (close to the donation date) as possible. It is not equivalent to leukoreduction and results in a loss of approximately 20% of RBCs from the unit.[11] A washed unit of RBCs must be transfused within 24 hours. The expiration date is modified because washing creates an open system with the attendant risk of bacterial contamination. In addition, the anticoagulant preservative solution has been removed; thus, the unit lacks the ability to support long-term RBC viability and function.[8]

Volume Reduction

Volume reduction of the RBC component is accomplished by removal of the suspending plasma. It is used to reduce the risk of circulatory overload in susceptible patients, such as those with congestive heart failure, children, and patients with plasma volume expansion. It is rarely necessary and not equivalent to washing for prevention of allergic reactions.

Irradiation

Inactivation of lymphocytes in RBC components is achieved by irradiation of the unit at 2,500 cGy. It is necessary for the prevention of transfusion-associated graft-versus-host disease. Directed donor components from a blood relative should be irradiated. Other indications are components to be transfused to allogeneic bone marrow transplant recipients, patients with immunodeficiency (congenital or immunosuppressive therapy induced), malignancies, intrauterine transfusion, and neonatal transfusion as well as other indications. Irradiation is not necessary for patients with HIV in the absence of other indications, or for those with aplastic anemia. The shelf life of an irradiated RBC unit is modified to 28 days or the date of expiration of the unit, whichever comes first.

Frozen Red Blood Cells

Long-term storage may be indicated for autologous units or, more commonly, for rare antigen-negative units. Cryopreservation is accomplished by freezing units in glycerol. Units are collected in CPD, CP2D, or CPDA-1, and are glycerolized and frozen within 6 days of collection. Units that have been stored at 1°C to 6°C may be rejuvenated up to 3 days after expiration using a solution to restore 2,3-DPG and ATP, then glycerolized and frozen. Storage life is 10 years at -80°C. Before transfusion, units must be thawed and deglycerolized. Complete removal of the glycerol solution is critical, as inadequately deglycerolized cells will hemolyze on contact with normal saline, serum, or plasma. Units prepared in an open system expire in 24 hours once thawed and deglycerolized. Closed-system preparation of units collected in CPDA-1 and frozen within 6 days of collection confers a post-thaw expiration of 2 weeks. Blood bank personnel and the transfusing physician should be advised as to which system, and therefore which expiration date, applies in their facility. Communication between the blood supplier, blood bank, and transfusing physician is critical to ensure rare units are not wasted. Units should only be thawed and deglycerolized when a definite decision to transfuse has been made. Units prepared and not transfused, but returned to the blood bank in the appropriate time period may be rejuvenated and refrozen. Due to the length of time required for thawing and deglycerolizing, frozen RBCs are not appropriate for emergent transfusion.[11]

Antigen-matched Red Blood Cells

Patients who have been alloimmunized and have developed clinically significant red cell alloantibodies require RBC units confirmed to be negative for the cognate antigen. Rare units may be necessary for patients with antibodies to high-frequency antigens or those with multiple alloantibodies. When such patients are identified, it is critical to consult with the blood supplier and the ordering physician to discuss availability and the time required to deliver rare units. When the patient requires transfusion more urgently than such units can be delivered, the ordering physician and transfusion service physician should consult to determine the best strategy for the patient.

PLATELETS

Indications

Platelets play a critical role in hemostasis and maintenance of vascular integrity. They have three important functions in the bleeding patient: adhesion, aggregation, and activation surface. When vessel injury occurs, subendothelial collagen is exposed. Primary hemostasis is achieved by platelet adherence, shape change, granule release, and aggregation resulting in formation of the "platelet plug." Platelets also provide a surface on which interactions in the coagulation cascade occur, leading to formation of the "definitive" or fibrin clot. Although they are usually considered in the context of vascular injury

or compromise and bleeding, a relatively fixed number (7,000 to $10,000/\mu L/day$) is required on a daily basis to repair minor endothelial defects.[12]

Platelet transfusions are indicated in the thrombocytopenic patient with active bleeding and in patients with platelet function defects when other therapies are not effective. They may also be administered prophylactically in thrombocytopenic patients with certain risk factors or who are about to undergo invasive procedures. As with RBCs, a definitive transfusion trigger is difficult to identify, and the individual clinical presentation and risk for bleeding must be considered. Nevertheless, several values have been established as being appropriate to guide the decision to transfuse in certain patient populations. Although a platelet count less than $100 \times 10^3/mm^3$ is thrombocytopenia by definition, numerous studies have established patients are not at risk for spontaneous bleeding until the platelet count falls much lower. In all cases, an effort to identify and treat the underlying etiology is of primary concern. Patients without additional risk factors usually do not undergo spontaneous bleeding until the platelet count falls to 5 to $10 \times 10^3/mm^3$.[13] Patients with concomitant fever, sepsis, or coagulation abnormalities (acute promyelocytic leukemia or disseminated intravascular coagulation) may require a higher threshold of $20 \times 10^3/mm^3$.[14] Transfusion to reach a platelet count of $50 \times 10^3/mm^3$ is recommended for invasive procedures such as liver biopsy and laparotomy. When operating on critical sites such as the brain or eyes, a preoperative platelet count of $100 \times 10^3/mm^3$ is desirable.[15]

Contraindications

Platelet transfusion in patients with thrombotic thrombocytopenic purpura (TTP) is relatively contraindicated, as their administration has sometimes been associated with rapid clinical deterioration and death. Although some authors have reported no adverse events with platelet transfusion in TTP patients receiving plasma exchange, this intervention is best reserved for those patients with severe bleeding. Platelet transfusion is not recommended in patients with heparin-induced thrombocytopenia (HIT) due to the risk of arterial and venous thrombosis.[16] Patients with idiopathic thrombocytopenic purpura (ITP) have accelerated platelet destruction that rapidly clears transfused platelets. In spite of this, the bleeding time in most patients is normal and platelet function is well maintained, due to the compensatory marrow response, which releases young, hyperfunctional platelets. Administration of corticosteroids is the preferred first-line therapy, followed by splenectomy in refractory patients. Platelet transfusion should be reserved for life-threatening bleeding, or perhaps during splenectomy once the splenic artery has been clamped.[17]

Dose and Administration

Platelets are usually administered as a ***single-donor apheresis unit*** (SDP) or as a pool of five to eight ***random donor concentrates*** (RDPs) derived from WB. RDPs may be pooled at the time of issue or may be prestorage pooled. A single apheresis unit must contain a minimum of 3.0×10^{11} platelets, while each unit in a random donor pool contains a minimum of 5.5×10^{10} platelets.[18] In either case, the dose usually corresponds to 50 to 100×10^9 platelets per 10 kg of the patient's body weight. Although the actual dose administered with a single-donor apheresis unit or random donor pool is highly variable, a rise in platelet count of 20 to 30×10^3 platelets/mm^3 can be expected.[19] If a more precise calculation is required, the following formula may be applied:

Dose in platelet units =

$$\frac{PI(mm^3) \times 1{,}000 \ mm^3/mL \times BV(mL) \times F^{-1}}{\text{Average number of platelets per unit}}$$

where PI represents the desired platelet increment, BV is the patient's blood volume (estimated by multiplying the patient's body weight in kilograms by 70 mL/kg in an adult), and F is a correction factor of 0.67, which allows for splenic pooling of approximately one third of the administered dose.[15]

Assessing Response to Transfusion

Effectiveness of platelet transfusion may be assessed by obtaining a posttransfusion platelet count from a specimen drawn 10 to 60 minutes following the transfusion. One may then consider the ***absolute platelet increment*** (API), calculated by subtracting the pretransfusion platelet count from the posttransfusion value. The posttransfusion platelet recovery (PPR) can then be expressed as the product of the estimated total blood volume and the API, divided by the number of platelets transfused. An appropriate response is a PPR >20% measured at 10 to 60 minutes post transfusion, or >10% when assessed 18 to 24 hours post transfusion. The ***corrected count increment*** (CCI) is similar to the PPR, but normalizes the posttransfusion platelet increment based on the patient's body surface area (BSA) expressed in meters squared, rather than weight in kilograms, when estimating blood volume. Thus, the CCI is calculated as BSA × API/(number of platelets transfused), where BSA is in m^2, and API is expressed as platelet number per microliter × 10^{11}. A response of 7,500 platelets × m^2 BSA per microliter is considered adequate.[11]

Platelet Refractoriness

Refractoriness to platelet transfusion is suggested when a patient's 1-hour posttransfusion CCI or PPR is below adequate response levels on two consecutive transfusions. A caveat must be applied to consider ABO compatibility, however, as transfusion of incompatible platelets with high-titer plasma anti-A or anti-B may cause destruction when soluble A or B antigens have adsorbed onto the platelet surface. It is most desirable to give ABO-identical units, but most platelets are usually ABO compatible due to inventory constraints. Sometimes minor incompatibility occurs. This is most significant when type O platelets are given to A or B recipients. High-titer anti-A can result in hemolysis. Except in neonates, the risk of thrombocytopenia is greater than the risk of platelet destruction or hemolysis caused by incompatible plasma. Since Rh antigens are not present on platelets, but may be present on contaminating red cells, Rh-negative RDPs should be administered to Rh-negative patients whenever possible, and the administration of Rh immunoglobulin (RhIg) should be considered in D-negative women of childbearing potential receiving D-positive RDPs. The red cell content in Rh-positive SDPs is below the immunizing dose; however, many still administer RhIg. It is not necessary to administer RhIg following transfusion of Rh-positive platelets to men or women with hematological malignancies, as these patients rarely make anti-D.[15] Patients who are significantly immunosuppressed are less subject to immunization.

Platelet refractoriness may be due to immune or nonimmune causes. Nonimmune causes include fever, sepsis, hypersplenism, DIC, massive hemorrhage, hemodilution, and drug effect, particularly amphotericin. Immune platelet destruction is usually due to alloimmunization resulting from HLA sensitization by transfusion or pregnancy. Less frequently it is due to the presence of platelet-specific antibodies. Such antibodies may be stimulated by pregnancy in women, or by the presence of leukocytes in transfusions to either gender. Provision of leukocyte-reduced products for patients requiring long-term transfusion may prevent or delay alloimmunization and resultant refractoriness.

Platelet Selection for Refractory Patients

Platelet selection for refractory patients depends upon whether a platelet-specific antibody or HLA antibody is identified. Many blood collection facilities maintain a cohort of platelet donors who have been HLA-A, B antigen typed, and are able to donate in response to a specific patient need. Donors who are negative for specific human platelet antigens may be recruited in the same way. Existing inventory may also be screened for compatibility by solid-phase red cell adherence assay (SPRCA) crossmatching. Compatible units for patients with antibodies to high-frequency antigens may be achievable only through recruitment of type-specific donors. The patient's blood relatives may also be screened to determine if they are suitable for directed donation.

Platelet Modifications

Irradiated

Indications for irradiation of platelet products are the same as those for RBCs.

CMV Seronegative

As with RBCs, leukocyte-reduced products are generally considered CMV reduced-risk (CMV "safe") and are equivalent to CMV-seronegative units for most patients. Since the virus is present in the transfused leukocytes, modern efficient leukoreduction ameliorates the risk of transmission from components with untested serostatus. Seronegative products should be reserved for patients known to be seronegative and at increased risk. Appropriate patients are those undergoing hematopoietic progenitor or solid organ transplant, those with HIV, pregnant women, and patients requiring intrauterine transfusions.

Volume Reduced

Volume reduction of platelet components is generally reserved for removal of ABO-incompatible plasma to prevent hemolysis in neonates when small total blood volume may confer a relatively larger dose effect.

Irradiated

Irradiation of platelet components is indicated for the prevention of transfusion-associated graft-versus-host disease in susceptible patients, applying the same criteria outlined for RBCs. Unlike RBCs, irradiation does not change the expiration date of platelet components.

GRANULOCYTE TRANSFUSIONS

Indications

Granulocyte transfusions remain a controversial intervention, due to the lack of sufficient evidence of efficacy as demonstrated by randomized controlled trials. However, case studies, anecdotes, and retrospective studies are reported in the literature, and as an aggregate generally support granulocyte transfusion in a select group of patients. In neutropenic patients (<0.5 granulocytes $\times 10^9$) with potential for marrow recovery, *granulocytes* may be an appropriate adjunct to antibiotics and antifungal agents in the face of refractory septicemia. Early studies demonstrated unimpressive results, but indicated a dose-dependent response, with better response in infants and children as compared to adults. This is likely due to the observation that at any given granulocyte dose, the dose per kilogram is much higher in neonates and children.[20] With improvements in collection technology and stimulation of donors, modern components contain a much higher number of granulocytes per collection. At a minimum, the product should contain 1×10^{10} granulocytes. Donors may be stimulated to increase neutrophil count by administration of corticosteroids, *granulocyte colony-stimulating factor* (G-CSF), or both. G-CSF produces higher yields than corticosteroids, and addition of corticosteroids to G-CSF increases the granulocyte yield by two- to threefold.[21] A minimum of a 12-hour interval is necessary in either case to achieve maximum granulocyte mobilization. Collection via apheresis may also include use of a sedimenting agent such as hydroxyethyl starch to maximize separation of RBCs and granulocytes. It is important to note, however, that even with maximum collection efficiency, the resultant product will still contain a significant number of RBCs, requiring the product to be ABO and crossmatch compatible with the recipient. Patients with concurrent thrombocytopenia may derive additional benefit from the fairly large number of platelets present in the granulocyte component.

Dosage and Administration

Granulocyte components must be transfused within 24 hours of collection, since neutrophils undergo rapid apoptosis. The product should be irradiated to prevent transfusion-associated graft-versus-host disease. Irradiation inactivates donor lymphocytes but does not interfere with neutrophil function. TRALI has been reported with granulocyte transfusions. It is prudent to obtain the patient's HLA and granulocyte antigen type when possible and transfuse compatible granulocyte concentrates. Following confirmation of ABO and crossmatch compatibility, they should be administered through a standard blood filter. A leukoreduction filter should not be used. Granulocytes are often administered daily for 5 to 7 days. Response should then be assessed prior to continuing transfusions. Administration of amphotericin B concurrently or within a short time frame of granulocyte transfusion should be avoided, due to the reported risk of adverse pulmonary reactions. It is not clear whether newer drugs such as the third-generation triazole voriconazole or liposomal formulations share the same risk.

PLASMA

Indications

Plasma is the noncellular fraction of blood and may be manufactured from WB or collected by apheresis. It is indicated for replacement of multiple coagulation factor deficiencies, or for single factor deficiencies for which no factor concentrate is available (i.e., factor V). Its use should be guided by clinical assessment in conjunction with appropriate coagulation testing. Plasma is indicated for the urgent reversal of warfarin when the clinical situation prohibits waiting for vitamin K to effect reversal. Historically prophylactic plasma transfusion before invasive procedures was considered appropriate with a prothrombin time (PT) of 1.5 times the geometric mean of the normal range, or a partial thromboplastin time (PTT) greater than 1.5 times the upper limit of the normal range. More recent studies demonstrate the futility of attempting to correct minor coagulation abnormalities by plasma transfusion. In fact, plasma transfusion has minimal benefit in correcting coagulation test results in patients with an international normalized ratio (INR) of less than 1.7 or a PT less than 1.7 times normal.[22] Plasma is also the replacement fluid of choice for plasma exchange in patients with TTP. It is also indicated in the setting of massive transfusion in combination with red cell and platelet products.

Contraindications

Plasma is not indicated for reversal of anticoagulant effects of warfarin therapy unless the patient is bleeding and/or emergent reversal is required. It should be used only in situations not allowing time for administration of vitamin K (orally or parenterally) to have the desired effect. Plasma is inappropriate for reversal of heparin anticoagulation. Protamine sulfate is the drug of choice. It should not be used solely for volume expansion, where crystalloids or colloids are adequate. It is ineffective as a source of protein in nutritionally deficient patients, especially since many are ICU patients, and thus likely to be sensitive to volume overload.

Available Plasma Products

Fresh Frozen Plasma

Fresh frozen plasma (FFP) must be frozen within 6 to 8 hours of collection, depending on the anticoagulant used. It is stored at $\leq -18°C$.

Plasma Frozen within 24 hours (FP24)

Due to the shift toward manufacture of transfusable plasma exclusively from males, many blood suppliers have converted to manufacture of FP24. Since FP24 can be frozen any time within 24 hours of collection, additional time is available to identify male units and also to receive blood from distant collection sites and mobiles beyond the 4 to 6 hours required for FFP. Labile coagulation factors (factors V and VIII) are slightly decreased in FP24 as compared to FFP, but maintain sufficient levels for hemostatic effect. Indications for FP24 are essentially the same as FFP.

Thawed Plasma

Thawed plasma (TP) is plasma prepared from FFP or FP24 and stored in the liquid state for up to 5 days. A TP policy allows the blood bank to reduce wastage of FFP or FP24 that has been thawed and not transfused and also allows a faster response time for urgent issue of plasma. There is a modest reduction in coagulation factors versus FFP, but factor levels are sufficient to support hemostasis. TP derived from FP24 also maintains hemostatic levels of labile factors.[23] Isolated factor deficiencies should be treated with factor concentrates when available.

Cryopoor Plasma

Cryopoor plasma is the remaining supernatant when *cryoprecipitate* has been removed from plasma. It is therefore depleted of those factors (FVIII [factor VIII], vWF [von Willebrand factor], FXIII [factor XIII], fibrinogen, cryoglobulin, fibronectin), but contains the remaining coagulation factors found in plasma. It is sometimes used as a replacement fluid in plasma exchange for the treatment of refractory TTP, where it was thought to be beneficial due to depletion of high molecular weight vWF. However, this benefit is equivocal, and FFP, FP24, or TP are all suitable for plasma exchange in TTP.[24]

Dose and Administration

If plasma is administered for replacement of coagulation factors, a dose of 10 to 20 mL/kg (three to six units in adult patient) will increase the factor levels by 20%. When administered to patients with severe liver disease, plasma dosing at the upper end of the range is usually required. The volume of plasma required as replacement fluid for TTP is calculated based on the patient's blood volume, using a standard formula for plasma exchange. When administering plasma prior to an invasive procedure, it is important to remember the short biologic half-life of factor VII (3–6 hours) and time transfusion appropriately so that effective levels will be present when the procedure is performed. It is noteworthy that factor VII concentrations of only 10% to 15% are usually adequate to achieve hemostasis.

CRYOPRECIPITATED ANTIHEMOPHILIC FACTOR (CRYOPRECIPITATE)

Indications

Cryoprecipitate is manufactured from plasma and is enriched in the cold, insoluble proteins FVIII, vWF, FXIII, fibronectin, and fibrinogen. Although historically indicated in the treatment of *hemophilia A*, virally inactivated factor concentrates are now available and are preferred. Likewise, in von Willebrand disease (vWD), the use of cryoprecipitate has been supplanted by the synthetic vasopressin analog desmopressin (*DDAVP*) as first-line therapy. The intermediate purity, virally inactivated FVIII concentrates Humate-P (Aventis Behring, Kankakee, IL) and Alphanate (Grifols Biologicals, Los Angeles, CA) contain adequate vWF to treat vWD and are preferred over cryoprecipitate. Currently cryoprecipitate is most commonly used to treat congenital and acquired hypofibrinogenemia or dysfibrinogenemia. The risk of severe bleeding complications is increased when fibrinogen levels fall below 80 to 100 mg/dL.

Contraindications

Cryoprecipitate should not be used to treat coagulation factor deficiencies other than fibrinogen or hemophilia A or vWD when virally inactivated factor concentrates are unavailable. It is poor source of vitamin K–dependent factors and is therefore not appropriate for the reversal of warfarin anticoagulation. Its use in treating vWD should be limited to severe cases unresponsive to treatment such as the synthetic vasopressin analog desmopressin (DDAVP) and when Alphanate and Humate-P are unavailable. In some cases of severe type III vWD, cryoprecipitate will only be effective if it is given together with platelets or DDAVP.[25]

Dose and Administration

Cryoprecipitate units are usually pooled to achieve adequate dose. Each unit of cryoprecipitate contains a minimum of 150 mg of fibrinogen (average 200 mg), 80 to 100 U of FVIII, 40% to 70% of the vWF from the original unit of plasma, and 40 to 60 U of FXIII suspended in 10 to 15 mL of plasma. Variable amounts of fibronectin, IgG, IgM, and albumin are also present.

Total milligrams of fibrinogen required (*R*) is calculated by multiplying the plasma (dL) by the desired fibrinogen increment (mg/dL). The number of cryoprecipitate units is estimated by dividing milligrams of fibrinogen from the previous calculation by 200 mg fibrinogen per unit of cryo.

$$\text{Units of cryoprecipitate} = R \times \frac{\text{Unit of cryoprecipitate}}{200 \text{ mg fibrinogen}}$$

In general, the fibrinogen level is expected to rise by a minimum of 5 to 10 mg/dL per unit of cryoprecipitate, with a half-life of 3 to 6 days. Factor concentrates are the preferred intervention for hemophilia A, but a similar calculation can be performed for FVIII replacement. Determining the desired FVIII increment and substituting 80 U FVIII per unit of cryoprecipitate for fibrinogen in the previous equation will indicate the number of units desired. One unit of FVIII per kilogram patient body weight usually raises the factor level by 2%, and FVIII levels required to achieve hemostasis depend upon the clinical situation and range from 20% to 100%, with higher levels required for severe bleeding. Since the half-life of FVIII is only 8 to 12 hours, cryoprecipitate transfusions are required every 8 to 12 hours to maintain levels. vWF concentrations in cryoprecipitate are similar and may be similarly calculated.[25]

Clotting Factor Concentrates

A variety of clotting factor concentrates have been developed for treatment of both acquired and inherited clotting factor deficiencies. Originally derived from pooled plasma products, the risk of transfusion-associated HIV and hepatitis C has led to the development of recombinant clotting factor concentrates as well as highly purified and virally inactivated human derived concentrates.

Recombinant Factor VIIa Concentrate

Recombinant factor VIIa (rFVIIa) concentrate is structurally similar to native activated factor VII and promotes coagulation by two proposed mechanisms. First, it directly binds tissue factor and forms an FVIIa–TF complex that activates factors IX and X.[26] Second, it directly activates factor X on activated platelets, including defective platelets in Glanzmann thrombasthenia.[27] rFVIIa is FDA licensed for treatment of inhibitors to factors VIII or IX and factor VII deficiency. FVIIa also effects primary hemostasis by generating thrombin, which is a potent platelet agonist. It has been used to treat infants with hemorrhage and in the treatment of coagulopathies in massively transfused trauma patients.[28] Post hoc analysis of two randomized placebo-controlled double-blind studies showed fewer blood products were required, with decreased incidence of multiorgan failure and respiratory distress syndrome versus placebo in severe trauma patients.[29] There is retrospective evidence that early administration of rVIIa reduces the number of transfused blood products by 22%.[30] Two cases of successful rFVIIa use in Jehovah's Witness patients undergoing cardiopulmonary bypass have been reported.[31] Such off-label use may be approved on an individual basis.

Factors VIII and IX Concentrates

Concentrates of clotting factors VIII and IX are indicated for the treatment of hemophilia A and B, respectively. There has been considerable progress in the manufacturing technology including viral inactivation since the early 1980s when several thousand hemophiliacs developed HIV and hepatitis C after exposure to pooled clotting factor concentrates. Recombinant factor VIII (rFVIII) is produced in a mammalian cell culture system using synthetic culture media and chromatographic purification. rFVIII can be produced in greater quantities than pooled human plasma techniques and has no documented viral transmission. High-purity factor IX fractionated from plasma and recombinant factor IX concentrates are currently available for the use in *hemophilia B.* Factor IX concentrates are associated with fewer complications than the previously used prothrombin complex concentrates derived from plasma that have been associated with thrombosis.[32]

Other Plasma Components

Albumin

Albumin is a plasma-derived colloidal solution. It serves to increase plasma oncotic pressure and thereby increase intravascular volume by fluid shift from the interstitial space. This fluid shift also reduces peripheral edema. Albumin is available in 5% and 25% solutions and is without risk of viral transmission. Hypersensitivity to albumin is uncommon. It may be used in volume replacement in nonhemorrhagic shock when crystalloids have failed, or in the presence of capillary leak syndromes. It is also indicated for volume replacement in patients with extensive burns or following removal of large amounts of ascitic fluid. Albumin is also used as a replacement fluid in plasma exchange.[33]

Plasma Protein Fraction

Plasma protein fraction (PPF) is similar to albumin in that it is a colloidal solution effective for volume expansion. It contains a greater amount of other PPFs in addition to albumin. Like albumin, it is without risk of transfusion-transmitted viruses.

Fibrin Sealant (Fibrin Glue)

Fibrin sealants may be prepared from large plasma pools ("commercial") or from a single autologous or allogeneic plasma donation ("blood bank"). The fibrinogen-rich concentrate is mixed with a thrombin concentrate at the time of use. The result is analogous to the final step of the coagulation cascade—formation of a fibrin clot that provides a fluid-tight seal while holding tissues and other materials in the desired position. Thus, fibrin sealants have hemostatic and sealing properties. They also promote wound healing. Unlike synthetic surgical glues, they are biocompatible, biodegradable, and do not promote inflammatory reactions or tissue necrosis. The fibrin clot is reabsorbed in days to weeks following the application of the sealant.[34]

Platelet Gel

Platelet gel is generated by combining platelet-rich blood fraction (*platelet concentrate* or platelet-rich plasma) from a single autologous or allogeneic component with calcified thrombin. Platelet activation results in formation of a gel-like biomaterial, as well as the release of growth factors from platelet granules (platelet-derived growth factor [PDGF], transforming growth factor beta [TGF-β], epidermal growth factor, and vascular endothelial growth factor). Peridontal regeneration is aided by PDGF, and cells associated with bone are stimulated by TGF-β. The fibrin-rich structure and growth factors allow molding and securing of graft material, as well as promote wound healing by cell migration and vascular invasion. Platelet gel is most commonly used in oral and maxillofacial surgery, and orthopedic and reconstructive surgery.[34]

Intravenous Immunoglobulin

Intravenous immunoglobulin (IVIG) is prepared from the pooled plasma of 3,000 to 60,000 donors. The γ-globulin fraction is separated by alcohol fractionation and variable anti-aggregation and stabilization techniques dependent upon the product. Pathogen inactivation steps reduce the risk of viral transmission. The result is a solution 95% to 99% IVIG. IVIG has an advantage over intramuscular preparations in that large volumes may be administered without the localized pain of injection. FDA-approved indications for

IVIG include replacement therapy for patients with primary immunodeficiency with hypogammaglobulinemia, chronic lymphocytic leukemia, Kawasaki syndrome, ITP, pediatric HIV infection, and allogeneic stem cell transplant. IVIG is also used in various neurologic diseases such as Guillan–Barré syndrome and chronic inflammatory demyelinating polyneuropathy, as well as hematologic, rheumatologic, dermatologic, and inflammatory conditions. Although generally well tolerated, adverse effects include hypersensitivity reactions, renal toxicity, hemolytic anemia, hemolysis, and cytopenia. The mechanism of action is not well understood, but in primary immunodeficiencies it may provide replacement antibody. In other disorders, it may serve as a "blocking" antibody, may inhibit B cell and complement activation, or may stimulate production of anti-inflammatory cytokines.[35]

MASSIVE TRANSFUSION

Massive transfusion has been variously defined as replacement of a patient's entire blood volume in 24 hours, replacement of 50% of the patient's blood volume in 3 hours, 10 or more RBC units per 70-kg adult per 24 hours, or administration of 4 or more RBC units in 4 hours with ongoing need for more blood. Often emergency uncrossmatched type O RBC units are transfused until type-specific crossmatched blood is available. Rapid administration of large volumes of RBCs combined with loss due to bleeding often results in a dilutional thrombocytopenia coupled with consumptive coagulopathy. Most patients require a combination of RBCs, platelets, cryoprecipitate, and plasma. Some facilities use a 1:1:1 fixed volume ratio of RBCs to SDPs and plasma. Combat experience with the use of FWB (generally not available in civilian settings) has suggested that a 1:1 transfusion of RBC to plasma may be beneficial in avoiding the "bloody vicious cycle" characterized by bleeding, resuscitation, hemodilution and hypothermia with depletion of procoagulant factors, and disruption of hemostatic plugs resulting in more bleeding.[14] Transfusion services should have massive transfusion protocols in place to guide emergency provision of blood in the setting of critical bleeding.

PEDIATRIC TRANSFUSION

When considering transfusion practice, children cannot be considered as merely small adults. Pediatric populations, especially neonates, require careful consideration of the risks and benefits of transfusion, particularly when weighed against the long posttransfusion life expectancy.

Whole Blood, Reconstituted Whole Blood, or Modified Whole Blood

WB storage requirements result in decreased activity of the labile clotting factors V and VIII. In addition, development of the platelet storage lesion is accelerated by refrigeration, as platelets lose their discoid shapes in colder environments. Some modern blood collection sets with in-line filters trap platelets and prevent their passage into the filtered blood collection bag. Mou and colleagues reported that the use of FWB for pump priming in cardiopulmonary bypass in infants had no advantage over use of a combination of *packed red blood cells* and FFP. In fact, patients whose circuits were primed with FWB had an increased length of stay in the intensive care unit, and experienced increased perioperative fluid overload.[36] These factors, in addition to the logistics of maximizing donations by component production, render WB either unavailable or available only by special request with advance notice. However, WB may be reconstituted by combining RBC and plasma (FFP or FP24) components. Such reconstitution does increase the number of donor exposures, and the benefit versus single-component therapy must be considered adequate to offset risk. Reconstituted blood may be appropriate for exchange transfusion necessitated by hemolytic disease of the newborn and fetus, following cardiopulmonary bypass, ECMO, or massive transfusion.[37]

Red Blood Cells

Although underlying clinical conditions may be responsible for anemia, a common cause of anemia in neonates and children is iatrogenic blood loss due to phlebotomy. Particularly for neonates, every effort should be made to maximize utilization of blood samples for diagnostic workup while minimizing the volume of blood removed. Transfusion of RBCs may be of benefit in neonates with hemoglobin <7.0 g/dL when reticulocyte count is low and symptoms are present. Transfusion at higher hemoglobin levels is appropriate when the patient requires supplemental oxygen due to severe pulmonary disease, cyanotic heart disease, or has significant apnea, bradycardia, tachycardia, or tachypnea. Transfusion at a hemoglobin level <8.0 g/dL can be considered in older children perioperatively, during chemotherapy or radiotherapy, or for acute blood loss unresponsive to colloid or crystalloid therapy. Higher hemoglobin thresholds may be considered in the presence of severe pulmonary disease. Children of any age on ECMO require RBCs. Those with disorders of RBC production (Diamond-Blackfan, β-thalassemia major) or SCD may be chronically transfused. Small-volume transfusions (5 to 15 mL/kg) do not usually require fresh RBCs. Although plasma potassium does rise during storage, the actual amount of bioavailable potassium is really quite small. The same holds true for additives found in some extended-storage media (mannitol, dextrose). Even though 2,3-DPG declines in older RBCs, even these provide an advantage over the infant's own cells, since 2,3-DPG increases rapidly in the transfused cells (but not the endogenous infant cells) following transfusion. Thus, consideration of fresh (<7 days old) blood should be reserved for large-volume transfusions (> 20 mL/kg) such as occurs with ECMO, cardiopulmonary bypass, or exchange transfusion. Alternatively, washing may be used for older units when fresh RBCs are not available.[37,38] Units that are leukocyte reduced (prestorage or bedside filter) should be transfused to mitigate the risk of CMV transmission. Gamma irradiation should be employed for cellular blood products (RBCs, platelets, and granulocytes) in neonates with cellular immunodeficiency, those receiving exchange transfusions or cellular components from blood relatives. Patients receiving hematopoietic progenitor cell transplants, HLA-matched cellular blood components, undergoing intense chemotherapy, or with hematologic malignancies should also receive irradiated products.

Platelets

Preterm infants are at risk for intracranial hemorrhage, especially in the presence of comorbid disease. Platelets should be transfused when the count is below $50 \times 10^9/L$ in a stable premature neonate, or below $100 \times 10^9/L$ in a sick patient if there is active bleeding or an invasive procedure planned. Full-term infants and other children may not require platelet transfusion until platelet count is as low as 5 to $10 \times 10^9/L$, provided there is no active bleeding. Transfusion is also indicated in the absence of thrombocytopenia when there is active bleeding associated with a qualitative platelet defect. Patients undergoing ECMO with a platelet count of $<100 \times 10^9/L$, or with active bleeding at higher platelet counts may also require transfusion. Children with unexplained excessive bleeding on cardiopulmonary bypass in the face of normal platelet counts may also benefit from transfusion. For children under 10 kg, 5 to 10 mL/kg from either an RDP or SDP unit yields a platelet count rise of 50 to $100 \times 10^9/L$. The same rise may be achieved in larger children with a dose of one random platelet unit per 10 kg. Since the recommended dose should produce an adequate rise, volume reduction is not necessary unless hemolysis due to ABO mismatch and incompatible plasma is likely. Very small premature infants with severely compromised renal or cardiac function may also benefit from volume reduction.[37]

Plasma

As in adults, plasma (as FFP, FP24, or TP) is indicated for replacement of coagulation factors when specific concentrates are unavailable, as a replacement fluid during plasma exchange for TTP, in the management of DIC, and to reverse warfarin anticoagulation emergently. A standard dose of 10 to 15 mL/kg is appropriate. Since coagulation assays are routinely abnormal in neonates (especially premature neonates), complete normalization cannot be used as a therapeutic goal.

Cryoprecipitate

The use of cryoprecipitate in children is primarily limited to replacement of fibrinogen in the setting of hypofibrinogenemia or dysfibrinogenemia with active bleeding. Cryoprecipitate may also be used to replace FXIII when there is active bleeding or an invasive procedure planned. A single unit of 10 to 15 mL is usually adequate for hemostasis in infants. Cryoprecipitate may be used in the preparation of fibrin sealant. Its use in the treatment of active bleeding in the patient with vWD is limited to circumstances where DDAVP is contraindicated or ineffective and virally inactivated concentrates are unavailable.

Granulocytes

As previously discussed, granulocyte (PMN) transfusions may benefit neonates or children with neutropenia or granulocyte dysfunction when there is bacterial sepsis unresponsive to appropriate antibiotics. Fungal infections unresponsive to antifungal therapy in neutropenic children may also be mitigated by granulocyte infusion. As with adults, efficacy appears dose related, with a minimum of 10 to 15 mL granulocyte concentrate per kilogram, which is approximately 1 to 2×10^9 PMN per kg for neonates and infants and 1 to 2×10^{10} PMN per infusion for older children required.

ALTERNATIVES TO ALLOGENEIC TRANSFUSION

Preoperative Autologous Donation

Autologous blood collection is the process of collecting blood or blood components from a prospective patient to be reinfused to the same individual. Such collections are usually made in anticipation of elective surgery, particularly orthopedic procedures. The patient/donor may donate autologous units no less than 72 hours prior to the surgery. Donation criteria are less stringent than for volunteer donors, as hemoglobin may be as low as 11 g/dL (hematocrit 33%), and some disease states that would result in deferral of volunteer donors do not impede autologous donation.[18] However, disease states such as unstable angina or severe aortic stenosis render donation unsuitable, since the benefits are not outweighed by the risks. Decisions on eligibility may be made on a case-by-case basis by the medical director in consultation with the ordering physician. Since some infectious diseases do not preclude donation, unused autologous units cannot be crossed over into the general blood supply. Bacteremia or sepsis is an absolute contraindication to preoperative autologous donation (PAD) for obvious reasons. Patients may be pretreated with oral iron supplementation to maximize iron stores prior to donation. Some patients request PAD due to concerns about the safety of the blood supply as it relates to infectious diseases. However, the cost-effectiveness and risk/benefit ratio of PAD has been questioned. Carless et al. performed a meta-analysis of studies related to PAD. Randomized controlled trials showed that autologous blood deposit reduced the probability of receiving an allogeneic blood transfusion by 63%. However, the outcome was different when the relationship of PAD to any transfusion, autologous or allogeneic, was considered. Overall, 80% of patients performing PAD required a blood transfusion, versus only 60% in control groups. Such studies suggest that PAD may merely decrease the patient's hemoglobin levels such that necessity for transfusion that might otherwise be avoided is actually ensured.[39] However, in patients with multiple alloantibodies or rare blood types, autologous donation may be the best way to ensure available blood components.

Intraoperative Blood Salvage (Cell Salvage)

Intraoperative blood salvage (IBS) is a process by which shed blood is recovered from the surgical wound for reinfusion. Although some programs use machines that neither wash nor concentrate shed blood, most machines collect, wash, and concentrate blood to produce a 225-mL unit of saline-suspended RBCs with a hematocrit of 50% to 60%.[11] Use of a microaggregate filter is necessary, since tissue debris, fragments, or blood clots may accompany blood suctioned from the operative field. Units may be stored in the operating room at room temperature for 4 to 6 hours depending on the collection method, or in the blood bank at 1°C to 6°C for up to 24 hours. Units must be appropriately labeled with patient identifiers, time, and date of collection and expiration, and marked "for autologous use only." Units stored in the blood bank should be handled according to procedures for autologous blood. Contraindications include presence of infection or malignancy at the operative site.[11] Meta-

analysis by Carless et al. demonstrated a reduction in allogeneic blood use by 42% to 65%, but an overall saving of less than one allogeneic unit of blood per patient.[39] Thus, the potential for benefit must be weighed against the risks of air embolism, infection, nephrotoxicity, and coagulation abnormalities.

Postoperative Blood Salvage

Postoperative blood salvage involves the collection of blood from surgical drains. It must be reinfused within 6 hours of collection, with or without additional processing. This process produces the least desirable autologous product, since it is dilute, partially hemolyzed, defibrinated, and cytokine rich. Like IBS, it is contraindicated when infection or malignancy of the surgical site is present.[11]

Acute Normovolemic Hemodilution

Acute normovolemic hemodilution (ANH) involves the removal of one or more units of WB immediately before surgery, and volume is maintained by 1:1 replacement with colloid solution, or 3:1 replacement of crystalloid to blood volume removed. Since this replacement effects hemodilution, any given volume of blood shed during surgery will have a lower hematocrit, thus reducing the total amount of red cell mass lost. The blood is kept in the operating room at room temperature, and then reinfused after cessation of major blood loss in surgery (or sooner if bleeding is substantial). Since the units are maintained as WB, reinfusion returns platelets and coagulation factors as well as RBCs to the circulation. Units are reinfused in the reverse order in which they have been collected, with the final unit (first collected) having the greatest hematocrit. Appropriate patients must be carefully selected and cannot have sepsis or preoperative anemia.[11] Meta-analysis demonstrated that overall the use of ANH reduced the rate of exposure to allogeneic blood transfusion by 31%, and on average a reduction of 1.9 units of allogeneic blood per patient was realized.[39]

SUMMARY

Component therapy enables the physician to address the specific need of the patient, while maximizing available blood products. The risks and benefits of transfusion for any given patient should be carefully considered, and unnecessary transfusions avoided. Blood bank personnel often have the opportunity to serve as consultants and educators for the facility's physicians, and play a vital role in the stewardship of an important and limited resource.

Review Questions

1. True or false? A liberal transfusion policy for red blood cells, utilizing a transfusion trigger of 10 g/dL should be utilized for all patients.

2. True or false? Transfusion of two units of packed red blood cells would be expected to raise a patient's hemoglobin from 7 to 9 g/dL.

3. True or false? Transfusion of HLA-matched platelets is indicated in a thrombocytopenic patient with refractoriness due to nonimmune causes.

4. True or false? The term "least incompatible" as applied to red blood cells assures the clinician that all of the units in the blood bank have been screened and the unit issued shows the lowest amount of reactivity on crossmatch with the patient's sample.

5. True or false? Leukocyte reduction reduces the risk of transfusion of Cytomegalovirus, and such products are considered "CMV safe."

6. True or false? Irradiation of blood products is performed to prevent transfusion-associated graft-versus-host disease.

7. True or false? Refractoriness to platelet transfusion is suggested when a patient's 1-hour posttransfusion CCI or PPR is below adequate response levels on two consecutive transfusions.

8. True or false? Granulocytes must be ABO and crossmatch compatible, irradiated, and transfused within 24 hours of collection.

9. True or false? A leukocyte reduction filter should be used when transfusing granulocytes.

10. True or false? Preoperative autologous blood donors must meet all of the same criteria as volunteer allogeneic blood donors.

11. Platelet transfusions are absolutely or relatively contraindicated in all of the following except:
    a. thrombotic thrombocytopenic purpura (TTP)
    b. idiopathic thrombocytopenic purpura (ITP)
    c. heparin-induced thrombocytopenia (HIT)
    d. a bleeding patient with a platelet count of $50 \times 10^3/mm^3$

12. Which of the following is the least-favored alternative to allogeneic transfusion?
    a. preoperative autologous donation
    b. intraoperative blood salvage
    c. postoperative blood salvage
    d. acute normovolemic hemodilution

13–20. **Matching.** Choose the component from Column B that is the choice for treatment of the condition in Column A.

Column A

13. Replacement fluid for plasma exchange in a patient with TTP
14. A 3-year-old profoundly neutropenic patient with leukemia and a bacterial infection unresponsive to antibiotics
15. A stable patient with a hemoglobin of 9 g/dL and asymptomatic
16. Patient with thrombocytopenia and active bleeding
17. Hypofibrinogenemia
18. Replacement fluid for plasma exchange for Guillan–Barré syndrome
19. Bleeding in hemophilia A patient
20. Exchange transfusion in patient with sickle cell disease

Column B

A. apheresis platelets
B. albumin
C. granulocytes
D. cryoprecipitate
E. packed red blood cells
F. plasma frozen within 24 hours (FP24)
G. no transfusion
H. recombinant factor VIII (rFVIII)

REFERENCES

1. Repine TB, Perkins JG, Kauvar DS, et al. The use of fresh whole blood in massive transfusion. *J Trauma.* 2006; 60: S59–S69.

2. Kauvar DS, Holcomb JB, Norris GC, et al. Fresh whole blood transfusion: a controversial military practice. *J Trauma.* 2006; 61: 181–184.

3. Carson JL, Hebert P. Anemia and red blood cell transfusion. In: Simon TL, et al., eds. *Rossi's Principles of Transfusion Medicine.* 3rd ed. Philadelphia: Lippincott Williams and Wilkins; 2002: 150–162.

4. Stehling LC, Doherty DC, Faust RJ, et al. Practice guidelines for blood component therapy: a report by the American Society of Anesthesiologists Task Force on Blood Component Therapy. *Anesthesiology.* 1996; 84: 732–747.

5. Hebert PC, Wells G, Blajchman MA, et al. A multicenter, randomized, controlled clinical trial of transfusion requirements in critical care. *N Engl J Med.* 1999; 340: 409–417.

6. Hebert PC, Yetisir E, Martin C, et al. Is a low transfusion threshold safe in critically ill patients with cardiovascular diseases? *Crit Care Med.* 2001; 29: 227–234.

7. Strauss RG. How I transfuse red blood cells and platelets to infants with the anemia and thrombocytopenia of prematurity. *Transfusion.* 2008; 48: 209–217.

8. Klein HG, Spahn DR, Carson JL. Red blood cell transfusion in clinical practice. *Lancet.* 2007; 370: 415–426.

9. Castro O, Sandler SG, Houston-Yu P, et al. Predicting the effect of transfusing only phenotype-matched RBCs to patients with sickle cell disease: theoretical and practical implications. *Transfusion.* 2002; 42: 684–690.

10. Josephson CD, Su LL, Hillyer KL, et al. Transfusion in the patient with Sickle cell disease: a critical review of

the literature and transfusion guidelines. *Transfus Med Rev*. 2007; 21: 118–133.

11. Brecher ME, ed. *Technical Manual*. 15th ed. Bethesda, MD: American Association of Blood Banks; 2005.

12. Hanson SR, Slichter SJ. Platelet kinetics in patients with bone marrow hypoplasia: evidence for a fixed platelet requirement. *Blood*. 1985; 66: 1105–1109.

13. Wandt H, Frank M, Ehninger G, et al. Safety and cost effectiveness of a $10 \times 10^9/L$ trigger for prophylactic platelet transfusions compared with the traditional $20 \times 10^9/L$ trigger: a prospective comparative trial in 105 patients with acute myeloid leukemia. *Blood*. 1998; 91: 3601–3606.

14. Shander A, Goodnough LT. Update on transfusion medicine. *Pharmacotherapy*. 2007; 27(9 pt 2): 57S–68S.

15. British Committee for Standards in Haematology, Blood Transfusion Task Force. Guidelines for the use of platelet transfusions. *Br J Hematol*. 2003; 122: 10–23.

16. Stroncek DF, Rebulla P. Platelet transfusions. *Lancet*. 2007; 370: 427–438.

17. Slichter SJ. Controversies in platelet transfusion therapy. *Ann Rev Med*. 1980; 31: 509–540.

18. Standards for Blood Banks and Transfusion Services. 25th ed. Bethesda, MD: American Association of Blood Banks; 2008.

19. Rebulla P. Revisitation of the clinical indications for the transfusion of platelet concentrates. *Rev Clin Exp Hematol*. 2001; 5.3: 288–310.

20. Price TH. Granulocyte transfusion therapy. *J Clin Apheresis*. 2006; 21: 65–71.

21. Atallah E, Schiffer CA. Granulocyte transfusion. *Curr Opin Hematol*. 2006; 13: 45–49.

22. Holland LL, Brooks JP. Toward rational fresh frozen plasma transfusion: the effect of plasma transfusion on coagulation test results. *Am J Clin Pathol*. 2006; 126: 133–139.

23. Smith D, et al. Comparison of Factor V and VIII concentrations in thawed FFP and P24. *Transfusion*. 2007; 47(S): 72A.

24. Raife TJ, Friedman KD, Dwyre DM. The pathogenicity of von Willebrand factor in thrombotic thrombocytopenic purpura: reconsideration of treatment with cryopoor plasma. *Transfusion*. 2006; 46: 74–79.

25. Pantanowitz L, Kruskall MS, Uhl L. Cryoprecipitate: patterns of use. *Am J Clin Pathol*. 2003; 119: 874–881.

26. Butenas S, Brummel KE, Branda RF, et al. Mechanism of factor VIIa-dependent coagulation in hemophilia blood. *Blood*. 2002; 99: 923–930.

27. Lisman T, Moschatsis S, Adelmeijer J, et al. Recombinant factor VIIa enhances deposition of platelets with congenital or acquired $\alpha_{IIb}\beta_3$ deficiency to endothelial cell matrix and collagen under conditions of flow via tissue factor-independent thrombin generation. *Blood*. 2003; 101; 1864–1870.

28. Brady KM, Easley RB, Tobias JD, et al. Recombinant activated factor VII (rFVIIa) treatment in infants with hemorrhage. *Pediatr Anesth*. 2006; 16: 1042–1046.

29. Rizoli SB, Boffard KD, Riou B, et al. Recombinant activated factor VII as an adjunctive therapy for bleeding control in severe trauma patients with coagulopathy: subgroup analysis from two randomized trials. *Crit Care*. 2006; 10: R178.

30. Perkins JG, Schreiber MA, Wade CE, et al. Early versus late recombinant factor VIIa in combat trauma patients requiring massive transfusion. *J Trauma*. 2007; 62: 1095–1101.

31. Sniecinski RM, Chen EP, Levy JH, et al. Coagulopathy after cardiopulmonary bypass in Jehovah's Witness patients: management of two cases using fractionated components and Factor VIIa. *Anesth Analg*. 2007; 104: 763–765.

32. Key NS, Negrier C. Coagulation factor concentrates: past, present and future. *Lancet*. 2007; 370: 439–448.

33. Vermeulen LC Jr, Ratko TA, Erstad BL, et al. A paradigm for consensus. The University Hospital Consortium guidelines for the use of albumin, nonprotein colloid, and crystalloid solutions. *Arch Intern Med*. 1995; 155: 373–379.

34. Burnouf T, Radosevich M, Goubran HA. Local hemostatic blood products: fibrin sealant and platelet gel. *Treat Hemophilia*. 2004; 36: 1–14.

35. Kumar A, Teuber SS, Gershwin ME. Intravenous immunoglobulin: striving for appropriate use. *Int Arch Allergy Immunol*. 2006; 140: 185–198.

36. Mou SS, Giroir BP, Molitor-Kirsch EA, et al. Fresh whole blood versus reconstituted blood for pump priming in heart surgery in infants. *N Engl J Med*. 2004; 351: 1635–1644.

37. Roseff SD, Luban NL, Manno CS. Guidelines for assessing appropriateness of pediatric transfusion. *Transfusion*. 2002; 42: 1398–1413.

38. Strauss RG. Data-driven blood banking practices for neonatal RBC transfusions. *Transfusion*. 2000; 40: 1528–1540.

39. Carless P, Moxey A, O'Connell D, et al. Autologous transfusion techniques: a systematic review of their efficacy. *Transfus Med*. 2004; 14: 123–144.

ADVERSE EFFECTS OF TRANSFUSION

STEVE GREGUREK AND MARLA TROUGHTON

OBJECTIVES

After completion of this chapter, the reader will be able to:

1. Describe the most common causes of transfusion-related fatalities.

2. List the steps of transfusion reaction investigation.

3. Compare and contrast TRALI versus TACO.

4. List two primary types of hemolytic transfusion reactions.

5. Differentiate between intravascular and extravascular hemolysis.

6. Describe nonhemolytic reactions including allergic, febrile, and septic.

7. Describe the primary types of delayed transfusion reactions.

8. Understand the indications for irradiating blood components.

9. Recognize HLA alloimmunization.

10. Understand the mechanism of the storage lesion.

11. Describe transfusion-related immunomodulation.

12. Understand the principles of reporting transfusion-related fatalities.

KEY WORDS

Air embolism

Alloimmunization

Anaphylactic reaction

Anaphylatoxins C5a and C3a

Bacterial contamination

Center for Biologics Evaluation and Research

Circulatory overload

Delayed hemolytic transfusion reaction

Disseminated intravascular coagulation

Febrile reaction

Hemolytic transfusion reaction

HLA alloimmunization

Hyperkalemia

Posttransfusion purpura

Posttransfusion sample

Pretransfusion sample

Storage lesion

Transfusion-associated graft-versus-host disease

Transfusion-related immunomodulation

Transfusion-associated iron overload

Vasoactive amines

*B*lood component transfusion is an essential and lifesaving necessity in modern medical practice. The principles of quality and good manufacturing practice at both collection centers and hospital settings have dramatically reduced the risk of patient exposure to viral pathogens such as HIV and hepatitis. Because of the great strides in reducing the risk of lethal viral transmission during transfusion, noninfectious adverse reactions are now the leading cause of transfusion-related death. Many of the noninfectious risks of transfusion are difficult to predict or prevent. Currently, intense efforts at both blood centers and hospitals have been created to reduce the occurrence of these reactions. For the 2008 fiscal year, the *Center for Biologics Evaluation and Research* (CBER) reported 46 transfusion-related fatalities related to transfusion-related acute lung injury (TRALI), *hemolytic transfusion reaction* (HTR) associated with ABO incompatibility, HTR not related to ABO incompatibility, microbial infection (nonviral), transfusion-associated circulatory overload (TACO), and anaphylaxis.

Appropriately trained nursing and bedside healthcare staff are of major importance in minimizing the severity and complications from transfusion reactions.

Strict adherence to the standard operating procedures regarding transfusion administration and frequent assessment of the symptoms and signs of adverse reactions during transfusions is crucial to a timely medical response. Although the majority of transfusion reactions are mild and self-limited, some may be life threatening. In many cases, it is difficult to distinguish the initial stages of a serious transfusion reaction from a mild reaction. For this reason, it is very important that all suspected transfusion reactions be treated as potentially life threatening, and the first action must be to STOP THE TRANSFUSION. After this point, the attending physician and the blood bank can be contacted for further action. In most cases, the transfusion of the component is discontinued for further workup. In some cases, however, the transfusion may be restarted after minimal intervention as is often the case with urticarial and allergic reactions.

Noninfectious causes of transfusion reactions are broadly classified as immediate or delayed. Immediate transfusion reactions manifest during transfusion or within several hours post transfusion. Delayed transfusion reactions can occur days to weeks after transfusion of the blood component. Both types of reactions can be subclassified as either immune or nonimmune. Many noninfectious transfusion reactions are preventable and often associated with error, as with most cases of ABO-incompatible transfusions. With TRALI, extensive strategies have been implemented by many collection centers to mitigate risk; however, no combination of interventions and laboratory testing is able to eliminate the risk of TRALI. To further complicate matters, the particular factors that predispose certain patients to this potentially life-threatening complication are not well understood. Fortunately, most severe transfusion reactions are rare. However, the more common mild transfusion reactions can often mimic the early signs and symptoms of the more serious adverse reactions. Examples include febrile nonhemolytic transfusion reactions (FNHTRs), mild TACO, and urticarial reactions. In summary, all transfusion reactions require prompt workup when detected, and HTR must always be considered in the differential diagnosis when new signs and symptoms appear in a patient receiving transfusion.

INVESTIGATION OF ADVERSE REACTIONS

Although transfusion reaction protocols may vary slightly between transfusion services, several specific steps are required in the recognition, investigation, and reporting of adverse events related to transfusion. In particular, the AABB standards require that there are processes and procedures in place for transfusion staff to recognize and immediately respond to possible transfusion reactions. The tranfusionist must realize the importance and urgency to STOP THE TRANSFUSION if the patient's symptoms and signs indicate a possible transfusion reaction since the initial presentation of acute HTR may be subtle or may lack the classic symptoms of back pain and feelings of impending doom. Some required steps when the transfusion is discontinued include: repeating patient identification; a check of the blood labels for identification errors; return of the blood container and associated tubing to the blood bank with the transfusion set and intravenous solutions attached; and analysis by the blood bank of a *posttransfusion sample* from the patient. Care must be taken to ensure that the patient's medical needs are addressed followed by notification of the transfusion service and the responsible physician. The transfusion reaction paperwork must be completed including patient identification, suspected unit identification, presenting signs and symptoms, approximate amount of component transfused, the start and stop time of the transfusion, and when the suspected reaction occurred. The pre-, 15-minute, and posttransfusion vital signs should also be recorded.[1]

Many clinical clues can guide the workup of a transfusion reaction. Increases in temperature of at least 1°C and/or chills may indicate HTR, TACO, *bacterial contamination*, or FNHTRs. Hypotensive changes and tachycardia often occur with HTRs, TACO, anaphylaxis, bacterial contamination, or air embolus. Hypertensive changes often occur with TACO, but may also be seen with transfusion-related acute lung injury (TRALI). Respiratory symptoms including coughing, shortness of breath, pain or difficulty with breathing, wheezing, and respiratory failure are not specific and may occur with HTR, acute lung injury (ALI) including transfusion-associated ALI, *circulatory overload* from any cause, anaphylaxis, bacterial contamination, air embolus, or hypothermia. Pain and anxiety can occur with HTRs, any type of *febrile reaction*, and citrate reactions. Renal failure, hemoglobinuria, and hematuria can occur with both immune and nonimmune HTRs. Hives and itching usually indicate an allergic or urticarial reaction. If respiratory distress is observed, a stat chest radiograph should be obtained. Sudden, bilateral pulmonary edema is seen in both transfusion-associated ALI and circulatory overload. ALI has many causes unrelated to transfusion, and a thorough medical history and assessment are often required. In fact, any of the above signs and symptoms may be coincidental and due to the patient's underlying condition.

Detecting delayed transfusion reactions can be especially difficult to discern in the days to weeks following the triggering transfusion, but should always be considered if patient experiences unexplained fevers or chills, decreasing hemoglobin, jaundice, hemoglobinuria, rash, nausea, diarrhea, pancytopenia, purpura, bleeding, thrombocytopenia, new antibody on screening test, or positive direct antiglobulin testing. In cases of delayed serologic transfusion reaction (DSTR), blood screening may be the only clue to the recognition of the hemolysis.

The blood bank or transfusion service is required to have procedures in place for evaluating and reporting of possible reactions. The first step is a prompt review of clerical information to confirm proper identification of patient and blood product. If a hemolytic reaction is suspected, the evaluation must include:

- Visual check for hemolysis in the pre- and post-transfusion samples.
- Repeat ABO group determination on the post-transfusion sample.
- Direct antiglobulin test (DAT) posttransfusion samples and if positive, a DAT on the most recent *pretransfusion sample*.

If any or all of these evaluations (clerical, visual, ABO, and DAT) indicate a possible reaction, there must be a process in place to determine what further investigation is necessary. Selection of further testing depends on the type of reaction the patient experienced. These tests may include repeating the compatibility testing; performing an antibody screen on the posttransfusion sample; an attempt to elute the antibody from the patient's red blood cells (RBCs) (even if the DAT is negative); bacteriologic studies; coagulation studies; plasma hemoglobin; bilirubin (performed within 5 to 12 hours after the reaction); and an evaluation of urine for products of hemolysis. The blood bank medical director must review and interpret the results of the investigation and a report must be recorded in the patient's chart. If bacterial contamination is suspected, a Gram stain and bacterial culture from both the returned blood bag and patient should be performed. If TRALI is suspected, access to radiographs and medical records should be obtained and blood samples collected in acid citrate dextrose tubes may be required for human leukocyte antigen (HLA) and HNA testing. The patient's treating physician should be contacted immediately if a serious transfusion reaction or adverse reaction occurs. Additional regulatory requirements govern the investigation and reporting of transfusion-related fatalities. Transfusion-related deaths must be reported by the blood bank to the Food and Drug Administration (FDA) within 24 hours with a final report submitted within 45 days.

TRANSFUSION-RELATED ACUTE LUNG INJURY

Respiratory compromise during or within 6 hours of transfusion raises the possibility of TRALI. Although this terminology was assigned by Popovsky and Moore in 1985, references to this syndrome appear in the literature as early as the 1950s.[2,3] TRALI presents as severe pulmonary compromise within a few hours of whole blood transfusion, and the most frequent findings include respiratory distress, acute pulmonary edema, hypotension, and fever. The typical findings of bilateral alveolar and interstitial infiltrates or classic "white-out" of lung fields on chest radiograph are the same as those seen in adult respiratory distress syndrome (ARDS). The National Heart, Lung and Blood Institute (NHLBI) working group's definition of TRALI incorporated the existing definition of

TABLE 14-1 NHLBI Definition of TRALI	
Definition in patients WITHOUT other ALI risk factor(s)	In a patient with no ALI before transfusion, the diagnosis of TRALI is made if there is: New ALI, and Onset of symptoms is within 6 hr after end of transfusion of one or more plasma-containing blood products.
Definition in patients WITH other ALI risk factors(s)	Same as above, however, based upon clinical course, the new ALI is either: TRALI related to the transfusion, or both the transfusion and other risk factor, or Not TRALI, and new ALI is related to the alternate ALI risk factor alone and the transfusion is coincidental.

Source: Toy P, Popovsky MD, Abraham E, et al. Transfusion-related acute lung injury: definition and review. *Crit Care Med.* 2005; 33: 721–726.

BOX 14-1

Risk Factors for Acute Lung Injury

Septic shock
Pneumonia
Aspiration of gastric contents
Multiple transfusions
Disseminated intravascular coagulation (DIC)
Burn

TABLE 14-2 FDA-reported Transfusion-related Fatalities by Complication

Total (FY2005 + 2006 + 2007 + 2008)

Complication	No.	%
TRALI	114	51
HTR (non-ABO)	34	15
Microbial infection	28	13
HTR (ABO)	22	10
TACO	17	8
Anaphylaxis	6	3
Other	2	1
Totals	223	100

Adapted from Food and Drug Administration. *Fatalities Reported to FDA Following Blood Collection and Transfusion, Annual Summary for Fiscal Year 2008.* Available at: http://www.fda.gov/BiologicsBloodVaccines/SafetyAvailability/ReportaProblem/TransfusionDonationFatalities/ucm113649.htm. Accessed July 1, 2009.

ARDS or ALI with distinction given to its occurrence in the presence of transfusion (Table 14-1).[4] Acute lung injury is defined as acute onset hypoxemia with bilateral infiltrates on chest radiograph, and with no evidence of circulatory overload. TRALI is ALI occurring within 6 hours of transfusion with no other risk factors for ALI present. See Box 14-1.

Case Study 1

A 59-year-old male in the operating room for removal of a meningioma received three units of RBCs and a unit of apheresis platelets during the procedure. During the platelet transfusion, the anesthesiologist noted the patient was becoming hypotensive and difficult to ventilate with increasing peak airway pressures. Central venous pressure was not elevated. Urine remained clear, no bleeding, fever, urticaria, or other abnormality was noted. Chest x-ray showed marked symmetrical edema. There was no laboratory evidence of red cell incompatibility between the donor and the recipient. After transfer to the neurosurgical intensive care unit, the patient required extremely high fluid volumes for resuscitation as well as aggressive mechanical ventilation. Over the subsequent 6 days, he was extubated and went on to recover.

Discussion

Over the last 10 years, this entity has become more widely recognized and the number of TRALI-related fatalities reported to the FDA has increased.[5] In FY2008, as in the previous 3 fiscal years, TRALI was the leading cause of transfusion-related death reported to CBER, representing 35% of total confirmed fatalities. For the last 4 years combined, TRALI represented 51% of total confirmed transfusion-related fatalities (see Table 14-2).

Data show the largest percentage of fatal TRALI cases are associated with female donors who have antibodies to neutrophils or HLAs.[6] In the case study above, the platelet donor was a female who did indeed have antibodies with specificity to type 2 HLA antigens DR 51 and 52. This donor had been pregnant three times. Evaluation of the recipient's HLA antigen type showed concordance in that he was HLA DR 51 and 52 antigen positive.

Etiology

TRALI causes respiratory compromise by increasing the permeability of the pulmonary microvasculature that allows fluid to move from the pulmonary vessels into the alveolar space of the lungs. This edema is also referred to noncardiogenic, as it is not a result of cardiac failure. Of the two proposed mechanisms, perhaps the most well recognized is that of donor antileukocyte antibodies causing aggregation and activation of WBCs with concordant antigen type in the recipient. The less-recognized mechanism is thought to involve biologically active substances such as lipids and cytokines, rather than antibodies, causing activation of neutrophils present within the lung due to an underlying clinical condition.[7,8] These lipids and cytokines accumulate within the component during storage of cellular blood products. Severity of reaction can range from mild to fatal; however, most events resolve within hours to several days. No specific treatment

TABLE 14-3	Adverse Transfusion Reactions by Symptom	

Symptom	Possible Reaction Type	Pertinent Differential Diagnostic Information
Hypertension	TACO Hemolytic	1. What has BP been in hours/days prior to transfusion 2. Back or other type of pain 3. Fluid status: volume of fluid in and out for 8–24 hr prior 4. Pulmonary wedge pressure ($n = 6-12$, >25 cardiogenic edema)
Hypotension	Hemolytic TRALI Anaphylactic Bacterial sepsis	1. Pulse: Slow—suggests vasovagal reaction Fast—suggests volume depletion or sepsis 2. Is patient on an ACE inhibitor 3. Was patient already on vasopressor medications 4. Was antihypertensive medication given prior to transfusion
Dyspnea	Anaphylactic TRALI TACO Sepsis Hemolytic Allergic	1. Did patient have rales vs. wheezing on lung exam 2. Did patient have coughing or bronchospasm 3. What was O_2 saturation and O_2 requirement 4. What was rate of blood product infusion 5. Fluid status: volume of fluid in and out for 8–24 hr prior 6. What was pulmonary wedge pressure ($n = 6-12$, >25 cardiogenic edema) or central venous pressure (CVP) 7. Were there abnormal CXR findings 8. Did symptoms improve with diuresis
Temperature increase	Hemolytic Febrile nonhemolytic Sepsis	1. Greater than 1°C change and temperature was greater than 38°C 2. What has temperature been in hours/days prior to transfusion 3. Were there signs of sepsis—hypotension, tachycardia, positive blood or urine cultures 4. Was patient post-op with lung atelectasis 5. Was patient premedicated with Tylenol
Hive/rash	Allergic Anaphylactic	1. What was extent and location of hives, rash, or swelling 2. Was patient premedicated with antihistamine or steroids 3. Does patient have any other known allergies 4. What other medications did patient receive

other than supportive care has been identified as therapeutic.

TRANSFUSION-ASSOCIATED CIRCULATORY OVERLOAD

The various types of transfusion reactions may have overlapping signs and symptoms (see Table 14-3). Thus, the differential diagnosis of suspected TRALI includes allergic/anaphylactic reaction, TACO, bacterial contamination, and even HTR. Perhaps the two most difficult to distinguish from each other are TRALI and TACO. Despite some very clear distinctions between these two entities, simultaneous occurrence of both events in the same patient is difficult to exclude. Circulatory overload may be defined as infusion of fluid volume beyond the capacity of an individual's cardiovascular system. Since transfusion of blood components occurs within and is maintained within the intravascular space, a corresponding expansion in intravascular volume occurs. Those at greatest risk have underlying conditions such as heart, lung, or kidney failure, which impair their ability to manage or tolerate increases in volume. Other risk factors include massive transfusion, pediatric patients, and severe anemia. Symptoms typically include shortness of breath, coughing, decreased oxygen saturation, wheezing, cyanosis, elevated blood pressure, decreased pulse rate, and peripheral edema. A chest radiograph often shows bilateral lung infiltrates and sometimes enlargement of the heart. To be transfusion related, a temporal relation within several hours to transfusion must exist. As with all transfusion reactions, if the symptoms occur during infusion then the transfusion must be stopped. Cases of TACO may respond to treatment with diuretics, and this response may guide confirmation of the diagnosis. Brain natriuretic peptide (BNP) and pre-BNP are diagnostic tests associated with heart failure and may be useful in ruling in the diagnosis. However, these tests are unlikely to be of diagnostic utility in distinguishing TACO from TRALI. In patients considered to be at risk for development of circulatory overload, transfusion should be administered slowly. Common practice in these individuals is to transfuse at 1 mL/kg body weight per hour.[9]

Case Study 2

An 83-year-old male with history of congestive heart failure (CHF), lower extremity osteomyelitis, and bilateral pedal wet gangrene was admitted for lower extremity angiogram. Reversal of the anticoagulant warfarin was required prior to the procedure. Two units of fresh frozen plasma (FFP) were transfused over 3 hours with a third unit also given several hours later. Shortly after completion, the patient became dyspneic, oxygen saturation dropped to 70%, and mechanical ventilation was required. Blood pressure was notably elevated but no fever, chills, or rash were reported. A pretransfusion chest x-ray showed an enlarged heart, emphysema, and mild interstitial edema. Posttransfusion radiograph showed worsening bilateral diffuse edema and pleural effusion. Improvement was immediately seen with diuresis and after several days of supportive care, his condition improved.

Discussion

Acute circulatory overload due to transfusion is similar in mechanism and presentation to other causes of CHF or pulmonary edema. Case Study 2 illustrates the typical findings of volume overload. Although the initial symptoms of shortness of breath, hypoxia, and infiltrates on the chest radiograph can also be seen with TRALI, other findings make volume overload a more likely explanation. The BNP of 540, a marker for CHF, was moderately elevated. Additionally, the patient's fluid balance was positive by 600 mL. The persistent pulmonary edema noted on radiograph, history of CHF with elevated BNP, and large volume infusion with rapid response to diuresis are consistent with transfusion-related circulatory overload.

Treatment and Prevention

If TACO is suspected, the transfusion should be immediately discontinued. Treatment is based upon symptoms and may include oxygen or ventilatory support as well as diuresis for reduction of the intravascular volume. Prevention of circulatory overload may be difficult in patients whose underlying condition makes them easily susceptible to volume overload. Infusion rate should be slow in settings other than acute blood loss, which require rapid volume and component replacement.

RED BLOOD CELL ANTIGEN–ANTIBODY REACTIONS

Intravascular and Extravascular Hemolysis

Historically, hemolytic reactions accounted for the majority of transfusion-related deaths; however, for the combined years 2005 to 2008, non-ABO HTRs were the second most common cause of transfusion-related death reported to the FDA after TRALI (see Table 14-4).[5] Potentially the most severe and life-threatening events remain the immediate (acute) hemolytic reactions that result in the intravascular destruction of transfused RBCs due to ABO incompatibility. The naturally occurring A and B antibodies, predominantly IgM with some small amounts of IgG, are potent activators of complement. Once activated, the complement cascade culminates with activation of the C5–9 membrane attack complex, which results in cell lysis and hemolysis. The ***anaphylatoxins C5a and C3a*** promote release of serotonin and histamine from mast cells that lead to smooth muscle contraction and dilation of the vasculature and bronchial tree. As these ***vasoactive amines*** prompt release of other cytokines, leukotrienes, and bradykinin, hypotension, chills, fever, back pain, and alterations in the coagulation system occur. Progression to shock, DIC, renal failure, and occasionally death may occur (see Fig. 14-1).[10]

TABLE 14-4   Hemolytic Transfusion Reactions by Implicated Antibody, FY2005 through FY2008

Antibody	FY2005	FY2005	FY2006	FY2006	FY2007	FY2007	FY2008	FY2008	Total	Total
	No.	%	No.	%	No.	%	No.	%	No.	%
ABO	6	27	3	25	3	60	10	59	22	39
Multiple antibodies[a]	6	27	4	33	1	20	1	6	12	21
Other[b]	3	14	0	0	0	0	0	0	3	5
Jk a	1	5	1	8	1	20	0	0	3	5
Jk b	3	14	0	0	0	0	2	12	5	9
Kell	1	5	1	8	0	0	2	12	4	7

[a]FY2005 antibody combinations included E + c, Fy^a + K, Fy^a + Jk^b, E + I + A^1, possible C + E + K, Wr^a + warm autoantibody.
FY2006 antibody combinations included E + c, S + K, Jk^b + cold agglutinin, unidentified auto- and alloantibodies.
FY2007: anti-M + C.
FY2008: anti-C + K + Fy^b + S + N + V + Js^a + Go^a + warm autoantibody.

[b]FY2005: Includes one report of nonimmune hemolysis, one report of an unidentified antibody to a low-incidence antigen, and one report of Cold Agglutinin Syndrome due to *Mycoplasma pneumonia* or Lymphoma.

Adapted from Food and Drug Administration. *Fatalities Reported to FDA Following Blood Collection and Transfusion, Annual Summary for Fiscal Year 2008.* Available at: http://www.fda.gov/BiologicsBloodVaccines/SafetyAvailability/ReportaProblem/TransfusionDonationFatalities/ucm113649.htm. Accessed July 1, 2009.

Non-ABO alloantibodies, which form after exposure to other red cell antigens, may also cause acute intravascular hemolysis if complement activation is complete. More typical, however, is an extravascular hemolysis directed by the removal of IgG or C3b coated red cells by phagocytes within the reticuloendothelial system. This removal may be brisk or slowly occurring over several days. Whether intra or extravascular, typical laboratory findings of hemolysis can be seen including hemoglobinemia, hemoglobinuria, elevated plasma hemoglobin, reduced serum haptoglobin, and elevated indirect bilirubin. The increase in bilirubin peaks around 4 to 6 hours and disappears within 24 hours if bilirubin excretion is normal. Haptoglobin binds to the free hemoglobin in an effort to remove it. Haptoglobin levels therefore decrease, but the measurement can vary so that post reaction values must be compared with the pretransfusion level. Determining a decline in haptoglobin has the most diagnostic value in the investigation of slow or subtle hemolysis.

Etiology

When ABO incompatibility is involved, the cause is most often a clerical or an identification error, which may include a sample being drawn from the wrong patient and being incorrectly labeled (e.g., sample is drawn from patient A, but labeled with patient B's identification) or the unit of RBCs being transfused to the wrong patient. Non-ABO antibody–related hemolysis may rarely result from antibody misidentification; however, a more common occurrence would be a drop in antibody titer below the level of detection. After primary immunization due to transfusion or pregnancy, antibody titers may decline with up to 40% of alloantibodies becoming undetectable over months to years. If reexposed to the antigen by subsequent transfusion, an anamnestic response occurs resulting in production of antibody. Certain blood group antigens such as those within the Kidd system are well known for this occurrence.[10] Hemolysis due to an anamnestic response and extravascular removal over days to weeks is referred to as a ***delayed hemolytic transfusion reaction* (DHTR)**. Although many studies that discuss hemolytic reactions do not differentiate between acute and delayed nor intravascular and extravascular reactions, the incidence of DHTR is estimated to be 5 to 10 times higher than that of acute HTR.[11]

Treatment and Prevention

As with any suspected acute reaction, the transfusion should be stopped immediately. An intravenous line should be kept open with only normal saline infusion.

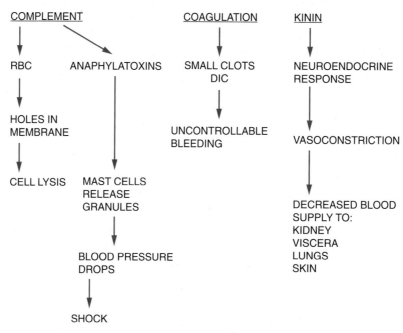

FIGURE 14-1   Acute hemolytic transfusion reactions. RBC, red blood cell; DIC, disseminated intravascular coagulation.

The patient should be closely monitored for shock, DIC, or renal failure with appropriate response as indicated. Further transfusion should be avoided if possible until the transfusion reaction investigation is complete and any previously undetected alloantibodies are identified. Prevention begins with strict adherence to well-established procedures in the laboratory and at the patient's bedside to reduce risk of sample, labeling, or patient identification error.

Case Study 3

A patient with metastatic cancer of unknown primary presented with abdominal pain. Perforation of the colon was identified and the patient was taken to the operating room for emergent exploratory lap. Transfusion of one unit of RBCs was initiated an hour into the surgery. After infusion of approximately 50 mL of RBCs, a discrepancy with the patient's name was noted by staff checking the bag tag of a second unit to be infused. The transfusion was immediately stopped and the unit checked for identification. The unit was A positive and the name on the bag tag did not match identification on the armband. The patient remained stable and surgery was completed. Post surgery the patient's creatinine increased and urine was positive for hemoglobinuria. Other clinical sequelae were minimal. The blood bank laboratory workup showed evidence of an HTR. The pre- and posttransfusion

samples labeled from the patient's armband both typed B positive. Plasma color was normal on pre and post samples. Pretransfusion blood DAT was negative, but the posttransfusion blood specimen revealed a weakly positive, mixed-field DAT. Anti-A was eluted off of the patient's red cells.

Discussion

In Case Study 3, the clerical check showed the name and medical record number (MRN) on the transmittal sheet and in the computer matched the name and MRN on the bag tag attached to the red cell unit. However, the name and MRN on the transmittal sheet did not match the patient's pre- and posttransfusion specimen information.

Investigation revealed several failures to follow standard procedure that resulted in this unit being transfused to the wrong patient. There were two patients in the OR with orders for transfusion. The transporter took this unit of red cells into the wrong OR and handed it to the anesthesiologist who immediately spiked and hung the blood without doing the required identification check against the patient's armband. The vital step of comparing the bag tag information with the patient's identification band was omitted. The patient's blood type was actually group B Rh positive, and he received 50 mL of ABO-incompatible type A Rh-positive RBCs. The mixed field seen on DAT reflected the presence of the patient's own type B cells as well as the transfused type A cells coated with Anti-A. Although a relatively small volume of the product was infused, hemolysis can result with as little as 10 mL of incompatible blood. Additionally, patients who are under anesthesia may not as readily demonstrate signs of hemolysis. Initial indications often include a change in the color of urine, increased oozing at the surgical site, or hypotension.

Identification errors resulting in ABO HTRs often involve two patients. Whether an error of administration to the wrong patient or mislabeling of the initial sample with another patient's demographic information, it is imperative to determine if another patient is in danger of receiving incompatible blood.

DELAYED EXTRAVASCULAR HEMOLYSIS

DHTR usually takes the form of delayed extravascular hemolysis that occurs days to weeks following transfusion. Like acute HTRs, these reactions are due to antibodies against transfused red cell antigens. The hemolysis is generally extravascular and the coated red cells are removed by the endothelial system. The symptoms may include unexplained fever and mild to moderate jaundice. Severe symptoms are usually absent. Helpful laboratory testing includes DAT, hemoglobin, bilirubin, and peripheral blood smear. Generally these reactions are self-limited and mild. Many cases do not require treatment, while others may require treatment of anemia with appropriately matched red cells that are negative for the newly discovered antibody. However, in all cases, the patient's physician and the blood bank physician should be notified since there are occasional reports of severe and life-threatening DHTRs including fatal delayed intravascular hemolysis.[12] The differential diagnosis for these symptoms includes underlying infection and, in rare cases, transfusion-associated *Babesia*.

DHTRs generally require presensitization to a prior foreign red cell antigen. This can occur from a prior transfusion, transplant, or pregnancy. Antibodies may take weeks to develop and usually the patient is asymptomatic during this time. The DHTR occurs on the subsequent exposure. Usually the antibodies are directed against antigens in the Kidd, Duffy, Kell, and MNS systems. These antigens may produce an anamnestic response in which the antibodies become serologically undetectable. For this reason, it is essential that an attempt to obtain a transfusion history should happen with every patient workup, and newly discovered antibodies must be recorded in the patient's transfusion and medical record. Rh alloimmunization is a form of DHTR, but is rare due to Rh

testing. DSTRs are similar to DHTR but present without clinical symptoms and are discovered during serologic testing. Since sickle cell patients are often frequently transfused, they are particularly vulnerable to developing alloantibodies, and the development of a DHTR may accelerate destruction of the patient's own cells.[13]

Case Study 4

A 54-year-old female patient presented to the emergency room in sickle cell chest crisis. Blood transfusion was requested due to a hemoglobin of 6.0 g/dL. The antibody screen was negative and three units were crossmatched then transfused. Within 36 hours of the red cell transfusion, the patient's eyes were icteric, respiratory function had deteriorated requiring mechanical ventilation, and the hemoglobin remained unchanged at 6 g/dL. A sample sent to the blood bank for evaluation revealed evidence of an HTR. The pretransfusion sample DAT was negative; however, posttransfusion DAT was positive. An antibody screen performed on the post reaction sample showed anti-Jk^b and anti-Fy^a. An eluate, performed to remove and identify antibody on the red cell surface, also showed anti-Fy^a and Jk^b.

Discussion

Review of this sickle cell patient's history revealed she had a known history of Fy^a, Jk^b, and E alloantibodies at another hospital in town where she typically received care. Although it was noted the patient had sickle cell disease and thus likely had prior transfusions, the transfusion and antibody history was not obtained prior to transfusion. Consequently, the transfused RBCs were positive for Fy^a and Jk^b, but coincidentally negative for E. Frequently transfused patients, particularly those with sickle cell disease have a higher rate of **alloimmunization**.[14] This case study illustrates how a thorough transfusion and antibody history may have reduced or eliminated the risk of HTR due to an anamnestic antibody response. Several AABB standards are aimed at identifying and reducing the risk of unexpected alloantibodies. A historical record check must be performed prior to issuing units for transfusion and once an antibody is identified, red cells negative for the corresponding antigen must always be provided if it is an alloantibody capable of causing clinically significant hemolysis. Additionally, specimens used for compatibility testing must be drawn within 3 days of scheduled transfusions if the patient has been transfused or pregnancy within the last 3 months. This is to detect rapidly developing antibodies.[1]

Etiology

Often seen in frequently transfused patients such as those with sickle cell disease, DHTR occurs within 7 to 14 days after transfusion and results most characteristically in extravascular removal by macrophages. Complement (activated only to the C3b stage) or a primary or secondary (anamnestic or memory) response of IgG antibody attach to the incompatible donor RBCs. The macrophages within the spleen and liver have IgG or C3b receptors, which recognize the antibody coated red cells and remove them from circulation. The patient may report a fever and dark urine, but most often, an unexplained drop in hematocrit occurs as the transfused RBCs are destroyed, and elevated bilirubin will be present. Renal impairment is a rare complication. A DSTR refers to production of an antibody that attaches to the red cell but does not result in lysis or removal of the cell. These are clinically benign, and usually, no treatment is required.

TRANSFUSION-RELATED BACTERIAL INFECTION

After TRALI and HTRs, bacterial contamination of blood products is the third most common cause of transfusion-related death reported to the FDA. Despite meticulous cleaning of the skin prior to collection, venipuncture may still introduce skin flora into the collection bag. Alternatively, donors may be asymptomatically bacteremic due to a subacute infection or chronic colonization of bacteria, often in the genitourinary tract. During storage, particularly of platelets that are stored at room temperature, bacteria proliferate within the collection bag.[15] When transfused, the recipient may experience a mild to severe, even fatal septic reaction.

Typical symptoms are those characteristic of sepsis, fever, and hypotension; however, if the patient is immunosuppressed, they may not manifest a typical febrile response. Other potential symptoms include shortness of breath, abdominal pain, and nausea. More severe cases may progress to DIC, renal failure, or death. Table 14-5 reports the most frequent organisms resulting in transfusion-related death as reported to the FDA from 2005 to 2008.

Case Study 5

A 35-year-old female in the bone marrow transplant unit received an apheresis platelet transfusion for a platelet count of 9,000. Ten minutes into the infusion,

TABLE 14-5	Microbial Infection by Implicated Organism	
Total (FY2005 + 2006 + 2007 + 2008)		
Organism	No.	%
Babesia[a]	10	36
Staphylococcus aureus	5	18
Escherichia coli	3	11
Serratia marcescens	2	7
Staphylococcus epidermidis	2	7
Staphylococcus lugdunensis	1	4
Eubacterium limosum	1	4
Morganella morganii	1	4
Yersinia enterocolitica	1	4
Group C Streptococcus	1	4
Klebsiella oxytoca	1	4
Total	28	100

[a]Four *Babesia microti* and one probable *Babesia MO-1* species.
Adapted from Food and Drug Administration. *Fatalities Reported to FDA Following Blood Collection and Transfusion, Annual Summary for Fiscal Year 2008.* Available at: http://www.fda.gov/BiologicsBloodVaccines/SafetyAvailability/ReportaProblem/TransfusionDonationFatalities/ucm113649.htm. Accessed July 1, 2009.

her blood pressure dropped to 60/40 and her temperature increased to 103°F. The infusion was immediately discontinued and blood cultures were drawn. The remaining platelet product was sent to the blood bank. An hour later on a different ward of the hospital, a 55-year-old male with acute myelogenous leukemia (AML) experienced a similar reaction 20 minutes after completion of a unit of apheresis platelets. He experienced rigors, shortness of breath, temperature elevation to 102.5°F, and hypotension. Likewise, blood cultures were immediately drawn and the platelet bag was retrieved and sent to the blood bank. Transfusion reaction investigation revealed no clerical discrepancy or evidence of hemolytic reaction. Gram stain of product in the two platelet components revealed gram-negative rods. Upon investigation, it was discovered these two platelet components were a split unit from one donor. Cultures of the remaining platelet products both grew *Escherichia coli*. Blood culture from one recipient was positive for *E. coli*, but was negative in the other patient who was already on broad-spectrum antibiotic coverage. Both patients successfully recovered from the events.

Discussion

In 2004, AABB and subsequently the CAP adopted a new standard that requires member blood banks and transfusion services to implement measures to reduce and detect bacterial contamination of platelets. Among the various methods available, microbial detection system cultures are now utilized by many blood manufacturers. The platelet product is held for 24 hours after collection, sampled, and the culture is then held for an additional 12 to 24 hours prior to release. After the product is released to the consignee, the culture is held until day 5 from collection. If the culture becomes positive after release, the consignee and patient's physician are notified. In Case Study 5, the initial cultures performed by the blood manufacturer were negative. The donor, a 55-year-old female, denied any symptoms at the time of donation. Posttransfusion donor blood cultures were negative; however, a urine culture was positive for *E. coli*.

Historically, the rate of bacterial contamination of platelets was estimated to be as high as 1 in 2,000.[16] With the implementation of screening, septic reactions have been reduced, but not completely eliminated.[14] Inadequate sampling, low concentration of organisms, and slower growth rates of some bacteria all contribute to false-negative culture results. Case Study 5 demonstrates such a case in which the required screening culture was negative; yet the patients experienced significant septic reactions due to bacteria within the platelet. As the platelet sits at room temperature during storage, even small amounts of bacteria within the product can proliferate to significant enough levels to produce a septic reaction in the patient.

Etiology

Microbial infections accounted for 13% of all transfusion-related deaths reported for the combined years 2005 through 2008. Of those, bacterial microorganisms represented the majority of offenders; however, the protozoa *Babesia microti* was implicated in a significant number of cases, 36% of all reported (Table 14-5). The more stable number of reported fatalities due to microbial infection of RBCs and platelets during the last 3 years is a decrease from numbers reported prior to 2006. Additionally, the number of fatalities reported due to bacterial infection of apheresis platelets has dropped from 8 cases reported in 2002 to only 2 per year for the last 3 years.[5]

Treatment and Prevention

When a platelet is discovered to be bacterially contaminated after the patient has already been transfused, the patient's physician should be notified immediately so they may evaluate for any signs of infection and put the patient on antibiotics if indicated. Patients who experience a transfusion-related septic event should be cultured and started on the appropriate antibiotic therapy.

Preventative measures include not only those directed at detecting the presence of microorganisms, but also at reducing the risk of contamination during the collection process such as using a meticulous arm scrub technique, diversion of the initial blood collection sample[17] and as always, strict adherence to process and procedure.

ALLERGIC AND ANAPHYLACTIC REACTIONS

The reported incidence of urticarial allergic reactions varies among different series ranging from 1% to 3%. Manifestations can be mild to severe with potential for life-threatening anaphylaxis. Although anaphylactic reactions only account for 3% of fatalities reported to the FDA from 2005 to 2008, the severity and mortality associated with them requires prompt recognition and treatment. The predominant pathophysiology is recipient antibody (IgE) to soluble antigens in the donor plasma. Plasma-containing platelet products have the highest incidence of allergic response compared to plasma and red cells. This finding has prompted the proposal that cytokines and/or platelet membrane–derived microparticles may be the nidus of reaction; however, studies thus far have not confirmed this theory.[18]

Case Study 6

A 34-year-old male with liver laceration sustained in a motor vehicle accident developed rash and itching during transfusion of a second unit of RBC. No other symptoms were noted and vitals remained stable. The transfusion was stopped and diphenhydramine administered. His symptoms resolved. Later that evening, a unit of FFP was initiated without additional premedication. Within 10 minutes, a pruritic rash developed and the patient became short of breath with wheezing with increased respiratory secretions. His BP, initially 112/68, dropped to 90/50, but other vitals remained unchanged. After stopping the transfusion, Benadryl and steroids were administered. Portable chest x-ray was within normal limits, and there was no evidence of incompatibility between the donor and the patient.

Discussion

The clinical findings of itching (pruritus), rash, wheezing, difficulty breathing, and hypotension

TABLE 14-6   Summary of Plasma Component Reaction Information

Allergic		Anaphylactic	
Cause	Recipient's IgE antibodies react to soluble antigens in the donor plasma	Cause	Selective IgA antibodies in an IgA-deficient patient react with the IgA normally found in the transfused plasma
Signs	Hives, urticaria, and severe itching	Signs	Profound hypotension, shock, respiratory distress, nausea, abdominal cramps, vomiting, diarrhea, laryngeal edema, bronchospasms, flushing of the skin, urticaria, and vascular instability

described in Case Study 6 are characteristic manifestations of an allergic transfusion reaction with subsequent anaphylaxis. The classic mechanism involves preformed IgE within the recipient reacting against foreign proteins from the donor. This could be the result of recipient allergies to food, plants, bee stings, etc. IgE attached to mast cells and basophils crosslinks with foreign antigen, resulting in the release of histamine and other vasoactive amines. Similar to the response seen when the complement cascade is activated, these reactive substances cause contraction of bronchial smooth muscle yielding wheezing and respiratory compromise, vasodilation and vascular permeability, and increased mucus secretion by glands in the lungs and nose.

A rare, but very severe type of *anaphylactic reaction* occurring with transfusion results from selective IgA deficiency. Anti-IgA antibodies in the recipient can be induced through pregnancy or transfusion and are directed against IgA or a subclass of IgA. The transfusion of only a small amount of plasma-containing IgA activates the complement cascade, releasing powerful anaphylatoxins. Again vasoactive amines released from mast cells lead to profound hypotension, shock, respiratory distress, nausea, abdominal cramps, vomiting, diarrhea, laryngeal edema, bronchospasms, flushing of the skin, and urticaria. See Table 14-6.

Treatment and Prevention

With severe anaphylaxis, whether due to IgA deficiency or other, the transfusion must be stopped immediately. Epinephrine may reverse the reaction while efforts are made to maintain blood volume and blood pressure. Diphenhydramine and intravenous steroids may be administered as well. If a patient repeatedly experiences allergic/anaphylactic transfusion reactions, additional actions beyond premedication with antihistamines may be indicated. Testing for anti-IgA should be performed and if identified, the patient should receive plasma and platelet products only from IgA-deficient donors. Washed or deglycerolized RBCs that are free of plasma are also potential options to prevent future reactions.

FEBRILE NONHEMOLYTIC TRANSFUSION REACTION

The most common of all adverse effects of transfusion, febrile nonhemolytic reactions are the least likely to be life threatening and are defined as a rise in patient temperatures of 1°C or more during or after transfusion unrelated to the patient's underlying condition. Several mechanisms for these reactions have been proposed, but the most widely accepted is that cytokines from WBC released into the blood product during storage initiate an inflammatory response in the recipient. Although related mortality is unlikely, significant discomfort can result from these reactions. Chills or severe rigors may precede or accompany the fever. Additional symptoms may include headache, nausea, and vomiting. It is of vital importance to closely evaluate these reactions as many of these symptoms may also be seen in other more life-threatening reactions (Table 14-3).

Treatment as well as prevention includes medicating with antipyretics. Some studies support the use of leukoreduction at bedside or prestorage as an effective means of reducing FNHTRs by decreasing the number of WBCs within the blood component.[19] Other interventions for persistent reactions may include use of washed or deglycerolized RBCs.

DELAYED TRANSFUSION REACTIONS

Delayed transfusion reactions can occur days to weeks after transfusion and are often difficult to diagnose clinically. Most cases are less severe than their acute counterparts. However, there are many case reports of fatal and life-threatening delayed reactions. The major immune-mediated delayed transfusion reactions include DHTR and DSTR discussed earlier, alloimmunization against HLA antigens or platelet antigens, *transfusion-associated graft-versus-host disease* (TAGVHD), *posttransfusion purpura* (PTP), and *transfusion-related immunomodulation* (TRIM). Nonimmune delayed reactions include infection, thrombophlebitis, and iron overload.

TRANSFUSION-ASSOCIATED GRAFT-VERSUS-HOST DISEASE

The great majority of patients who develop TAGVHD will die within weeks of their diagnosis. The initial symptoms are nonspecific and may include a rash, fever, nausea, vomiting, or diarrhea occurring days to weeks following transfusion. A complete blood count often reveals pancytopenia, and there are usually abnormalities with liver function tests. Immunosuppressed patients on chemotherapy, with congenital disorders, and newborns are at the greatest risk for TAGVHD. The pathophysiology is believed to be related to an attack from the donor T-cell lymphocytes against the patient. The donor cells recognize the recipient as foreign, but the recipient does not recognize the donor cells as foreign. The donor lymphocytes engraft, proliferate, and generate cytokines directed against the recipient's cells. The greatest risk for TAGVHD occurs when the donor and recipient share common HLA alleles as is often seen with directed donations from related family members or donations within homozygous populations. Leukoreduction has been shown to reduce the risk of TAGVHD, but irradiation is the only method to ensure destruction of the function of the donor lymphocytes. Irradiation does induce some cellular damage and irradiated components have a shorter outdate. Irradiation needs to occur in an approved irradiator with 25 Gy applied to the center of the unit and no less than 15 Gy to the periphery. Any patient at risk for TAGVHD should receive irradiated units, as well as any donation from a blood relative or a product that was processed to be HLA compatible.[20]

Case Study 7

A 52-year-old man with prior history of chronic lymphocytic leukemia sustained multiple fractures of his lower extremities as a passenger in a motor vehicle collision. He was transported to the hospital in stable condition by ambulance. During orthopedic surgery, he required six units of crossmatch-compatible packed leukoreduced red cells, three units of apheresis platelets, and four units of thawed plasma. He was healing well until 2 weeks after admission when he developed severe diarrhea and a rash on his chest and back. Laboratory workup showed anemia, thrombocytopenia, and abnormal liver function testing. A review of his medical history revealed that he had received fludarabine for his leukemia several years prior. A bone marrow biopsy showed a paucity of bone marrow cells, and a skin biopsy showed changes consistent with graft-versus-host disease. His clinical course deteriorated, and he died from sepsis 2 weeks later.

Discussion

AABB standards require that a blood component be irradiated if it is HLA compatible to the donor or from a blood relative. Blood components must also be irradiated if the recipient has a history of bone marrow transplant, Hodgkin lymphoma, and/or treatment with fludarabine or similar chemotherapeutics. Irradiation is also required for all neonates requiring exchange transfusion, intrauterine fetal transfusions, and patients with congenital defects of their T-cell population.[1] At-risk patients should carry an identification card, wrist bracelet, or necklace indicating their requirement for irradiated blood products. An appropriate transfusion history should be attempted even with trauma and critical patients. If a chronic immunodeficient state is suspected then irradiated products should be used. Many hospitals have additional indications for irradiation of blood components. There is no effective treatment for TAGVHD and nearly all cases are fatal.

POSTTRANSFUSION PURPURA

PTP is a rare transfusion-related adverse event that is potentially life threatening. The patient manifests a sudden onset of severe thrombocytopenia that usually occurs 1 to 2 weeks following transfusion of red cell components. Often PTP is associated with red to purple discolorations on the skin, approximately the size of a pencil eraser, which do not blanch when pressed. Since similar symptoms can occur with heparin-induced thrombocytopenia (HIT), a thorough history of anticoagulation use must be obtained. PTP is thought to be related to preformed platelet-specific alloantibodies in the patient's serum that were induced through prior pregnancy, blood, or tissue exposure. Usually the patient is negative for platelet antigen HPA-1a located on the platelet glycoprotein complex GPIIb/IIIa and present in approximately 98% of donors. After reexposure to the antigen through transfusion, the antibody causes destruction of both donor and patient platelets. The exact mechanism that the patient's platelets are destroyed is unknown but is thought to be related to production of platelet-specific autoantibodies that are immune complexes formed with donor blood that attach to the patient's platelets, or donor platelet antigens that combine to the patient's platelets inducing destruction. Patients suspected of having PTP should have testing for platelet antibodies using SPRCA/MPHA, flow cytometry/monoclonal antibody methods, or a monoclonal antibody-specific immobilization of platelet assay (MAIPA). The patient should also be tested for the absence of HPA-1a antigen after recovery. Alternatively, molecular genetic testing can also determine the lack of HPA-1a. The transfusion record should record these results and future transfusion should be from HPA-1a-negative donors. Treatment is accomplished by removing the offending antibody by IVIG. Transfusion of platelets is contraindicated. Antigen-negative platelets are sometimes given in urgent situations, but often have significantly decreased survival.[21]

ALLOIMMUNIZATION TO HLA ANTIGENS

Alloimmunization to foreign HLAs occurs in approximately 10% of transfused patients and is also common in women with previous pregnancies and transplant recipients. In addition to being present on leukocytes, HLA antigens are also found on platelets. Because of this, patients requiring frequent transfusion are prone to develop refractoriness to platelet transfusion. For this reason, platelet counts should be obtained 1 and 24 hours post transfusion to assess the response to transfusion. The 1-hour corrected count increment (CCI) is a useful test to address refractoriness and can be calculated by first multiplying the platelet count increment by the body surface area in meters squared. The product is then multiplied by 10^{11} and divided by the total number of platelets (not components) transfused (Box 14-2). A result of less than 7,500 may indicate alloimmune refractoriness. Patients with platelet refractoriness secondary to *HLA alloimmunization* often respond to irradiated HLA-matched or crossmatched platelets. However, these units may take considerable time and expense to procure. Use of leukoreduced products and ABO-matched platelets has shown to reduce the rates of HLA alloimmunization.[22]

BOX 14-2

Corrected Count Increment (CCI)

$$CCI = \text{Platelet Increment} \times \text{Body Surface Area} \times 10^{11} / \text{Number of Transfused Platelets}$$

Case Study 8

A 48-year-old woman on the bone marrow transplant unit with a history of multiple blood transfusions for pancytopenia received an ABO-compatible apheresis platelet transfusion for a platelet count of 4,000. Her 1-hour platelet count was 5,000. Her body surface area was 1.6 meters squared. The platelet component contained approximately 4×10^{11} platelets. Her CCI was calculated at 457, which indicated platelet refractoriness that was likely secondary to alloimmunization. There was no significant rise in the platelet count after two additional apheresis platelet transfusions. A request for HLA-matched platelets was initiated. After antibodies to HLA antigens were confirmed, two crossmatched platelets were available by the next day. After transfusion of both units, the 1-hour platelet count was 55,000. The platelet count decreased to 9,000 by the next day, which was related to nonimmune mechanisms of refractoriness due to her underlying illness. The local blood center was able to locate HLA-matched donors within several days to provide additional product.

Discussion

HLA alloimmunization may decrease over weeks to months and platelet antibody testing should be repeated in patients with chronic platelet requirement. If levels decrease, ABO-matched platelets from the inventory may be used. The CCI can be very useful in monitoring refractoriness. Up to one third of HLA-matched or crossmatched platelet components will still be refractory due to nonimmunogenic mechanisms. Factors that can worsen nonimmune refractoriness include splenomegaly, fever, bleeding, *disseminated intravascular coagulation*, and heparin use.[23]

MISCELLANEOUS REACTIONS

Out-of-type Plasma Reactions

FFP, plasma frozen within 24 hours, thawed plasma, platelet concentrates, cryoprecipitate, and whole blood are rich in plasma. Plasma that is not ABO appropriate may introduce donor antibodies that can attach to the recipient's red cells and lead to either extravascular or intravascular hemolysis. Type O donors may contain anti-A,B antibodies with reactivity to IgG. With transfusion of a small volume of plasma, these antibodies are usually clinically insignificant. However, during massive transfusion and pediatric transfusion, exposure to ABO-inappropriate plasma may cause some hemolysis. In infants, plasma must be ABO compatible and many times an AB unit is selected.[24]

Hypothermia

Since packed red cells are stored cold, massive transfusion of red cells can lead to hypothermia, which is a clinically significant decrease in the core body temperature. Hypothermia can inactivate the proteins within the coagulation cascade, induce heart failure or respiratory distress, and cause neurologic disturbances. The use of approved, inspected blood warmers has decreased the incidence of hypothermia secondary to transfusion. An approved blood warmer usually consists of a warming drum in which the plastic tubing of the infusion set is coiled around. The blood warming device must be appropriately tested and certified for use. Excessive, improper warming or use of a nonapproved warming device could lead to severe hemolysis of the transfused cells.

Potassium Abnormalities

Potassium is the most abundant intracellular cation. However, extracellular potassium is much lower in concentration and must remain in the narrow range of 3.5 to 5.5 mEq/L to prevent cardiac failure. Serious abnormalities in potassium concentration can often be detected on electrocardiogram. During storage, some of the intracellular potassium leaks into the small extracellular volume. Red cell components near their outdates can contain approximately 7 mEq of potassium at a relatively high concentration within the blood bag. In most situations, this is clinically insignificant. However, in some patients receiving massive transfusion, neonates, and patients with renal failure, the quick introduction of potassium may lead to transient *hyperkalemia*, which can cause cardiac arrhythmia or arrest. Some centers have advocated the use of blood components less than 7 to 14 days old, but this practice remains controversial. Paradoxically, hypokalemia occurs more frequently during massive transfusion than hyperkalemia and may be related to reabsorption of potassium by the citrate in additive solution packed red cells. Potassium abnormalities may also occur due to factors intrinsic to the patient's underlying disease.[25,26]

Transfusion-related Immunomodulation

Allogeneic transfusion has been associated with chronic changes in the immune system of certain recipients termed transfusion-related immunomodulation. This phenomenon appears to have either beneficial or detrimental effects depending on conditions specific to the patient. Kidney transplants have increased survival if the recipient has had prior transfusion. Patients with Crohn disease have fewer flare-ups if exposed to prior transfusion. Although unproven, current research and speculation suggests that a history of prior transfusion may be associated with an increased recurrence rate of malignancies, increased risk of infection after surgery, and increased short-term mortality. The etiology of TRIM is unknown but is thought to be related to donor leukocytes in the component bag. Leukoreduction may be associated with a decrease in TRIM.[27]

Transfusion-associated Iron Overload

There is approximately 1 g of iron in 4 units of packed red cells. Given the lack of efficient mechanisms to remove excess iron from the human body, patients requiring frequent transfusions, including patients with myelodysplastic syndrome and sickle cell disease, are at considerable risk for iron overload. Iron is normally stored and bound to the intracellular protein ferritin, if this system is overwhelmed, free iron causes cellular damage to the heart, liver, pancreas, and endocrine glands in a process called hemochromatosis. Treatment consists of iron chelation therapy and is usually indicated for patients receiving over 50 red cell transfusions.[28]

Air Embolism

Air embolism during transfusion is a very rare adverse event that is associated with equipment malfunction or improper setup of the infusion set and has been reported during perioperative blood recovery. Infusion with as little as 100 mL of air within the intravascular compartment can be fatal. Air bubbles can interfere with blood flow through the circulation, and, if the air reaches the lungs or heart, can drastically reduce the heart's pumping efficiency. Symptoms are usually related to the impact on the cardiovascular system and include cough, difficulty breathing, choking, and potentially death. This complication can be avoided by ensuring strict adherence to standard operating procedures and adequate, timely training for all health-care personnel involved with infusions.[29]

STORAGE LESION

Current standards allow packed red cells to be stored at 1°C to 6°C for up to 42 days when using additive solutions. In most cases of transfusion, this 42-day storage period is considered to be safe and clinically efficacious. Although stored red cells have different physiologic characteristics than red cells in the circulation, there is much debate over the clinical significance of these changes. These changes are termed the *storage lesion*. Stored red cells undergo a change from a biconcave disk to a shape resembling an echinocyte, and this physical change often persists when transfused. There are also many biochemical changes including depletion of ATP, depletion of 2,3-DPG, loss of deformability, and blister formation on the red cell. Some studies suggest that these changes may reduce the efficiency of the stored red cells from unloading oxygen in the end-organ microcirculation, even though most of the depleted ATP content in stored red cells is replenished after transfusion. The first changes in stored red cells are reversible and include the depletion of ATP and leak of intracellular potassium into the additive solution. This causes the progressive shape change and the minor decreases in oxygen-carrying capacity. This damage becomes irreversible as cells are stored beyond their expiration dates. The increased extracellular potassium content in the blood bag may pose a cardiac risk during massive transfusion or pediatric heart surgery. The possible clinical significance of the storage lesion has recently emerged for debate with the appearance of three retrospective clinical studies. In one study, critically ill patients had decreased mortality when a restrictive transfusion strategy was implemented. In another study, there was a small but significant increase in morbidity and mortality in cardiac surgery patients who received red cell components exclusively stored for over 14 days compared to patients receiving red cells stored for less than 14 days. The final study showed worse outcomes in critical care patients when exposed to red cells that were nearer to their expiration. These findings are suggestive, but not conclusive, and further multicenter, prospective studies will be needed to elucidate the true significance of the storage lesion.[30–32]

MORBIDITY AND MORTALITY ASSOCIATED WITH TRANSFUSION

The CBER, a component of the FDA, states that, "the blood supply is safer today than at any time in history." Between 2005 and 2008, there were 223 fatal transfusion reactions out of approximately 60 million units. Eighty-seven percent of cases are caused by noninfectious transfusion reaction, and almost 60% of these cases are due to TRALI. It is no surprise that mitigation of TRALI has become central to many of the risk-reduction strategies in blood centers and hospitals across the country. Approximately 10% of

transfusion-related fatalities are attributed to HTR due to ABO antibodies with many of these due to errors in clerical checks or identification. Approximately 15% of deaths are from non-ABO antibodies causing HTR. Multiple antibodies are most common followed by antibodies in the Kidd, Kell, Duffy systems and also including antibodies to the E and I antigens.[33]

Febrile and urticarial reactions are the most common acute reactions and occur at a frequency of 1% to 3% of transfusions. Many of these reactions are underreported so the true incidence is unknown. Febrile reactions are becoming less common with the widespread use of leukocyte reduction. TACO occurs less than 1% of the time and is usually mild and treated with conservative medical therapy. TRALI, non-fatal HTR, and anaphylaxis tend to occur once per several thousand transfusions. Among the delayed transfusion reactions, alloimmunization of HLA antibodies is very common and may occur in greater than 10% of exposed patients. HLA alloimmunization to RBC components occurs about 1% of the time, and progression to DHTR occurs once in several thousand transfusions. Other transfusion reactions and adverse events are rare and many are unrecognized or underreported.[9]

RECORDS OF ADVERSE TRANSFUSION EVENTS

The AABB standards require that a process be developed and implemented for transfusion reactions and adverse events associated with transfusion. The procedure must contain a mechanism to recognize immediate and delayed transfusion reactions. Relevant medical information including pertinent symptoms and patient vital signs must be reported to the blood bank. Mild transfusion reactions such as urticarial reactions do not need to be reported under the current standards. However, most hospital policies require the reporting of all transfusion reactions to the blood bank. The transfusion reaction procedure must include specific instructions as when and how to stop the transfusion and ensure that the patient's clinical needs are met during the workup. In the event of a transfusion-related fatality, CBER, the Center for Biologics Evaluation and Research, must be contacted as soon as possible by phone or e-mail. Their web address is http://www.fda.gov/BiologicsBloodVaccines/SafetyAvailability/ReportaProblem/TransfusionDonationFatalities/default.htm. Relevant information to gather includes the date and time of the call, the name of the reporting person, facility fax number and phone number, facility e-mail, facility name and address, facility FDA registration if available. The following patient information is required: the age, gender, date and time of death, suspected cause of death, pertinent medical history, if an autopsy will be conducted, and the facility where the death occurred. The following must be reported on the implicated components: transfusion dates, blood components, unit numbers, names, and address of providers of implicated components. A written report must be submitted within 7 days including a summary of the case by the transfusion medicine physician.[34]

Patient-specific records pertaining to adverse transfusion events and transfusion reactions must be kept for a minimum of 10 years with safeguards in place to protect patient privacy. This includes records relating to the transfusion reaction workup, donor unit information, amount transfused, appropriate identification of personnel, details of the adverse event, pre- and posttransfusion vital signs, consent records, and other pertinent medical information. Documents specific to the laboratory investigation must be kept for a minimum of 5 years including records of supervisor review. A peer-review process must be in place to monitor and review adverse events of transfusion and usually occurs through the hospital transfusion committee.[1]

Review Questions

1. True or false? Two of the biologic systems that may be activated by an immediate hemolytic reaction are complement and coagulation.
2. True or false? When an ABO-mediated hemolytic reaction occurs a testing error in the blood bank is the most common cause.
3. True or false? A reaction due to ABO incompatibility results in extravascular hemolysis.
4. True or false? ABO antibodies are generally IgG.
5. True or false? An anamnestic response of antibody may result in a delayed transfusion reaction.
6. True or false? Pulmonary edema that occurs in TRALI is due to cardiac failure.
7. True or false? Febrile nonhemolytic reactions are the most frequent in occurrence, but least life threatening.
8. True or false? Among the most severe and life threatening of reactions is the extremely rare anaphylactic reaction in patients who have selective IgA deficiency.
9. If a hemolytic reaction is suspected the evaluation must include:
   a. visual check for hemolysis in the pre- and posttransfusion samples
   b. repeat ABO group determination on the posttransfusion sample
   c. direct antiglobulin test (DAT) posttransfusion samples and if positive, a DAT on the most recent pretransfusion sample
   d. all of the above
10. Administration of multiple units of red cells and FFP to a patient with cardiac insufficiency would most likely result in which of the following?
    a. extravascular hemolytic
    b. allergic
    c. anaphylactic
    d. circulatory overload
11. Allergic reactions may be prevented or reduced by:
    a. washing
    b. filtration
    c. irradiation
    d. a and b

12. Which combination of the following can be seen if a patient is experiencing an intravascular transfusion reaction?
    a. hemoglobinuria, increased haptoglobin, decreased bilirubin, hemoglobinemia
    b. decreased haptoglobin, hemoglobinuria, hemoglobinemia, increased bilirubin
    c. decreased haptoglobin, hemoglobinuria, hemoglobinemia, decreased bilirubin
    d. none of the above
13. Which of the following involves hemolysis of RBCs through removal by the reticuloendothelial system?
    a. extravascular hemolysis
    b. intravascular hemolysis
    c. anaphylaxis
    d. none of the above
14. Which of the following does NOT occur days to weeks following transfusion?
    a. transfusion-associated graft-versus-host disease
    b. hemolytic transfusion reaction
    c. transfusion-related acute lung injury
    d. posttransfusion purpura
15. Which of the following is most effective at reducing the risk of transfusion-related graft-versus-host disease?
    a. irradiate components at 15 Gy for susceptible patients
    b. universal leukoreduction
    c. provision of fresh units for immunosuppressed patients
    d. use of an approved irradiator on red cell components for newborn babies
16. All fatal transfusion reactions need to be reported within 24 hours to which agency?
    a. Center for Biologics Evaluation and Research
    b. Center for Drug Evaluation and Research
    c. Center for Disease Control
    d. Serious Hazards of Transfusion Agency
17. The red cell component storage lesion may show changes with all of the following except
    a. changes in the shape of the red cell
    b. decrease in extracellular potassium

(continued)

REFERENCES

1. Standards for Blood Banks and Transfusion Services. 25th ed. Bethesda, MA: AABB; 2008.

2. Popovsky MA, Moore SB. Diagnostic and pathogenic considerations in transfusion related acute lung injury. *Transfusion*. 1985; 25: 573–577.

3. Barnard R. Indiscriminate transfusion: a critique of case reports illustrating hypersensitivity reactions. *N Y State J Med*. 1951; 51: 2399–2402.

4. Toy P, Popovsky MD, Abraham E, et al. Transfusion-related acute lung injury: definition and review. *Crit Care Med*. 2005; 33: 721–726.

5. Food and Drug Administration. *Fatalities Reported to FDA Following Blood Collection and Transfusion, Annual Summary for Fiscal Year 2008*. Available at: http://www.fda.gov/BiologicsBloodVaccines/SafetyAvailability/ReportaProblem/TransfusionDonationFatalities/ucm113649.htm. Accessed July 1, 2009.

6. Eder A, Herron R, Strupp A, et al. Transfusion-related acute lung injury surveillance (2003–2005) and the potential impact of the selective use of plasma from male donors in the American Red Cross. *Transfusion*. 2007; 47: 599–607.

7. Silliman CC, Bjornsen AJ, Wyman TH, et al. Plasma and lipids from stored platelets cause acute lung injury in an animal model. *Transfusion*. 2003; 43: 633–640.

8. Silliman CC, Mclaughlin NJ. Transfusion-related acute lung injury. *Blood Rev*. 2006; 20: 139–159.

9. Li G. The accuracy of natriuretic peptides (brain natriuretic peptide and N-terminal pro-brain natriuretic) in the differentiation between transfusion-related acute lung injury and transfusion-related circulatory overload in the critically ill. *Transfusion*. 2009; 49: 13–20.

10. Roback JD, ed. *Technical Manual*. 16th ed. Bethesda, MD: AABB; 2008.

11. Davenport RD. Hemolytic transfusion reactions. In: Popovsky MA, ed. *Transfusion Reactions*. 2nd ed. Bethesda, MA: AABB Press; 2001.

12. Tormey C, Stack G. Delayed intravascular haemolysis following multiple asymptomatic ABO-incompatible red blood cell transfusions in a patient with hepatic failure. *Vox Sang*. 2008; 95(3): 232–235.

13. Schonewille H, van de Watering LM, Loomans DS, et al. Red blood cell alloantibodies after transfusion: factors influencing incidence and specificity. *Transfusion*. 2006; 46(2): 250–256.

14. Josephson CD, Su LL, Hillyer KL, et al. Transfusion in the patient with sickle cell disease: a critical review of the literature and transfusion guidelines. *Transfus Med Rev*. 2007; 21(2): 118–133.

15. Anderson KC, Lew MA, Gorgone BC, et al. Transfusion-related sepsis after prolonged platelet storage. *Am J Med*. 1986; 81: 405–411.

16. Brumit MC, Brecher ME. Bacterial contamination of platelet transfusions. In: McLeod BC, Price TH, Weinstein R, eds. *Apheresis: Principles and Practice*. 2nd ed. Bethesda, MD: AABB Press; 2003.

17. Benjamin RJ, Kline L, Dy BA, et al. Bacterial contamination of whole blood-derived platelets: introduction of sample diversion and prestorage pooling with culture testing in the American Red Cross. *Transfusion*. 2008; 48(11): 2348–2355.

18. Gilstad CW. Anaphylactic transfusion reactions. *Curr Opin Hematol*. 2003; 10(6): 419–423.

19. King KE, Shirey RS, Thoman SK, et al. Universal leukoreduction decreases the incidence of febrile nonhemolytic transfusion reactions to RBCs. *Transfusion*. 2004; 44(1): 25–29.

20. Triulzi D, Duquesnoy R, Nichols L, et al. Fatal transfusion-associated graft-versus-host disease in an immunocompetent recipient of a volunteer unit of red cells. *Transfusion*. 2006; 46: 885–888.

21. Woelke C. Post-transfusion purpura in a patient with HPA-1a and GPIa/IIa antibodies. *Transfus Med*. 2006; 16(1): 69–72.

22. Slichter SJ. Evidence-based platelet transfusion guidelines. *Hematology Am Soc Hematol Educ Program*. 2007; 2007: 172–178.

23. Slichter SJ, Davis K, Enright H, et al. Factors affecting post-transfusion platelet increments, platelet refractoriness, and platelet transfusion intervals in thrombocytopenic patients. *Blood*. 2005; 105: 4106–4114.

24. Duguid JKM. Incompatible plasma transfusions and haemolysis in children. *BMJ*. 1999; 318: 176–177.

25. Smith HM, Farrow SJ, Ackerman JD, et al. Cardiac arrests associated with hyperkalemia during red blood cell transfusion: a case series. *Anesth Analg*. 2008; 106(4): 1062–1069.

26. Carmichael D, Hosty T, Kastl D, et al. Hypokalemia and massive transfusion. *South Med J*. 1984; 77(3): 315–317.

27. Vamvakas E, Blajchman M. Transfusion-related immunomodulation (TRIM): an update. *Blood Rev.* 2007; 21(6): 327–348.

28. Dreyfus F. The deleterious effects of iron overload in patients with myelodysplastic syndromes. *Blood Rev.* 2008; 22(suppl 2): S29.

29. Palmon SC, Moore LE, Lundberg J, et al. Venous air embolism: a review. *J Clin Anesth.* 1997; 9(3): 251–257.

30. Hebert PC, Wells G, Blajchman MA, et al. A multicenter, randomized, controlled clinical trial of transfusion requirements in critical care. Transfusion Requirements in Critical Care Investigators, Canadian Critical Care Trials Group. *N Engl J Med.* 1999; 340: 409–417.

31. Koch CG, Li L, Sessler DI, et al. Duration of red-cell storage and complications after cardiac surgery. *N Engl J Med.* 2008; 358: 1229–1239.

32. Tinmouth A, et al. Clinical consequences of red cell storage lesion in the critically ill. *Transfusion.* 2006; 46: 2014–2027.

33. Food and Drug Administration. *Fatalities Reported to the FDA Following Blood Collection and Transfusion, Annual Summary for Fiscal Years 2005 and 2006.* Available at: http://www.fda.gov/cber/blood/fatal0506.htm.

34. Code of Federal Regulations, Title 21, Volume 7, Sec. 606.170 Adverse reaction file; 2008.

TRANSFUSION-TRANSMITTED DISEASES

EVA D. QUINLEY

WITH ASSISTANCE FROM SUSAN STRAMER AND ROGER DODD

OBJECTIVES

After completion of this chapter, the reader will be able to:

1. Describe measures taken to ensure that infectious disease is not transmitted by transfusion.
2. Categorize the infectious diseases that can be transmitted by transfusion (e.g., viruses, bacteria, and parasites).
3. Name the diseases and their etiologic agents that can be transmitted by transfusion.
4. Discuss the pathology of the diseases transmitted by transfusion.
5. Discuss the incidence of the diseases transmitted by transfusion.
6. Describe the serologic testing used to screen donor blood for evidence of infectious disease markers.

KEY WORDS

Acquired immunodeficiency syndrome
Babesiosis
Chagas disease
Chikungunya
Chronic hepatitis
Creutzfeldt–Jakob disease
Cytomegalovirus
Delta hepatitis
Dengue

Epstein–Barr virus
Hepatitis A
Hepatitis B
Hepatitis B vaccine
Hepatitis C
Human immunodeficiency virus
Human T-cell lymphotropic virus
Lyme disease

Non-A, non-B hepatitis
O variants
Parvovirus
Retrovirus

Syphilis
Toxoplasmosis
Yersinia enterocolitica

The number of infectious disease markers for which blood is screened has continued to increase over the years. Before 1984, there were only two diseases for which blood was tested—hepatitis B and syphilis. By the late 1990s, blood had to be tested for nine different infectious disease markers. Soon there may be additional required tests.

Viruses, parasites, and bacteria can all be transmitted through blood. Box 15-1 lists some of the diseases that may be acquired through transfusion of blood or blood components. Donor interviewing techniques combined with sensitive testing methods have drastically reduced the risks for acquiring such infections. However, the possibility of transfusion-transmitted disease still remains a constant threat for all blood banks and transfusion facilities. This chapter presents a brief overview of the infectious agents that have the potential to be transmitted by blood transfusion.

VIRAL INFECTIONS

A large percentage of the transfusion-transmitted disease complications known today have a viral etiology. Viruses are intracellular organisms, often using cells of the host to reproduce. Because effective

Infectious Complications of Blood Transfusion

Hepatitis A
Hepatitis B
Hepatitis C
Hepatitis D
Cytomegalovirus infection
Epstein–Barr virus infection (mononucleosis)
Acquired immunodeficiency syndrome
Tropical spastic paraparesis
Adult T-cell leukemia
Babesiosis
Lyme disease
Chagas disease
West Nile Virus
Creutzfeldt–Jakob disease
Syphilis
Malaria
Toxoplasmosis
Parvovirus infection
Leshmaniasis
Chikungunya
Dengue

Viruses That Are Transmissible by Blood Transfusion

VIRUSES FOUND IN PLASMA

- Hepatitis B virus
- Delta agent
- Hepatitis C?
- Hepatitis A (rarely)
- Non-A, non-B, non-C virus
- Parvovirus B19
- Human immunodeficiency virus, type 1 (HIV-1)
- HIV-2
- West Nile Virus

VIRUSES ASSOCIATED WITH CELLULAR ELEMENTS

- Cytomegalovirus?
- Epstein–Barr virus?
- Human T-lymphotropic virus, type I (HTLV-I)
- HTLV-II
- HIV-1
- HIV-2

antiviral agents are still not available for most viral infections, blood banks rely heavily on donor history, testing, and donor self-exclusion to keep the blood supply safe.

Transmission of viruses can be associated with cellular components or with plasma alone. Box 15-2 lists the plasma- and cell-associated viruses that may be transmitted by blood. Untreated blood products, especially those prepared from large pools of plasma derived from many donors, have a high incidence of viral transmission. For a virus to infect a person, a number of factors, such as the person's age, nutritional status, and previous exposure to the virus (immune status), must be considered. For ease of discussion, the viruses are divided into four groups: (1) hepatitis viruses, (2) retroviruses, (3) herpesviruses, and (4) other.

Hepatitis Viruses

Viral hepatitis denotes infections caused by viral agents that attack the liver and include five different types of diseases caused by at least five different viruses: (1) hepatitis A, (2) hepatitis B, (3) hepatitis D, (4) hepatitis C, and (5) hepatitis E.

Viruses such as *cytomegalovirus* (CMV) and *Epstein–Barr virus* can cause hepatitis, but are discussed in a later section of this chapter. Table 15-1 lists

some of the terminology used to describe the markers found in the various forms of hepatitis.

Transfusion-transmitted hepatitis is a common major complication of blood transfusion. All of the viruses mentioned earlier can be transmitted by transfusion of cellular and acellular products. Only those products that are specially treated to inactivate viruses, such as plasma protein fraction, are considered safe from hepatitis. Although the incidence of transfusion-transmitted hepatitis has decreased dramatically, the residual risk for hepatitis C is 1 in 103,000 and that for hepatitis B is 1 in 63,000. Obviously, the risk of acquiring hepatitis is directly proportional to the number of transfusions received.

Hepatitis A

History

The first epidemics of jaundice recognized to be hepatitis were reported in the writings of Hippocrates. Large epidemics, often associated with military campaigns, were reported during the 17th to 19th centuries. During the United States' Civil War, in excess of 70,000 cases of what was thought to be *hepatitis A* were recognized. By the mid-1940s, two distinct forms of hepatitis infection were recognized—one known as infectious hepatitis and the other known as serum hepatitis. In 1973, Feinstein and associates discovered the hepatitis A virus (HAV) in fecal extracts. Infectious

TABLE 15-1	Currently Accepted Terminology Used to Describe Hepatitis Viral Markers
Hepatitis A	
HAV	Hepatitis A virus
Anti-HAV (IgM)	Antibody to hepatitis A seen in recent infection
Anti-HAV (IgG)	Antibody to hepatitis A indicating immunity
Hepatitis B	
HBV	Hepatitis B virus
Dane particle	Entire hepatitis B particle, infective
HBsAg	Hepatitis B surface antigen; exists with intact infective virion and alone in tubular, spherical, and filamentous forms
Anti-HBs	Antibody to the hepatitis B surface antigen
HBeAg	Hepatitis B e antigen, which is part of the core antigen
Anti-HBe	Antibody to hepatitis B e antigen
HBcAg	Hepatitis B core antigen
Anti-HBc (IgM)	Antibody to hepatitis B core antigen indicating recent infection
Anti-HBc (IgG)	Antibody to hepatitis B core antigen indicating immunity
Delta Hepatitis	
HDV	Delta virus
Delta antigen	Delta viral antigen seen in early infection
Anti-HDV	Antibody to delta antigen
Hepatitis C	
HCV	Hepatitis C virus
Anti-HCV	Antibody to hepatitis C virus
Hepatitis E	
HEV	Hepatitis E virus, agent of nontype A enterically transmitted hepatitis; also sometimes noted as ET-NANB

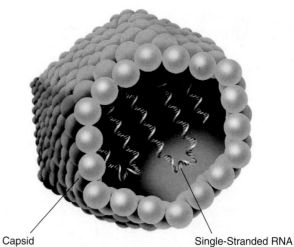

Capsid   Single-Stranded RNA

FIGURE 15-1 Hepatitis A virus; Picornavirus. (Adapted with permission from *Hepatitis Learning Guide*. Abbott Park, IL: Abbott Diagnostics Educational Services; 2008.)

and at physiologic pH retains its physical integrity and biologic activity at 60°C for 30 minutes.

Incidence

Infection is sometimes seen in outbreaks, often of epidemic proportion. Based on serosurveys, approximately 40% to 45% of adults have evidence of prior exposure. The percentage of children infected is less than 10%. Those at risk include people who may live in conditions of overcrowding or poor sanitation, travelers to endemic areas, military personnel, inhabitants of adult and child care facilities, and people in prisons.[1]

Transmission

Hepatitis A is usually spread by the fecal–oral route. Crowded conditions and poor hygiene contribute to its spread. Less than 10% of the cases are associated with food or water, and in about 50% of the cases, there is no known source of infection. Hepatitis A is rarely spread by transfusion because no chronic carrier state occurs, although in rare incidents, a transient viremia may be seen. For the disease to be spread by a blood transfusion, the blood donor would need to be in the incubation phase of the infection, which is limited from 2 to 6 weeks. In addition, many adults who receive transfusions are not susceptible to hepatitis A because of immunity from a past exposure to the virus. Further evidence of the lack of transmission by blood transfusion is seen in the fact that multiply transfused patients have no greater incidence of antibody to hepatitis A than do normal, healthy blood donors.[2]

Pathology

The incubation period of hepatitis A ranges from 14 to 45 days, with a median of 28 days. Viral replication occurs in the liver, and the virus is excreted through the

hepatitis is now known to be caused by this virus and is referred to as hepatitis A.

Etiologic Agent

HAV is a small (27 nm) RNA virus that belongs to the picornavirus class. The structure is that of a simple, nonenveloped virus with a nucleocapsid. Figure 15-1 is an artist's sketch of the virus. HAV is very stable biliary system into feces. There is a very brief period of viremia. Symptoms of the disease are usually mild. They may include nausea, vomiting, loss of appetite, malaise, and diarrhea. Jaundice is often present. Rarely does fulminant disease occur, and mortality rates are very low.

Serology and Laboratory Testing

In the laboratory, hepatitis A markers (Fig. 15-2) can be used to identify current or past infections. Usually, if hepatitis A is suspected, a test for immunoglobulin M (IgM) antibody is performed. In the absence of IgM antibody, a positive total or IgG antibody to HAV will indicate a past infection. Figure 15-3 indicates the serologic testing used in the diagnosis and staging of HAV infection.

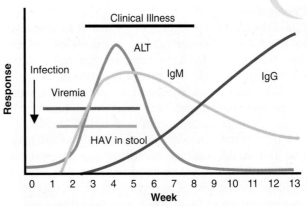

FIGURE 15-2 Clinical and serologic course of a typical case of hepatitis A. (Adapted with permission from *Hepatitis Learning Guide*. Abbott Park, IL: Abbott Diagnostics Educational Services; 2008.)

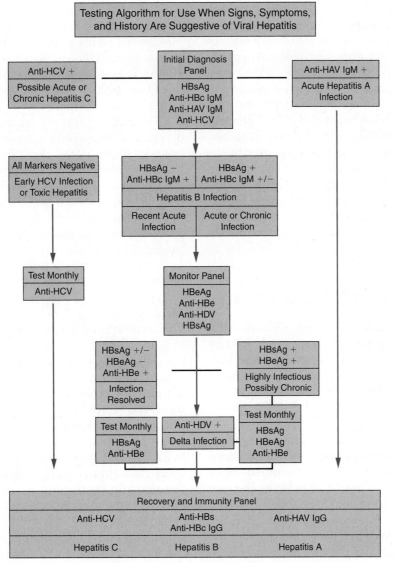

FIGURE 15-3 Serologic tests used to diagnose and stage hepatitis infections.

Prevention

Blood donations are not routinely tested for antibody to hepatitis A. Donor interview questions are designed to detect physical symptoms that may indicate general illness, including that of hepatitis A.

If a blood donor subsequently develops hepatitis A, the recipients of products from this donor may be given immune serum globulin prophylactically. Although the immunoglobulin does not prevent infection, it does decrease the severity of the symptoms of the disease. It is recommended that travelers to areas endemic for hepatitis A be given hepatitis A vaccine or immune serum globulin to prevent infection.

Hepatitis B

History

The transmission of a form of hepatitis through blood was documented in the late 1800s, but the modern history of *hepatitis B* began in the 1930s, when it was recognized that hepatitis could be transmitted through human serum. This serum was being used in an attempt to prevent measles and mumps. Outbreaks of hepatitis associated with yellow fever vaccines yielded even more convincing evidence of parenteral transmission. Human volunteer studies using filtered plasma from lots of yellow fever vaccine implicated in the outbreaks established the viral etiology of blood-borne hepatitis.[3]

Viral hepatitis research was further spurred by the discovery of Blumberg et al., who found an antigen in the blood of Australian aborigines that was later shown to be related to the hepatitis B virus (HBV).[4] The discovery of this Australian antigen, now known as the hepatitis B surface antigen (HbsAg), resulted in the full characterization of the virus, the definition of various antigen and antibody systems, and the development of assays to detect components of hepatitis viruses. All this was accomplished in a short period of time.

Today, the results of hepatitis research have virtually eliminated hepatitis B as a disease transmitted by transfusion. In addition, the licensing of hepatitis vaccines, as discussed later in this chapter, has introduced the potential for eradication of the disease.

Etiologic Agent

With a diameter of 42 nm, HBV is a member of the virus family Hepadnaviridae. The inner core contains partially double-stranded DNA surrounded by a surface coat composed of lipid and protein. The core contains, in addition to the double-stranded DNA, an enzyme known as DNA polymerase. Four genes are present within the HBV DNA: the *S* gene encodes the HbsAg; the *C* gene encodes the core antigen and the antigen; the *P* gene encodes polymerase; and the *X* gene encodes a protein that promotes viral replication.[2]

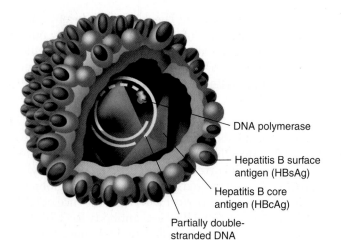

FIGURE 15-4   Hepatitis B virus. (Adapted with permission from *Hepatitis Learning Guide*. Abbott Park, IL: Abbott Diagnostics Educational Services; 2008.)

The hepatitis B e antigen (HBeAg) is associated with infectivity of HBsAg-positive blood. The hepatitis B core antigen (HBcAg) is not seen in the blood, but HBsAg is associated with the intact virion, known as the Dane particle, and independent, noninfectious forms, as seen in Figure 15-4.

The surface antigen can be serotyped into four different subtypes: adr, adw, ayr, and ayw. The presence of HBsAg in the blood indicates HBV infection but does not determine the state of the disease without further evaluation (see section on Serology in the text). Sensitive to heat and chemicals such as sodium hypochlorite, the virus is absent from heat-treated products, such as plasma protein fraction and heat-treated albumin. The virus has, however, been shown to survive and remain infective for at least 1 month when stored at room temperature or frozen.[5]

Incidence

The incidence of hepatitis B varies worldwide; the highest incidence is found in China, Southeast Asia, sub-Saharan Africa, parts of the Middle East, and South America. In more developed areas of the world, such as North America, Western Europe, Australia, and temperate South America, the incidence of infection with hepatitis B is low, with chronic carrier rates of less than 1% and overall infection rates of 5% to 7%.[6] At-risk populations can be identified in these areas. Such groups include male homosexuals, intravenous drug users, health-care workers, institutionalized people, and heterosexual contacts with cases or carriers.

Infants born to HBV carrier mothers who test positive for the HBeAg have a 70% chance of becoming infected through perinatal transmission. Ninety percent of these children become chronic carriers of hepatitis B.[7]

Transmission

The virus is spread through contact with blood (parenterally), sexual contact, and perinatally. In countries where the virus is endemic, the primary mode of transmission is perinatally and horizontally among children during the first 5 years of life. In more developed countries, the infection is primarily found in adults. High rates of transmission are found in homosexuals, heterosexuals with multiple sexual partners, and intravenous drug users. There are also documented cases of transmission to health-care workers through needle sticks from infected patients or mucous membrane contact with infected blood. Transmission from health-care worker to patient also has been documented.

Before testing, a high incidence of infection was found among those who were transfused. Today, the chances of receiving a transfusion infected with hepatitis B are extremely low with a residual risk of 1 in 63,000. Box 15-3 summarizes those at risk for HBV infection.

Pathology

The virus gains entrance to the circulation through direct inoculation, mucous membrane contact, or breaks in the skin. From here, the virus travels to the liver, where it enters the liver cells (hepatocytes) and repli-

> **BOX 15-3**
>
> ## Individuals at Risk for Hepatitis B Infection
>
> Intravenous drug users
> Male homosexuals
> Prostitutes
> Recipients of transfusions of blood components
> Sexual partners of the above
> Infants born to infected mothers
> Health-care workers

cates. Although the exact mechanism of injury to liver cells is not known, it is believed that the primary damage occurs due to an immune reaction.[6] The virus itself does not seem to destroy the hepatocytes.

The onset of the disease is often insidious. Symptoms include fever, loss of appetite (anorexia), malaise, weakness, nausea and vomiting, and abdominal pain. A rash, jaundice, dark urine, and light-colored stools also may be seen. The incubation period for hepatitis B is much longer than that for hepatitis A, ranging from 2 weeks to 6 months. Liver enzymes, aspartate aminotransferase and ALT, characteristically increase. Figure 15-5 depicts the possible outcomes of

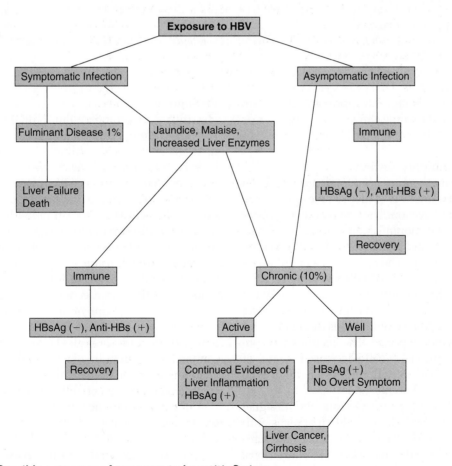

FIGURE 15-5   Possible outcomes of exposure to hepatitis B virus.

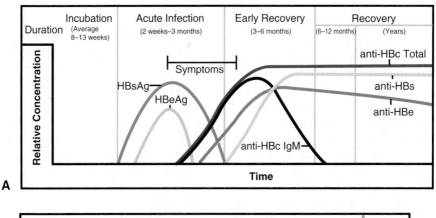

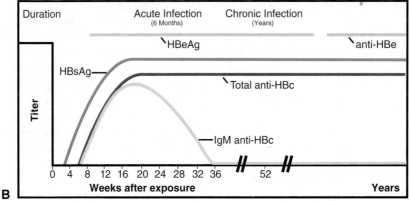

FIGURE 15-6   A: Acute hepatitis B diagnostic profile. (Adapted with permission from *Hepatitis Learning Guide*. Abbott Park, IL: Abbott Diagnostics Educational Services; 2008.) B: Progression to chronic HBV infection typical serologic course. (Adapted with permission from *Hepatitis Learning Guide*. Abbott Park, IL: Abbott Diagnostics Educational Services; 2008.)

hepatitis B infection. Note that approximately 5% to 10% of those infected become chronic carriers, whereas 1% to 3% contract fulminant hepatitis and die.[8]

Serology and Laboratory Testing

Several serologic markers are used to identify infection with hepatitis B. Figure 15-6A,B depicts the appearance of these markers in infection. The first marker to appear is HBsAg. Millions of noninfectious forms of the surface antigen can be found in the blood along with entire virions that are infective. The appearance of HBsAg is followed by the appearance of HBeAg. The first antibody to appear is the core antibody. Remember that the core antigen itself is not detectable in blood. There is a period when only IgM core antibody is detectable; this is known as the window period. The institution of core testing by blood banks has greatly decreased the risk of transfusion of an HBV-infected unit from a donor who is in the window period of infection.

Antibody to HBeAg appears next and should signal the loss of HBeAg. The last detectable marker is antibody to HBsAg, anti-HBs. Figure 15-3 depicts the serologic tests used to diagnose and stage HBV infections.

Prevention

Hepatitis B immunoglobulin (HBIG) is prepared from plasma with high titers of antibody to the surface antigen (anti-HBs). This product is screened for antibody to *human immunodeficiency virus* (HIV), and during the fractionation process, HIV is inactivated. This eliminates the chance of the preparation passing HIV infection. HBIG is given when an individual is believed to have had a direct parenteral exposure to hepatitis B. It does not provide permanent protection from HBV.

Hepatitis B vaccine was first developed from the sera of people who were infected with HBV. It was made from the noninfectious HBsAg particles in the sera using both biophysical and biochemical procedures. These procedures have been shown to inactivate representatives of all classes of viruses found in human blood, including HIV. Plasma-derived vaccine is no longer made in the United States but is still used to vaccinate people with allergy to yeasts.

Hepatitis B vaccine is now made from recombinant technology. *Saccharomyces cerevisiae*, which is common baker's yeast, is used. A plasmid containing the gene for HBsAg is inserted into the yeast, and HBsAg is obtained by lysing the yeast cells and separating HBsAg by biochemical and biophysical techniques. The product has 5% residual yeast protein and is therefore contraindicated for people with allergies to yeast.

Recombinant hepatitis B vaccine is given in a series of three intramuscular injections. Optimal levels of protection are not seen until after the third dose. It has been found to induce anti-HBs in greater than 90% of those vaccinated. The vaccine does not harm people who are carriers of HBV, nor does it cause ill effects in people who have already developed anti-HBs. If desired, people may be tested before receiving the vaccine for evidence of anti-HBc to see if prior exposure to HBV has occurred. Box 15-4 lists people who may benefit from hepatitis B vaccination.

Delta Hepatitis

History

Delta hepatitis virus (HDV) was discovered by Rizzetto in Italy in 1977. It was later discovered that the agent depended on the presence of an acute HBV infection. HDV is found in two circumstances—as a superinfection in an HBV carrier and as a coinfection of HDV/HBV in a susceptible individual.

Etiologic Agent

HDV is a 35- to 38-nm enveloped particle that contains a small, circular, single-stranded RNA, a unique internal protein, and an outer coat of the HBsAg (Fig. 15-7).[6] Without surface antigen coating, HDV is an incomplete virus that cannot survive, multiply, or infect. The delta antigen is readily detectable in hepatocytes by immunofluorescence, but mature particles that contain the antigen are not easily detectable in blood.

Incidence

Little is known about the incidence of HDV infection. Most of the data are inferred from studies of the incidence of hepatitis B. The prevalence of HDV worldwide correlates with that of HBV. In the United States, the highest incidence of HDV is found in certain high-risk groups for HBV—drug abusers and hemophiliacs.

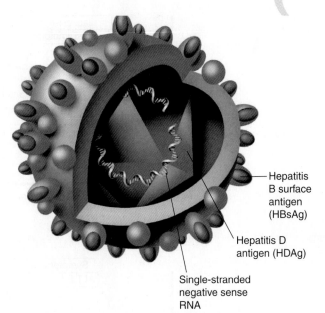

Hepatitis B surface antigen (HBsAg)

Hepatitis D antigen (HDAg)

Single-stranded negative sense RNA

FIGURE 15-7   Hepatitis D virus. (Adapted with permission from *Hepatitis Learning Guide*. Abbott Park, IL: Abbott Diagnostics Educational Services; 2008.)

Transmission

Transmission of HDV, like HBV, occurs through percutaneous exposure to blood containing the virus. Direct blood-borne transmission appears highly efficient, as defined by the high risk in parenteral drug abusers and hemophiliacs.[6] Sexual contact has been shown to transmit the infection but is considered to be less efficient than the transmission of HBV. Infection from mother to infant occurs only when the mother is HBeAg positive.[9]

Pathology

The course of infection with HDV depends on whether the infection is a coinfection with HBV or a superinfection of an HBV carrier (Fig. 15-8A,B). The incubation period for HDV in coinfection is believed to be approximately 6 to 12 or more weeks, like that of HBV. The resolution of HBV infection, which occurs in most hepatitis B cases, limits the replication of HDV. Anti-HBs, formed in response to exposure to HBV, yields permanent protection from HDV reinfection.

A superinfection occurs when an HBV carrier is exposed to HDV. The incubation period of the virus in this case is only 2 to 6 weeks. HDV can begin to replicate rapidly because of the presence of HBV within liver cells. The inflammation is acute, and signs of hepatitis appear rapidly. In most cases, the HDV infection persists indefinitely owing to HBV chronicity.

The disease may present as a subclinical, acute, or fulminant infection. The disease often is severe, with 10% of the coinfections and 20% of the superinfections presenting as fulminant cases.[6] Most HDV infections

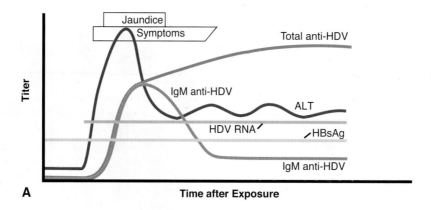

A   Time after Exposure

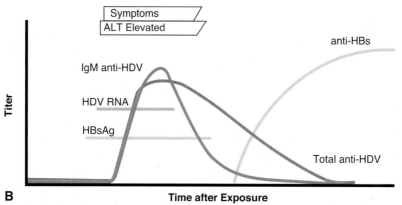

B   Time after Exposure

FIGURE 15-8   A: Typical sequence of markers in hepatitis delta superinfection. (Adapted with permission from *Hepatitis Learning Guide*. Abbott Park, IL: Abbott Diagnostics Educational Services; 2008.) B: Typical serologic course in hepatitis D coinfection. (Adapted with permission from *Hepatitis Learning Guide*. Abbott Park, IL: Abbott Diagnostics Educational Services; 2008.)

result in jaundice. It also has been found that the presence of HDV greatly increases the chances of chronic liver disease.

Prevention

Measures taken to prevent infection with hepatitis B should prevent infection with HDV. Preexposure and postexposure to HBV-infected people should be avoided. HBsAg carriers are at high risk of HDV infection and should avoid participation in behaviors that put them at high risk for repeated exposure to HBV. At present, there are no products that might prevent HDV infection in HBV carriers before or after exposure.

Hepatitis C

History

Hepatitis C, formerly known as *non-A, non-B hepatitis*, has been recognized since the 1970s and is the primary transfusion-transmitted form of viral hepatitis today. It was considered a disease of exclusion—non-A, non-B hepatitis was present if serologic testing revealed the absence of hepatitis A or hepatitis B (see Fig. 15-9).

Today, because the etiologic agent has been identified and a serologic test exists to detect exposure to this agent, the term "non-A, non-B" is used to refer to

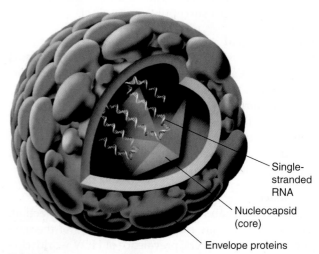

FIGURE 15-9   Hepatitis C virus. (Adapted with permission from *Hepatitis Learning Guide*. Abbott Park, IL: Abbott Diagnostics Educational Services; 2008.)

other hepatitis infections, such as those caused by Epstein–Barr virus, CMV, or some undiscovered agent.

Etiologic Agent

Much of the progress that has been made in studying the hepatitis C virus (HCV) is the result of the work of Michael Houghton and colleagues at Chiron Corporation. Although much remains to be learned about the HCV, it is believed to be approximately 30 to 60 mm in diameter and to have an envelope, and is probably a flavivirus, which is the family of arboviruses that includes the yellow fever and dengue viruses. It is known to have a single-stranded molecule of RNA. The virus is sensitive to chloroform and has the ability to form cytoplasmic tubular ultrastructures in the liver of experimentally infected chimpanzees.

Incidence

The Centers for Disease Control (CDC) estimates that the number of new cases of acute HCV infection in the United States has fallen from approximately 230,000 per year in the 1980s to its current level of about 19,000 cases per year. The overall incidence in 2006 was estimated to be 0.3 to 100,000.[10] The decline relates primarily to reduced infections in injection drug users, a probable consequence of changes in injection practices motivated by a concern for HIV risk. The number of cases of transfusion-associated acute hepatitis C decreased significantly after 1985 and has been reduced almost to zero.[11]

Transmission

Hepatitis C is believed to be spread much in the same way as hepatitis B, that is, through parenteral exposure and sexual contact. Many intravenous drug abuse groups show an 80% to 90% seropositivity. Because the virus is seen much less frequently in homosexuals than hepatitis A or hepatitis B, it appears that sexual transmission is not as predominant for HCV as for those viruses.

The fact that approximately 50% of the cases of hepatitis C do not have known risk factors suggests that the disease also may be spread in ways different from that of hepatitis B. Some would suggest that insect vectors may be a factor, but there is no evidence at this time for vector transmission.

Pathology

Disease due to HCV appears to be relatively serious. The incubation period is usually 5 to 12 weeks, with a mean of 7 weeks. In the acute phase, symptoms are mild. Jaundice is seen in about 75% of the cases, and the ALT levels are not extremely elevated. Widely fluctuating ALT levels are characteristic of HCV infection; elevations persist in up to 50% of infected people for 1 year or more.[2] In many patients, chronic hepatitis develops, and cirrhosis develops in approximately 10%.

Serology

The implementation of testing for anti-HCV in 1990 provided a way to decrease the incidence of transfusion-transmitted hepatitis C. Figure 15-10 shows the serologic response associated with HCV infection. The studies performed thus far show that the HCV core and envelope proteins, as well as other nonstructural proteins, are immunogenic. As yet, the exact chronology of appearance of various serologic markers has not been fully developed. Two generations of anti-HCV tests have been developed. The first-generation test used a single protein of HCV, the c100–3 antigen, whereas the second-generation test makes use of three

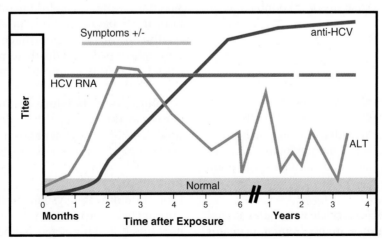

FIGURE 15-10   Serologic pattern in acute HCV infection with progression to chronic infection. (Adapted with permission from *Hepatitis Learning Guide*. Abbott Park, IL: Abbott Diagnostics Educational Services; 2008.)

proteins—one structural protein, the c22–3, and two nonstructural proteins, the c100–3 and the c33c. The second test is more sensitive and more specific. Recombinant immunoblot assay (RIBA) testing is used to provide additional information related to HCV infection.

A close correlation exists between the finding of an elevated ALT level or an anti-HBc in the blood and anti-HCV. This has been well documented in many studies. As a result, before anti-HCV testing, these two tests were used as surrogate indicators of potential HCV infection.

Prevention

Because HCV has not been completely described, vaccination does not exist. Preventive measures rely on careful screening of blood donors and testing. Currently, two enzyme immunoassays (EIAs) and one automated chemiluminescent assay for anti-HCV are licensed and available in the United States. (Additional tests and formats are available outside the United States.) A strip immunoassay is available and licensed for confirmatory testing. Even using the most sensitive assays for anti-HCV, there is a substantial infectious window period. In the United States and a number of other countries, nucleic acid amplification tests (NAT) are used to detect HCV RNA and thus reduce this window period. This testing is done in addition to the immunologic testing. Currently, this is achieved largely through pooled testing using duplex (HIV/HCV) or triplex (HIV/HCV/HBV) test systems. It may be noted that a positive test for HCV RNA in a seropositive individual obviates the need for a serologic confirmatory test. A test that is capable of detecting HCV viral antigens has also been developed, but was never used in the United States. This approach has been developed into a combination assay capable of detecting both antibodies and the antigen and is in limited use in some countries as an alternative to NAT.

Hepatitis E

History

Enterically transmitted non-A, non-B hepatitis was recognized in the late 1970s from epidemics that had occurred 20 years earlier in India. The disease is probably an ancient one that is common in many countries where standards of hygiene and sanitation are poor.

Etiologic Agent

The hepatitis E virus (HEV) particle was characterized through laboratory studies in nonhuman primates and by electron microscopy. In partially purified stool extracts, the particle appears to be 27 to 34 nm. Unlike HAV, the virus is relatively unstable to purification procedures. Current virologic and molecular properties suggest a classification similar to caliciviruses.

Incidence

Epidemic and sporadic forms of hepatitis E have been observed in Asia, Africa, and Central and South America. There is a high attack rate among young adults that distinguishes HEV from HAV. Usually, an enteric disease would be expected to be equal in children and adults. In developed countries, some imported cases have been seen. Without a serologic test to identify the virus, it is difficult to determine the exact percentage of non-A, non-B hepatitis due to hepatitis E.

Transmission

The spread of hepatitis E is associated with some of the same conditions as hepatitis A, with the fecal–oral route being the mode of infection. Contamination of the water supply has been implicated as a causative factor in many areas where large outbreaks have occurred. This particularly has been noted during heavy rainy seasons. It is not believed that hepatitis E is transmitted through blood or sexual contact.

Pathology

Hepatitis E has an incubation period of 1 to 10 days, which is much less than the incubation period for hepatitis A. Symptoms of the disease include nausea, dark urine, abdominal pain, vomiting, and diarrhea. Jaundice is also present (only symptomatic cases with jaundice have been studied because no serologic test is available). A cholestatic form of viral hepatitis occurs. Liver cell necrosis varies from a single-cell degeneration to more severe forms with necrosis.

Hepatitis E results in a great deal of mortality among pregnant women. This is a consistent finding, and the average mortality rate is 30%. The risks to pregnant women for fulminant hepatitis and death appear to be highest in the third trimester. Most deaths are due to hemorrhage. Although there is a high rate of perinatal death, termination of pregnancy does not appear to improve the woman's condition.

Serology and Laboratory Testing

Serologic tests for hepatitis E do not exist. Most diagnoses of this form of hepatitis are based on ruling out acute hepatitis A and hepatitis B.[12]

Prevention

Protection of water systems from fecal contamination appears to be the most important means of preventing hepatitis E. Boiling water is known to prevent transmission. It is not known whether immunoglobulin prophylaxis is beneficial.

Chronic Hepatitis

Chronic hepatitis infection is referred to as persistence of evidence of hepatic inflammation for more than 6 months. Approximately 5% to 10% of patients with hepatitis B become chronic, whereas 40% to 60% of patients with hepatitis C may become chronic. Chronic hepatitis may be active or inactive. In active cases, the disease may progress to liver cell necrosis and fibrosis and eventually to cirrhosis. The chances that liver cancer will develop in a chronically infected individual are great. Hepatoma, or hepatocellular carcinoma, is causally related to chronic hepatitis B infection and possibly to hepatitis C. Although rare in North America, it is the most common cancer in sub-Saharan Africa, where carrier rates for hepatitis B are as high as 15%.[6]

Summary

Serologic testing for the agents of viral hepatitis has greatly decreased the chances of infection being acquired through transfusion. The chance for transmission during early infection or by yet to be discovered viruses remains a problem for blood banks. Table 15-2 shows a summary of information known about the major hepatitis viruses.

Retroviruses

Retroviruses are characterized by a common morphology, the presence of reverse transcriptase, and the presence of two identical strands of RNA. The reverse transcriptase allows the viruses to produce DNA that is complementary to the viral RNA. This proviral DNA can then be integrated into the DNA of the host.

Retroviridae, the family retroviruses, includes Oncovirinae, Lentivirinae, and Spumavirinae. Figure 15-11 depicts the life cycle of a retrovirus.

Human Immunodeficiency Virus

History

First reported in 1981, the disease now known as the *acquired immunodeficiency syndrome* (AIDS) has totally changed the blood banking world. AIDS includes a diverse group of clinical manifestations that are the result of a loss of immunocompetence. The clinical entity was defined by the CDC in 1982 as "a case of a disease at least moderately predictive of a defect in cell-mediated immunity occurring in a person with no known cause for diminished resistance to that disease."[1]

In 1981, in a cluster of young men who had no known reason for immune dysfunction, *Pneumocystis carinii* pneumonia developed, an opportunistic infection usually seen only in immunosuppressed people, such as those on chemotherapy. The only thing these young men had in common was that they were all homosexuals; thus, AIDS was stigmatized as being a disease of homosexuals. Cases of Kaposi sarcoma, a rare cancer, also began to be detected in homosexual men and drug addicts. This form of Kaposi sarcoma, however, was different than that in Africa and in elderly men

TABLE 15-2 Comparison of the Human Hepatitis Viruses					
	HAV	**HBV**	**HCV**	**HDV**	**HEV**
Nucleic acid	RNA	DNA	RNA	RNA	RNA
Strands	Single	Double	Single	Single	Single
Classification	Picornavirus	Hepadnavirus	Flavivirus	Satellite	Calicivirus
Size (nm)	27	42	30–60	35–38	27–34
Incubation period (days)	15–45	40–150	20–90	30–50	22–60
Viremia	Transient	Prolonged	Prolonged	Prolonged	Transient
Transmission	Fecal–oral	Parenteral, sexual, perinatal	Parenteral, sexual, perinatal	Parenteral, sexual, perinatal	Fecal–oral
Carrier state	No	Yes	Yes	Yes	No
chronicity	No	Yes	Yes	Yes	No
Mortality	Low	Low	Low	High	Low
Existence of vaccine	No	Yes	No	No	No

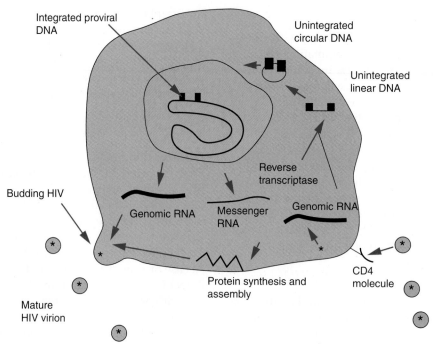

FIGURE 15-11   Life cycle of human immunodeficiency virus (HIV).

from the Mediterranean regions, the major places where Kaposi sarcoma had previously been seen. The tumors were much more aggressive, and there was visceral involvement. In addition, the Kaposi sarcoma was often accompanied by other opportunistic infections.

Even before the etiologic agent was known, it was recognized that the disease could be transmitted by sexual contact with infected people, by exposure to infected blood or blood products through transfusion or contaminated needles, and perinatally from mother to child. In 1982, the condition was found in hemophiliacs who were not homosexual and who did not participate in intravenous drug use. The death of an infant who experienced numerous opportunistic infections later in that same year led researchers to believe that the agent causing the disease was transmitted by transfusion, because the only factor these people had in common were multiple transfusions of blood components.

In 1983, a virus was isolated in France from the serum of a person with a generalized lymphadenopathy that was thought to be associated with AIDS. This virus was named lymphadenopathy-associated virus by French researchers. At the same time, researchers in the United States discovered a similar virus and named it *human T-cell lymphotropic virus* type III (HTLV-III). When it was found that these viruses were essentially the same and that AIDS resulted from infection with either, an international committee on viral nomenclature named the virus HIV.

In 1986, another virus that caused AIDS was discovered in western Africa. This virus shared only approximately 40% nucleic acid homology with the original HIV, and as a result, the original virus came to be called HIV-1, and the new virus was called HIV-2.[6,13] In 1985, an antibody screening test began to be used. This test was originally designed to detect evidence of the exposure to HIV in blood donors. It was found that the virus could be cultured from most people with positive results on this test.

The disease began to be studied retrospectively, and many theories exist as to the origin of HIV. Researchers have learned a great deal about how HIV is spread, how to detect it early, what it does to the immune system, and the opportunistic infections that are seen in those with full-blown cases of AIDS.

Etiologic Agents

HIV belongs to the family of Retroviridae, which includes HTLV-I and HTLV-II, two other viruses that are discussed in the next section of this chapter. Figure 15-12 shows the physical structure of HIV. Three important components of the virus should be noted: (1) the RNA, (2) the reverse transcriptase, and (3) a protein within the viral core known as p24. A retrovirus carries its genetic information in the form of RNA and uses reverse transcriptase to replicate.

The HIV genome possesses three genes that are common to other retroviruses. These are the *env*, which encodes the glycoproteins of the viral envelope; the *gag*, which encodes the core proteins in the virus, including p24; and the *pol*, which encodes enzymes necessary for replication, such as reverse transcriptase.

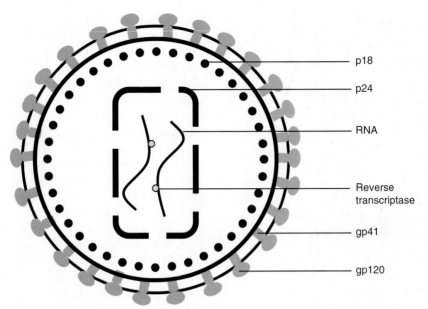

FIGURE 15-12   The human immunodeficiency virus.

There are two recognized forms of HIV: HIV-1 and HIV-2. The genomes of the viruses are very similar and both cause AIDS. HIV-1 is responsible for most of the infections in the United States.

Subtypes of HIV

The strains of HIV-1 that have caused the worldwide pandemic of AIDS have been designated as group M viruses. A group of HIV-1 viruses that also cause AIDS but that have extensive genetic divergence from group M strains has been identified; these viruses are classified as group *O variants*. Reports of group O infection are primarily from inhabitants of West and Central Africa and from individuals from these areas who have emigrated to other countries. EIAs are being modified to detect the antibody response to group O; as with current assays, the antibody response to group O is not consistently detected.[14]

Incidence

Although the disease was not seen with any significance until the late 1970s, it is believed to have existed much earlier. Approximately 40,000 new HIV infections occur each year in the United States, about 70% to 75% among men and 25% to 30% among women. Those at high risk for infection with HIV are listed in Box 15-5.

Transmission

HIV-1 and HIV-2 are spread primarily through contact with blood or other body fluids containing the virus. The virus has been isolated in a number of body fluids, as listed in Box 15-6. Transmission from mother to unborn child is also a means of spread. Most people who are infected with HIV have acquired the virus through sexual contact. The presence of other sexually transmitted diseases may facilitate the transmission of the virus by providing openings (ulcerations) in the skin through which the virus can enter. Although in the United States the primary spread has been male to male, there

---

BOX 15-5

Individuals at Risk for Infection with HIV

Homosexuals
Bisexuals
Prostitutes
Intravenous drug users
Recipients of transfusions of blood components
Sexual partners of the above
Health-care workers
Infants born to infected mothers

BOX 15-6

Fluids from Which HIV Has Been Isolated

RELATIVELY HIGH CONCENTRATION

Blood
Semen

VERY LOW CONCENTRATION

Vaginal fluid
Tears
Sweat
Breast milk

is an increase of male-to-female and female-to-male transmissions, indicating that the virus has permeated the heterosexual population to a great extent. Box 15-7 summarizes the routes of transmission for HIV.

Although with sensitive testing and extensive donor questioning, the risk of acquiring HIV through transfusion has decreased, there is little chance of transmission of HIV through transfusion even when the blood is tested, especially if the donor is in the window period of infection (see section on Serology for explanation).

Pathology

Early Infection. A brief, flulike illness occurs a few weeks after acquiring HIV in approximately 25% of those infected. Symptoms may include fever, rash, lymphadenopathy, headache, and sore throat. Most infected people, however, have no symptoms at all. Within 2 to 6 weeks, there is usually evidence of seroconversion, and antibody to the virus can be detected in the infected person's serum.

This initial period is followed by a latent time, which may last for many years. Some people have been infected for as long as 10 years and are not clinically symptomatic of AIDS.

Replication of the Virus. The latent period is followed by a time of replication of the virus within the T4 cell, also referred to as the T-helper cell. Investigations into

the mechanism of the disease pathology have shown that the virus infects the T4 (CD4+) lymphocyte. Once inside the cell, HIV inserts its own genetic information and turns the T4 cell into an HIV factory. As the virus replicates and buds from the T4 cell, the T4 cell is destroyed. As the number of T4 cells decreases, the ability of the person's immune system to respond adequately and appropriately is lessened.

Other cells of the body also have CD4 receptors and may serve as reservoirs for the virus. Included in these cells are monocytes, macrophages, and some brain and skin cells. HIV is not cytopathic for some of these cells; however, the reason for this is not yet understood.

Occasionally, in the second phase of HIV infection, the infected individual experiences a slight and continual swelling of the lymph nodes. Some general signs of poor health, such as chronic headache, unexplained weight loss, fatigue, and persistent diarrhea, also may be noted.

Early AIDS. As the virus replicates and destroys the T4 cell population, the symptoms of infection become more prevalent. This phase of infection usually means that the development of full-blown AIDS is near. The infected individual is now extremely susceptible to opportunistic infection. Generalized lymphadenopathy is usually evident, and the other "constitutional" symptoms, such as persistent diarrhea and weight loss, intensify. The individual may also experience night sweats and hair loss.

AIDS. Once the T-cell count has fallen to less than 200, opportunistic infections are able to overwhelm the almost defenseless immune system. Box 15-8 lists some of the opportunistic infections seen in cases of full-blown AIDS. Once an individual acquires these infections, the mean time of duration of the disease is 2 years. Life expectancy for people with AIDS has increased considerably, however, with the advent of new treatments for the opportunistic infections and with the new and experimental antiviral drugs now available.

Serology and Laboratory Testing

HIV infects the immune system, and eventually all elements of the system are affected. Although the most noticeable defects occur with the T-cell population, problems are evident with B-cell and monocyte functions as well. Antibody to the virus usually appears within 3 months after infection. Although neutralizing antibody is developed, the virus is able to escape owing to its constant transfer from cell to cell.

In 1985, EIAs to HIV-1 (HIV-2 was not recognized at this time) were licensed and were found useful in screening blood donors, diagnosing infected people, and conducting epidemiologic studies. It is almost always true that the virus can be cultured from antibody-positive people. The specificity and sensitivity of these tests approach 99.9%. A combination test exists for the detection of HIV-1 and HIV-2 as well as assays for the individual viruses.

The EIA procedure used usually involves viral lysates or may use synthetic or recombinant antigen. The antigen is coated to the wells of a microtiter plate or on plastic beads that are placed into microtiter wells. The serum sample is then placed into the microtiter wells and allowed to incubate. After washing, an enzyme-labeled conjugate (antihuman antibody) is added. Finally, enzyme substrate is added, and the intensity of color development is directly proportional to the amount of antibody present. Interpretation of the test is based on comparison of the results to a cutoff value. If a specimen is reactive, the test should be repeated in duplicate on the same specimen. Figure 15-13 diagrams the typical EIA tests for HIV antibody.

An EIA test that will detect the p24 antigen was required on all donor blood as of 1995 in an effort further to close the window period. This test was eliminated when NAT testing for HIV was implemented.

Confirmatory/Supplemental Testing. Because some people have nonspecific reactions with the EIA procedure, it is necessary to perform a confirmation test on all repeatedly reactive tests. The test most commonly used is the Western blot. This procedure involves immunoelectrophoresis and immunoblot technology. In this test, viral proteins are electrophoresed through a gel. The protein is then transferred to nitrocellulose paper, and the paper is cut into thin strips. Each strip

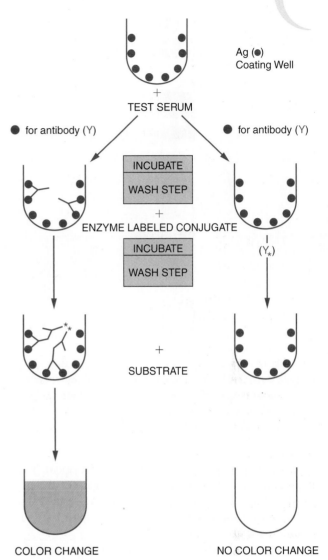

FIGURE 15-13 Diagram of enzyme immunoassay for human immunodeficiency virus antibody testing. The basic principle of this test is used for many infectious disease screening procedures.

contains a full complement of HIV antigen bands. The strip is then used as a solid support (analogous to the plastic bead) for an enzyme assay. Serum is overlaid onto the strip. After incubation and washing, enzyme-labeled conjugate is added, followed by enzyme substrate. Insoluble colored bands appear on the strip, representing the antibodies present in the sample.

An HIV-positive sample produces a characteristic banding pattern, as seen in Figure 15-14. Bands can be found to a number of proteins, and different interpretive schemes have been developed.[15] Table 15-3 lists the criteria of four different groups. If a definite pattern does not exist (bands are missing), the sample is called indeterminate. It is usually recommended that such a sample be retested in several weeks. If truly HIV

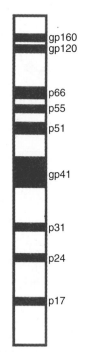

gp160
gp120

p66
p55
p51

gp41

p31

p24

p17

FIGURE 15-14   Drawing of Western blot banding pattern detectable in human immunodeficiency virus type 1–positive sample. Not all these bands must be present for a sample to be called reactive. (See interpretative criteria in Table 15-3.)

positive, a full banding pattern should appear. It is also possible to determine by the intensity of the p24 band if antigenemia is returning. This is demonstrated by a weak or fading p24 band. Western blot tests are available for HIV-1 and HIV-2.

There is also an immunofluorescence assay for HIV antibody that can be used as a confirmatory test.

TABLE 15-3	Interpretive Criteria for Western Blot Tests for HIV-1
Organization	**Band Requirements for Reactive Pattern**
American Red Cross group	At least one band from each gene product *gag* and *pol* and *env*
ASTPHLD/CDC	Any two of p24, gp41, or gp120/160
Consortium for Retrovirus Serology Standardization	p24 and p31 and one of gp41 or gp120/160
DuPont	p24 and p31 and gp41 or gp120/160

From Centers for Disease Control and Prevention. Interpretive criteria used to report Western blot results for HIV-1 antibody testing: United States. *MMWR Morb Mortal Wkly Rep.* 1991; 40: 692.

This test is a standard indirect assay, and although it is relatively easy to perform, the interpretation of results is subjective and requires experience. Immunofluorescence assay has been used to resolve indeterminate Western blot results.

New Testing Methodologies. Nucleic acid testing (NAT) is the next step in further reduction of the window period in HIV infection. The requirement to test for p24 antigen was dropped with the advent of NAT testing. NAT, which is very sensitive and specific, involves detection of the viral protein itself.

Prevention

The best method of preventing the spread of HIV is education. Such education must be directed at infected and noninfected people, informing them of how HIV is spread and how to prevent that spread. Although vaccine research is ongoing, estimates are that an effective vaccine is years away. Screening of all blood donors for HIV has virtually eliminated the transmission of HIV by transfusion. The use of self-deferral for donors at high risk for HIV infection and temporary exclusion of donors from malaria-endemic regions offers additional protection against divergent HIV strains. Even with NAT testing, however, there is still a small chance that an infected unit might pass screening procedures.

Treatment

A number of treatments have been tried with HIV-infected people who have progressed to full-blown AIDS, most with little or no success. There have been advances, however, in preventing progression from the HIV-positive status to AIDS. Many of the efforts have been directed toward prevention of viral replication. The drugs azidothymidine (AZT, zidovudine), dideoxycytidine (ddC), and dideoxyinosine (ddI) have been found to be effective in slowing the replication of the virus. Often, "cocktails," combinations of these and other drugs, are most effective in achieving the desired effect. It is not within the scope of this text to discuss treatment modalities, and the interested reader should consult "Additional Readings" section for further reading.

Human T-lymphotropic Virus Types I and II

History

HTLV-I and HTLV-II were the first human retroviruses identified.[16,17] HTLV-I was isolated in 1978 from a patient with a cutaneous T-cell lymphoma. The association of HTLV-I with disease was at first uncertain. However, the discovery of adult T-cell leukemia or lymphoma (ATL) did provide an epidemiologic link because most ATL cases were positive for antibodies to HTLV-I. HTLV-I antibodies also were found in West Indian patients, with the disease known as tropical spastic paraparesis.

HTLV-II was first identified from a patient with a T-cell variant of hairy cell leukemia. This virus showed extensive homology with HTLV-I. The association of this virus with disease is under continuing study.

Etiologic Agent

HTLV-I and HTLV-II are members of the retrovirus family and are considered oncoviruses. Both HTLV-I and HTLV-II carry single strands of RNA. These viruses are known to be leukemogenic and cause cell proliferation. HTLV-I is 80 to 110 nm in diameter and is enveloped. The virus is sensitive to organic solvents, detergents, and heat but resistant to ultraviolet light and x-rays.

Incidence

HTLV-I is endemic in areas of Japan, the Caribbean, Africa, South America, Southeast Asia, and Europe. Owing to the cross-reactivity between HTLV-I and HTLV-II antibodies, most prevalence reports for nonendemic areas are given in terms of HTLV-I/II. In volunteer blood donors in the United States and Canada, the seroprevalence of HTLV-I/II is approximately 0.03%.[7] The seroprevalence among paid donors is 10 times higher than this. This difference is possibly explained by the high seroprevalence rate among intravenous drug users.

Transmission

Human T-cell lymphotropic viruses are transmitted much in the same way as HIV. A difference does exist, however, in that HTLV transmission is associated almost exclusively with cells. Transmission of HTLV-I has been shown to occur parenterally, sexually, and perinatally. It also has been transmitted through infected lymphocytes in breast milk, which is a rare mode of HIV transmission. Little is known at this time about HTLV-II transmission. However, a high seropositivity for HTLV-II exists among intravenous drug users, which would suggest parenteral transmission.

Pathology

Adult T-cell Leukemia or Lymphoma. It is estimated that ATL will develop in approximately 5% of HTLV-I–infected people in their lifetime. In the preleukemic stage, the infected individual is asymptomatic, HTLV-I seropositive, and capable of transmitting the infection to others. In the acute phase of ATL, a clone of aggressive T cells is present. Lymphadenopathy, hepatosplenomegaly, elevated lactate dehydrogenase, hyperbilirubinemia, and hypercalcemia are seen.

Tropical Spastic Paraparesis and Human T-lymphotropic–associated Myelopathy. This disease, present in all parts of the world endemic for HTLV-I, is characterized by an onset of weakness of the legs, which progresses to a spastic paraparesis. Neurologic findings include weakness and spasticity of the extremities, hyperreflexia, urinary or fecal incontinence, and mild peripheral sensory loss.

HTLV-II and Disease. The association between HTLV-II and disease is not certain. Although there have been reports of HTLV-II associated with T-cell malignancy, investigation was not complete enough to give definitive evidence of linkage of the virus and the disease.

Serology and Laboratory Testing

Antibodies to the various proteins of HTLV-I/II have been found in people with the conditions previously described and in asymptomatic carriers of the virus. In the United States, serologic screening is performed by an EIA technique, whereas in Japan, a particle agglutination assay is used. Supplemental Western blot and sometimes immunofluorescent assays are used to confirm seroreactivity. Most assays for HTLV-I detect both HTLV-I and HTLV-II because of the strong similarities in the viruses. Some assays do incorporate a separate HTLV-II antigen as a part of the test. PCR testing can be used to distinguish between HTLV-I and HTLV-II. New peptide- and recombinant protein-based serologic assays that can more easily differentiate the two have also been developed.[18]

Prevention

As with HIV, prevention of spread involves education and screening of blood donors. People should avoid behaviors that put them at high risk for infection, such as intravenous drug use and multiple sexual partners. Pregnant women who are HTLV-I positive should not nurse their children.

Herpesviruses

CMV

History

First recognized in infants who had symptoms of congenital syphilis but no serologic evidence of syphilis, CMV was so named owing to the presence of large, swollen cells in infants who had died. These cells had expanded cytoplasm, and thus the term "cytomegalic" described them well. The virus was successfully isolated in tissue culture in 1954.

Etiologic Agent

CMV is a member of the herpes family of viruses, which includes seven large, enveloped DNA viruses that cause infections that remain for the lifetime of the host. The hallmark of these infections is the existence of periods of latency and intermittent reactivation. The reactivation of the virus may or may not present with the same symptoms as the primary infection. In the case of CMV, the actual site where the virus lies dormant is not exactly known, although it is believed to be in the peripheral blood lymphocytes.

CMV is the largest of the herpesviruses. It is composed of a core of double-stranded DNA enclosed by an icosahedral capsid surrounded by an envelope derived from the membrane of the host cell. Lipid solvents readily inactivate the virus, as does storage at a pH less than 6.0. High heat also has been shown to inactivate CMV. CMV has marked species specificity. The features distinct to each virus–host system cannot be applied directly to humans and human CMV. The use of human subjects in clinical situations and human cell culture lines has therefore been necessary.

CMV can survive for hours on surfaces and on the skin. The virus is sensitive to lipid solvents because of the lipid-containing viral envelope. It can survive storage at 4°C for a few days, but infectivity is lost at −20°C.

Incidence

CMV is ubiquitous in the human population. It is the most common cause of congenital infection in the United States. The infection is pandemic and nonseasonal. Prevalence of the virus increases with age and is inversely proportional to socioeconomic status. The prevalence in adults is high, with a significant geographic variability, ranging from a low of 40% to a high of 100%.[2]

Transmission

The virus is transmitted through contact with infectious body secretions. Urine, oropharyngeal secretions, breast milk, blood, semen, and cervical secretions are all known to spread the virus. Close or crowded conditions enhance the chances for spread.

Pathology

CMV is a lifelong infection in which there are periods of viral shedding and latency after the primary infection. Most primary infections go unnoticed, usually with no overt symptoms. It is only when the host is immunocompromised that disease can be severe.

TABLE 15-4	Individuals at Risk for Cytomegalovirus Infection	
At-risk Individuals	**Pathology**
Premature infants	Atypical lymphocytosis, hepatosplenomegaly, pneumonia, death
Recipients of organ/ tissue transplants from cytomegalovirus-positive donors	Interstitial pneumonia, high rate of mortality
Immunosuppressed individuals	Disseminated multisystem involvement with pneumonitis, hepatitis, gastrointestinal ulceration, retinitis, arthralgias

Reactivation in the healthy host is seldom symptomatic as well, but in the individual with immune dysfunction, symptoms are often evident.

When a primary infection occurs during pregnancy, the congenitally infected infant may experience severe disease, and death may result. Symptoms in these infants include fever, jaundice, rash, low platelets, and neural defects, such as mental retardation and deafness. CMV infection is a major cause of these conditions.

The disease is particularly serious in immunosuppressed, CMV-seronegative people who become infected with the virus. Table 15-4 summarizes those at risk for CMV infection. Such people may experience a primary infection or a reactivation of a past infection. Also, existing evidence links the progression of HIV with a simultaneous infection with CMV. Three associations have been cited that lend evidence to this theory: (1) more than 90% of people with HIV infection are CMV seropositive, (2) CMV and HIV infect the same cell types in vitro, and (3) CMV possesses genes that are capable of increasing the expression of the HIV genome by transactivation.[2]

Often, CMV infection presents with mononucleosis-like symptoms. Almost any organ can become infected with CMV. The most commonly infected ones are the liver, the lung, the central nervous system, and the gastrointestinal tract. Malaise and arthralgia also are seen. Hematologic involvement can include leukopenia, thrombocytopenia, and anemia.

Serology and Laboratory Testing

Humoral and cell-mediated immunities are seen with CMV infection. Antibodies of the IgG, IgA, and IgM classes appear after the onset of viral excretion in the

TABLE 15-5	Laboratory Tests Used to Detect Cytomegalovirus Infection

Test	Immunoglobulin Detected
Complement fixation	Primarily IgG
Indirect hemagglutination	IgG and IgM
Neutralization	IgG and IgM
Indirect immunofluorescence	IgG or IgM
Enzyme-linked immunosorbent assay	IgG or IgM
Radioimmunoassay	IgG or IgM
Latex agglutination	IgG and IgM

urine and saliva. Numerous tests have been developed to detect CMV infection. Table 15-5 lists the types of laboratory tests performed, and Table 15-6 lists interpretations of the laboratory tests performed.

Blood donors are screened for the presence of IgM CMV antibody because there is the danger that neonates and immunosuppressed people might receive CMV-positive blood components.

Prevention

It is important that certain people be protected from exposure to CMV, including premature neonates, CMV-seronegative pregnant women, and bone marrow transplant recipients. Screening methods to detect CMV-positive blood donors are helpful in this endeavor. The filtration of blood products to remove leukocytes also has been described as a method of preventing CMV transmission.

Epstein–Barr Virus

History and Etiologic Agent

First discovered in 1964 as the cause of infectious mononucleosis, Epstein–Barr virus is an infrequent transfusion-transmitted disease. The virus is a human herpes DNA virus and is found in association with blood leukocytes. In the carrier state, the virus is found in the B lymphocyte.

Transmission

The virus is transmitted primarily by contact with oropharyngeal secretions. It also has been reported to be transmitted by blood transfusion, organ transplantation, and transplacentally. People who do not have antibodies to the virus are at risk for infection. Because the virus is common, most people have developed antibody to it by adulthood. The incidence of the Epstein–Barr virus ranges from 35% to 47%.[8] Interestingly, more than 90% of blood donors have antibodies to Epstein–Barr virus and thus are carriers of the virus.

Pathology

Infectious mononucleosis is seldom life threatening. Most of the time the disease is a self-limiting, acute infection. The incubation period is from 2 to 6 weeks, and the symptoms of the disease may persist for up to 1 month. Splenomegaly is seen in approximately half of the cases, and hepatitis is the most common complication of the infection. The infection is often a serious problem in the immunocompromised individual.

Serology and Laboratory Testing

Along with the symptoms and abnormal hematologic findings (e.g., elevated white count, increased lymphocytes, and atypical lymphocytes), heterophil antibodies are seen in infectious mononucleosis. These

TABLE 15-6	Laboratory Testing for Cytomegalovirus

Antibody Titers			
IgG	IgM	Interpretation	Clinical Status
−	−	No evidence of infection	Susceptible individual
+	−	Infection, not recent if culture negative	Immune individual or passive immunity through placental transfer or transfusion from immune individual
−	+	Recent primary infection	CMV mononucleosis, reactivation in transplant patients, congenital CMV
+	+	Recurrent infection, possible recent primary infection	Reaction in normal or immunocompromised patient or congenital CMV

antibodies are present in low titer normally, but the titer during acute infection rises sharply. Tests also are available for IgM and IgG antibodies to Epstein–Barr virus. These antibodies appear approximately 2 weeks after the onset of disease. One of the antibodies formed is an alloanti-i, which has been known to cause immune hemolytic anemia.

Prevention

Prevention of transfusion-transmitted Epstein–Barr virus infection may be aided by the use of leukocyte-depleted products. Excellent filters are available that remove most of the white blood cells.

Other Virus Transmitted by Blood

Parvovirus

Human B19 *parvovirus* has been shown to be transmitted by blood transfusion. This virus is the common cause of a childhood disease called erythema infectiosum, or fifth disease. In adults, a polyarthralgia is seen. It is also associated with a number of other conditions, including chronic hemolytic syndromes, acute lymphocytic leukemia, and hydrops fetalis.

The virus is a single-stranded DNA virus discovered in 1975 in the serum of normal blood donors. Infection and replication of the virus occur in the marrow's erythroid progenitor compartment. This results in a reticulocytopenia, a common finding in infection with B19 parvovirus. Neutropenia and thrombocytopenia may occur as well. Approximately 50% of adults have evidence of past infection with the B19 parvovirus. The incubation period of the virus is 1 to 2 weeks. Antibodies to the virus appear, and the disease usually clears rapidly.

At this time, testing for the B19 parvovirus is available only at a few research sites and through the CDC. The presence of antibody does not indicate infectivity, and most people have antibody by adulthood. With this in mind, the routine screening of donors for antibody to the virus is not recommended.[2]

West Nile Virus

West Nile Virus (WNV) is a mosquito-borne flavivirus that apparently entered the Americas for the first time in 1999, as evidenced by an outbreak centered on Queens, New York. The route of entry is unknown but was likely associated with the transport of an infected human, bird, or even mosquito by jet aircraft. The virus causes acute infection in most cases, and the majority of such infections are asymptomatic. A relatively mild febrile illness may occur, but severe neurologic disease (meningoencephalitis) is the most significant outcome, occurring once in approximately

150 infections. Such disease can be fatal. WNV spread remarkably rapidly across North America, infecting up to 400,000 individuals in the United States in 2002, by which time it had appeared in almost every state and a number of Canadian provinces.

From the outset, it was recognized that WNV offered a risk of transfusion transmission and the first estimate of such risk, based upon the Queens outbreak, was published in 2002.[19]

Shortly afterwards, the first such transmission was recognized and a total of 23 cases were reported in 2002. As a result of cooperative work by industry, blood establishments, public health agencies, and regulators, NAT tests for WNV RNA were in place for all donations by July 2003. Initially, all testing was performed in minipools, but it became apparent that this approach failed to detect infectious donations with low levels of circulating RNA. Therefore, programs to trigger individual donor testing in periods and areas of high incidence were developed and refined.

Dengue

Dengue virus is a flavivirus and is responsible for the greatest number of arboviral infections globally. It is endemic throughout the tropics and is transmitted by *Aedes* spp. (particularly *A. aegypti*) mosquitos. Unlike WNV, it can be transmitted human–mosquito–human, without need for an amplifying intermediate host. There are four serotypes, which do not confer mutual immunity. The disease associated with infection varies from asymptomatic dengue fever to the much more severe and potentially fatal dengue hemorrhagic fever. The pattern of infection is very similar to that of WNV, and it would be anticipated that transfusion transmission would be possible, and indeed likely, although only two clusters of such transmission have been definitively documented. It seems likely that, in the face of huge epidemics, particularly in developing countries, transfusion transmission would not necessarily be differentiated from the background cases. Recent studies, however, have shown that viremic blood donors may be detected at appreciable rates in Brazil, Honduras, and Puerto Rico. It will be important to remain alert to the potential for transfusion transmission and of the potential need to implement interventions, such as NAT. It should be noted that dengue outbreaks in Northern Queensland, Australia, have led to measures to halt blood collection during epidemic periods.

Chikungunya

Chikungunya virus is another arbovirus of the alphavirus group, with many characteristics similar to those of dengue virus. In particular, it is a primarily tropical virus, transmitted human to human by *Aedes* mosquitoes without the need for an intermediate host. Of note, it has recently caused explosive outbreaks, particularly in the Indian Ocean; the outbreak in the French island of La Reunion is particularly well described, with more than a third of the population infected. Likely contributing to the outbreak is a viral mutation that results in effective transmission by the almost ubiquitous mosquito *Aedes albopictus* (the Asian tiger mosquito). There is a potential threat of outbreaks in areas where this mosquito is present, as illustrated by an outbreak in Italy, attributed to a traveler from India.[20]

Although no case of transfusion transmission has been reported, there is clear risk, and French authorities took extensive precautions in la Reunion, including provision of all red cells from the mainland and implementation of NAT and pathogen reduction for apheresis platelets collected on the island. It is also interesting that chikungunya was explored as a biologic weapon.[21]

Prions

Prions are small, proteinaceous, infectious particles that do not invoke immune responses. These are believed to be the transmissible agents of a disease known as *Creutzfeldt–Jakob disease*, which is a worldwide disorder with an incidence of about 1 death per 1 million population per year.[2] The disease appears to be related to other encephalopathies, such as kuru.

It is believed that recipients of human growth hormone could possibly transmit Creutzfeldt–Jakob disease through their blood. As a result, people who have received injections of human growth hormone should be permanently deferred. Recombinant DNA technology now is used to produce growth hormone.

BACTERIAL INFECTIONS

Blood can become contaminated at the time of collection owing to technical problems or because the donor has bacteria in his or her bloodstream at the time of donation. In past history, it was estimated that approximately 2% of stored blood is contaminated with bacteria. With the advent of diversion pouches for blood collection, this percentage is much lower. Most organisms do not survive storage; the cold temperature of storage and the citrate in the anticoagulant are not conducive to the growth of many bacteria. Organisms that do survive are primarily gram-negative bacilli. Such organisms may multiply rapidly in the blood and produce endotoxins, which can reach dangerously high concentrations within 14 to 21 days.

Platelets can be a particular problem because they are stored at room temperature. The literature contains many reported cases of sepsis induced by the transfusion of contaminated platelet units. As a result, the American Association of Blood Banks (AABB) introduced a standard in 2004 to require bacterial testing of platelet products prior to transfusion. Currently, there are several available methods to screen for bacterial contamination of platelets. Some of these tests can be done at the bedside prior to transfusion whereas others require incubation periods for samples from the collection prior to release of the platelets.

Syphilis

History

At one time, **syphilis** was a major medical disease with a host of different manifestations. The advent of penicillin in 1943 changed this. Adequate treatment meant that infected people would not develop all possible outcomes of the disease. After World War II, the reported incidence of syphilis declined each year until the late 1950s, when it began to rise again. Today, the disease is one of the most common sexually transmitted diseases in the United States.

Etiologic Agent

The etiologic agent of syphilis is *Treponema pallidum*, a spiral bacterium (spirochete). The organism does not survive in blood stored at 4°C for more than 72 hours, but does remain viable when frozen.

Transmission

Syphilis is transmitted primarily through sexual contact. For *T. pallidum* to be spread by transfusion, the donor would have to be in the short period of time when the spirochete can be found in the blood, and the blood would have to be transfused within 72 hours. When vein-to-vein transfusions were performed, transmission in this manner was much more possible. Only one case of transfusion-transmitted syphilis has been recorded since modern storage techniques have been developed.[2,22]

Incidence

The availability of antibiotics and education was believed to have brought syphilis under control. Until 1986, the national rate of infectious syphilis was low, approximately 10 cases per 100,000 population. Since that time, the rate has increased dramatically. In 1987, the rate increased by 31%, and in many areas the rise continues. Illicit drug use has been cited as a factor in the increase because men and women have admitted to the exchange of sex for drugs.

Pathology

Syphilis infection can be divided into stages. During the primary stage, a chancre sore develops. The sore is painless and resolves within a few weeks. If the individual is not treated, the infection moves into the secondary stage. This stage may present with a generalized rash and is followed by a period of latency without symptoms in the untreated individual. Tertiary syphilis is the final stage of infection and may take on one of three forms: neurosyphilis, cardiovascular syphilis, or a form that involves skin, bones, and viscera.

Serology and Laboratory Testing

Using darkfield microscopy, it is possible to detect *T. pallidum* in direct smears from lesion material. Serologic detection is also possible because specific and nonspecific antibodies develop during the course of syphilis infection. The common abbreviation used for such tests is STS (serologic test for syphilis).

Nontreponemal serologic tests detect an antibody-like substance found in infected people. These include the rapid plasma reagin and the Venereal Disease Research Laboratory test. Most screening tests detect reagin, the name by which the antibody-like substance is known. The basic antigen in these tests is an extract called cardiolipin. Screening tests may be negative in early and latent syphilis infections and are not specific. Treponemal antibody tests are used to confirm positive screening tests because there are several causes of biologic false-positive results with the screening tests, including pregnancy and the presence of autoimmune disease, such as rheumatoid arthritis. Although screening tests should become negative with adequate treatment, the treponemal tests usually remain positive indefinitely. Box 15-9 lists the tests used in diagnosing syphilis.

Blood donors are screened using one of the methods described. An automated method, the PK-TP, is commonly used in blood centers. Donor samples that test positive on the screening test are then subjected to a confirmatory test. Such testing, however, does not prevent transmission of syphilis because the serologic tests do not become positive until after the period of infectivity has already passed.

Through the years, a great deal of controversy has arisen over the need for syphilis testing of blood donors. Although the AABB dropped its recommendation that

> **BOX 15-9**
>
> ## Tests Used to Detect Syphilis
>
> **NONTREPONEMAL SCREENING TESTS**
> - Rapid plasma reagin (RPR)
> - Venereal Disease Research Laboratory (VDRL)
> - PK-TP (Olympus automated test)
>
> **TREPONEMAL CONFIRMATORY TESTS**
> - Fluorescent antibody test absorbed for *Treponema pallidum*
> - Microhemagglutination test for *Treponema pallidum*

donors be tested in 1978, the Food and Drug Administration kept its requirement. This decision was reinforced by the Presidential Commission on the Human Immunodeficiency Virus Epidemic, which recommended that surrogate testing, including syphilis testing, be done to prevent those at risk for HIV from donating blood. The AABB has now reinstated syphilis testing in the most recent *Standards for Blood Banks and Transfusion* Services as a result of this recommendation.

Prevention

Blood donors are questioned about personal infection or contact with people who have been diagnosed with venereal disease and are deferred for a specified amount of time after such exposure. As with most sexually transmitted diseases, education is a key factor in prevention of syphilis infection. Tougher laws on prostitution and drugs also may play important roles in decreasing its spread.

Lyme Disease (Borreliosis)

History

As people from the city have made trips to the country, there has been an increase in the incidence of borreliosis. Cases have been reported from 41 states, and the disease is now the primary tick-transmitted infection in the United States.

Etiologic Agent

The causative agent of borreliosis is *Borrelia burgdorferi*, a spirochete. The organism survives storage in blood components and in studies has been found to live in blood stored at 1°C to 6°C, in frozen plasma, and in platelet concentrates.

Transmission

B. burgdorferi is spread by the deer tick, *Ixodes dammini*. Transmission by blood transfusion is possible.[23]

Pathology

Lyme disease is very difficult to identify and not all cases report a tick bite. Infection is associated with a host of symptoms, which range from malaise, fever, and fatigue early in the disease to severe arthritic, neurologic, and cardiac manifestations in untreated cases.

Serology and Laboratory Testing

Although antibody does develop to *B. burgdorferi*, the test that detects this antibody is unreliable. Isolation of the organism through culture is also difficult because a special medium is required.

Prevention

Because no reliable test for detection of infection exists, the AABB and the American Red Cross have made some recommendations regarding prevention of transfusion-transmitted Lyme disease[2]:

- Because people with Lyme disease are symptomatic, specific questions to detect infection with *B. burgdorferi* are not necessary.
- Testing for evidence of infection with *B. burgdorferi* is not recommended.
- Health-care workers should take note as to whether an individual diagnosed with Lyme borreliosis has donated blood; if so, the collection or transfusion facility should be notified.
- After adequate treatment, people who have been diagnosed with Lyme disease may resume donating.

Yersinia Enterocolitica

History

One of the few organisms that flourishes in the environment of stored blood is **Yersinia enterocolitica**, a gram-negative bacillus. Between April 1987 and May 1989, seven cases of transfusion-associated *Y. enterocolitica* sepsis were investigated by the CDC.[21] All seven cases involved the transfusion of red blood cells (RBCs), occurred in seven different states, and were unrelated. None of the contaminated units was visibly tainted. As a result of these initial cases and several more that have been reported since 1989, blood donor centers have had to reevaluate the procedures for donor screening, blood collection, and blood storage.

Etiologic Agent

Y. enterocolitica is a facultative anaerobic, gram-negative bacillus. Although it grows best at higher temperatures, the organism is known to grow well in refrigeration. In addition, the growth of some strains of the organism is enhanced in an iron-rich environment. As the organism grows, it produces a deadly endotoxin, which can reach dangerous levels at 21 or more days' storage.[24–26] The organism has been isolated from humans in many countries of the world but is most prevalent in cooler climates.

Transmission

Transmission of *Y. enterocolitica* to humans is believed to occur by a common vehicle or by the fecal–oral route, primarily from animal to humans. Person-to-person transmission through transfusion is well documented. Vehicles of transmission include milk, water, tofu, bean sprouts, and turkey chow mein.[24]

Pathology

Illness with *Y. enterocolitica* is usually short lived, lasting 5 to 14 days, but may persist for several months. The organism can be isolated from the stool for 2 to 14 weeks after detection. Enterocolitis is seen with diarrhea, low-grade fever, and abdominal pain. Most cases are not associated with bacteremia. Asymptomatic infection also is seen. Bacteremia, when present, is associated with a reported case-fatality rate of 34% to 50%. The fact that the organism can be spread by blood transfusion from apparently healthy donors lends evidence to support the existence of an asymptomatic bacteremia as well.

Prevention

The primary way to prevent transmission of *Y. enterocolitica* transmission is through careful donor questioning about recent illness. A number of other suggestions have been proposed, as listed in Box 15-10, but none of these is reasonable at this time.

BOX 15-10

Proposals to Lessen Risk of Transfusion-transmitted *Yersinia* Infection

Screening of all blood donors by questioning about recent gastrointestinal illness

Reduction of the dating period of blood to 21 days

Testing all donor units older than 25 days for the presence of endotoxin or for the presence of bacteria

PARASITIC INFECTIONS

Malaria

History

The transmission of malaria through blood was demonstrated in 1884, and the first case of transfusion-transmitted malaria was recorded in 1911. Although the disease is endemic in tropical areas and is rarely seen in the United States, the incidence of transfusion-transmitted malaria has risen. Factors contributing to this rise are the ease of travel and immigration.[2,27]

Etiologic Agent

There are four important species of malaria: *Plasmodium vivax*, *Plasmodium falciparum*, *Plasmodium malariae*, and *Plasmodium ovale*. These species are the only ones known to infect humans. The life cycles of the plasmodium take place both in the mosquito and in humans.

There appear to be species-specific receptors that allow plasmodia to enter RBCs. In studies it has been shown that $En(a^-)$ RBCs and Duffy-negative $(Fy([a^-b^-]))$ RBCs are resistant to infection.

Incidence

Malarial organisms have a worldwide distribution and are endemic in areas with the *Anopheles* mosquito and human reservoirs. Transfusion-transmitted malaria is particularly high in Bangladesh, Brazil, India, Iran, and Mexico. In the United States, close to three cases of transfusion-transmitted malaria are reported per year.

Transmission

The plasmodia are transmitted to humans through an infected female *Anopheles* mosquito. Other types of transmission include accidental transfusion of infected blood or blood components or transplantation of infected organs, reuse of needles contaminated with the organism, and congenital transmission. *P. falciparum* malaria has been transmitted by blood stored for 19 days and parasites may even survive well in frozen blood.[28] The frequency of posttransfusion malaria has been estimated to vary from less than 0.2 cases per million in nonendemic countries to 50 or more cases per million in endemic countries.[29]

Pathology

Infection by way of the vector usually is not evident until the organism has gone through several life cycles. The rupture of RBCs that results from an asexual phase of the plasmodia life cycle releases toxic products and produces the fever and chills that are characteristic of malarial infection. The infected person's temperature may spike to as high as 105°F. These symptoms may last for 4 to 6 hours and recur at regular intervals.

The morbidity and mortality associated with malarial infections are particularly severe in splenectomized patients, immunosuppressed patients, and patients under treatment for malignancies, sometimes with early cerebral involvement or even death.

Transfusion-transmitted malaria compared with natural infection often has a short incubation period because there is no preerythrocytic phase.

Serology and Laboratory Testing

Routine serologic screening of asymptomatic people, such as blood donors, is impractical, as is direct examination of blood smears from these people. There are, however, serologic tests that can be used to identify infection. These include indirect hemagglutination, enzyme-linked immunosorbent assay (ELISA), and indirect fluorescent antibody tests.

In recent years, flow cytometry has been used to identify infected RBCs. DNA in infected cells will stain, whereas normal RBCs that do not contain DNA will not.

Prevention

Although much research has gone into the development of a malarial vaccine, one has not yet been developed. Travelers to endemic areas usually take prophylactic drugs (i.e., quinine, chloroquine); however, strains resistant to these drugs have emerged. A deferral of 6 months or 3 years is indicated for travel or living in a malarial area. Policies recommended by the AABB include the following:

- Travel in an endemic area, as defined by the CDC, indicates a need for a 12-month deferral after return to a nonendemic area, provided that the person is symptom free and has not taken antimalarial drugs. People diagnosed with malaria may donate 3 years after becoming asymptomatic or after cessation of treatment.
- People who have taken antimalarial drugs must wait 3 years after cessation of therapy, provided that they have not returned to an endemic area and have been asymptomatic in the interim.
- Immigrants or visitors from an endemic area may donate 3 years after departure from the endemic area, provided that they have been asymptomatic in the interim.

In the United States, to prevent malaria from entering the blood supply, donors are questioned about travel and prophylactic medication. In countries where malaria is endemic, different methods must be used to find blood donors. In these countries, serologic methods play a much more important role, as does pretreatment with antimalarial drugs.

Chagas Disease

History

Chagas disease, also known as *Trypanosoma cruzi infection*, is found only in the western hemisphere. It is important that it not be confused with other forms of trypanosomiasis, such as African sleeping sickness. Trypanosomiasis is normally found in rural areas, but as more people move into urban areas to seek employment, the disease is appearing in these locales. Imported and indigenous cases of Chagas disease have been reported in the United States.

Etiologic Agent

T. cruzi is a parasitic blood and tissue protozoan. The organism can be found in the cells of cardiac muscle and other tissues, as well as in the blood in the form of a trypanosome. *T. cruzi* is a 15- to 20-mm protozoan and is propelled by a flagellum. *T. cruzi* can be found in many kinds of wild and domestic animals. In the United States, the most important reservoirs are opossums and raccoons.

Incidence

In excess of 12 million people live in areas endemic for *T. cruzi*.[30] Approximately one third of those living between northern Argentina and southern Mexico are infected with the organism. The disease is most commonly seen in children younger than 5 years of age. The infection is often severe in these people. The organism can survive for at least 10 days in refrigerated, citrated blood and has been recovered from frozen plasma.

Transmission

The organism is transmitted to humans from infected animals by the bite of the reduviid bug (bedbugs). Genera of reduviids include *Triatoma* and *Rhodnius*. These insects are bloodsucking, and while feeding, they deposit infected feces. *T. cruzi* is able to penetrate the skin and infect the bitten individual. Reduviid bugs are associated with dirty and crowded conditions.

Transmission also may occur by needle stick and congenitally. Blood transmission is the second most important mechanism of transmission. Risks of becoming infected after transfusion from a seropositive donor vary from 12% to 50%.[2] This is a real problem in some parts of the western hemisphere, given that in these areas seroprevalence may reach as high as 60%.

Pathology

Infection with *T. cruzi* is lifelong, and clinical symptoms appear eventually. At the site of infection, erythematous areas known as chagomas are produced. Incubation is from 4 to 116 days.[8] Organisms appear in the blood at about 10 days. General malaise, chills, high fever, muscular aches and pains, and exhaustion are symptoms of infection. Later in the disease, lymphadenopathy and splenomegaly may be seen. Cure is possible with early treatment; without such treatment, a chronic infection may ensue.

Serology and Laboratory Testing

Infection with *T. cruzi* results in a strong immune response. IgM antibodies are formed, which can serve as serologic markers of infection. Procedures such as complement fixation, indirect hemagglutination, and ELISA have been used to diagnose Chagas disease. The Machado test is a test used to diagnose Chagas disease and uses as antigen an extract of the spleen of puppies severely infected with *T. cruzi*.

Prevention

Obviously, eradication of the reduviid bug as vector would help in preventing the spread of the disease. In addition, living in close contact with animal reservoirs should be avoided. To prevent the transmission of *T. cruzi* in endemic areas, serologic testing of blood donors is necessary. Those with positive serology should be permanently deferred as blood donors.

Toxoplasmosis

History

The organisms causing *toxoplasmosis* were first discovered in a North African rodent and have been observed in numerous birds and mammals around the world, including humans. In the United States, it is not uncommon to see a high rate of seropositivity.

Etiologic Agent

Toxoplasmosis is caused by *Toxoplasma gondii*, a parasite of cosmopolitan distribution. It is able to develop in a wide variety of hosts, including the domestic cat and certain other feline animals. The organism exists in three forms: trophozoite, cyst, and oocyst. The trophozoite is the invasive form that is responsible for the acute symptoms of the disease. Infection occurs from the ingestion of the oocyst.[30]

Incidence

Seropositivity in the United States varies from 20% to 70%, and congenital toxoplasmosis is estimated to occur in 0.5 to 5 cases per 1,000 live births.[3] The highest rate of infection is found in Parisian women who eat undercooked or raw meat. Approximately 50% of the children of these women are infected as well.

Transmission

Domestic cats are the source of the disease, and they are the only animal in which the entire life cycle of the organism takes place. Oocysts are deposited into the feces of the animal. Humans become infected when they ingest meat that is contaminated with feline fecal material. The organism also may be ingested through contaminated water or raw milk. Transplacental transmission also occurs; however, congenital infection is only found in women who acquire the primary infection during pregnancy. The earlier the mother becomes infected, the more serious the sequelae are for the fetus. Infection is also possible through blood transfusion or organ transplantation.

Pathology

Local or generalized lymphadenopathy is the most common clinical manifestation of infection with *T. gondii*. Fever, malaise, and a rash may occur. The symptoms are mononucleosis like, but asymptomatic adenopathy is the most common clinical symptom in adults. Spontaneous resolution usually occurs within a few months.

   Infection is a special problem in immunosuppressed people, and the infection may be fatal. AIDS patients are particularly susceptible to reactivation of a latent infection.

Serology and Laboratory Testing

Testing for the organism can be accomplished by indirect fluorescent antibody, hemagglutination, and ELISA. The antibodies are detectable in approximately 2 weeks and rise to a high level that persists for many months.

Prevention

Although the transmission of *T. gondii* is not frequent, screening of blood donors for antibody to the organism would aid in preventing transmission of the organism. At this time, such screening does not seem warranted. Prevention of infection during pregnancy is very important, and pregnant women are advised to refrain from any contact with cat feces, such as would occur when cleaning a litter box.

Babesiosis

History

Babesiosis in humans was first recognized and reported in Yugoslavia in 1957.[8] Cases have since been reported in North America. The first transfusion-transmitted case was reported in 1979, although a suspected transmission was seen in 1976 in Georgia.[31,32]

Etiologic Agent

In the United States, *Babesia microti* is responsible for babesiosis, whereas in Europe, *Babesia divergens* is the primary agent. *B. divergens* is a parasite of cattle, and *B. microti* is found in rodents.

Incidence

Babesiosis in Europe has occurred primarily in people who were splenectomized, but this has not been the case in the United States. Cases in the United States have been associated with people living in or visiting the Cape Cod area. There also have been cases reported in Georgia and in California.

Transmission

The organisms are transmitted by ticks. In the United States, the principal vector is the northern deer tick, *I. dammini*. The European vector is the *Dermacentor* species; this tick has been eliminated from the United States.

   Transmission through blood transfusion also is possible. The organisms can remain infective in blood drawn from donors with subclinical disease even after 14 days of storage. In the two documented cases of transfusion-transmitted babesiosis, the donors had been in the Cape Cod area before the donations.

Pathology

Babesiosis has an incubation period of approximately 1 month and can be found in the blood for 4 to 6 months. Most cases are asymptomatic in nonsplenectomized patients. When symptoms are seen, they include malaise, fever, headache, chills, sweating, fatigue, myalgia, and weakness. Splenectomy and administration of corticosteroids and immunosuppressive drugs contribute to the morbidity and mortality of the infection.[33]

Serology and Laboratory Testing

Antibodies to *Babesia* occur and can be detected by indirect immunofluorescent antibody tests. Specific testing, however, is limited by the availability of the *B. microti* antigen. Antibody titers begin to decrease after a few months.

Prevention

It is not feasible to screen blood donors for infection with *Babesia* either through examination of blood smears or antibody testing. Excluding donors from endemic areas also has been shown not to be reasonable because seropositivity rates from endemic areas are not necessarily greater than those from nonendemic areas.

Leishmaniasis

Leishmania tropica is a common parasite in the Middle East. Its usual host is the desert gerbil, and it is spread by the bite of the sandfly (*Phlebotomus*). The organism normally causes cutaneous infection, but in 1991, soldiers returning form the Gulf War were found to have visceral leishmaniasis. As a result, a deferral was instituted for those who had traveled to or visited Saudi Arabia, Kuwait, Iraq, Oman, Yemen, Qatar, Bahrain, or the United Arab Emirates on or after August 1, 1990. They were deferred from donating until January 1, 1993.[34,35] Further study may result in additional guidelines for donor deferral.

Although transmission of *L. tropica* by blood transfusion had not been reported in 1990, cases of transmission of *Leishmania donovani*, resulting in an infection known as kalaazar, had been documented. Because a great number of military personnel donate, the deferral was instituted because the blood banking community wanted to do everything possible to protect the blood supply from donors infected with *L. tropica*.

SUMMARY

Transmission of disease by transfusion presents a significant problem. The risk of contracting an infection (or of some other type of reaction) must always be weighed against the benefit. The blood supply is safer than it has been in many years; however, the small chance of infection by transfusion continues to spur research into better screening and testing procedures, as well as techniques for purifying blood once collected.

A serious side effect of increased testing with more sensitive tests is the number of healthy donors who are lost because of false-positive test results. Considering an already shrinking donor population, this has had a profound impact on many blood centers. In addition, the expense of more testing is ultimately reflected in additional and higher costs to blood centers, hospitals, and patients.

There almost certainly will be other infectious agents in the future that will threaten the safety of the blood supply. One must remember that a little more than 20 years ago, no one had heard of HIV-1 or HIV-2, HTLV-I or HTLV-II, or HCV. Blood banks must continue to strive to do whatever is possible to detect such agents and to eliminate or reduce the potential for their transmission by blood.

Review Questions

1. Which of the following plays an important part in prevention of transfusion-transmitted disease?
   a. donor history
   b. testing
   c. self-exclusion
   d. all of the above

2. Which of the following is not usually spread parenterally?
   a. hepatitis A
   b. hepatitis B
   c. hepatitis C
   d. hepatitis D

3. Blood banks began testing for the hepatitis B core antibody and performing ALT levels as a surrogate test for:
   a. hepatitis A
   b. hepatitis B
   c. hepatitis C
   d. hepatitis D

4. Which of the following is an incomplete virus and is present only when hepatitis B infection is present?
   a. hepatitis A
   b. hepatitis B
   c. hepatitis C
   d. hepatitis D

5. Which of the following is true of hepatitis B vaccination?
   a. the vaccine is made in a bacterium
   b. the vaccine is made in a yeast
   c. the vaccine can transmit HIV
   d. the vaccine is given in a single-shot dose

6. Which of the following tests is positive during the window period of infection with hepatitis B?
   a. hepatitis B surface antigen
   b. hepatitis B surface antibody
   c. hepatitis B core antibody
   d. hepatitis C antibody

(continued)

REVIEW QUESTIONS (continued)

7. HIV is pathogenic for which of the following cells?
   a. T4 cell
   b. T8 cell
   c. monocytes
   d. nerve cells

8. Which of the following products does not transmit hepatitis?
   a. packed red cells
   b. fresh frozen plasma
   c. platelets
   d. plasma protein fraction

9. HIV seropositivity is highly prevalent in all of the following except:
   a. intravenous drug users
   b. homosexuals
   c. hemophiliacs
   d. health-care workers

10. Which of the following is not true of retroviruses?
    a. they contain reverse transcriptase
    b. they contain identical strands of RNA
    c. they contain identical strands of DNA
    d. they include oncoviruses and lentiviruses

11. Which of the following tests are used to supplement a reactive enzyme-linked immunosorbent assay test for HIV?
    a. Western blot
    b. immunofluorescent assay
    c. rapid plasma reagin
    d. both a and b

12. Most individuals infected with HIV acquired it through:
    a. blood transfusion
    b. sexual contact
    c. perinatally
    d. none of the above

13. Cytomegalovirus-positive blood is dangerous for which of the following?
    a. pregnant women who are seronegative
    b. immunosuppressed individuals
    c. neonates
    d. all of the above

14. Individuals who have received injections of human growth hormone are permanently deferred from blood donation because of the possible transmission of an agent responsible for which of the following diseases?
    a. AIDS
    b. hepatitis
    c. Creutzfeldt Jakob–disease
    d. infectious mononucleosis

15. Which of the following organisms grows well in the cold and especially likes the iron-rich environment of stored blood?
    a. *Escherichia coli*
    b. hepatitis B virus
    c. malarial organisms
    d. *Yersinia enterocolitica*

16. Which of the following explains why bacterial contamination of blood is rarely a problem?
    a. the cold storage temperature of blood is not conducive to bacterial growth
    b. the citrate in the anticoagulant is not conducive to bacterial growth
    c. the arm preparation ensures that most bacteria are removed
    d. all of the above

17. Lyme disease is spread by:
    a. a mosquito
    b. a tick
    c. water
    d. none of the above

18. Donor history is the primary way the United States excludes units that may be infected with which of the following?
    a. HIV
    b. HTLV-I
    c. syphilis
    d. malaria

19. Chagas disease can be transmitted by blood infected with:
    a. *Treponema pallidum*
    b. *Mycoplasma pneumoniae*
    c. *Yersinia enterocolitica*
    d. *Trypanosoma cruzi*

20. Which of the following has dramatically reduced the likelihood of window period transmission?
    a. donor questioning
    b. implementation of NAT
    c. Western blot testing
    d. none of the above

REFERENCES

1. Lennette EH. *Laboratory Diagnosis of Viral Infections.* 2nd ed. New York: Marcel Dekker; 1992.
2. American Red Cross Home Page. https://crossnet. redcross.org/home/virus.htm. November 1997.
3. Jaundice following yellow fever vaccination [editorial]. *JAMA.* 1942; 119: 110.
4. Blumberg BS, Alter HJ, Visnich S. A new antigen in leukemia sera. *JAMA.* 1965; 191: 541.
5. Kobayashi H, Tsuzuki M, Koshimizu K, et al. Susceptibility of hepatitis B virus to disinfectants or heat. *J Clin Microbiol.* 1984; 20: 214.
6. Evans AS, ed. *Viral Infections of Humans: Epidemiology and Control.* New York: Plenum Medical Book Company; 1989.
7. Stevens CE, Taylor PE, Long MJ, et al. Yeast-recombinant hepatitis B vaccine: efficacy with hepatitis B immune globulin in prevention of perinatal hepatitis B transmission. *JAMA.* 1987; 257: 2612–2616.

8. Turgeon ML. Transfusion acquired infectious diseases. In: *Fundamentals of Immunohematology*. Philadelphia: Lea and Febiger; 1989.

9. Zanetti AR, Ferroni P, Magliano EM, et al. Perinatal transmission of hepatitis B virus and the HBV associated delta antigen from mother to offspring in northern Italy. *J Med Virol*. 1982; 9: 139.

10. Wasley A, Grytdal S, Gallagher K. Surveillance for acute viral hepatitis—United States, 2006. *MMWR Surveill Summ*. 2008; 57: 1.

11. Alter MJ. Epidemiology of hepatitis C. *Hepatology*. 1997; 26: 62S.

12. Gust ID. Enterically transmitted non-A, non-B hepatitis A virus infections. In: *Testing in the Blood Bank*. Raritan, New Jersey: Ortho Diagnostics; 1988.

13. Obrien TR, George JR, Holmberg SD. Human immunodeficiency virus type 2 infection in the United States: epidemiology, diagnosis, and public health implications. *JAMA*. 1992; 267: 2775.

14. Center for Disease Control and Prevention. *CDC National AIDS HIV/AIDS Surveillance Report*. Atlanta, Georgia: Center for Disease Control and Prevention; June 1997; 9(1).

15. Centers for Disease Control and Prevention. Interpretive criteria used to report Western blot results for HIV-1 antibody testing: United States. *MMWR Morb Mortal Wkly Rep*. 1991; 40: 692.

16. Poiesz BJ, Ruscetti FW, Gazdar AF, et al. Detection and isolation of type-C retrovirus particles from fresh and cultured lymphocytes of a patient with cutaneous T-cell lymphoma. *Proc Natl Acad Sci U S A*. 1980; 77: 7415.

17. Kalyanaraman VS, Sarngadharan MG, Robert-Guroff M, et al. A new type of subtype of human T-cell leukemia virus (HTLV-II) associated with a T-cell variant of hairy cell leukemia. *Science*. 1982; 218: 571.

18. Lal RB, Heneine W, Rudolph DL, et al. Synthetic peptide-based immunoassays for distinguishing between human T-cell lymphotrophic virus type I and type II infections in seropositive individuals. *J Clin Microbiol*. 1991; 29: 2253.

19. Calisher CH. West Nile virus in the New World: appearance, persistence, and adaptation to a new econiche—an opportunity taken. *Viral Immunol*. 2000; 13(4): 411–414.

20. http://www.cdc.gov/eid/content/13/8/1264.htm. 2009.

21. *Chemical and Biological Weapons: Possession and Programs Past and Present*. James Martin Center for Nonproliferation Studies, Middlebury College; April 9, 2002.

22. van der Sluis JJ, ten Kate FJ, Vuzevski VD, et al. Transfusion syphilis, survival of *Treponema pallidum* in stored donor blood. *Vox Sang*. 1985; 49: 390.

23. Johnson SE, Swaminathan B, Moore P, et al. *Borrelia burgdorferi*: survival in experimentally infected human blood processed for transfusion. *J Infect Dis*. 1990; 162: 557.

24. Woernle CH, et al. Update: *Yersinia enterocolitica* bacteremia and endotoxin shock associated with red blood cell transfusion—United States. *MMWR Morb Mortal Wkly Rep*. 1991; 40: 176.

25. Tipple MA, Bland LA, Murphy JJ, et al. Sepsis associated with transfusion of red cells contaminated with *Yersinia enterocolitica*. *Transfusion*. 1990; 30: 207.

26. Centers for Disease Control (CDC). Update: *Yersinia enterocolitica* bacteremia and endotoxin shock associated with red blood cell transfusion—United States, 1991. *MMWR*. 1991; 40: 176–178.

27. Harmening D. *Modern Blood Banking and Transfusion Practices*. 2nd ed. Philadelphia: FA Davis; 1989.

28. DeSilva M, Contreras M, Barbara J. Two cases of transfusion-transmitted malaria (TTM) in the UK [letter]. *Transfusion*. 1988; 28: 86.

29. Kark JA. Malaria transmitted by blood transfusion. In: Tabor E, ed. *Infectious Complications of Blood Transfusion*. New York: Academic Press; 1982: 93.

30. Bruce-Chwatt LJ. Transfusion associated parasitic infections. In: Dodd RY, Barker LF, eds. *Infection, Immunity and Blood Transfusion*. New York: Alan R. Liss; 1985: 101.

31. Bell DR. *Manson's Tropical Diseases*. 19th ed. London: Bailliere-Tindall; 1987.

32. Marcus LC, Valigorsky JM, Fanning WL, et al. A case report of transfusion-transmitted babesiosis. *JAMA*. 1982; 248: 465.

33. Smith RP, Evans AT, Popovsky M, et al. Transfusion-acquired babesiosis and failure of antibiotic treatment. *JAMA*. 1986; 256: 2726.

34. American Association of Blood Banks: CDC issues update on leishmaniasis. *Blood Bank Week*. 1992; 9: 3.

35. Centers for Disease Control and Prevention. *Leishmania in military personnel returning from the Persian Gulf* [memo]. Washington, DC; 1991.

ADDITIONAL READINGS

Allain JP. *Retrovirus Learning Guide*. Abbott Park, IL: Abbott Diagnostics Educational Services; June 1988.

Alter HJ. *The Universe of Non-A, Non-B Hepatitis, Update: Testing in the Blood Bank*. Raritan, New Jersey: Ortho Diagnostics; 1988.

Badon SJ, Fister RD, Cable RG. Survival of *Borrelia burgdorferi* in blood products. *Transfusion*. 1989; 29: 581.

Barbara JA, Contreras M. Infectious complications of blood transfusion: viruses. *Br Med J*. 1990; 300: 450.

Bradley DW. *Editor's Note, Update: Testing in the Blood Bank*. Raritan, New Jersey: Ortho Diagnostics; 1989.

Busch MP, Eble BE, Khayam-Bashi H, et al. Evaluation of screened blood donations for human immunodeficiency virus type 1 infection by culture and DNA amplification of pooled cells. *N Engl J Med*. 1991; 325: 1.

Carson JL. The risks of blood transfusion: the relative influence of acquired immune deficiency syndrome and non-A, non-B hepatitis. *Am J Med*. 1992; 92: 45.

Centers for Disease Control (CDC). Transfusion malaria: serologic identification of infected donors—Pennsylvania, Georgia. *MMWR Morb Mortal Wkly Rep*. 1983; 32: 222.

Centers for Disease Control (CDC). The HIV/AIDS epidemic: the first 10 years. *MMWR Morb Mortal Wkly Rep*. 1991; 40: 357.

Centers for Disease Control (CDC). Update: serologic testing for human T-lymphotropic virus type 1—United States, 1989 and 1990. *MMWR Morb Mortal Wkly Rep*. 1992; 41(15): 259.

Coslett GD, Hojvat S, eds. *Hepatitis Learning Guide*. Abbott Park, IL: Abbott Diagnostics Educational Services; 1988.

Cotton P. Immune boosters disappoint AIDS researchers [Medical News and Perspectives]. *JAMA*. 1991; 266: 1613.

Dodd RY. Screening for hepatitis infectivity among blood donors: a model for blood safety? *Arch Pathol Lab Med*. 1989; 113: 227.

Hadler SC. Vaccines to prevent hepatitis B and hepatitis A virus infections. *Infect Dis Clin North Am*. 1990; 4:29.

Hoffman SL. Prevention of malaria [editorial]. *JAMA*. 1991; 265: 398.

Howard RJ. *Infectious Risks in Surgery*. Norwalk, CT: Appleton and Lange; 1991.

Koff RS. *Viral Hepatitis*. New York: John Wiley & Sons; 1978.

Lackritz EM. Imported *Plasmodium falciparum* malaria in American travelers to Africa. *JAMA*. 1991; 265: 383.

Nadelman RB, Sherer C, Mack L, et al. Survival of *Borrelia burgdorferi* in human blood stored under blood banking conditions. *Transfusion*. 1990; 30: 298.

Perrillo RP. *Perspectives on Viral Hepatitis, Hepatitis Information Center*. Abbott Park, IL: *Abbott Laboratories, Diagnostics Division*; 1981.

Polesky HF, Hanson MR. Transfusion associated hepatitis C virus (non-A, non-B) infections. *Arch Pathol Lab Med*. 1989; 113: 232.

Prentice M, Cope D. Infectious complications of blood transfusion [letter]. *Br Med J*. 1990; 300: 678.

Purcell RH, *Blood-borne Non-A, Non-B Hepatitis, Update: Testing in the Blood Bank*. Raritan, New Jersey: Ortho Diagnostics; 1988.

Sloand EM, et al. HIV testing: state of the art. *JAMA*. 1991; 266: 2861.

Tegtmeier FE. Posttransfusion cytomegalovirus infections. *Arch Pathol Lab Med*. 1989; 113: 236.

HEMOLYTIC DISEASE OF THE FETUS AND NEWBORN

SUZANNE H. BUTCH

OBJECTIVES

After completion of this chapter, the reader will be able to:

1. Describe the cause of hemolytic disease of the fetus and newborn (HDFN).

2. Identify the antibodies most responsible for severe HDFN.

3. Describe serologic testing for determining fetal risk for HDFN.

4. Describe nonserologic methods of monitoring fetal risk for HDFN.

5. Describe the attributes of blood components used for perinatal transfusions.

6. Describe cord blood testing.

7. List two reasons that ABO HDFN is usually mild.

8. Explain the four goals of an exchange transfusion in the neonate.

9. Identify the indications for administration of Rh immune globulin (RHIG) in the prevention of HDFN.

10. Describe two methods of quantitating a massive fetomaternal hemorrhage.

11. Identify two causes of perinatal thrombocytopenia.

12. Describe the treatment of perinatal thrombocytopenia.

KEY WORDS

Amniocentesis
Bilirubin
Cord blood
Cordocentesis
Critical titer
Exchange transfusion
Fetomaternal hemorrhage
Flow cytometry
Hemolytic disease of the fetus and newborn (HDFN)
Hydrops fetalis
Immune thrombocytopenic purpura
Intrauterine transfusion
Jaundice
Kernicterus
Kleihauer–Betke
Middle cerebral artery (MCA) Doppler
Neonatal alloimmune thrombocytopenia
Percutaneous umbilical cord blood sampling
Rh immune globulin
Rosette test

In 1609, the popular press published the first report of a Paris midwife's description of twins with hemolytic disease of the newborn.[1] One infant was grossly edematous (hydropic) and still born. The second was severely jaundiced (kernicterus), developed neurologic symptoms, and died a few days later. Levine et al. determined that D of the Rh system was a major cause of the disease.[2] Once the cause was identified, risk assessment, treatments, and prevention strategies were developed. A list of significant events in the detection and management of *hemolytic disease of the fetus and newborn (HDFN)* is shown in Box 16-1. Today, HDNF due to anti-D can be prevented by the use of Rh immune globulin. In addition, there are less invasive methods of determining the risk for HDFN. Improvements in treatment have made intrauterine and *exchange transfusion* uncommon. However, these lifesaving procedures continue to be needed for those with severe HDFN.

BOX 16-1

Significant Events in HDFN

Description of HDFN, 1609

Rh system identified, Landsteiner and Weiner, 1940

Anti-D identified as cause of most HDFN, Diamond, 1941

Neonatal exchange transfusion, Wallerstein, 1946

Early delivery, Armitage and Mollison, 1953

Acid elution method for identifying fetal red cells in maternal blood, Kleihauer, Braun, and Betke, 1957

Phototherapy for hyperbilirubinemia, Cremer and Perryman, 1958

Graph of bilirubin in amniotic fluid and intrauterine transfusion, Liley, 1961–1963

Postpartum Rh immune globulin, Freda, Gorman, and Polack; Clarke et al., 1963–1964

Ultrasonography, Donald and Abdulla, 1967

Antepartum Rh immune globulin, Bowman, 1978

Rosette screening test for fetomaternal hemorrhage, Sebring and Polesky, 1982

Extended Liley curve to 14 to 40 weeks gestation, Queenan et al., 1993

DNA from amniocytes used for fetal RHD determination, Bennett et al., 1993

Maternal plasma used for fetal RHD determination, Lo et al., 1998

Measure risk of anemia by cerebral artery blood flow by Doppler, Marl et al., 2000

MATERNAL ALLOIMMUNIZATION

Antibodies that cause hemolytic disease of the newborn are IgG antibodies made in response to red cell transfusion or exposure to fetal red cells during a prior or current pregnancy. As early as 38 days gestation (D antigen), antigens develop on the fetal red cells.[3] As the pregnancy progresses, small amounts of fetal cells can be found routinely in the amniotic fluid and in the maternal blood stream. Color Plate C-5 shows a fetus and placenta. Color Plate C-6 shows the fetal and maternal circulation. Maternal exposure to fetal red cells can occur throughout a pregnancy, and variable amounts of fetal red cells can be transferred to the maternal circulation during abortion, amniocentesis, chorionic villus sampling, trauma, and at delivery. Color Plate C-7 displays how fetal cells can gain access to maternal circulation through tears in the placenta. The exact amount of red cells needed to cause alloimmunization is not known, but as little as 0.1 mL of D-positive fetal cells have been shown to cause alloimmunization.[4] Because the risk of exposure to a significant number of fetal red cells to cause sensitization usually occurs later in the pregnancy, the fetus is most often not affected in the first pregnancy.

Currently, the most common antibodies found to cause HDN are anti-D, anti-K anti-c, anti-C, and anti-Fy[a].[5] However, any IgG antibody is capable of crossing the placenta and harming fetal red cells. The presence of maternal antibodies may cause no HDFN or the effect may range from a weakly positive direct antiglobulin test (DAT) to the need for exchange transfusion. Table 16-1 lists common antibodies and to their likelihood of causing HDFN.

Approximately 85% of D-negative individuals exposed to 200 mL of D-positive red cells will produce anti-D. Even after repeated challenges, approximately 7% of D-negative individuals will not produce anti-D when exposed to D-positive red cells.[6] Because the maternal exposure to fetal red cells is likely to be very small (<0.1 mL), the immunization rate in the first pregnancy is approximately 16%. From 1.5% to 2% of D-negative women with D-positive infants will develop anti-D at the time of their delivery, another 7% will be sensitized by 6 months, and alloimmunization will be detected in the next pregnancy for another 7%.[6] When the infant and mother are ABO incompatible, the rate of sensitization is reduced to 1% to 2%.[4] This is likely due to the destruction of fetal red cells by maternal anti-A and anti-B.

PATHOPHYSIOLOGY OF HDFN

When the mother has IgG antibodies to red blood cell antigens and the antigens are present in the fetus, the IgG antibodies cross the placenta and the maternal antibody on the fetal red cells attaches to the Fc receptors of the macrophages in the fetus's spleen. The red cell is hemolyzed causing fetal anemia. As the fetus's anemia worsens, the fetus accelerates red cell production. Red cells are produced in the liver and spleen and the organs increase in size. As a result, portal hypertension occurs causing the liver to reduce its albumin production. This, in turn, results in edema (an abnormal accumulation of fluid beneath the skin) and ascites (fluid in the peritoneal cavity). This condition in the fetus is known as *"hydrops fetalis."* If untreated, fetal death can occur from heart failure.

The IgG subclass of the maternal antibody affects the amount of hemolysis. IgG1 and IgG3 are more effective than IgG2 and IgG4 in causing hemolysis. In addition, IgG1 subclass antibodies cross the placenta earlier and in greater amounts than the other subclasses. This results in more hemolysis and an increase in the severity of the disease.[7]

TABLE 16-1   Clinical Significance in HDFN of Common Antibodies

Blood Group System	ABO	MNS	P	Rh	Lu	Kel	LE	FY	JK
Mild				C E e	Lu^b			Fy^b	
No to mild					Lu^a				Jk^b Jk^3
No to moderate	A B			C^w		Kp^b Ku			
Mild to moderate									Jk^a
No to severe		S s		G					
Mild to severe		U		D c		K k Kp^a Js^a Js^b		Fy^a	
Generally not significant	A1	M N	P1				Le^a Le^b		

Hemoglobin from fetal red cell destruction is broken down into bilirubin. During gestation, bilirubin passes through the placenta and is processed by the maternal liver. At delivery, with the maternal liver no longer available, the bilirubin must be processed by the immature liver of the newborn. The newborn's inability to bind all the unconjugated bilirubin to albumin to produce conjugated bilirubin results in the unconjugated bilirubin increasing and crossing the blood–brain barrier. The unconjugated bilirubin attaches to neurons in the brain stem and basal ganglia causing death of the neuron cells. This results in the condition known as *"kernicterus"* and possible permanent brain damage.

ASSESSING THE RISK FOR HEMOLYTIC DISEASE

Prenatal Evaluation

A number of methods of assessing fetal risk of HDFN are listed in Box 16-2, which combine patient history, serology, DNA testing, ultrasound, and *amniocentesis*. The evaluation begins with a history of previous pregnancies and transfusions. A maternal history of an affected fetus or infant increases the likelihood that there will be a problem with the current pregnancy. Because amniocentesis and *cordocentesis* (also known as PUBS—*percutaneous umbilical cord blood sampling*) are associated with fetal loss and maternal morbidity, less invasive assessment techniques are used when possible.[8]

BOX 16-2

Risk Assessment Strategy

Maternal history
    Previously affected fetus or infant
Serologic studies—maternal specimens
    ABO
    Rh
    Antibody screen
    Antibody identification
    Titration of IgG antibodies
    Serial titrations with saved specimens
Genetic studies
    Paternal antigen testing
    Antigen testing of the fetus
Amniocentesis
    Queenan chart
Percutaneous umbilical cord sampling (PUBS)
    Fetal antigen typing
Middle cerebral artery (MCA) Doppler

Initial screening for potential HDFN begins at the first prenatal visit. Maternal ABO, Rh, and antibody screening tests are performed. When there is no previous history of the mother's Rh type, a second sample should be collected at a subsequent visit to detect an erroneous Rh conclusion.[9] If an Rh-negative woman is mistakenly concluded to the Rh positive, RHIG may not be administered if needed. Testing for a maternal weak D antigen is not required and could lead false-positive results if performed following a massive *fetomaternal hemorrhage* (FMH).[9] Judd recommends that the direct reaction with anti-D be ≥2+ by the tube method to conclude the patient as Rh positive.[9] This is based on the premise that the red cells of women with partial D antigens will react weakly with anti-D. However, not all red cells with partial D antigens react weakly with antisera. Because women with partial D antigens are capable of making anti-D directed against the portions of the D antigen they lack, it is theoretically possible that administration of RHIG would prevent this sensitization. However, not all practitioners believe that this is a significant risk and would consider a woman who has a positive test for weak D to be Rh positive and not a candidate for Rh immune globulin.[8] Recently, bioarray assays are available to determine Rh genes and identify those women who may have missing parts of the D antigen.

Antibody screening should be performed with anti-IgG antihuman globulin and without antibody enhancement by using enzyme-treated cells to prevent the detection of antibodies that do not cause HDNF.[9] If the antibody screen is positive, the antibody should be identified using methods that detect clinically significant IgG antibodies (see Chapter 6).

Not all antibodies directed against red cell antigens cause HDNF. For example, the antigens Le^a, Le^b, I, and P_1 are poorly developed on fetal red cells, and antibodies to these antigens generally do not cause HDNF. Some antibodies may be primarily IgM and not cross the placenta. When the immunoglobulin class of the antibodies such as anti-M, anti-E, or anti-S is of interest, 2-mercaptoethanol (2-ME) or dithiothreitol (DTT) may be used to determine if the antibody is IgM, IgG, or a mixture. These substances inactivate IgM antibodies by cleaving the disulfide bonds in these antibodies leaving only the IgG component active. When the antibody is initially found to be IgM, it may be of value to repeat this testing periodically to ensure that the antibody remains IgM. Testing to determine the IgG subclass of an antibody is not available in most laboratories. Thus, if IgG antibodies are known to cause HDFN, titration studies may be indicated.

Performing Antibody Titration Studies

In order to provide an assessment of the strength of the antibody and its likelihood of causing significant hemolysis, a titration is usually performed. Maternal serum is diluted in doubling dilutions (2, 4, 8, 16, etc.). The undiluted (neat) serum and the dilutions are incubated with reagent red cells containing the antigen against the maternal antibody. The method used is one known to work well with IgG antibodies. Although various methods can be used, the serum cell mixtures are incubated at 37°C for a specified period of time (30 minutes to 1 hour) and the reactions are read at the antiglobulin phase by using IgG antihuman globulin. For anti-D, R_1R_1 cells are most often used as indicator cells as there is less variation in the expression of the D antigen. However, other indicator cells can be used. When multiple Rh antibodies are detected, it is not necessary to perform separate titrations using different indicator cells except when anti-G (anti-C + anti-D) is suspected.[9] The titration may be performed in various media including saline, using an enhancement media or gel cards, different incubation times, and temperatures as well as differences in the antigens on the indictor cells. In addition, the titer is somewhat dependent on the individual reading the results. To minimize these effects, the current specimen is tested in parallel with the specimen used to perform the previous titration study.

The titer has traditionally been the reciprocal of the dilution that contains the last 1+ reaction. Recent attempts to provide a standardized method for performing titrations has suggested using a weak positive (w+ or +/−) reaction as the end point.[10] Because of the inherent error in manual titrations, a two-tube increase between the specimens is considered significant. Because of the biological and method variables, titer results from different facilities are generally not comparable.

In the initially affected pregnancy, titers are performed initially at 18 to 20 weeks and every 4 weeks thereafter.[11] The titer is used to determine when additional more invasive procedures should be performed to assess fetal risk. There is no consensus concerning the exact cutoff or *"critical titer."* Rh antibody titers of 8, 16, or 32 have been used as the institutional cutoff depending on the method used and experience of the center.[8] An increase of two tubes is considered significant. Table 16-2 shows the results obtained from a current sample and the previous sample. Note that the interpretation of the change in titer depends on the end point used by the facility. There are very limited data on the critical titers for non-Rh antibodies. The severity of HDNF generally increases with subsequently affected pregnancies. Titration studies are

TABLE 16-2	Antibody Titration Comparing Results								
Specimen	Neat	1/2	1/4	1/8	1/16	1/32	1/64	1/128	1/256
Current specimen	3+	2+	2+	1+	1+	±	0	0	0
Previous specimen	3+	2+	1+	1+	0	0	0	0	0

most predictive in the first affected pregnancy. Thus, it may not be necessary to perform these studies in subsequently affected pregnancies. Antigens in the Kell blood group system appear on fetal red cells earlier than Rh proteins. Anti-Kell is known to suppress red cell production by facilitating phagocytosis before cells produce hemoglobin. This leads to anemia and hydrops without a significant antibody titer.[9,12]

Repeat Antibody Screening

The need for repeat antibody screening for the development of antibodies during a pregnancy is controversial. Some practitioners suggest that both Rh-positive and Rh-negative patients should be tested at the initial patient visit and at approximately 28 weeks gestation.[9] Alloimmunization due to anti-D will occur between the first trimester and the 28th week of gestation in about 0.18% of cases. The American College of Obstetricians and Gynecologists (ACOG) believes that such testing is not cost-effective for Rh-positive patients since antibodies developed during a pregnancy are uncommon, few cases would require medical intervention, and fetal distress will be identified by routine ultrasound procedures that are used to monitor pregnancies.[13]

Amniocentesis

Since the 1950s, amniocentesis was the technique used to provide a specimen to assess the severity of fetal hemolytic disease. In amniocentesis, a needle is introduced through abdomen and the uterus and into the amniotic sac. A small amount of amniotic fluid is removed for testing.

In 1961, Liley published the concept of using the level of bile pigment in the amniotic fluid to measure hemolysis in the fetus.[14] The optical density of the amniotic fluid is measured at wavelengths between 350 and 650 nm, and the absorbance is plotted against the wavelength. The *bilirubin* peaks at 450 nm. The difference (change) between the expected optical density at 450 nm and the peak at 450 nm is marked on a graph designed to predict the seriousness of the

disease. The Liley graph interpreted the results from 27 weeks gestation to term and had three levels. Queenan et al.[15] expanded the graph from 14 to 40 weeks, added a fourth zone, and improved the accuracy of the prediction. A Queenan curve for the change in optical density is shown in Figure 16-1. In general, the higher the change in optical density, the more likely the risk of fetal distress or demise. With a change in optical density of 0.35 to 0.7, the fetus is likely to deteriorate; at 0.7, fetal demise is imminent.

Because of the inherent inaccuracy of the measurement, serial amniocenteses are performed every 10 to 12 days. However, there are some risks associated with the procedure including infection, puncture of the placenta, FMH, induction of labor, and fetal loss, and less invasive methods of estimating fetal risk of hemolytic disease and fetal hemoglobin are now used.

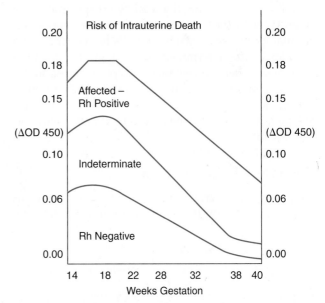

FIGURE 16-1 Queenan curve for ΔOD 450 for Rh. (Adapted from Queenan JT, Tomai TP, Ural SH, King JC. Deviation in amniotic fluid optical density at a wavelength of 450 nm in Rh-immunized pregnancies from 14 to 40 weeks of gestation: a proposal for clinical management. *Am J Obstet Gynecol.* 1993:168:1370–1376, with permission from Elsevier.)

NONSEROLOGIC METHOD OF ASSESSING FETAL RISK

Ultrasonography is used to examine the fetus starting at 16 weeks gestation. At 18 weeks gestation, Doppler ultrasonography allows the measurement of the velocity of blood flow to various fetal vessels (Fig. 16-2). The peak velocity increases with the severity of the anemia. It also increases with gestational age and can be plotted on the graph shown in Figure 16-3. It can also be expressed as multiples of the median (MOM) by using an online web-based calculator such as the one found at www.perinatology.com. *Middle cerebral artery (MCA) Doppler* has become the preferred method of assessing fetal anemia. MCA peak velocity has shown to correlate well with fetal hemoglobin and the change in optical density of amniotic fluid 450 nm (ΔOD 450).[16] Signs of fetal distress, fetal anemia, and hydrops are indications for more invasive studies such as amniocentesis and potential intrauterine transfusion.

OBTAINING A FETAL BLOOD SPECIMEN

With increased clarity of ultrasound, it is possible to introduce a needle into the umbilical vein and obtain a fetal blood specimen. If a fetal blood specimen is to be used for further testing, it must not be overly contaminated with maternal blood. The hematocrit of the sample can be determined or serologic testing for *i* antigen or other red cell antigen typing found on the fetal cells and not maternal cells can be performed at the bedside. Differences in red cell size or the presence of fetal hemoglobin can be determined in the hematology laboratory.

Predicting Fetal Antigens

Predicting whether the fetus is likely to carry an antigen is based on the determination of the father's

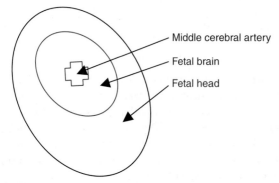

FIGURE 16-2   Location of the middle cerebral artery

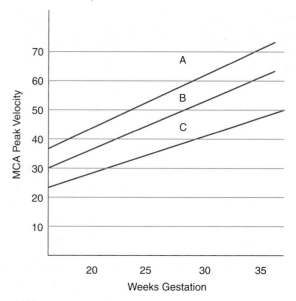

FIGURE 16-3   MCA Doppler. Zone A 1.5 MOM moderate to severe anemia; Zone B 1.29 MOM mild anemia; Zone C Median. (Adapted with permission from Moise KJ Jr. Management of rhesus alloimmunization in pregnancy. *Obstet Gynecol.* 2008;21:170.)

probable genotype. Through mapping of the human genome, the two-gene theory (RHD and RHCE) replaced the Fisher Race three-gene theory (D, C/c, and E/e) of the encoding Rh genes.[17] The expression of C rather than c results from a one nucleotide difference of cytosine to thymine in exon 2 of the RHCE gene that produces a single amino acid change of serine to proline. A change of cytosine to guanine in exon 5 of the RHCE gene produces e rather than the E antigen to be expressed. This change in theory modified the charts used to predict the probability that the father was heterozygous or homozygous for the Rh antigen. Most charts of paternal probability take into consideration the serologic typing results and the ethnic background of the father. Moise published a chart (Table 16-3), which added the number of previously affected D-positive offspring to the evaluation to improve its accuracy.[8] For example, a father with serology indicating that he expresses the DCce antigens would be 90%, 41%, and 85% likely to be heterozygous for the D antigen depending on his ethnicity of White, Black, and Hispanic descent, respectively. However, after the fifth pregnancy, each producing an Rh-positive infant, the probability that the same individual is heterozygous is reduced to 22%, 2%, and 15%, respectively. Fathering an Rh-negative infant confirms heterozygosity.

DNA techniques have been developed that determine if there are one or two paternal RHD genes present. Polymerase chain reactions (PCRs) signal intensities of the RHD exons 5 and 7 have been

TABLE 16-3   Predicting Paternal Zygosity for D Considering Phenotype, Ethnicity, and the Number of Previous Rh-positive Infants

White

# Rh+ Infants	DCce	DCe	DCEe	DcE	DCcEe	Dce
	Rh Phenotype					
0	90	9	90	13	11	94
1	82	5	82	7	6	89
2	69	2	69	4	3	80
3	53	1	53	2	2	66
4	36	0.6	36	0.9	0.8	50
5	22	0.3	22	0.5	0.4	33

Black

# Rh+ Infants	DCce	DCe	DCEe	DcE	DCcEe	Dce
0	41	19	37	1	10	54
1	26	11	23	0.5	5	37
2	15	6	13	0.3	1	23
3	8	3	7	0.1	0.7	13
4	4	1	4	0.1	0.3	7
5	2	0.7	2	0	12	4

Hispanic

# Rh+ Infants	DCce	DCe	DCEe	DcE	DCcEe	Dce
0	85	5	85	2	6	92
1	74	2	74	0.9	3	85
2	59	1	59	0.5	2	74
3	42	0.6	42	0.2	0.8	59
4	26	0.3	26	0.1	0.4	42
5	15	0.1	15	0.1		26

Adapted with permission from Moise KJ Jr. Management of rhesus alloimmunization in pregnancy. *Obstet Gynecol* 2002;100;600–611.

compared with the RHCE gene on exon 7 (used as an internal control) to determine paternal zygosity.[18]

The predictive value of a positive test for RHD using fetal DNA obtained from amniotic fluid is reported to be 100%, and the predictive value of a negative test is 96.9%.[19] Using free fetal DNA in a maternal serum specimen to detect the fetal RHD gene is a recent development in assessing fetal heterozygosity. Free fetal DNA can be found in maternal

plasma.[20] Müller et al. reported sensitivities from 99.7% to 99.8% and specificities of 98.1% to 99.7% by using two slightly different methods.[21] A reverse transcriptase PCR test is currently available in the United States, but its accuracy is limited to confirming the RHD gene. In the case of an Rh-negative fetus, the results cannot be verified because there is no internal control. It is anticipated that as PCR methods of testing improve, it will be used in place of obtaining a sample of amniotic fluid by amniocentesis.[8] It is probable that this testing also could be expanded to test for the other antigens most often causing HDFN.

INTRAUTERINE TRANSFUSIONS

Transfusion of the fetus allows the fetal lungs to mature and delivery to occur after 35 weeks gestation decreasing the risk to the infant. In the first *intrauterine transfusions*, fetal anemia was treated by injecting blood into the abdomen of the fetus.[22] Because of the increased clarity of modern ultrasound, fetal anemia can be treated in utero using cordocentesis or PUBS. Intrauterine transfusion is most often administered through the umbilical vein. When that is not possible due to placental or fetal placements or the size of the infant, the infusion can be given in the fetal peritoneal cavity. However, it will take several weeks for the red cell to be absorbed in the fetal circulation. Intrauterine transfusion may cause fetal loss in 1% to 2% of cases.

Red Blood Cell Selection and Preparation

Red blood cells prepared for intrauterine transfusion should be as fresh as possible group O units and be negative for the antigens in the maternal serum. Box 16-3 lists the requirements for units used for intrauterine transfusions or during PUBS. Some centers attempt to match the major antigens of the mother to prevent additional sensitization of the mother to additional antigens. The unit should be irradiated to prevent graft-versus-host disease. The unit should be either seronegative for cytomegalovirus (CMV) or leukocyte reduced to reduce the risk of CMV infection of the fetus. Testing for hemoglobin S is generally performed to reduce the risk of the transfused cells sickling under low oxygen tension.[23]

BOX 16-3

Red Cell Selection for Intrauterine and Exchange Transfusion

Group O
Rh negative or appropriate for the causative antibody
Freshest available
Irradiated
CMV seronegative or leukocyte reduced
~75% hematocrit for intrauterine transfusions
40–60% for exchange transfusions
Compatible antiglobulin crossmatch with maternal
  specimen

Several processing methods have been used to remove the supernatant anticoagulant and products of red cell metabolism in the fluid that suspends the red blood cells. Red blood cells may be centrifuged and the supernatant fluid removed or washed using manual centrifugation and supernatant removal or automated instruments. Deglycerolized red cells may be used to provide rare antigen-negative red cells. In rare circumstances, washed maternal red blood cells may be used if it is the only source antigen-negative blood available. Fresh frozen plasma or albumin is generally used to reconstitute the red cells to a final hematocrit of approximately 75% to 85%.[8] The hematocrit is high to prevent volume overload.

The volume to be administered is dependent on the size of the fetus, gestational age, initial hematocrit, the final intended hematocrit, and the hematocrit of the unit. For intrauterine transfusions, the volume to be transfused is calculated by subtracting 20 from the gestational age in weeks and multiplying by 10 mL. The target is a hematocrit of 40% to 50%.[8] The frequency of intrauterine transfusion is variable based on the condition of the fetus and the anticipated 1% decline in fetal hematocrit per day. The transfusion may be repeated every 12 to 14 days until there is suppression of fetal erythropoiesis. Then less frequent transfusions are needed.

CORD BLOOD TESTING

A *cord blood* specimen should be collected and labeled with two unique identifiers of the infant. There must be a method to match the infant and the fetus. Some centers label the cord blood specimen with the mother's identifying information as well as the infant's, but this is best done on a requisition or computer query. The preferred method of collecting a cord blood specimen is using a needle to puncture the umbilical vein. Milking the cord will lead to contamination of the specimen with a substance known as Wharton's jelly that can interfere with serologic testing. The cord blood specimen may be held in the birthing unit or sent to the transfusion service for storage and used for testing as needed.

There are many causes of neonatal *jaundice* including dehydration, breast-feeding, genetic disorders, and HDNF. Routine testing of the cord blood is not indicated unless the infant becomes severely jaundiced or the mother has antibodies known to cause HDNF. Routine serologic testing of the cord blood specimen includes typing the infant cells for ABO, Rh, and performing a DAT using IgG antihuman globulin serum. Table 16-4 lists testing performed on cord and maternal specimens.

TABLE 16-4 Postpartum Testing	
Criteria	**Testing**
Cord blood	
Cord blood—qualifying mother for RHIG	Rh including test for weak D
Cord blood—mother has known antibodies	ABO, Rh, and DAT
Cord blood—infant has severe jaundice	ABO, Rh, and DAT, determination of ABO incompatibility with mother
Maternal specimen	
Specimen from Rh-negative mother	Test for massive fetomaternal hemorrhage
Maternal specimen—mother has antibodies	Reserve to be used if needed for antibody identification

If the DAT is positive, HDNF could be due to ABO or other blood group incompatibility. An eluate can be prepared using the infant's red cells and the eluate can be tested against a panel of red cells to identify the antibody. It may be helpful to use a maternal specimen to identify the antibody as there is generally more specimen available to test. When the infant's DAT is positive and the maternal antibody screen is negative, HDFN may be due to ABO incompatibility or due to a low-incidence antigen not generally present on reagent red cells. In the latter case, a sample of paternal red cells is needed to test against the infant's eluate or maternal serum.

If the infant's DAT is negative, there is still the possibility of ABO HDFN. When the infant is A, B, or AB, and the mother is ABO incompatible, serologic testing for ABO HDFN could be performed using a sample of the infant's cord blood or serum. The serum or plasma can be incubated with several examples of A1 and/or B and O reagent red cells and tested at the antiglobulin phase with anti-IgG to identify maternal anti-A or anti-B in the infant. In some centers, serologic testing for passive anti-A and anti-B has been eliminated in most cases in favor of reporting the potential for ABO incompatibility between the mother and infant (Table 16-5).

COMPATIBILITY TESTING FOR TRANSFUSION AFTER BIRTH

Although uncommonly performed because the use of bililights prevents kernicterus in most cases, exchange transfusions can be used to treat anemia and remove antibody-coated red cells bilirubin and maternal antibody. In addition, small-volume transfusions to maintain the infant's hematocrit may be needed after delivery. When the mother is known to have antibodies that cause HDFN, the cord blood is tested for bilirubin and hematocrit or hemoglobin. The level of

TABLE 16-5 Reporting ABO Potential for ABO HDN		
Maternal ABO	**Infant ABO**	**Report**
O	O	Infant ABO compatible with mother
A	O, A	
B	O, B	
AB	O, A, B, AB	
O	A, B, AB	Maternal/infant ABO incompatibility.
A	B, AB	Potential exists for ABO HDN
B	A, AB	

BOX 16-4

Indications for Administration of RHIG

Fetal death
Spontaneous or therapeutic abortion
Amniocentesis
Chorionic villus sampling
Antepartum hemorrhage
Molar pregnancy
Ectopic pregnancy
Abdominal trauma
External version
28 weeks gestation
Delivery

---

unconjugated bilirubin in the cord blood coupled with the rate of rise in the unconjugated bilirubin levels are used to predict the need for exchange transfusion of the newborn.[8]

Unit Selection

If transfusion is necessary, the red cells used are usually group O and should be negative for the antigen(s) directed against the causative antibody(ies). The Rh can match the type of the infant unless the antibody is anti-D. The freshest available red cell unit that is negative for the necessary antigens is centrifuged, the supernatant fluid removed, and the red cells mass is reconstituted to a hematocrit of 40% to 50% with fresh frozen plasma or 5% albumin. Box 16-4 is a formula that can be used to calculate the proportion of red cells and plasma needed for reconstitution of a unit. CMV-seronegative red cells or leukocyte-reduced red cells are used to prevent transfusion transmission of CMV. Irradiation of the unit is required to prevent graft-versus-host disease.

Serologic Testing

ABO testing is performed using anti-A and anti-B antisera. Some centers also use anti-A,B antisera to pick up weak A and B antigens frequently found on neonatal red cells. Previous intrauterine transfusion can mask the patient's actual blood type. Testing the newborn's serum for anti-A and anti-B should not be performed on cord blood or peripheral blood specimens. If these antibodies are present, they are of maternal origin.

A serologic crossmatch should be performed using either the newborn's peripheral blood specimen or a maternal sample. There is generally a larger volume of maternal specimen but it may contain antibodies that are not the cause of HDFN. Testing of cell panels to identify the antibody(ies) and antiglobulin crossmatches may be performed to provide crossmatch-compatible red cells.

When the mother has an antibody to high-incidence antigens, there may be no compatible blood available. When recognized early enough in the pregnancy, maternal red cells can be collected and frozen, or siblings and other close relatives of the mother could be tested. If maternal red cells are collected at the time of delivery, the red cells should be washed to remove maternal antibody. The last alternative is to perform an exchange transfusion of the infant with red cells that contain the antigen. Antibodies will attach to the fetal red cells resulting in removal from circulation or hemolysis. It is likely that additional exchange transfusions will be needed to remove the red cells coated with maternal antibody and reduce the amount of unconjugated bilirubin caused by hemolysis.

Due to the suppression of erythropoiesis related to transfusion, infants affected with HDFN may require additional red cell transfusion for 1 to 3 months after delivery. Periodic testing of hemoglobin and reticulocyte production is performed to monitor the infant's need for transfusion.

PREVENTION OF HDNF DUE TO ANTI-D

During 1963 and 1964 prevention of anti-D using postdelivery administration of *Rh immune globulin (RHIG)* was described by Clarke et al. in Britian[24] and Freda et al. in the United States.[25] While the actual mechanism is not known, the suppression of anti-D is probably the result of anti-D coating the fetal Rh-positive red cells and preventing the cells from being recognized as foreign thus preventing primary immunization. A few cases of HDFN still occur because RHIG was not administered when indicated.

The original source of RHIG was women sensitized by pregnancy. Currently, the source is individuals who have been actively sensitized with Rh-positive red cells. An effective RHIG using multiple monoclonal antibodies is not yet available. The standard dose of RHIG is 300 μg (1,500 IU) in the United States and 100 μg (500 IU) in Britain. A dose of 50 μg is available for pregnancies that end within the first trimester of pregnancy, but most hospitals in the United States stock only the 300-μg dose. The 300-μg dose of RHIG will prevent immunization to anti-D for up to 15 mL of red cells and 30 mL of whole blood. The 50-μg dose provides protection for up to 2.5 mL of red cells. The first commercial preparation of RHIG available in the United States was administered postpartum intramuscularly (IM). Preparations are now available that can be administered either intravenously (IV) or IM.

In 1978, Bowman et al. recommended antepartum RHIG administration to prevent alloimmunization that occurred during pregnancy.[26] Because 92% of women who develop anti-D during pregnancy do so at or after 28 weeks gestation, an antepartum dose is given at approximately 28 weeks gestation.[13] Because the amount of anti-D in the maternal circulation falls due to the approximate 21-day half-life of IgG antibodies, repeat doses of RHIG may be administered every 12 weeks.

To prevent unnecessary serologic testing to identify the cause of the positive antibody screen that will occur after the injection is given, RHIG should be administered after the 28-week antibody screening specimens are collected. Reagent red cell panels of four to six cells are now available to identify anti-D and screen for other clinically significant antibodies when RHIG has been administered and an antibody screen is needed.

SEROLOGIC TESTING

If the mother is known to be Rh negative, the infant's cord blood should be tested for the D antigen. If the infant is Rh positive, including testing for weak D, the mother is a candidate for RHIG. False-positive and false-negative Rh testing results can occur. In the case of intrauterine transfusions with Rh-negative red cells, there may be too little Rh-positive blood in the infant's circulation to be detected in routine testing. To prevent this misinterpretation, the infant's transfusion history including any intrauterine transfusions is needed.

Another cause of false-negative results in routine direct testing for the D antigen is exhibited when so much maternal anti-D is coating the fetal cells that agglutination is blocked because the antibodies cannot bridge between cells linking them together. This problem is detected during weak D testing when the Rh control is positive. It is likely that the infant has a positive DAT and the results of the weak D test cannot be interpreted. False-positive results also can occur when high-protein anti-D reagents cause spontaneous agglutination. The use of an Rh control along with the anti-D reagent will identify this problem.

QUANTIFYING FETAL–MATERNAL HEMORRHAGE

RHIG is indicated during pregnancy if the mother has an event that may cause fetal red cells to leak into the maternal circulation (Box 16-4). If the pregnancy is terminated at less than 20 weeks, a single 300-μg dose of RHIG will be protective as the fetal blood volume is less than 30 mL. At or after 20 weeks gestation, screening for massive FMH is indicated. The screening test that is most often used is the *rosette test* using a maternal specimen collected within 1 hour of delivery.[27] Anti-D is mixed with a sample of maternal red cells. After incubation, the anti-D is washed away and Rh-positive indicator cells are added. A rosette is formed by Rh-positive indicator cells attaching to the anti-D-coated Rh-positive fetal cells. This test is positive if about 10 mL of Rh-positive fetal cells are in the maternal circulation.

If the rosette test is positive or the fetus is weak D positive, additional testing to quantify the amount of the FMH should be performed by a *Kleihauer–Betke (K–B)* acid elution or *flow cytometric analysis*.[23] K–B is based on the resistance of fetal hemoglobin to be eluted from red cells. Fetal cells stain brightly, while cells with adult hemoglobin are seen as ghosts. There are many technical concerns and the test has poor precision and accuracy, and a safety margin is generally included in the dose calculation. The percentage of stained cells is determined and the mother's weight is obtained. Box 16-5 illustrates the calculation of the number of vials of RHIG needed in a massive fetal–maternal hemorrhage. Because of the inherent error in a K–B test, some centers add an additional vial of RHIG. When more than one 30-μg dose is indicated, the manufacturer's administration instructions should be followed for number of doses administered at one time and the spacing of the doses.

BOX 16-5

RHIG Dose Calculation Based on Whole Blood

Count of 2,000 cells and the percentage of fetal cells is determined.
Maternal blood volume (based on weight)

$$\frac{\text{Fetal cells} \times \text{maternal blood volume (mL)}}{\text{Total cells counted}} = \text{fetal hemorrhage (mL)}$$

$$\frac{16 \text{ cells} \times 4,500 \text{ mL}}{2,000} = 36 \text{ mL}$$

36/30 mL per vial = 1.2 vials
Round up to 2 vials

Previously Sensitized Women

Since RHIG will not suppress anti-D in a sensitized patient, RHIG is not administered to women who are already immunized. Therefore, upon occasion, it may be necessary to determine if the maternal anti-D was passively acquired or through active immunization as a result of previous transfusion or pregnancy. Passive anti-D is IgG and generally has a titer ≤4. Anti-D from alloimmunization has an IgM component and is likely to have a higher titer. If there is any doubt as to the mother's Rh type or whether the anti-D present is active or passive, RHIG should be administered.

Administer RHIG Within 72 Hours

Unless the mother is known to be sensitized to anti-D, RHIG should be administered with 72 hours of delivery or sensitizing event. This time limit was set by the criteria used in the original clinical trials. However, if 72 hours have elapsed, ACOG recommends that RHIG be administered as soon as possible and as late as 28 days.[13]

NEONATAL THROMBOCYTOPENIC PURPURA

Neonatal Alloimmune Thrombocytopenic Purpura (NAITP) is due to maternal IgG antibodies directed against fetal platelet antigens that can begin to cross the placenta as early as 17 weeks gestation. Unlike alloimmunization to red blood cells, NAITP may involve first pregnancies. These antibodies may result in platelet counts of <50,000 at birth. Intracranial hemorrhage can occur in utero and after delivery.

HPA-1 (PLA1) accounts for approximately 80% of cases, HPA-5b accounts for 10%, HPA-1b for 4%, HPA-3a for 2%, and a variety of others make up 6%. The incidence of NAITP is approximately 1 per 1,500 to 2,000 births.[28]

In subsequent pregnancies, the mother and father should be tested for platelet antigens and the mother should be tested for platelet alloantibodies. Zygosity of the father may be determined through genetic testing. PUBS may be performed at approximately 20 weeks gestation to determine the status of the infant. Once it has been determined that the fetus is affected, intravenous immune globulin may be administered to the mother to reduce antibody production.[23]

If ongoing monitoring indicates the need for platelet transfusion, irradiated, leukocyte-reduced, or CMV-seronegative, antigen-negative platelets may be transfused to prevent hemorrhage. Some blood centers have identified HPA-1-negative donors and apheresis platelets may be obtained. Whole-blood–derived platelets may be used if antigen-negative units are not available. The transfusion goals are to maintain the platelet count above 50,000/μL for vaginal delivery and above 20,000/μL after birth.[23] Washed maternal platelets may be used for transfusion. The decrease in platelet count resolves in approximately 2 to 3 weeks after birth.

In rare instances the mother may have IgG antibodies to their own platelets that cross the placenta and affect the fetus. This is known as *immune thrombocytopenic purpura* (ITP). ITP is usually less severe than NAITP with only 10% of newborns having a platelet count of less than 50,000/μL. Treatment of the mother with prednisone or IVIG has been shown to be effective in increasing the maternal platelet count. However, the maternal and fetal platelet counts do not correlate well.[29]

SUMMARY

While the frequency of HDNF due to anti-D has decreased significantly due to RHIG prophylaxis, there are cases of RHIG failures and alloimmunization to other antigens. Less invasive techniques have improved the diagnosis and treatment of HDNF. However, serologic testing remains an important part of the risk assessment process. And for those severely affected infants, intrauterine and exchange transfusions significantly improve the outcome for these infants.

Review Questions

1. The most common type of HDFN is due to antibodies of the
   a. Kell system
   b. Kidd system
   c. Lewis system
   d. Rh system

2. Which class of antibodies causes HDFN?
   a. IgA
   b. IgD
   c. IgG
   d. IgM

(continued)

REVIEW QUESTIONS (continued)

3. In HDFN, the greatest risk to the fetus prior to birth is due to
   a. anemia
   b. hyperbilirubinemia
   c. an enlarged head
   d. bleeding

4. After birth, the infant with severe HDFN is at risk for which of the following?
   a. bleeding
   b. brain damage
   c. anemia
   d. enlarged head

5. The most common method of determining fetal anemia is
   a. amniotic fluid analysis
   b. cordocentesis
   c. middle cerebral artery Doppler
   d. analysis of maternal serum

6. Since mapping of the human genome, the theory of Rh inheritance is based on
   a. one gene—Rh
   b. two genes—RHD and RHCE
   c. three genes—D, C/c, and E/e
   d. five genes—D, C, c, E, and e

7. Titration studies are most predictive of the severity of hemolytic disease
   a. during the first affected pregnancy
   b. when the antibody is anti-K
   c. when there is a one tube difference between the current and most recent past specimen
   d. if the titration is done using enzyme enhanced indicator cells

8. The primary intent of an intrauterine transfusion is to
   a. prevent kernicterus
   b. prevent graft-versus-host disease
   c. increase the albumin in the fetus to prevent hemolysis
   d. increase the fetal hematocrit to prevent hydrops

9. The rosette test is used to
   a. screen for fetal lung maturity
   b. screen for massive fetomaternal hemorrhage
   c. screen for IgG antibodies
   d. quantitate massive fetomaternal hemorrhage

10. The principle of the K–B test is resistance
    a. of fetal hemoglobin to acid solutions
    b. of fetal hemoglobin to alkaline solutions
    c. adult hemoglobin to alkaline solutions
    d. adult hemoglobin to acid solutions

11. Cellular blood components for infants who have had an intrauterine transfusion are irradiated to prevent
    a. sickle cell formation
    b. CMV transmission
    c. graft-versus-host disease
    d. high potassium in the product

12. The test that may not be positive in ABO HDNF is
    a. direct antiglobulin test
    b. rosette test
    c. Kleihauer–Betke
    d. Antibody-screening cells

13. A paternal specimen is most useful in identifying HDNF cause by antibodies directed against
    a. Low-incidence antigens
    b. Rh antigens
    c. High-incidence antigens
    d. antiplatelet antibodies

14. The K–B result is 15 cells. The dose of Rh immune globulin needed to prevent sensitization to anti-D in an Rh positive woman is
    a. none
    b. 1 vial
    c. 2 vials
    d. 3 vials

15. NAITP is a condition in which a
    a. mother develops specific platelets antibodies that destroy fetal platelets
    b. mother develops nonspecific antibodies to platelets that destroy fetal platelets
    c. fetus develops anti-Pl^{A1}
    d. fetus develops nonspecific platelet antibodies

REFERENCES

1. Bowman J. Thirty-five years of Rh prophylaxis. *Transfusion.* 2003;43:1661–1666.
2. Levine P, Katzin EM, Burnham L. Isoimmunization in pregnancy: its possible bearing on the etiology of erythroblastosis fetalis. *JAMA.* 1941;116:825–827.
3. Bergstrom H, Nilsson LA, Ryttinger L. Demonstration of Rh antigens in a 38-day-old fetus. *Am J Obstet Gynecol.* 1967;99:130–133.
4. Bowman JM. The prevention of Rh immunization. *Transfus Med Rev.* 1988;2:129–150.
5. Klein HG, Anstee DJ. The Rh group system. In: *Mollison's Blood Transfusion in Clinical Medicine.* 11th ed. Oxford: Blackwell;2005:496–545.
6. Bowman JM. Controversies in Rh prophylaxis. Who needs Rh immune globulin and when should it be given? *Am J Obstet Gynecol.* 1985;151:289–294.
7. Firan M, Bawdon R, Radu C, et al. The MHC class I-related receptor, FcRn, plays an essential role in the maternal fetal transfer of gamma-globulin in humans. *Int Immunol.* 2001;13:993–1002.
8. Moise KJ Jr. Management of rhesus alloimmunization in pregnancy. *Obstet Gynecol.* 2008;112:164–176.
9. Judd WJ. *Guidelines for Prenatal and Perinatal Immunohematology.* Bethesda, MD: AABB; 2005.
10. AuBuchon JP, de Wildt-Eggen J, Dumont LJ. Biomedical Excellence for Transfusion Collaborative, Transfusion Medicine Resource Committee of the College of American Pathologists. Reducing the variation in performance

of antibody titrations. *Arch Pathol Lab Med*. 2008;132: 1194–1201.

11. AGOC Educational Bulletin. Management of isoimmunization in pregnancy. American College of Obstetrics and Gynecologists. *Int J Gynaecol Obstet*. 1996;55(2): 183–190.

12. Daniels G, Hadley A, Green CA. Causes of fetal anemia in hemolytic disease due to anti-K [letter]. *Transfusion* 2003;43:115–116.

13. ACOG Practice Bulletin No. 4. Prevention of Rh alloimmunization. American College of Obstetrics and Gynecologists. *Int J Gynaecol Obstet*. 1999;66(1):63–70.

14. Liley AW. Liquor amnii analysis in the management of the pregnancy complicated by Rhesus sensitization. *Am J Obstet Gynecol*. 1961;82:1359–1370.

15. Queenan JT, Tomai TP, Ural SH, et al. Deviation in amniotic fluid optical density at a wavelength 450 nm in Rh-immunized pregnancies from 14 to 40 weeks' gestation: a proposal for clinical management. *Am J Obstet Gynecol*. 1993;168:1370–1376.

16. Moise KJ Jr. Management of rhesus alloimmunization in pregnancy. *Obstet Gynecol*. 2002;100:600–611.

17. Cherif-Zahar B, Mattei MG, Le Can Kim C, et al. Localization of the human Rh blood group gene structure to chromosome region 1p34.3–1p36.1 by in situ hybridization. *Hum Genet*. 1991;86:398–400.

18. Pirelli K, Pietz B, Johnson S, et al. Molecular determination of RhD zygosity. *Am J Obstet Gynecol*. 2006;195: S1723.

19. Van den Veyver IB, Moise KJ Jr. Fetal RhD typing by polymerase chain reaction in pregnancies complicated by rhesus alloimmunization. *Obstet Gynecol*. 1996;88: 1061–1067.

20. Müller SP, Bartels I, Stein W, et al. The determination of the fetal D status from maternal plasma for decision making on Rh prophylaxis is feasible. *Transfusion*. 2008; 48:2292–2301.

21. Harper TC, Finning KM, Martin P, et al. Use of maternal plasma for noninvasive determination of fetal RhD status. *Am J Obstet Gynecol*. 2004;191:1730–1732.

22. Liley AW. Intrauterine transfusion of foetus in haemolytic disease. *Br Med J*. 1963;2:1107–1109.

23. Roback JD, Combs MR, Grossman BJ, et al. *Technical Manual*. 16th ed. Bethesda, MD: American Association of Blood Banks; 2008:629–636.

24. Clarke CA, Donohoe WT, McConnel RB, et al. Further experimental studies on the prevention of Rh hemolytic disease. *Br Med J*. 1963;1:979–984.

25. Freda VJ, Gorman JG, Pollack W. Successful prevention of experimental Rh sensitization in man with an anti-Rh gamma2-globulin antibody preparation: a preliminary report. *Transfusion*. 1964;4:26–32.

26. Bowman JM, Chown B, Lewis M, et al. Rh isoimmunization during pregnancy: antenatal prophylaxis. *Can Med Assoc J*. 1978;118:623–627.

27. Sebring ES, Polesky HF. Detection of fetal–maternal hemorrhage in Rh immune globulin candidates. A rosetting technique using enzyme-treated Rh_2Rh_2 indicator erythrocytes, *Transfusion*. 1982;22:468–471.

28. Williamson LM, Hackett G, Rennie J, et al. The natural history of fetomaternal alloimmunization to the platelet-specific antigen HPA-1a (PL^{A1}, Zw^2) as determined by antenatal screening. *Blood*. 1998;92:2280–2287.

29. Webert KE, Mittal R, Sigouin C, et al. A retrospective 11-year analysis of obstetric patients with idiopathic thrombocytopenic purpura. *Blood*. 2003;102:4306–4311.

AUTOIMMUNE HEMOLYTIC ANEMIAS AND DRUG-INDUCED IMMUNE HEMOLYTIC ANEMIA

REGINA M. LEGER AND PATRICIA A. ARNDT

OBJECTIVES

After completion of this chapter, the reader will be able to:

1. Define autoantibody.

2. Compare the immunoglobulin class, thermal amplitude, and common autoantibody specificities for warm autoimmune hemolytic anemia, cold agglutinin syndrome, and paroxysmal cold hemoglobinuria.

3. Discuss the serologic problems encountered, and procedures for resolution, when testing samples containing warm autoantibodies.

4. Discuss the serologic problems encountered, and procedures for resolution, when testing samples containing potent cold agglutinins.

5. Describe the use of autologous adsorption and allogeneic adsorption procedures.

6. Describe the Donath-Landsteiner test.

7. List the drugs most commonly associated with DIIHA.

8. Describe the different classification types of DIIHA.

9. Discuss methods used to investigate the presence of drug-dependent antibodies.

KEY WORDS

Adsorption
Allogeneic
Autoantibody
Autologous
Cold autoantibodies
Cold agglutinin syndrome
Donath-Landsteiner test
Drug-dependent antibodies
Drug-independent antibodies
Drug-induced immune hemolytic anemia

Hemoglobinemia
Hemoglobinuria
Immune hemolysis
Nonimmunologic protein adsorption
Paroxysmal cold hemoglobinuria
Thermal amplitude
Warm autoantibodies
Warm autoimmune hemolytic anemia

*H*emolytic anemia is the shortening of the length of time red blood cells (RBCs) survive in the circulation. Normal RBCs circulate approximately 90 to 120 days; about 1% of RBCs are removed by the reticuloendothelial system each day. In healthy individuals, this normal destruction is matched by production of new RBCs in the bone marrow. When the destruction exceeds RBC production, anemia can develop.

TABLE 17-1	Classification of Immune Hemolytic Anemias

Autoimmune hemolytic anemia (AIHA)
Warm AIHA
Cold AIHA
  Cold agglutinin syndrome (CAS)
  Paroxysmal cold hemoglobinuria (PCH)
Mixed-type AIHA

Alloimmune hemolytic anemia
Hemolytic transfusion reaction
Hemolytic disease of the fetus and newborn

Drug-induced immune hemolytic anemia (DIIHA)
Drug-dependent
Drug-independent
Nonimmunologic adsorption of protein

In immune hemolytic anemia (IHA), the RBC destruction is due to an immune response. However, hemolytic anemia is not always mediated by an antibody. Nonimmune-mediated hemolytic anemia can be caused by toxins (e.g., snake venom), infections (e.g., malaria, septicemia), and membrane disorders (e.g., paroxysmal nocturnal hemoglobinuria).

IHA can be classified in various ways. One classification is shown in Table 17-1. Autoimmune hemolytic anemia (AIHA) and *drug-induced immune hemolytic anemia (DIIHA)* are the subjects of this chapter.

IMMUNE HEMOLYSIS

In previous chapters, the formation of antibodies in response to transfusion or pregnancy has been discussed. These antibodies (alloantibodies) are directed against RBCs that are foreign to an individual. Autoantibodies are directed against an individual's own RBCs. Production of autoantibodies is not clearly understood, but it probably occurs as a result of some failure in the control mechanism of immune response. Not all autoantibodies will result in destruction of RBCs.

Destruction of RBCs that occurs within the blood vessels is called intravascular hemolysis. The characteristic features of this rare type of hemolysis are *hemoglobinemia* and *hemoglobinuria,* and the serum haptoglobin level will be low.[1] Hemoglobinemia is the release of free hemoglobin into the plasma; when the plasma hemoglobin is markedly raised, the plasma becomes pink or red. If the level of plasma hemoglobin exceeds the renal threshold, hemoglobin appears in the urine (hemoglobinuria) and the urine may be pink, red,

brown, or almost black. Urine from a patient with hematuria (RBCs in the urine) can also be red, but is typically cloudy (vs. clear for hemoglobinuria) and numerous intact RBCs would be seen on microscopic exam of the sediment. Hemoglobinemia is almost always accompanied by hemoglobinuria.[1]

Extravascular hemolysis, on the other hand, results when RBCs (sensitized by antibody or complement) are damaged or destroyed by macrophages in the reticuloendothelial system, for example, in the spleen or liver. Spherocytes are formed when a portion of the RBC escapes the macrophage. The characteristic feature of extravascular hemolysis is increased serum bilirubin (and bilirubin-degradation products in the urine and stool). This distinction between intravascular and extravascular hemolysis is a simplification, however, because hemoglobin can also be released into the plasma following extravascular destruction, particularly if hemolysis is brisk.[1]

Immune-mediated intravascular hemolysis is associated with ABO hemolytic transfusion reactions, paroxysmal nocturnal hemolytic anemia, paroxysmal cold hemolytic anemia, and IHA caused by some drugs. In the context of this chapter, intravascular hemolysis is caused by complement-mediated destruction of RBCs in the blood stream. Most alloantibodies other than anti-A or -B are not capable of destroying RBCs intravascularly; exceptions are anti-Jk^a, anti-PP_1P^k, and anti-Vel. Other than in *paroxysmal cold hemoglobinuria (PCH)*, intravascular hemolysis is not common in AIHA. Extravascular hemolysis is characteristic in immune destruction by alloantibodies and in warm and cold AIHA.

Clinical and Laboratory Indicators of Hemolysis

The diagnosis of hemolytic anemia rests on a combination of the clinical history and exam, and laboratory results. Symptoms of anemia, jaundice, and splenomegaly are nonspecific manifestations. Laboratory indicators of hemolysis are listed in Table 17-2. A rapid decrease in the hemoglobin or hematocrit can be due only to bleeding or hemolysis. Thus, an acute drop in hemoglobin without evidence of blood loss points to a possible diagnosis of hemolysis. Spherocytes are often seen on the peripheral blood smear, and agglutination can be seen in cases of *cold agglutinin syndrome (CAS)* if the blood was not warmed to 37°C prior to making the film. An elevated reticulocyte count reflects compensated erythropoiesis by the bone marrow and is an indirect indicator of shortened RBC life span. Bilirubin is a breakdown product of heme from hemoglobin; the direct or conjugated fraction is excreted in the bile but the indirect or unconjugated

TABLE 17-2 Laboratory Indicators of Hemolysis
Decreased hemoglobin and hematocrit
Morphology on peripheral blood film (e.g., spherocytes, agglutination)
Increased reticulocytes
Increased bilirubin (indirect)
Decreased haptoglobin
Increased LDH

fraction cannot be excreted. When there is a rapid destruction of RBCs, the indirect fraction of bilirubin elevates. Hyperbilirubinemia is usual in hemolytic anemia, but it is not a constant, so its absence does not exclude the diagnosis. Haptoglobin binds free hemoglobin as RBCs are destroyed, so when large amounts of hemoglobin–haptoglobin complexes are formed and cleared, the plasma haptoglobin is depleted. Low haptoglobin can be an indicator of hemolysis, but it is not specific. Lactic dehydrogenase (LDH) is also used as an indicator of hemolysis because RBCs have a high content of the enzyme. Intravascular hemolysis produces a marked elevation in LDH.

Classification of Autoimmune Hemolytic Anemias

The AIHAs are subdivided into two major types based upon the characteristics of the causative antibody: *warm autoimmune hemolytic anemia (WAIHA),* associated with antibodies reacting optimally at 37°C, and cold AIHA, associated with antibodies reacting optimally in the cold, for example, CAS and PCH. Primary or idiopathic AIHA is not associated with an underlying disorder. Secondary AIHA has been associated with lymphoproliferative, autoimmune, and immunodeficiency disorders; tumors; and infections. Drugs (discussed in a later section of this chapter) may also induce *immune hemolysis*; autoantibodies that are drug-induced are serologically indistinguishable from idiopathic WAIHA.

Serologic Tests to Investigate Autoimmune Hemolytic Anemia

Serologic tests performed in the blood bank (e.g., direct antiglobulin test [DAT], eluate, antibody detection) help determine whether hemolysis has an immune basis and, if so, what type of IHA is present. This is important because the treatment for each type is different.

The Direct Antiglobulin Test

The DAT is a simple test used to determine if RBCs have been coated in vivo with immunoglobulin, complement, or both. A positive DAT, however, may or may not be associated with immune-mediated hemolysis; there are many causes for a positive DAT (Table 17-3).

The DAT should be performed on every patient in whom the presence of hemolysis has been established to help determine if the hemolysis has an immune basis. The predictive value of a positive DAT is 83% in a patient with hemolytic anemia, but only 1.4% in a patient without hemolytic anemia.[2] Small amounts of IgG and complement, generally below the threshold of detection in the routine DAT, appear to be present on RBCs from all individuals.[1] Healthy individuals, blood donors, and hospitalized patients can have a positive DAT with no obvious signs of hemolytic anemia.

While a positive DAT in a patient with hemolytic anemia indicates that the most likely diagnosis is one of the IHAs, the DAT can be positive, coincidentally, in patients with hemolytic anemia that is not immune-mediated. Interpretation of a positive DAT should include the patient's history, clinical data, and the results of other laboratory tests.

The DAT is performed by testing freshly washed RBCs directly with antiglobulin reagents such as anti-IgG and anti-C3d. The DAT can initially be performed with a polyspecific antihuman globulin reagent capable of detecting both IgG and C3d but if the test is positive, tests with monospecific reagents (e.g., anti-IgG and anti-C3d) should be performed for appropriate characterization of the immune process involved. The RBCs need to be washed to remove globulins and complement that are present in the surrounding plasma; otherwise the antiglobulin reagent can be neutralized, resulting in a false-negative test. The RBCs should be

TABLE 17-3 Some Causes of a Positive DAT
Autoantibodies to intrinsic red cell antigens
Hemolytic transfusion reactions
Hemolytic disease of the fetus and newborn
Drug-induced antibodies
Alloantibodies passively acquired
Nonspecifically adsorbed proteins
Complement activation due to bacterial infection, autoantibodies, or alloantibodies
Alloantibodies produced by passenger lymphocytes

tested immediately after washing to prevent false-negative results due to the potential elution of IgG. EDTA-anticoagulated blood samples are preferred for testing because the EDTA prevents in vitro fixation of complement. RBCs from a clotted blood sample could have a positive DAT due to complement bound in vitro.

When the DAT is positive with both anti-IgG and anti-C3d, the RBCs should be tested with an inert control reagent, for example, 6% albumin or saline. Lack of agglutination of the RBCs in the control reagent will provide some assurance that the test results are accurately interpreted. RBCs strongly coated with globulins (e.g., in WAIHA) have the potential to be spontaneously agglutinated after centrifugation (in other words, no antiglobulin reagent is needed for the agglutination to occur); strong *cold autoantibodies* (e.g., as in CAS) can cause autoagglutination (see later sections). If the control is reactive, the DAT result is invalid and additional procedures would be required to obtain a valid DAT result.

Elution

An eluate should be prepared from immunoglobulin-coated RBCs and tested to determine if the coating protein has RBC antibody activity. Elution frees antibody from sensitized RBCs by physical or chemical means and recovers the antibody in a usable form.[3] When the only coating protein is complement, eluates are frequently nonreactive.

A nonreactive eluate prepared from IgG-coated red cells may have several causes (see later section on DIIHA). Commercial acid elution kits are suitable to recover antibody in most cases; however, no single elution method is ideal in all situations.[4] Use of an alternative elution method may be indicated when a nonreactive eluate is not in agreement with clinical data. Pursuing the cause of a nonreactive eluate for patients with no evidence of hemolysis is usually not indicated. Toy et al. showed that 79% of pretransfusion patients with a positive DAT have a nonreactive eluate.[5]

Antibody Detection and Characterization

Routine antibody detection and identification testing can help to determine if allo- and/or autoantibodies are present. Cold agglutinins may not be apparent in these studies if the only test performed is the indirect antiglobulin test (IAT), though cold agglutinins may be suspected because of ABO or DAT results. If a cold agglutinin is present at room temperature and the patient has evidence of hemolytic anemia, a titer and *thermal amplitude* study may be indicated. *Adsorptions* to remove warm or cold autoantibodies may be necessary to detect underlying alloantibodies. If PCH is a possibility, for example, in a child with hemoglobinuria and a positive DAT due to complement, a *Donath-Landsteiner test* should be performed.

Before testing is even begun, it is important to consider the sample. Samples to be used for thermal amplitude studies and the Donath-Landsteiner test ideally need to be maintained at 37°C prior to separating the plasma or serum. Also, serum rather than plasma is the required specimen when hemolysis is the endpoint (e.g., Donath-Landsteiner test).

Table 17-4 shows the typical serologic characteristics of the AIHAs. If the DAT is positive but both the serum and eluate are nonreactive, there is evidence of immune hemolysis, and the patient has received a drug previously reported to have caused immune

TABLE 17-4	Serologic Characteristics of the Autoimmune Hemolytic Anemias			
	DAT	Immunoglobulin Class	Eluate	Serum Reactivity
WAIHA	IgG (20%) IgG + C3 (67%) C3 (13%)	IgG	IgG antibody	IAT; 35% agglutinate untreated red cells at 20°C
CAS	C3 only	IgM	Nonreactive	IgM agglutinating antibody; titer ≥1,000 (60%) at 4°C; react at ≥30°C
PCH	C3 only	IgG	Nonreactive	Routine IAT negative; IgG biphasic hemolysin in Donath-Landsteiner test

hemolysis, testing to demonstrate drug-related antibodies should be considered (see later section).

WARM AUTOIMMUNE HEMOLYTIC ANEMIA

The majority (80%) of AIHA cases are caused by warm-reactive autoantibodies, optimally reactive with RBCs at 37°C. The *autoantibody* is usually IgG (but can be IgM or IgA).

Corticoid steroids are the standard therapy for patients with WAIHA. Splenectomy has been a traditional second-line approach, but other pharmaceutical options, for example, rituximab, are now available.[6,7]

Serologic Characteristics

In WAIHA, the DAT may be positive due to IgG plus complement (67%), IgG only (20%), or complement only (13%).[1] The presence of an IgG autoantibody on the RBCs can be confirmed by elution. Typically, the eluate reacts with all RBCs tested. The eluate will usually be nonreactive if the only protein coating the RBCs is complement.

Circulating autoantibody is continuously being adsorbed by the patient's RBCs. The serum will contain free antibody after all the specific antigen sites on the RBCs have been occupied and no more antibody can be bound in vivo. The DAT in such cases is usually strongly positive. Autoantibody in the serum typically reacts by the IAT with all RBCs tested. Approximately 60% to 90% of patients with WAIHA have detectable serum antibodies depending on the testing method used. Agglutination at room temperature can be seen in about one-third of patients with WAIHA, but the cold agglutinins have normal titers at 4°C and are usually nonpathogenic (i.e., nonreactive at 30°C and 37°C).[1]

Some patients with clinical and hematologic evidence of WAIHA have a negative DAT. There are three common causes for WAIHA associated with a negative DAT: the RBC-bound IgG is below the threshold of the routine DAT, IgM or IgA is the RBC-bound protein, or the IgG is low affinity and is washed off the RBCs during the washing phase for the DAT.[1,8] Several assays have been used for these cases, including flow cytometry, enzyme-linked antiglobulin tests, solid-phase, direct Polybrene test, column agglutination, or concentrated eluates.[8] Reagents that react with RBC-bound IgA or IgM are not routinely available and require standardization.[1] One easier test for detection of low-affinity IgG antibodies involves washing with ice cold (e.g., 4°C) saline, which may help

retain antibody on the RBCs; a control (e.g., 6% albumin) is necessary to confirm that cold autoagglutinins are not the cause of positive results.[1]

Serologic Problems

Warm autoantibodies can cause technical difficulties for RBC testing. Spontaneous agglutination can occur if the RBCs are heavily coated with IgG and the reagent contains a potentiator such as albumin. This is not commonly observed with the lower protein ABO and anti-D typing reagents currently in use; however, other monoclonal antisera may give problems due to a potentiator in the reagent and results should be suspect if the observed reactivity is weaker than expected or fragile.[9]

When the DAT is positive due to IgG, antiglobulin-reactive typing reagents cannot be used unless the IgG is first removed.[4] An alternative is to use low-protein antisera (e.g., monoclonal reagents) that do not require an antiglobulin test (AGT).

The presence of autoantibody in the serum increases the complexity and the time needed to complete pretransfusion testing, which may require hours. The challenge is to determine if alloantibodies are also present. Some alloantibodies may make their presence known by reacting more strongly than the autoantibody, but quite often the presence of alloantibodies is masked by the autoantibody reactivity.[10,11]

Methods to detect alloantibodies in the presence of warm-reactive autoantibodies attempt to decrease or eliminate the autoantibody reactivity. Autoantibody reactivity is typically enhanced by techniques such as polyethylene glycol (PEG), enzymes, column agglutination (e.g., gel), or solid-phase red cell adherence. Using a low–ionic-strength saline (LISS) or saline tube method may still allow for detection of most clinically significant alloantibodies but circumvent autoantibody reactivity. Some samples may require an adsorption procedure to remove the autoantibody; two widely used approaches are *autologous* and *allogeneic* adsorptions.

Autologous Adsorption

Autologous adsorption uses the patient's own RBCs to remove autoantibodies and is the best way to detect alloantibodies in the presence of warm autoantibodies in a patient who has not been recently transfused. Only autoantibodies will be removed and alloantibodies, if present, will rem   orp-
tion should not b   peen
transfused in the   nple
used for adsorp   BCs
that could adsor   have
shown that <10   apa-
ble of removing

Autoadsorption requires some initial preparation of the patient's RBCs. The IgG coating the autologous RBCs will block further adsorption of autoantibody in vitro. A gentle heat elution at 56°C for 5 minutes can dissociate some of the RBC-bound IgG. This can be followed by treatment of the autologous RBCs with proteolytic enzymes to increase their capacity to adsorb autoantibody. Treatment of the RBCs with ZZAP, a mixture of papain or ficin and dithiothreitol (DTT) accomplishes both the increased ability to adsorb the autoantibody and removal of immunoglobulin and complement from DAT-positive autologous RBCs in one step.[13-15] Usually, 1 mL of the patient's serum or plasma is adsorbed with 1 mL of the patient's treated, packed RBCs.[4] Multiple sequential autoadsorptions with new aliquots of RBCs may be necessary. Once autoantibody has been removed, the adsorbed serum is tested for alloantibody reactivity.

Allogeneic Adsorption

Allogeneic RBCs (i.e., RBCs from another individual) can be used for adsorption when the patient has been recently transfused or when insufficient autologous RBCs are available. Because the allogeneic RBCs are not identical to the patient's (autologous) RBCs, the potential to remove alloantibody exists. RBCs of one to three known phenotypes are used; these are often treated with enzyme or ZZAP reagent. The selected cells need only demonstrate those few antigens to which alloantibodies of clinical significance are likely to be present. These include the common Rh antigens (D, C, E, c, and e), K, Fy^a and Fy^b, Jk^a and Jk^b, and S and s. Enzyme treatment of the RBCs prior to use in the adsorption will destroy Fy^a, Fy^b, and S antigens, making the RBC selection easier.[4] Likewise, the K antigen is destroyed by the DTT in ZZAP reagent. Antibodies to high-incidence antigens cannot be excluded by allogeneic adsorptions because the adsorbing cells will be expected to express the antigen and adsorb the alloantibody along with autoantibody.

When the patient's phenotype is not known, group O RBC samples of three different Rh phenotypes (R_1R_1, R_2R_2, and rr) are selected. One should lack Jk^a, another Jk^b, and one should lack s. If enzyme-treated RBCs are used, at least one of the three RBC samples should also lack K. Untreated RBCs may be used, but antibody may be more difficult to remove and the adsorbing RBCs must, at a minimum, include at least one negative for the S, s, Fy^a, Fy^b, and K antigens in addition to the Rh and Kidd requirements. If the patient's RBC phenotype is known, adsorption with a single sample of phenotype-similar RBCs may be possible.

The serum may need to be adsorbed two or three times to remove all the autoantibody. The adsorbed aliquots are then tested against reagent RBCs, for example, antibody detection RBCs. If an adsorbed aliquot is reactive, the aliquot should be tested against more reagent RBCs to identify the antibody. The adsorbed serum from each of the RBC adsorptions (e.g., from the R_1R_1, R_2R_2, and rr aliquots) provides a separate set of "panel" results, which taken together, create a complete picture. For example, if the aliquot adsorbed with Jk(a−) RBCs subsequently reacts only with Jk(a+) RBCs, alloanti-Jk^a is identified in that aliquot. Occasionally autoantibody will not be removed by three sequential adsorptions. Further adsorptions can be done, but multiple adsorptions have the potential to dilute the serum and a weak antibody could be missed.

Due to the phenotype requirements of the adsorbing RBCs, the volume of RBCs needed for allogeneic adsorptions, and the time required, transfusion services often refer samples that require allogeneic adsorptions to an immunohematology reference laboratory.

Specificity of Autoantibody

In many cases of WAIHA, the patient's serum reacts with all RBC samples tested and no autoantibody specificity is apparent. If testing is performed with RBCs of rare Rh phenotypes, the autoantibody often appears to have broad specificity in the Rh system. Apparent specificity for simple Rh antigens (D, C, E, c, and e) is occasionally seen, especially in saline or LISS tube IATs. A "relative" specificity may also be seen, based on stronger reactivity with cells of certain phenotypes or in adsorbed aliquots. Apart from Rh specificity, warm autoantibodies with many other specificities have been reported, for example, specificities in the LW, MNS, Gerbich, Kell, Kidd, Duffy, and Diego systems.[16,17]

Tests against RBCs of rare phenotype and by special techniques have limited clinical or practical application. Compatible donor blood is unlikely to be available and there is little point in determining the specificity. Blood of rare phenotypes, if available, should be reserved for patients with uncommon phenotypes who are alloimmunized.

Transfusion of Patients with Warm-reactive Autoantibodies

The most important determination for any transfusion candidate is to exclude the presence of potentially clinically significant alloantibodies *before* selecting RBCs for transfusion. Patients who have warm autoantibodies in their serum have a higher rate of alloimmunization (e.g., 12% to 40% with a mean of

32%); only about 5% of multitransfused patients without warm autoantibodies develop alloantibodies.[10,18–21] The technical difficulty in working with these samples is that autoantibodies that react with all reagent RBCs, even weakly, are capable of masking alloantibody reactivity. The exclusion of newly formed alloantibodies is of primary concern in patients with warm autoantibodies that have been transfused. Due to the presence of autoantibodies, all crossmatches will be incompatible. This is unlike the case of clinically significant alloantibodies without autoantibodies, where a compatible crossmatch with antigen-negative RBCs can be obtained. Monitoring for evidence of RBC destruction due to *alloantibodies* is difficult in patients who already have AIHA; the transfused RBCs as well as the patient's own RBCs will have shortened survival due to the autoantibody.

If no alloantibodies are detected in adsorbed serum, random units of the appropriate ABO and Rh type may be selected for transfusion. If clinically significant alloantibodies are present, the transfused RBCs should lack the corresponding antigen(s). If the autoantibody has apparent and relatively clear-cut specificity for a single antigen (e.g., autoanti-e) and there is active ongoing hemolysis, there is some evidence that blood lacking that antigen may survive better than the patient's own RBCs.[1] However, it is undesirable to expose a D− patient to the highly immunogenic D antigen, especially in females who may bear children later, merely because e–RBCs, for example, are serologically compatible with the autoantibody (e−RBCs, if available, will probably be D+; D−e− RBCs are extremely rare).

The adsorbed serum may be used to screen and select nonreactive units for transfusion (antigen negative for clinically significant alloantibodies, if detected). Using the adsorbed serum may provide some assurance that the correct unit is selected and avoid incompatibility, but this practice can also provide a false sense of security for the transfusion of these patients. The unit is still incompatible with the patient's circulating autoantibody.

Resolving these serologic problems is important; however, a delay in transfusion for these patients because of serologic incompatibility may cause greater harm. Transfusion of patients with AIHA is a decision made by the patient's physician, after evaluating the risks and benefits. Ongoing communication with the patient's physician is critical.[22]

Patients with warm-reactive autoantibodies may or may not have apparent hemolysis or severe anemia. Patients with little or no evidence of significant hemolysis tolerate transfusion quite well. Survival of the transfused RBCs (compatible with any alloantibodies that are present) is about the same as the survival of the patient's own RBCs.

In patients who have active hemolysis, transfusion may increase the hemolysis and the transfused RBCs may be destroyed more rapidly than the patient's own RBCs. This may be due to the increased RBC mass available from the transfusion.[1] Hemoglobinemia and hemoglobinuria may be increased due to the destruction of the transfused RBCs; disseminated intravascular coagulation (DIC) can develop in patients with severe hemolysis.[1]

COLD AGGLUTININ SYNDROME

CAS is less common than WAIHA and constitutes about 18% of all AIHAs.[1] It is the hemolytic anemia most commonly associated with autoantibodies that react preferentially in the cold. CAS can be an acute or chronic condition, idiopathic or secondary. The acute form is often secondary to infection (e.g., *Mycoplasma pneumoniae*). The chronic form, often seen in elderly patients, has been associated with lymphoma and chronic lymphocytic leukemia. Almost always, the cold agglutinins in the chronic form are IgM monoclonal proteins with kappa light chains. In the acute form induced by *Mycoplasma* or viral infections, the antibody is polyclonal IgM with normal kappa and lambda light-chain distribution. Anemia is most commonly chronic with mild-to-moderate severity. Cold weather can exacerbate acrocyanosis and hemoglobinuria. The RBCs in EDTA specimens from these patients are often agglutinated; the RBCs on a peripheral smear may also appear to be agglutinated unless the smear is prepared after warming the blood sample.

Therapy for CAS is avoidance of cold and many patients can be managed without transfusion.[6]

Serologic Characteristics

The DAT is typically positive with anti-C3 only and no reactivity will be found in the eluate. If IgG is detected, a negative control for the DAT, for example, 6% albumin or saline, should be tested to ensure that the cold autoagglutinin is not causing a false-positive test. The cold-reactive autoagglutinin is usually IgM, which binds to RBCs in the lower temperature of the peripheral circulation and causes complement components to attach to the RBCs. As the RBCs circulate to warmer areas, the IgM dissociates, but the complement remains. Similarly, in vitro, autoagglutination should disperse when the EDTA RBCs are warmed at 37°C and/or 37°C saline is used to wash the RBCs for the DAT.

The autoagglutinin in CAS generally has a titer of greater than 1,000 at 4°C and has a high thermal amplitude, reacting in vitro at 30°C or higher. Occasionally, pathologic cold agglutinins will have a lower titer (i.e., <1,000 at 4°C), but these will have a high thermal amplitude (i.e., reactive at ≥ 30°C); agglutination in the presence of 30% albumin at 30°C has been associated with pathogenicity.[1]

To determine the true thermal amplitude or titer of the cold autoagglutinin, the specimen must be maintained at 37°C after collection until the sample is sufficiently clotted to allow separation of the serum and RBCs, to avoid in vitro autoadsorption of the cold antibody. Alternatively, plasma can be used from an EDTA-anticoagulated specimen that has been warmed for 10 to 15 minutes at 37°C (with repeated mixing) and then separated from the RBCs without delay. This should release autoadsorbed antibody back into the plasma.

Serologic Problems

Problems with ABO and Rh typing and other tests can be encountered in samples from patients with CAS. Maintaining the EDTA blood sample at 37°C immediately after collection and washing the RBCs with warm (37°C) saline before testing usually resolves the problem. Alternatively, an EDTA sample can be warmed to 37°C for about 10 minutes, followed by washing the RBCs with warm saline. It is helpful to perform a parallel control test with 6% bovine albumin, or other control as directed by the reagent manufacturer, to determine if the cold autoagglutinin is interfering with results. If the control test is nonreactive, the results obtained with anti-A and anti-B are usually valid. If autoagglutination still occurs, it may be necessary to treat the RBCs with sulfhydryl reagents.[4]

When the serum agglutinates group O reagent RBCs, ABO serum (reverse typing) tests are invalid. Repeating the tests using prewarmed serum/plasma and group A_1, B, and O RBCs and allowing the RBCs to "settle" after incubation at 37°C for 1 hour (instead of centrifuging the test) will often resolve any discrepancy. By eliminating the centrifugation step, interference by cold-reactive autoantibodies may be avoided; a disadvantage of this method is that anti-A and/or -B in some patients' sera may be too weak to react at 37°C. Alternatively, adsorbed serum (either autoadsorbed or adsorbed with allogeneic group O RBCs) can be used. Rabbit erythrocyte stroma should not be used for ABO serum tests because it may adsorb anti-B or anti-A_1, thus affecting the correct interpretation of the ABO group.[23,24]

Detection of Alloantibodies in the Presence of Cold-reactive Autoantibodies

Most cold autoagglutinins do not react at 37°C so if serum tests are conducted at 37°C (e.g., without centrifugation for agglutination) and if anti-IgG is used for the AGT, there is rarely a difficulty in detecting clinically significant alloantibodies. Potentiators (e.g., albumin, PEG) are not recommended as these may increase the reactivity of the autoantibodies. In rare cases, it may be necessary to perform an autoadsorption at 4°C; complete removal of the autoagglutinin is very time-consuming and is usually unnecessary. Sufficient removal of cold autoagglutinins can be facilitated by treating the patient's RBCs with enzymes or ZZAP reagent before adsorption. One or two cold autoadsorptions should remove enough of the cold autoantibody for alloantibody detection. Alternatively, allogeneic adsorption as for WAIHA can be performed at 4°C. Rabbit erythrocyte stroma, used to remove autoanti-I and -IH from sera, should be used with caution as clinically significant alloantibodies, (e.g., anti-D, -E, -Vel) have been removed by this method.[25,26]

Specificity of Autoantibody

The agglutinin specificity in CAS is usually anti-I, and less commonly anti-i; other specificities are seen on rare occasions. The specificity may not be apparent unless dilutions of the patient's serum are tested at various temperatures. Determining the specificity of the cold autoagglutinin is of academic interest only and is not diagnostic for CAS. Autoanti-I may also be seen in healthy individuals. However, the nonpathologic forms of autoanti-I rarely react to titers above 64 at 4°C, and are usually nonreactive with I− (cord i and the rare adult i) RBCs at room temperature. In contrast, the autoanti-I of CAS usually reacts quite strongly with I− RBCs in tests at room temperature, while equal or even stronger reactions are observed with I+ RBCs (e.g., group O reagent RBCs). Autoanti-i reacts in the opposite manner, demonstrating stronger reactions with I− RBCs than with RBCs that are I+. Procedures to determine the titer and specificity of cold-reactive autoantibodies are found elsewhere.[4]

MIXED-TYPE AIHA

About one-third of patients with WAIHA have nonpathologic cold agglutinins that react at room temperature. Another group of patients with WAIHA have "mixed"[27] or "combined warm and cold"[28] AIHA, with IgG 37°C reactive antibodies and cold agglutinins reacting at or above 30°C. The cold agglutinin can be high titer (as in CAS) or normal titer (<64 at 4°C) with a high thermal amplitude.[1] The serum from patients with mixed-type AIHA can be reactive in all phases of testing.

Serologic Characteristics

Both IgG and C3 are usually detectable on the patient's RBCs in mixed-type AIHA; however, either C3 or IgG (or IgA) alone may be detectable on the RBCs.[1] A warm-reactive IgG autoantibody will be detected in an eluate.

Both warm-reactive IgG autoantibodies and cold-reactive, agglutinating IgM autoantibodies are present in the serum. The agglutinating autoantibody reacts at 30°C or above. If adsorptions are done to detect alloantibodies, it may be necessary to perform adsorptions at both 37°C and 4°C.

Specificity of Autoantibody

The cold-reactive IgM agglutinating autoantibody often has no apparent specificity but can be anti-I. The warm-reactive IgG autoantibody often appears serologically indistinguishable from typical autoantibodies encountered in WAIHA.

Transfusion in Mixed-type AIHA

Procedures for exclusion of alloantibodies and selection of blood for transfusion are identical to those described for patients with WAIHA.

PAROXYSMAL COLD HEMOGLOBINURIA

PCH is very rare and accounts for only about 2% of all IHAs. Historically, PCH has been associated with tertiary syphilis, but PCH more frequently presents, particularly in young children, as an acute transient condition secondary to viral infections. PCH can also occur as an idiopathic chronic disease in older individuals.

Serologic Characteristics

The DAT is usually only positive for complement. IgG is usually not detected unless the RBCs have been washed with cold saline and tested with cold anti-IgG (keeping the test system close to the optimal temperature for the causative antibody).[1] Eluates are almost always nonreactive.

The causative antibody in PCH, classically referred to as a biphasic hemolysin, is a cold-reactive IgG complement-binding antibody. The autoantibody reacts with RBCs in colder areas of the body (e.g., the extremities) and causes complement to bind to RBCs. Hemolysis does not occur until the RBCs circulate to warmer parts of the body where the complement is activated.

The diagnostic test for PCH is the Donath-Landsteiner test.[4] Serum, rather than plasma, is the required sample, preferably from a specimen allowed to clot at 37°C prior to separation. This is done to prevent the cold-reactive antibody that causes PCH from adsorbing to the patient's RBCs and thus not be detected when the patient's serum is tested. Classically, 1 drop of a 50% suspension of P+ RBCs is added to 10 drops of the patient's serum. The test is set up in duplicate. One tube set up as the "test" is first incubated in a melting ice bath (0°C), which is the temperature for the cold-reacting IgG antibody to attach to the RBCs. After 30 to 60 minutes, this tube is gently mixed and moved to 37°C for 30 minutes. The control tube is incubated only at 37°C. Another set of tubes with the patient's serum plus fresh normal serum as a source of complement is set up the same way. The tubes are then centrifuged and observed for hemolysis. The Donath-Landsteiner test is positive if the tube that was incubated in the ice bath and moved to 37°C showed lysis and the tube that was maintained at 37°C did not show lysis.

Because the antibody rarely reacts above 10°C and does not cause agglutination, pretransfusion antibody detection tests are usually nonreactive and the serum is usually compatible with random donor cells by routine procedures.

Specificity of Autoantibody

Anti-P is the most common specificity of the biphasic hemolysin in PCH. To determine the antibody specificity, the Donath-Landsteiner test needs to be performed with the rare RBCs of individuals with the P− or p phenotype. Rarely, other specificities reacting in the Donath-Landsteiner test have been described.

Transfusion in PCH

Adult patients with PCH rarely need transfusion; treatment includes keeping the patient warm. In young children, transfusion may be required if the hemolysis is life threatening. While P− RBCs survive better than P+ (P_1+ or P_1−) RBCs; RBCs of the p phenotype are very rare. Transfusion of random donor blood should not be withheld.[1]

DRUG-INDUCED IMMUNE HEMOLYTIC ANEMIA

Therapeutic drugs are widely used. Only rarely do individuals develop antibodies as a result of receiving one of these drugs, which then are capable of causing immune cell destruction (hemolytic anemia, thrombocytopenia, and/or neutropenia). This chapter will focus on IHA; many of the principles are similar for drug-induced immune thrombocytopenia and neutropenia.[29,30] It has been estimated that DIIHA occurs with an incidence of about one in a million people.[1]

The first drug suspected as causing IHA was mephenytoin (an anticonvulsant) in 1953; the patient had a positive DAT but no other serologic studies were performed.[31] Three years later, antibodies to stibophen (an anthelminthic drug) were serologically demonstrated in a patient with hemolytic anemia.[32] Since then, numerous drugs have been described as causing IHA; not all reports are supported by serologic evidence. Table 17-5 lists 120 drugs that have been described with reasonable evidence as having caused IHA and/or a positive DAT. The majority of the drugs fall into three therapeutic categories: antimicrobial (43%), nonsteroidal anti-inflammatory (16%), and antineoplastic (14%). Thirty-three percent of the drugs listed in Table 17-5 have been described as being associated with IHA only once in the literature. In the 1970s, the drugs most commonly associated with DIIHA were penicillin (an antibiotic) and methyldopa (an antihypertensive). Recently, the drugs most commonly associated with DIIHA have been cefotetan, ceftriaxone, and piperacillin (all antibiotics).[34]

TABLE 17-5 Drugs Described as Causing Immune Hemolytic Anemia and/or Positive DAT Listed by Therapeutic Category[33]

Antimicrobial
Amoxicillin[a,b]
Amphotericin B[b]
Ampicillin[b]
Cefamandole[a,b]
Cefazolin[b]
Cefixime[a,b]
Cefotaxime[b]
Cefotetan[b,d]
Cefoxitin[b]
Cefpirome[a,b]
Ceftazidime[b]
Ceftizoxime[b]
Ceftriaxone[b]
Cefuroxime[b]
Cephalexin[b]
Cephalothin[b,d]
Chloramphenicol[b]
Ciprofloxacin[b]
Clavulanate potassium[d]
Cloxacillin[a,b]
Erythromycin[b]
Ethambutol[a,b]
Fluconazole[a,b]
Isoniazid[b]
Latamoxef[a,b]
Levofloxacin/ofloxacin[b]
Mefloquine[b]
Minocycline[a,b]
Nafcillin[b]
Nitrofurantoin[a,b]
Norfloxacin[a,b]
p-Aminosalicyclic acid[b]
Penicillin G[b]

Piperacillin[b]
Pyrazinamide[a,b]
Pyrimethamine/pirimetamine[b]
Quinidine[b]
Quinine[b]
Rifabutin[a,b]
Rifampin[b]
Stibophen[b]
Streptomycin[b]
Sulbactam sodium[d]
Sulfamethoxazole[b]
Sulfisoxazole[a,b]
Tazobactam sodium[d]
Teicoplanin[a,b]
Temafloxacin[b]
Tetracycline[b]
Ticarcillin[b]
Trimethoprim[b]
Vancomycin[a,b]

Nonsteroidal anti-inflammatory
Aceclofenac[a,b]
Acetaminophen/paracetamol[b]
Aminopyrine/pyramidon[a,b]
Aspirin[a,b]
Azapropazone/apazone[b]
Diclofenac[b]
Dipyrone[b]
Etodolac[a,b]
Fenoprofen[a,b]
Ibuprofen[b]
Mefenamic acid[c]
Nabumetone[a,b]
Naproxen[b]

Phenacetin[b]
Propyphenazone[a,b]
Sulindac[b]
Suprofen[a,b]
Tolmetin[b]
Zomepirac[a,b]

Diuretic/antihypertensive
Butizide[a,b]
Furosemide[b]
Hydralazine[a,b]
Hydrochlorothiazide[b]
Methyldopa[c]
Triamterene[b]

Antidiabetic
Chlorpropamide[b]
Insulin[b]
Tolbutamide[b]

Antineoplastic
Carboplatin[b]
Cisplatin[b,d]
Cladribine/2-chloro-
  deoxyadenosine[c]
Diglycoaldehyde/INOX[d]
Fludarabine[c]
Fluorouracil[b]
Glafenine[b]
9-Hydroxy-
  methyl-ellipticinium[b]
Imatinib Mesylate[b]
Melphalan[a,b]
6-Mercaptopurine[a,b]
Methadone[b]

Methotrexate[b]
Oxaliplatin[b,d]
Sulfasalazine[b]
Teniposide[a,b]

Others
Acyclovir[a,b]
Antazoline[b]
Carbimazole[b]
Carbromal[a,b]
Catechin/catergen/
  cianidanol[b]
Chlorinated hydrocarbons[b]
Chlorpromazine[b]
Cyclofenil[b]
Cimetidine[a,b]
Cyclosporine[b]
Dexchlorpheniramine
  maleate/chlorpheniramine[a,b]
Diethylstilbestrol[b]
Fluorescein[a,b]
Levodopa[c]
Hydrocortisone[a,b]
Metrizoate-based
  Radiographic contrast media[b]
Nomifensine[b]
Phenytoin/fenitoine[a,b]
Probenecid[b]
Procainamide[c]
Ranitidine[b]
Sodium pentothal/thiopental[a,b]
Streptokinase[a,b]
Tartrazine[a,b]
Trimetallic anhydride[a,b]

[a]Only a single report in the literature.
[b]Drug-dependent antibody (may have drug-independent antibody also).
[c]Drug-independent antibody only.
[d]Associated with nonimmunologic protein adsorption.

TABLE 17-6 Serologic and Clinical Findings Associated with Different Drug Antibodies

Classification	Serology DAT	Eluate	Serum	Clinical
Drug-dependent antibodies Antibodies that react with drug-treated RBCs and are inhibited by drug	IgG ± C3	Reacts with drug-treated RBCs but not with untreated RBCs	Reacts with drug-treated RBCs but not with untreated RBCs	Hemolysis of moderate severity, usually extravascular
Antibodies that react in the presence of drug and are not inhibited by drug	C3 ± IgG (sometimes IgM is detected)	Usually nonreactive in presence of drug	Reactive only when drug solution, RBCs and serum are mixed	Severe hemolysis, often intravascular and often with renal failure
Drug-independent (auto) antibodies, e.g., methyldopa	IgG ± C3	Reacts with normal cells in absence of drug	Reacts with normal cells in absence of drug	Hemolysis of moderate severity, usually extravascular
Nonimmunologic protein adsorption	IgG, C3, IgM, IgA, albumin, fibrinogen, etc.	Nonreactive with drug-treated RBCs	Reactive with drug-treated RBCs (normal sera are also reactive)	Extravascular

Serologic Classification

The mechanisms by which drugs cause IHA are unclear and not proven but clinical and serologic characteristics can be classified into four types (Table 17-6): *drug-dependent antibodies* (antibodies that require the presence of drug in the test system for their detection by in vitro serologic methods; these antibodies can be further subdivided into those that react with drug-treated RBCs and those that only react in the presence of drug), *drug-independent antibodies* (antibodies that do not require the in vitro addition of drug for their detection), and *nonimmunologic protein adsorption* (the drug causes plasma proteins, including antibodies, to be adsorbed nonimmunologically onto the RBC membrane).

Drug-dependent Antibodies

Drug-dependent antibodies are only detected when drug is present in the test system. This usually involves addition of the drug to the test system in the laboratory. Drug-dependent antibodies can be divided into two subtypes: (1) those that react with drug-treated RBCs and are inhibited by the addition of drug, and (2) those that react in the presence of drug and are not inhibited by the addition of drug.

Antibodies That React with Drug-treated RBCs
The best-studied example of an antibody that reacts with drug-treated RBCs is anti-penicillin, which was first described in 1958.[35] Penicillin binds firmly to RBC membranes in vivo and in vitro (e.g., forms covalent bonds with proteins on the RBC membrane that withstand washing); thus, penicillin-coated RBCs can be easily prepared in the laboratory. Penicillin antibodies will react with penicillin on penicillin-coated RBCs (Fig. 17-1); if serum containing anti-penicillin is first incubated with a solution of penicillin, the antibody will be inhibited by the drug, thus preventing it from reacting with penicillin-coated RBCs. This type of reactivity is sometimes referred to as the "penicillin-type" or "drug-adsorption type." "Hapten-type" should not be used to describe this particular type of reactivity because all drugs are haptens (small molecules that can elicit an immune response only when attached to a large carrier such as a protein). Other drugs that have been associated with antibodies that react with drug-treated RBCs include some drugs in the penicillin family (e.g., ampicillin, nafcillin) and some cephalosporins (e.g., cephalothin, cefotetan).

DIIHA due to penicillin only occurs in patients who have received high doses of intravenous penicillin (>10 million units per day) for at least a week or more. The plasma antibody that reacts with penicillin-coated RBCs in IHA cases due to penicillin is typically a high-titer (>1,000) IgG antibody. Low-titer IgM penicillin antibodies are found in the plasma of some people but are not associated with IHA. Patients with DIIHA due to penicillin typically will have a positive DAT due to IgG coating with or without complement (Table 17-6); an eluate prepared from these RBCs should contain anti-penicillin and react with penicillin-treated RBCs but not with untreated

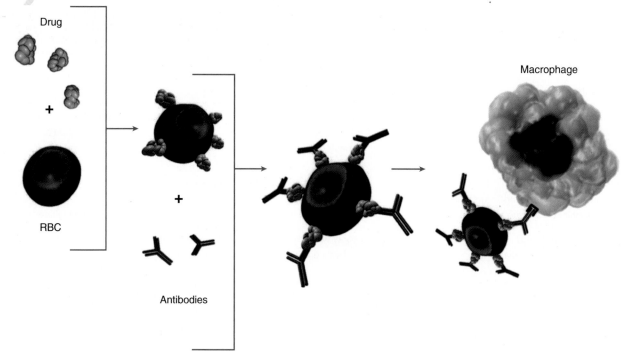

FIGURE 17-1   Drug-coated RBCs. Drug covalently bonds to RBCs in vivo or in vitro. Antibody binds to the drug on the RBCs. RBC-bound antibody is recognized by receptors on macrophages, for example, in the spleen. (Illustrator: Adrienne B. Mendoza.)

RBCs. Clinically, these patients have hemolysis (usually extravascular) of moderate severity. Patients recover completely after the drug has been stopped, but hemolysis of weakening severity may persist for several weeks (until the in vivo penicillin-coated RBCs have cleared from the circulation).

Antibodies That React in the Presence of Drug

Most drugs that cause DIIHA do not bind firmly to RBCs and thus drug-coated RBCs cannot be prepared in vitro (i.e., drug is washed off after incubation with RBCs). Antibodies to these drugs can only be detected by incubating the patient's serum, a solution of the drug, and the test RBCs together at the same time; this reactivity is not inhibited (and may be enhanced) by preincubation of the serum with the drug. It has been suggested that during the incubation of serum + drug + RBCs, the drug and the antibody (often IgM) form immune complexes that attach nonspecifically to "innocent bystander" RBCs and activate complement (Fig. 17-2). Although clinical and serologic findings fit this theory, it has not been proven (and there is some evidence against it) and thus is usually referred to as the "immune complex" theory (in quotes) or as the so-called immune complex theory.[1] Another theory that has been proposed to explain antibodies that are detected by this method is that the drug binds loosely (noncovalently) to RBCs (in vivo and in vitro) and the

antibody reacts with a compound antigen that is part drug and part RBC membrane (Fig. 17-3B).

The first antibodies detected using this method were directed against the drug stibophen[32]; the most commonly reported drugs associated with antibodies that react by this method are ceftriaxone, phenacetin, and tolmetin. Patients with IHA due to these drugs typically have complement on their RBCs (sometimes IgG with or without IgM is also present) and often have acute, severe complement-mediated hemolysis. This hemolysis is often intravascular (associated with hemoglobinemia and hemoglobinuria) and some of these patients have renal failure; a number of deaths, especially in children, have been associated with ceftriaxone antibodies. IHA may occur after receiving only a small amount of the drug (e.g., phenacetin) or after receiving the drug multiple previous times (e.g., ceftriaxone). Once the drug is stopped, hematologic remission is often rapid.

Drug-independent Antibodies

Drug-independent antibodies are those that do not require the addition of drug in the laboratory for their detection. Serologically, they react similarly to autoantibodies found in WAIHA, that is, antibodies that react by the AGT with all RBCs, including the patient's own, that are found in the patient's serum and

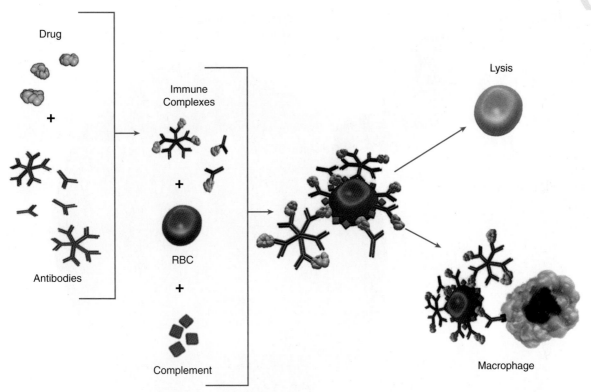

FIGURE 17-2   The "immune complex" theory. Drug and antibodies form immune complexes. Immune complexes bind nonspecifically to RBCs and activate complement. RBCs are destroyed intravascularly (via complement-mediated hemolysis) or extravascularly (via macrophages). (Illustrator: Adrienne B. Mendoza.)

in an eluate prepared from the patient's RBCs. There is no way to distinguish a drug-independent antibody from an idiopathic warm autoantibody in the laboratory and thus prove that the antibody is due to a drug. The only way to suggest that a drug-independent antibody is due to a drug is by in vivo means, for example, demonstrate that the antibody and IHA are present while the patient is receiving the drug and absent when the patient is no longer receiving the drug. To confirm that this is not coincidence the patient needs to be restarted on the drug that was suspected of causing IHA; as this is usually not desirable, the association of the drug with the IHA in the patient is often unproven. There are two types of drug-independent antibodies: (1) those that are found alone ("true" autoantibodies), and (2) those that are found in combination with drug-dependent antibodies.

Drug-independent Antibodies That Are Found Alone
The best-studied drug associated with this type of drug-independent antibody is methyldopa.[36,37] Patients who developed these autoantibodies typically had been taking methyldopa for at least 3 to 6 months. About 10% to 30% of patients who took methyldopa this long developed a positive DAT (IgG with or without C3), but only a few (0.5%) went on to

develop IHA. Within 2 weeks of stopping methyldopa, the patients with IHA recovered hematologically but the DAT could continue to be positive for up to 2 years. The most popular theory, to explain these types of autoantibodies, is that the drug directly affects the patient's cellular immune system, for example, inhibits suppressor T-cell activity.[38] This theory is consistent with the prolonged time period before autoantibody is detectable but has not been definitively proven.

Clinical features associated with this type of autoantibody are similar to those associated with WAIHA, for example, extravascular RBC destruction. Another well-studied drug that causes this type of AIHA is procainamide. Currently, the drug most commonly associated with this mechanism is fludarabine; other drugs with convincing evidence that they cause DIIHA by this mechanism are cladribine, levodopa, and mefenamic acid.

Drug-independent Antibodies That Are Found in Combination with Drug-dependent Antibodies
Some drugs that cause DIIHA, for example, cefotetan, can be shown to be associated with both detectable drug-dependent antibodies and drug-independent antibodies. In the case of cefotetan, the drug-dependent

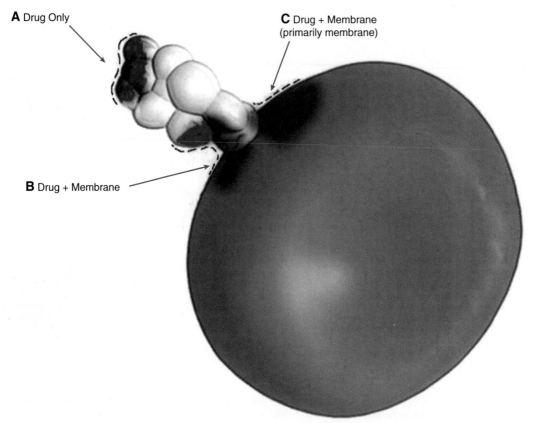

FIGURE 17-3   A unifying hypothesis to explain the concurrent presence of drug-dependent and drug-independent antibodies. Antibodies can be produced to (a) the drug alone, (b) a combination of the drug and RBC membrane, (c) a combination of the drug and RBC membrane that consists largely of RBC membrane. A combination of a, b, and/or c can occur. (Illustrator: Adrienne B. Mendoza.)

antibodies react to a very high titer, for example, median AGT titers of 16,000 versus drug-treated RBCs and 64 versus untreated RBCs in the presence of cefotetan, but the drug-independent antibody reacts to a much lower titer, for example, AGT titers of 1 to 4 versus untreated RBCs.[39] These drug-independent antibodies are not believed to be caused by alterations in the immune system (as seen with methyldopa) but rather are thought to be due to the presence of a spectrum of drug-related antibodies, some that react with the drug alone and some that react with the drug + RBC membrane (see Fig. 17-3).[16,40] If some of the latter antibodies are directed primarily against the RBC membrane, then they may react (although less optimally) without the drug being present.

Sometimes patients appear to have drug-independent antibodies, for example, antibodies that are detected without adding drug in vitro, but reactivity is due to the presence of in vivo circulating drug (or drug–antibody immune complexes) in the patient's blood sample and not due to a true drug-independent antibody. If the drug has a short half-life, the presence or absence of a drug-independent antibody can be demonstrated by obtaining a new blood sample from the patient a few days after stopping the drug, when it is no longer circulating. A few days after stopping a drug with a short half-life, a sample containing a drug-independent antibody will still react while one containing a drug-dependent antibody will no longer react without the in vitro addition of drug. Alternatively, in vitro methods (e.g., chromatography and/or dialysis) could be used to detect and/or remove drug from a patient's blood sample.

Nonimmunologic Protein Adsorption (NIPA)

NIPA was first described in the 1960s with the first-generation cephalosporin, cephalothin.[41,42] It was noted that a significant percentage of patients receiving cephalothin developed a positive DAT. One theory, with serologic evidence to support it, proposes that drugs that cause NIPA change the RBC membrane and that plasma proteins (immunoglobulins, complement, albumin, fibrinogen, etc.) are then

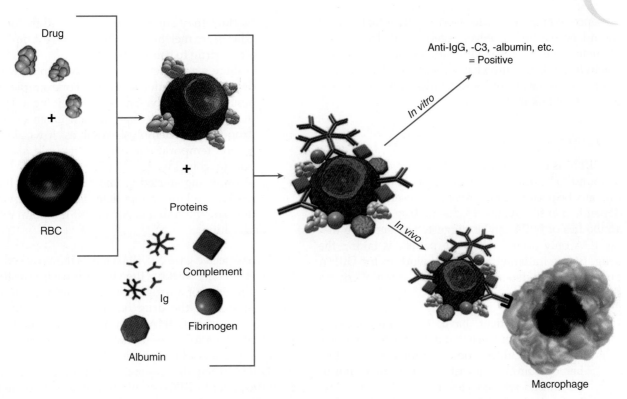

FIGURE 17-4 Nonimmunologic protein adsorption. Certain drugs that bind to RBC membranes cause a change in the membrane. This change makes the RBC membrane "sticky" so that plasma proteins (immunoglobulins, complement, albumin, fibrinogen, etc.) will bind nonspecifically. In vitro, this can cause positive antiglobulin tests. In vivo, this can lead to macrophage-mediated RBC destruction. (Illustrator: Adrienne B. Mendoza.)

nonimmunologically adsorbed onto the changed RBC membrane (Fig. 17-4).[43] When RBCs coated with one of these drugs in vitro are incubated with serum/plasma, either from a patient suspected of having DIIHA or a normal donor, the IAT will be positive due to nonspecifically adsorbed complement and/or IgG. This may also occur in vivo, explaining the presence of a positive DAT (due to nonspecifically bound IgG and complement) in patients taking a drug that causes NIPA. Positive reactions with an antihuman albumin reagent would provide evidence for this type of reactivity; antihuman albumin is not routinely available but could be obtained from a manufacturer of immunology reagents and standardized for use with RBCs for research purposes.

When NIPA was first described and for many years after, it was thought that NIPA could only be the cause of positive serologic results but that it was clinically unimportant. In the last 10 years, there has been in vivo and in vitro evidence[44,45] indicating that NIPA may be associated with IHA, for example, in patients with increased plasma IgG levels.[46] Other drugs that have been associated with NIPA include some other cephalosporins (e.g., cefotetan), cisplatin, diglycoaldehyde, oxaliplatin, suramin, and the β-lactamase

inhibitors, clavulanate, sulbactam, and tazobactam. The β-lactamase inhibitors are found in combination with β-lactam antibiotics, for example, in Timentin (ticarcillin + clavulanate), Unasyn (ampicillin + sulbactam), and Zosyn or Tazocin (piperacillin + tazobactam). Some of the drugs that cause NIPA (e.g., cefotetan and oxaliplatin) are also associated with drug-dependent antibodies (with or without drug-independent antibodies). Similar to IHA due to drug-independent antibodies, IHA due to NIPA cannot be proven in the laboratory (all sera, including that from normal donors, will react by the AGT with RBCs treated with drugs that cause NIPA). Showing that the IHA only occurs when the patient is taking the drug could lend support to the presence of IHA due to NIPA.

Management of DIIHA

If a patient is suspected of having IHA due to a drug, then the drug should be stopped. If the IHA resolves, then that is evidence that the IHA may have been due to the drug but it could also be coincidental, especially if the patient was started on some other treatments (e.g., steroids, intravenous immunoglobulin) at the same time.[47] If serologic studies demonstrate the presence of an antibody to the drug, then that patient should be warned to never receive that drug again. There have been some in vitro studies looking at cross-reactivity of drug antibodies with other related drugs, but the relationship of these results to in vivo cross-reactivity is unknown.[48]

Laboratory Investigation of DIIHA

As DIIHA is rare, many cases of suspected DIIHA will be found to be due to other causes. Laboratory testing can only be performed to prove the presence of a drug-dependent antibody; DIIHA due to drug-independent antibodies or NIPA can be suggested by showing that the IHA only occurs when the patient is taking the drug. Before initiating a serologic workup for DIIHA due to a drug-dependent antibody, certain criteria should be met.

1. Does the patient have an acquired IHA? Laboratory evidence that indicates the presence of IHA includes some combination of low hemoglobin/hematocrit, raised indirect bilirubin, raised reticulocytes, raised LDH, and low haptoglobin level. The presence of hemoglobinemia and hemoglobinuria is evidence that the hemolysis is likely intravascular in nature, especially if signs of renal failure are present.

2. Is the patient's DAT positive? For a drug-related antibody to cause IHA, the drug-dependent antibody and/or complement must be bound to the patient's RBCs in vivo at the time of the IHA. An eluate prepared from a patient's DAT-positive RBCs, containing drug-dependent antibody, should only react with drug-treated RBCs or untreated RBCs in the presence of a solution of drug, that is, untreated RBCs should not react. However, if a patient presents with a positive DAT and an eluate that is nonreactive with untreated RBCs, a drug antibody should not be the first thing to suspect. Other more likely reasons for a positive DAT with a nonreactive eluate are that the patient's RBCs are (a) nonimmunologically coated with IgG due to high plasma IgG levels or (b) coated with anti-A or anti-B from an out-of-group platelet or plasma transfusion (which would not be detected if the eluate is only tested vs. group O RBCs).

3. Has the patient recently received a drug that has been previously described as causing IHA? Table 17-5 lists drugs that have been associated with DIIHA and/or a positive DAT. If the suspected drug is not on the list, a serologic workup may still be warranted if all the other criteria are met, as it may be the first example of a new drug to cause IHA.

4. Is there a good temporal relationship between drug administration and IHA? For example, if a nonhemolyzing patient starts receiving a drug, then starts hemolyzing, is then taken off the drug and the hemolysis resolves, it would be a good temporal relationship (it could also be due to coincidence). If the patient had IHA before being started on the drug or if the IHA resolves while the patient is still receiving the drug, then that is not a good temporal relationship.

If a suspected case of DIIHA meets the above criteria for a serologic workup, then the approach to testing for the presence of a drug-dependent antibody needs to be decided. If the drug has been previously described as causing DIIHA, then the reported methods used to detect antibodies to that drug should be used. If the drug has not been previously described as causing DIIHA, then the patient's serum and an eluate from the patient's RBCs should be tested by two methods: (a) against drug-treated RBCs and (b) against untreated and enzyme-treated RBCs in the presence of drug. If the patient has one or more RBC alloantibodies, then the test RBCs need to be negative for those antigens. Detailed step-by-step procedures for the detection of drug-dependent antibodies are given in the *AABB Technical Manual*[4] and in *Immune Hemolytic Anemias* by Petz and Garratty.[1] Some general considerations follow.

Preparation of Drug Solutions

The first step of a serologic investigation to detect a drug-dependent antibody, after obtaining the drug (usually from a pharmacy), is to prepare a solution of the drug. The drug solution needs to be compatible with RBCs and thus the first choice for a solvent is normal saline, for example, phosphate-buffered saline (PBS). Information about a drug's solubility can be obtained from a variety of sources: the *Merck Index*,[49] the *Physicians' Desk Reference*,[50] the pharmacy, and/or the drug's manufacturer. If the drug is in powder form and is soluble in water, then it is simply a matter of adding a measured amount of the drug powder to PBS to make a solution of the desired concentration. Drugs that come in tablet (which requires grinding) or capsule form contain inactive ingredients, for example, dyes and/or fillers, in addition to the therapeutic drug. These inactive ingredients often do not go completely into the solution but the supernatant can be used after centrifugation to remove the precipitate (the concentration of drug in this type of solution is unknown). If the drug is not soluble in water, a number of different methods have been described to help increase solubility; these include vortexing the drug solution and/or heating it to 37°C, and the use of different solvents, for example, organic solvents or those that contain bovine albumin or have a low pH. The final solution should be compatible with RBCs.

If a drug antibody is detected after testing with a drug solution that contains inactive ingredients, further testing with the pure drug is needed in order to prove that the antibody was directed against the drug and not an inactive ingredient.[51] Pure drug can sometimes be obtained from a commercial chemical company (e.g., Sigma-Aldrich, St. Louis, MO) or the drug's manufacturer. Some drugs are found in combination with other drugs, for example, Bactrim = trimethoprim + sulfamethoxazole and Zosyn = piperacillin + tazobactam. When testing combination drugs like these, it is important to test the individual drugs separately. Some drug antibodies are only detected by testing metabolites (breakdown products) of the drug.[40] Well-characterized drug metabolites can sometimes be obtained from a drug's manufacturer; uncharacterized drug metabolites can sometimes be obtaining by collecting samples (serum and/or urine) from individuals who have recently taken the drug. The latter are referred to as "ex vivo" drug preparations.

Preparation and Testing of Drug-coated RBCs

Drug-coated RBCs are prepared in vitro by incubating fresh, group O RBCs with a solution of drug, for example, 40 mg/mL. If the patient has one or more alloantibodies (e.g., anti-K, anti-Jk[a], etc.), then RBCs negative for the appropriate antigen(s) should be used. If the patient has an autoantibody detectable, the possible approaches include: (1) use serum/plasma that has been adsorbed to remove autoantibody, (2) use a dilution of serum/plasma at which the autoantibody (which is typically of a low titer) no longer reacts knowing that a weak drug antibody could be missed, or (3) if the autoantibody has a specificity use antigen-negative test RBCs if available, for example, for autoanti-e use e- test RBCs.

The patient's serum/plasma and an eluate from the patient's RBCs should be tested against the drug-treated RBCs and the same RBCs that were incubated with the solvent alone (control RBCs). This testing should include examinations for hemolysis (if serum is used) and agglutination after a 37°C incubation, and

sensitization via the AGT. A positive control containing antibody that reacts with the drug should be tested, if available, to show that the drug-treated RBCs are indeed coated with drug; without this control a negative result with the patient's serum is difficult to interpret. Negative controls should include PBS and a pool of sera/plasma from normal donors. If the pool of normal sera/plasma reacts with the drug-treated RBCs then there are two likely explanations: (1) if the AGT is positive with all normal sera/plasma, then the drug may cause NIPA and the testing should be repeated using serum/plasma diluted 1 in 20 in PBS to decrease the protein levels (eluates are low protein by nature and should not be reactive due to NIPA), or (2) if there is direct agglutination after the 37°C incubation with some normal sera/plasma, then some normal individuals may have low titer IgM antibodies to the drug or a structurally similar chemical. The presence of low titer IgM antibodies in some normal sera/plasma has been demonstrated with penicillin, cefotetan, and piperacillin but the antibodies found in patients with IHA due to these drugs have different characteristics. Patients with IHA due to penicillin and cefotetan typically have drug antibodies in their serum/plasma that react to high titers by the AGT and in eluates prepared from their RBCs. Patients with IHA due to piperacillin have antibodies to piperacillin that are detected by testing in the presence of drug (see next section).

Testing RBCs in the Presence of Drug

Most drugs associated with IHA do not bond firmly with RBCs and antibodies to these drugs can only be detected by mixing serum and drug and RBCs together at the same time (the "immune complex" method). Antibodies that are detected by this method often cause in vitro hemolysis that can only be detected if *serum* (containing complement) is used for these tests. The addition of fresh normal inert serum as a further source of complement, the use of a 6% to 10% (v/v) suspension of test RBCs, and the use of enzyme-treated RBCs often enhances the detection of in vitro hemolysis. Agglutination and AGT results are also often stronger with enzyme-treated RBCs. The drug is usually prepared as a 1 mg/mL solution or as a saturated solution; in control tests PBS is added instead of the drug solution. After incubation at 37°C for 1 to 2 hours, tests are examined for hemolysis, agglutination, and sensitization by the AGT (using anti-IgG + anti-C3).

Eluates from patients' RBCs can be tested by this method but are often nonreactive. If the PBS control (patient's serum + PBS + RBCs) is reactive, the presence of in vivo circulating drug or drug-immune complexes in the patient's sample should be considered. This can be demonstrated by removing the drug from the sample (via dialysis) or testing a new sample obtained from the patient several days after stopping the drug, which should no longer contain in vivo circulating drug or drug-immune complexes (unless the drug has a very long half-life); the dialyzed sample or a new sample should no longer react without added drug in vitro. If the patient's serum still reacts without the in vitro addition of drug, then an autoantibody is most likely present and the same approaches mentioned under preparation and testing of drug-coated RBCs for testing in the presence of autoantibody should be used.

Clinical and Serologic Features of DIIHA Due to Cefotetan, Ceftriaxone, and Piperacillin

Cefotetan

Recently the most common drug associated with DIIHA has been cefotetan. Cefotetan is a second-generation cephalosporin that started being used in the United States in 1985 (available as Cefotan until 2006 and as the generic form starting in 2007). The first case of IHA due to cefotetan was reported in 1989[52]; since then over a 100 cases have been described in the literature. Patients with DIIHA due to cefotetan typically have high titer antibodies to cefotetan (in some cases the AGT titer vs. cefotetan-coated RBCs has been reported to be as high as 200,000) and unlike DIIHA due to penicillin, may have only received a single dose of cefotetan for the first time. Most patients receive cefotetan prophylactically (e.g., in surgery), often for obstetric/gynecologic procedures (e.g., cesarean section delivery).[53,54] The hemolytic anemia usually becomes apparent 1 to 2 weeks after receiving the drug; in contrast to penicillin, signs of intravascular hemolysis (hemoglobinemia and hemoglobinuria) are not uncommon in DIIHA due to cefotetan, and a number of deaths have occurred. Patients with DIIHA due to cefotetan have drug-dependent antibodies in their serum that react with both cefotetan-coated RBCs and untreated RBCs in the presence of cefotetan; in about a third of cases weak drug-independent antibodies are also detectable (and cefotetan has been shown to cause NIPA).[39] Eluates from these patients' RBCs are strongly reactive with cefotetan-coated RBCs; the last wash control may also be reactive.[55]

A patient with DIIHA due to cefotetan who presents with IHA, a positive DAT and a drug-independent antibody could be misdiagnosed with WAIHA instead of cefotetan-induced IHA. If a patient receives cefotetan and a blood transfusion during surgery, and presents 1 to 2 weeks later with IHA and a positive DAT, both a delayed hemolytic transfusion reaction and IHA due to cefotetan need to be considered. Some investigation may be needed to discover that a patient received cefotetan in surgery, that is, this information may be in the anesthesiologist's notes and not on the patient's medication list. Unfortunately, sometimes a patient presents (e.g., to the emergency room) with IHA 1 to 2 weeks postsurgery but is initially suspected of having a postsurgical infection and receives more cefotetan (with disastrous results—e.g., death and/or renal failure). RBC-bound cefotetan can be detected in vivo for a median of 67 days, which may explain why IHA due to cefotetan can persist longer than expected after the drug is stopped.[56]

Ceftriaxone

After cefotetan, the most common drug currently causing IHA is ceftriaxone. Ceftriaxone is a third-generation cephalosporin that was introduced in the United States in 1984 (as Rocephin and now is also available as a generic). It was first described as causing DIIHA in an adult in 1988[57]; since then over 30 cases of DIIHA due to ceftriaxone have been reported with at least half of these occurring in children or adolescents. The patients' RBCs are usually coated with C3 and often with IgG as well, but anticeftriaxone cannot usually be demonstrated in eluates prepared from these RBCs. Ceftriaxone antibodies can only be detected by testing serum in the presence of the drug (i.e., by the "immune complex" method)[39]; the antibodies are often IgM and directly agglutinate RBCs as well as bind complement. In vitro hemolysis is generally seen when testing serum, especially with enzyme-treated RBCs. These patients often have severe intravascular hemolysis associated with renal failure and death (particularly in children/adolescents). Typically, patients with IHA due to ceftriaxone have previously received multiple doses of ceftriaxone with no obvious ill effects. When hemolysis does occur, it is often acute and dramatic, typically occurring within a very short time after receiving ceftriaxone (minutes) in children versus a longer time (days) in adults.

Piperacillin

In our laboratory, piperacillin is now the third most common cause of DIIHA due to a drug-dependent antibody. Piperacillin (a semisynthetic penicillin) was first approved by the FDA in 1981 and in the United States was available as Pipracil until 2002 and as a generic starting in 2004. A combination of piperacillin with tazobactam (a β-lactamase inhibitor) was approved by the FDA in 1993 (trade name is Zosyn in the United States and Tazocin outside the United States). The first case of DIIHA due to piperacillin was described in 1994[58]; since then at least 10 other cases have been reported. Patients with DIIHA due to piperacillin have drug-dependent antibodies that react in the presence of piperacillin (the "immune complex" method); their serum may also react with piperacillin-coated RBCs but many normal donors have IgM piperacillin antibodies that react with piperacillin-coated RBCs, thus rendering these results noninformative.[59] The patients' RBCs are usually coated with IgG with or without C3 but eluates have not been shown to contain antipiperacillin reactive with piperacillin-coated RBCs. Clinically, some patients have been described with signs of intravascular hemolysis and there have been a couple of deaths. Similar to cefotetan, cases of IHA due to piperacillin have been initially confused with WAIHA (due to the presence of circulating drug) and hemolytic transfusion reactions.

If a patient receiving the combination drug of piperacillin + tazobactam (e.g., Zosyn) presents with IHA, both piperacillin and tazobactam need to be considered as possible causes of the IHA and each drug should be tested separately by the "immune complex" method only. Tazobactam has been described as causing IHA due to NIPA; thus, tests with tazobactam-treated RBCs will not be informative.

SUMMARY

The AIHAs can be broadly classified serologically according to the optimal temperature of reactivity of the autoantibody, for example, warm-reactive or cold-reactive. The role of the blood bank is to characterize the serologic reactivity and determine if alloantibodies are also present along with the autoantibodies.

Free autoantibodies in the serum of patients with WAIHA and CAS can interfere with pretransfusion testing; approaches to deal with these serologic issues diminish or remove the autoantibody reactivity so that test results can be interpreted with confidence. For most cases of PCH, pretransfusion testing is not affected because the causative antibody does not generally cause agglutination at room temperature or above; the biphasic hemolysin is demonstrated by the Donath-Landsteiner test.

Drugs are a rare cause of IHA. The serologic and clinical characteristics of DIIHA fall into four types: drug-dependent antibodies (those that react with drug-treated RBCs and those that only react in the presence of the drug), drug-independent antibodies, and NIPA. The presence of DIIHA due to drug-independent antibodies or NIPA can only be suggested by showing a temporal relationship between drug administration and in vivo hemolysis. Methods are available for detection of drug-dependent antibodies in the laboratory. A good clinical history is important for deciding if a laboratory workup for DIIHA is warranted.

Review Questions

1. Warm autoimmune hemolytic anemia is characterized most frequently by which of the following serologic patterns?
   a. DAT positive (IgG and C3) and a reactive eluate
   b. DAT positive (IgG only) and a nonreactive eluate
   c. DAT positive (C3 only) and a reactive eluate
   d. DAT positive (IgG and C3) and a nonreactive eluate

2. In cold agglutinin syndrome, the DAT is usually positive for:
   a. C3 only
   b. IgG only
   c. IgG plus C3
   d. neither IgG nor C3

3. Which of the following is characteristic of paroxysmal cold hemoglobinuria?
   a. the autoantibody is usually IgM
   b. the antibody is biphasic
   c. the antibody is usually detected in pretransfusion tests
   d. the antibody has a high titer at 4°C

4. Autologous adsorptions should not be used when:
   a. the patient has never been transfused
   b. the patient has a history of anti-Jk[a] but has not been transfused within the last 3 months
   c. the patient received two units of RBCs last month
   d. none of the above

(continued)

REVIEW QUESTIONS (continued)

5. A child with clinical signs of hemolytic anemia was admitted to the emergency room. He had a viral infection last week and his mother noticed that his urine was red. The DAT is positive with anti-C3 only and the antibody detection test was negative. Which of the following is a possible diagnosis?
   a. WAIHA
   b. CAS
   c. PCH
   d. none of the above

6. Which of the following is the least encountered reason for a positive IgG DAT with a nonreactive eluate?
   a. drug-dependent antibody
   b. anti-A or anti-B from plasma-containing product(s)
   c. nonimmunologic IgG uptake due to increased plasma IgG
   d. none of the above

7. A patient presents with hemolytic anemia and a history of receiving Zosyn (piperacillin + tazobactam) just prior to the start of hemolysis. The DAT is positive (IgG + C3). What testing should be performed?
   a. test serum versus piperacillin-treated RBCs
   b. test serum versus untreated RBCs and enzyme-treated RBCs in the presence of piperacillin
   c. test serum versus tazobactam-treated RBCs
   d. test serum versus untreated RBCs and enzyme-treated RBCs in the presence of tazobactam
   e. both b and d.

8. A patient receiving ceftriaxone develops hemolytic anemia. The DAT is positive (IgG+C3). The patient's serum reacts with all test RBCs (no drug added) by the indirect antiglobulin test, but an eluate prepared from the patient's RBCs is nonreactive. Which is the most likely explanation for these results?
   a. idiopathic warm autoantibody
   b. drug-independent antibody (e.g., due to fludarabine)
   c. circulating drug (or drug-immune complexes) in the patient's sample
   d. Nonimmunologic protein adsorption

9. In 2008, cefotetan was the most common reported cause of DIIHA. True or false?

10. A patient is suspected of having hemolytic anemia due to a drug that has not been previously described as causing DIIHA. Drug-treated RBCs are prepared in the laboratory and tested with the patient's serum and an eluate from the patient's RBCs. Which of the following is *not* true of results with drug-treated RBCs?
    a. nonreactive results with the patient's samples proves that no drug antibody is present
    b. antiglobulin test reactivity with all normal sera indicates the possibility of nonimmunologic protein adsorption
    c. direct agglutination after the 37C incubation with some normal sera indicates the possibility of IgM antibodies to the drug (or a structurally similar chemical)
    d. reactivity of the patient's serum and eluate and nonreactive results with normal sera indicates the presence of an antibody to the drug

REFERENCES

1. Petz LD, Garratty G. *Immune Hemolytic Anemias.* 2nd ed. Philadelphia, PA: Churchill Livingstone; 2004.

2. Kaplan HS, Garratty G. Predictive value of direct antiglobulin test results. *Diagnostic Med.* 1985; 8: 29–32.

3. Judd WJ. Elution—dissociation of antibody from red blood cells: theoretical and practical considerations. *Transfus Med Rev.* 1999; 13: 297–310.

4. Roback JD, Combs MR, Grossman BJ, et al., eds. *Technical Manual.* 16th ed. Bethsda: AABB, 2008.

5. Toy PT, Chin CA, Reid ME, et al. Factors associated with positive direct antiglobulin tests in pretransfusion patients: a case control study. *Vox Sang.* 1985; 49: 215–220.

6. King KE, Ness PM. Treatment of autoimmune hemolytic anemia. *Semin Hematol.* 2005; 42: 131–136.

7. King KE. Review: pharmacologic treatment of warm autoimmune hemolytic anemia. *Immunohematology.* 2007; 23: 120–129.

8. Garratty G. Immune hemolytic anemia associated with negative routine serology. *Semin Hematol.* 2005; 42: 156–164.

9. Rodberg K, Tsuneta R, Garratty G. Discrepant Rh phenotyping results when testing IgG-sensitized RBCs with monoclonal Rh reagents [abstract]. *Transfusion.* 1995; 35(suppl): 67S.

10. Leger RM, Garratty G. Evaluation of methods for detecting alloantibodies underlying warm autoantibodies. *Transfusion.* 1999; 39: 11–16.

11. Church AT, Nance SJ, Kavitsky DM. Predicting the presence of a new alloantibody underlying a warm autoantibody [abstract]. *Transfusion.* 2000; 40(suppl): 121S.

12. Laine EP, Leger RM, Arndt PA, et al. In vitro studies of the impact of transfusion on the detection of alloantibodies after autoadsorption. *Transfusion.* 2000; 40: 1384–1387.

13. Branch DR, Petz LD. A new reagent (ZZAP) having multiple applications in immunohematology. *Am J Clin Pathol.* 1982; 78: 161–167.

14. Branch DR. Blood transfusion in autoimmune hemolytic anemias. *Lab Med.* 1984; 15: 402–408.

15. Leger RM, Garratty G. A reminder that ZZAP reagent removes complement in addition to IgG from coated RBCs [letter]. *Immunohematology.* 2006; 22: 205–206.

16. Garratty G. Target antigens for red-cell-bound autoantibodies. In: Nance SJ, ed. *Clinical and Basic Science Aspects of Immunohematology*. Arlington, VA: American Association of Blood Banks; 1991: 33–72.

17. Garratty G. Specificity of autoantibodies reacting optimally at 37°C. *Immunohematology*. 1999; 15: 24–40.

18. Branch DR, Petz LD. Detecting alloantibodies in patients with autoantibodies [editorial]. *Transfusion*. 1999; 39: 6–10.

19. Young PP, Uzieblo A, Trulock E, et al. Autoantibody formation after alloimmunization: are blood transfusions a risk factor for autoimmune hemolytic anemia? *Transfusion*. 2004; 44: 67–72.

20. Maley M, Bruce DG, Babb RG, et al. The incidence of red cell alloantibodies underlying panreactive warm autoantibodies. *Immunohematology*. 2005; 21: 122–125.

21. Ahrens N, Pruss A, Kähne A, et al. Coexistence of autoantibodies and alloantibodies to red blood cells due to blood transfusion. *Transfusion*. 2007; 47: 813–816.

22. Petz LD. A physician's guide to transfusion in autoimmune haemolytic anaemia. *Br J Haematol*. 2004; 124: 712–716.

23. Waligora SK, Edwards JM. Use of rabbit red cells for adsorption of cold autoagglutinins. *Transfusion*. 1983; 23: 328–330.

24. Dzik WH, Yang R, Blank J. Rabbit erythrocyte stroma treatment of serum interferes with recognition of delayed hemolytic transfusion reaction [letter]. *Transfusion*. 1986; 26: 303–304.

25. Mechanic SA, Maurer JL, Igoe MJ, et al. Anti-Vel reactivity diminished by adsorption with rabbit RBC stroma. *Transfusion*. 2002; 42: 1180–1183.

26. Storry JR, Olsson ML, Moulds JJ. Rabbit red blood cell stroma bind immunoglobulin M antibodies regardless of blood groups specificity [letter]. *Transfusion*. 2006; 46: 1260.

27. Sokol RJ, Hewitt S, Stamps BK. Autoimmune haemolysis: an 18 year study of 865 cases referred to a regional transfusion centre. *Br Med J*. 1981; 282: 2023–2027.

28. Shulman IA, Branch DR, Nelson JM, et al. Autoimmune hemolytic anemia with both cold and warm autoantibodies. *JAMA*. 1985; 253: 1746–1748.

29. Aster RH, Bougie D W. Drug-induced immune thrombocytopenia. *N Engl J Med*. 2007; 357: 580–587.

30. Stroncek DF. Drug-induced immune neutropenia. *Transfus Med Rev*. 1993; 7: 268–274.

31. Snapper I, Marks D, Schwartz L, et al. Hemolytic anemia secondary to mesantoin. *Ann Intern Med*. 1953; 39: 619–623.

32. Harris JW. Studies on the mechanism of a drug-induced hemolytic anemia. *J Lab Clin Med*. 1956; 47: 760–775.

33. Garratty G, Arndt PA. An update on drug-induced immune hemolytic anemia. *Immunohematology*. 2007; 23: 105–119.

34. Arndt PA, Garratty G. The changing spectrum of drug-induced immune hemolytic anemia. *Semin Hematol*. 2005: 42: 137–144.

35. Ley AB, Harris JP, Brinkley M, et al. Circulating antibody directed against penicillin. *Science*. 1958; 127: 1118–1119.

36. Carstairs K, Worlledge S, Dollery C, et al. Methyldopa and haemolytic anaemia [letter]. *Lancet*. 1966; 1: 201.

37. Worlledge SM, Carstairs KC, Dacie JV. Autoimmune hemolytic anemia associated with alpha-methyldopa therapy. *Lancet*. 1966; 2: 135–139.

38. Kirtland HH, Mohler DN, Horwitz DA. Methyldopa inhibition of suppressor-lymphocyte function: a proposed cause of autoimmune hemolytic anemia. *N Engl J Med*. 1980; 302: 825–832.

39. Arndt PA, Leger RM, Garratty G. Serology of antibodies to second- and third-generation cephalosporins associated with immune hemolytic anemia and/or positive direct antiglobulin tests. *Transfusion*. 1999; 39: 1239–1246.

40. Mueller-Eckhardt C, Salama A. Drug-induced immune cytopenias: a unifying pathogenetic concept with special emphasis on the role of drug metabolites. *Transfus Med Rev*. 1990; 4: 69–77.

41. Gralnick HR, Wright LD Jr, McGinniss MH. Coombs' positive reactions associated with sodium cephalothin therapy. *JAMA*. 1967; 199: 725–726.

42. Molthan L, Reidenberg MM, Eichman MF. Positive direct Coombs tests due to cephalothin. *N Engl J Med*. 1967; 277: 123–125.

43. Garratty G, Leger R. Red cell membrane proteins (CD55 and CD58) are modified following treatment of RBCs with cephalosporins [abstract]. *Blood*. 1995; 86: 68a.

44. Garratty G, Arndt PA. Positive direct antiglobulin tests and haemolytic anaemia following therapy with beta-lactamase inhibitor containing drugs may be associated with nonimmunologic adsorption of protein onto red blood cells. *Br J Haematol*. 1998; 100: 777–783.

45. Arndt P, Garratty G. Can nonspecific protein coating of RBCs lead to increased RBC destruction? Drug-treated RBCs with positive antiglobulin tests due to nonspecific protein uptake give positive monocyte monolayer assays [abstract]. *Transfusion*. 2000; 40: 29S.

46. Broadberry RE, Farren TW, Bevin SV, et al. Tazobactam-induced haemolytic anaemia, possibly caused by non-immunological adsorption of IgG onto patient's red cells. *Transfus Med*. 2004; 14: 53–57.

47. Petz LD, Gitlin N, Grant K, et al. Cimetidine-induced hemolytic anemia: the fallacy of clinical associations. *J Clin Gastroenterol*. 1983; 5: 405–409.

48. Arndt PA, Garratty G. Cross-reactivity of cefotetan and ceftriaxone antibodies, associated with hemolytic anemia, with other cephalosporins and penicillin. *Am J Clin Pathol*. 2002; 118: 256–262.

49. O'Neil MJ, ed. *The Merck Index: An Encyclopedia of Chemicals, Drugs, and Biologicals*. 14th ed. Whitehouse Station, NJ: Merck Research Laboratories; 2006.

50. Physicians' Desk Reference. 62nd ed. Oradell, NJ: Medical Economics; 2008.

51. Law IP, Wickman CJ, Harrison BR. Coombs'-positive hemolytic anemia and ibuprofen. *South Med J*. 1979; 72: 707–710.

52. Eckrich RJ, Fox S, Mallory D. Cefotetan-induced immune hemolytic anemia due to the drug adsorption mechanism [abstract]. *Transfusion*. 1989; 29: 17S.

53. Garratty G, Leger RM, Arndt PA. Severe immune hemolytic anemia associated with prophylactic use of

cefotetan in obstetric and gynecologic procedures. *Am J Obstet Gynecol.* 1999; 181: 103–104.

54. Viraraghavan R, Chakravarty AG, Soreth J. Cefotetan-induced haemolytic anaemia. A review of 85 cases. *Adverse Drug React Toxicol Rev.* 2002; 21: 101–107.

55. Arndt PA, Leger RM, Garratty G. Reactivity of "last wash" elution controls in investigations of cefotetan antibodies [abstract]. *Transfusion.* 1999; 39: 47S.

56. Davenport RD, Judd WJ, Dake LR. Persistence of cefotetan on red blood cells. *Transfusion.* 2004; 44: 849–852.

57. Postoway N, Schwellenbach J, McMahill PC, et al. A fatal case of cephalosporin-induced immune hemolytic anemia with clinical and serological characteristics usually associated with an immune-complex mechanism [abstract]. *Transfusion.* 1988; 28: 35S.

58. Johnson ST, Weitekamp LA, Sauer DE, et al. Piperacillin-dependent antibody with relative e specificity reacting with drug treated red cells and untreated red cells in the presence of drug [abstract]. *Transfusion.* 1994; 34: 70S.

59. Leger RM, Arndt PA, Garratty G. Serological studies of piperacillin antibodies. *Transfusion* 2008;48:2429–2434.

QUALITY ASSURANCE AND SAFETY IN IMMUNOHEMATOLOGY

MARY LIEB AND EVA QUINLEY

OBJECTIVES

After completion of this chapter, the reader will be able to:

1. Define quality assurance.
2. Describe the role of quality assurance in a blood center or transfusion service.
3. Identify and define key words of a successful quality assurance process.
4. Understand the value of standard operating procedures.
5. Know the components of an error management system.
6. Describe the process for performing a quality assurance audit.
7. Know the purpose of internal audits.
8. Discuss the relationship of quality assurance to quality control and continuous quality improvement.
9. Explain the relationship between the systems, processes, inputs, and outputs.
10. Describe the problem-solving process.
11. Describe the hazardous exposure risks.
12. Define the elements of a biosafety program.
13. Discuss the factors involved in waste management.

KEY WORDS

Audits
Biohazards
Calibration
Continuous quality improvement
Corrective action
Customer
Inputs
Outputs
Performance indicators
Problem solving
Process
Quality assurance
Quality assurance program
Quality control
Quality improvement process
Quality management
Quality system essentials
Standard operating procedure
Supplier
Systems
Trends
Universal precautions
Validation

The *quality improvement process* is a style of management that puts quality first in all activities. According to W. Edwards Deming, improving the quality of our products and services improves productivity by reducing rework, waste, and inefficiencies. This way, companies do less and spend less to achieve the same outcomes. It leads to lower operating costs, making our organizations more competitive.[1,2]

During the 1990s, increased regulatory scrutiny has played a major role in forcing changes in the way blood establishments operate. The Food and Drug Administration (FDA) began to more strictly enforce sections of the Code of Federal Regulations (CFR) known as the good manufacturing practices (GMPs). A special emphasis was placed on compliance with the 200 series of GMPs. Also, in 1995, the FDA released the *Guideline for Quality Assurance in Blood Establishments.*[3] This document provides guidance for the content of a *quality assurance* program. It states that a quality assurance program must include steps to prevent, detect, and correct deficiencies that may compromise blood product quality.[3]

Quality management plays an important role in the management of any blood establishment. Quality management is seen as a way to increase the quality of health care and reduce costs, to become efficient. Quality assurance plays a major role in quality management. Because organizations work through *processes* and *systems*, improvements are made as the result of reengineering processes and systems and removal of non–value-added steps.

There are many business reasons for establishing a quality assurance program within a blood establishment. Quality assurance functions not only assure the quality of the services and products provided but also identify the customers and suppliers of a process, their needs, and how well these needs are being met.

Customers include internal and external people such as patients, donors, fellow employees, hospitals, doctors, the community, and regulatory agencies. A person, department, or organization that provides input (e.g., information, materials) to any process is a *supplier*. A person, department, or organization that receives the output of any process is a *customer*. External customers purchase the final products and services. Internal customers are employees who receive work from other employees within the organization.

Once we realize how customers and suppliers relate internally and externally, the idea of quality management becomes clearer. The focus should then be on the processes or systems that need to be improved in order to improve the service or products provided by a supplier to a customer.

The FDA's *Guideline for Quality Assurance in Blood Establishments* and AABB's *The Quality Program*[4] provide examples of defined blood banking systems. The original guidance provided in developing a Quality Program for Blood Banks and Transfusion Services indicated systems were broken down into critical control points and their associated key elements. Within each system, the critical control points of the process were identified. These are the areas that may affect the safety and the quality of work being done if the key elements are not performed correctly. The key elements are the individual steps within the critical control points. Many times the key elements are addressed by written *standard operating procedures* (SOPs). *Performance indicators* can be established to monitor the key elements, critical control points, and systems of the organization. This terminology although still found to be used in many quality plans has been updated to address systems as *Quality System Essentials*. These systems can be broken down into individual *processes* that support each system. Each process includes specific *inputs* to provide an *output*, which may result in a test result, report, or product. The *Quality System Essentials* (QSEs) address specific processes that must be present in a blood bank and transfusion service.

QUALITY ASSURANCE

A *quality assurance program* is defined in the FDA's *Guidelines for Quality Assurance in Blood Establishments* as a system designed and implemented to ensure that manufacturing is consistently performed in such a way as to yield a product of consistent quality.[3]

Quality assurance is the combination of activities necessary for blood centers and transfusion services to ensure quality products and services for their customers. These activities include compliance with GMPs as stated in the CFR as one part of the quality assurance program.

Quality assurance is part of the broader quality improvement process, which ensures that quality continually benefits the organization and its customers (Fig. 18-1). Areas of concern in the quality assurance process include personnel, training, policies and procedures, documentation and records, error reporting, audits, inspections, validation and quality control, supplier qualification, and label control.

As stated in the FDA's *Guideline for Quality Assurance in Blood Establishments*, the goals of quality assurance are to significantly decrease errors, ensure the credibility of test results, implement effective manufacturing processes and system controls, and ensure continued product safety and quality. Quality assurance includes

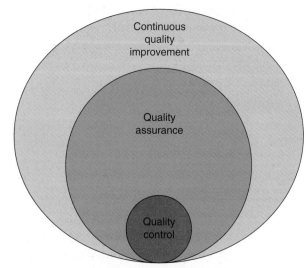

FIGURE 18-1 Relationship of continuous quality improvement, quality assurance, and quality control.

measures to prevent, detect, investigate, assess, prioritize, and correct errors.[3] The emphasis is on preventing errors rather than detecting them retrospectively.

Quality assurance is the responsibility of everyone in the organization. Quality is everyone's job. One person or one department cannot be responsible for the quality of the entire organization. It takes teamwork, with everyone aware of and responsible for their share of the quality assurance activities, to improve the quality of blood banking services.

Quality Assurance Department

Each blood establishment should have a designated set of people responsible for developing, implementing, and monitoring its quality assurance activities. This quality assurance department may consist of one or more people. This department may perform strictly quality assurance functions or it may have other responsibilities in the organization. Ideally, quality assurance personnel should report directly to top management independent from operations.

Quality assurance is charged with taking immediate, proactive, and preventive actions before systems and process go out of control.[5] To do this, quality assurance must review and analyze data and reports to look for *trends* that may indicate a system is going out of control.

Responsibilities of the quality assurance department include the following:

The review and approval of:

- procedures and policies,
- training program content,
- validation protocols and results,
- document control,
- record-keeping systems,
- corrective action plans,
- suppliers,
- product specifications,
- error reports,
- job descriptions,
- lot release,
- performing audits,
- analyzing for trends,
- monitoring corrective actions,
- maintaining current SOPs,
- providing summary reports of findings.

Personnel

Qualifications

The most important part of any quality improvement or quality assurance process is the people involved. Well-trained, knowledgeable personnel are responsible for the quality of the work produced and the services provided by any blood center or transfusion service.

Ensuring the quality of personnel begins with the selection process, which starts with properly written job descriptions and performance standards. The job description should list the duties and responsibilities the employees are expected to perform. The continuing education requirements of the position should also be specified in the job description.

Performance standards should address how each duty and responsibility is to be measured. These performance standards should be developed with input from all personnel for their particular position. The performance standards should offer an understanding of the extent to which the job is to be performed. These standards should be written for every position within an organization. The orientation of new employees should include a review and explanation of the performance standards required by the organization.

When interviewing a job candidate, relevant education and work experience should be obtained from his or her resume. The personal interview is used to evaluate the behavior of the candidate. The interviewer should ask for specific examples of how the candidate reacted in certain situations in the past, which may give insight as to the candidate's ability to handle similar situations in the future.

Well-selected employees increase the quality of the work performed. Hiring people who are best qualified for a particular job increases the cooperation and teamwork between coworkers. Thus, the quality of the work performed improves. Also, good employee selection increases job satisfaction and decreases turnover and related personnel problems.

Periodically, the job description and performance standards should be reviewed with each employee. Discussions should focus on the employee's progress, with the development of action plans to improve performance as necessary.

Training and Continuing Education

All personnel should be encouraged and allowed to participate in continuing education and training activities. These activities may include outside professional meetings and seminars, in-house meetings, written exercises, journal clubs, presentations, reading assignments, audio- or videotapes, computer-assisted learning, and self-instruction.

Records of all training and continuing education activities attended by or presented by any staff should include date, topic, objectives, presenter, location, and length of the activity. These records are to be maintained and made available for review by any of the regulating agencies or organizations. Information obtained by attending any educational activities should be shared with the rest of the staff in a written or oral format.

The quality assurance department should be involved in the development, review, and approval of training programs before they are implemented. This review includes training programs in the areas of

- new employee orientation,
- policy and procedures,
- computers,
- technical issues,
- management issues,
- quality assurance,
- GMPs.

The quality assurance department must also be involved in identifying areas where refresher training may be necessary. Quality assurance should approve retraining programs before they are implemented.

Proficiency Testing

Proficiency testing is used to monitor and compare the performance of laboratories. Proficiency testing specimens should be treated and tested the same as any routine patient or donor specimen. Testing of these specimens should be rotated among all personnel who perform the procedures being evaluated. All observations, results, and interpretations of this testing must be recorded. Supervisory review of results and interpretations should be recorded. In cases when proficiency testing results are unacceptable, *corrective action(s)* taken should be documented.

Proficiency tests can be developed internally using patient or donor specimens or situations. Such prepared tests are more frequently obtained, however, from outside sources. External proficiency testing programs are available through organizations such as the College of American Pathologists (CAP). These programs offer comparison of one laboratory with all other laboratories participating in testing.

The quality assurance department should review and monitor the results of proficiency testing for trends that suggest problems with the testing methods or equipment. A corrective action plan should be written by operations and submitted to quality assurance for review, approval, and monitoring for any failed proficiency testing.

Competence Assessment

Competence assessment documents the performance abilities of the personnel performing the various tasks in a blood center or transfusion service. It ensures that

personnel are adequately trained and maintain their competency to perform their assigned functions.

Competence assessment programs should test technical skills and knowledge. This testing may include direct observation of performance, review of production and quality control and other records for completeness and accuracy, written tests, and practical or demonstrable testing. These tests should be administered on a routine basis and include all personnel on all shifts. Competence assessment should be administered by the operational management staff for the department.

The quality assurance department should regularly review the competence assessment program to determine its adequacy and to determine if any trends exist, suggesting performance problems.

Standard Operating Procedures

One of the most important documents in any blood bank or transfusion service is the SOP manual. The SOP manual must be up to date, with procedures for all tasks to be performed in the collection and processing of blood, component preparation, compatibility testing, and storage, distribution, and disposition of all blood and blood components. Each procedure should provide detailed instructions on how a particular task is to be performed. The manufacturer's directions for use of reagents and equipment must be strictly followed when developing the procedures. The procedure manual must be complete, accessible to all staff, strictly adhered to, and understandable.

An SOP should include examples of any forms for recording and interpreting test results as well as any labels used. Any symbols or abbreviations used should be defined. Where applicable, instructions on how to read, score, record, and interpret test results are required for each procedure. The maintenance and retention of all records should be described. SOPs should contain sections on troubleshooting and corrective actions to be taken if quality control testing does not fall within acceptable limits. Instructions for recording results in a computer system should be included in the SOPs if a computer is used at the facility.

A uniform format should be followed for each written procedure. A suggested SOP format is given in Box 18-1. Other suggested SOP formats include the one given in the AABB *Transfusion Service Manual of Standard Operating Procedures, Training Guides and Competence Assessment Tools.*[6]

SOPs must be revised as new regulations and standards are issued and as problems with the existing procedures are discovered and resolved. They must also be revised when changes are made to manufacturers' package inserts. Personnel who use the

---

BOX 18-1

Procedure Format

- Name and location of the facility
- Title
- Document ID number
- Original, effective, and revision dates
- Principle of purpose
- Scope
- Specimen requirements
- Material requirements (supplies, reagents, equipment)
- Quality control
- Step-by-step procedure
- Interpretation of test results
- Documentation
- Procedural notes
- References
- Author's and reviewer's signatures

---

procedures should be involved in writing, revising, and validating them. As users of this information, they have a better knowledge of the problems and special situations to be addressed.

Validation of a procedure involves at a minimum reading the procedure to see if it is understandable and complete. If at all possible, the new or revised procedure should be performed to assess if the procedural steps can be performed as written.

Documentation must exist to show that personnel are aware of and have been trained on procedures. This training must occur before a new or revised procedure can be implemented. Training for new SOPs or for complicated changes to existing SOPs should consist of more than reading, initialing, and dating the procedure.

All procedures must be reviewed at least annually by individuals who are familiar with the task. It is helpful to establish a schedule for reviewing certain procedures throughout the year. This avoids the necessity to review all procedures at one time, as well as providing a more thorough review of each procedure. A written procedure should explain how and when this review is to occur. The procedure should describe how revisions or changes to any procedure are to be handled. It also should describe how the rationale for the revision or modification is to be documented. This documented rationale is to be filed with the removed procedure for future reference.

As part of the quality assurance function, all revised or newly written procedures should be reviewed and approved in writing by the quality assurance department for adherence to regulations and

for impact the SOPs may have on other areas/departments. These concerns should he addressed and resolved before the procedure is implemented. A quality assurance review of an SOP should determine if

- the procedure is clear, complete, and logical,
- SOP format use followed,
- SOP reflects what is being done,
- personnel and supervisory responsibilities are delineated,
- staff accountability is addressed,
- instructions for documenting on forms and logs are given,
- records maintenance and retention are addressed,
- quality control requirements are stated,
- training plan is written and approved by quality assurance,
- any required validation has been performed and approved by quality assurance.

Standard Operating Procedure Document Control

Document control systems are needed to ensure that procedures and changes to procedures are received and distributed properly, and that obsolete versions are retrieved and archived. The document control system should be developed and maintained by operations for the distribution, retrieval, and archiving of all procedures, forms, and documents related to each procedure.

Quality assurance should review and evaluate this document control system on a periodic basis to determine if the system is operating as described and effectively. This review should include determining if

- documents are appropriately distributed,
- a master list of all documents is available,
- departmental copies of SOPs are current, in the appropriate manual, and the table of contents is current,
- all obsolete versions of procedures are retrieved when a new or revised procedure is implemented.

The purpose is to track and trace all SOPs from implementation through all revisions to its current state or archival of the document.

Documentation and Records

Documentation must be maintained for all of the steps involved in donor recruitment and the collection, processing, testing, labeling, storage, distribution, compatibility testing, administration, and final disposition of all components. Documentation must be performed to allow both traceability and trackability.

Trackability means having an audit trail that allows a process to be followed sequentially. Traceability refers to the ability to identify what was done, who did it, when it was done, what was used to do it, and so forth.

Records must include dates and initials of personnel performing each critical step. These records should be reviewed for completeness and accuracy before components are released from the blood center for distribution or from the transfusion service for transfusion. These records should be well maintained so that a unit of blood can be traced from its donor to the final disposition of each component.

Good record keeping is necessary as proof of proper performance and to show that requirements were met. Also, it helps to recreate a problem situation and determine what went wrong. Corrective action can then be taken to prevent similar errors and problems in the future.

A review of records is very important at the blood establishment. For example, a final review step at the blood bank should include a physical check that the components from units with reactive tests for any of the infectious disease markers are quarantined before the day's work is released for labeling or for distribution.

All results are to be recorded as the work is being performed. Records are to be completed appropriately with dates and initials as they are created. A daily review by designated personnel is necessary to ensure that all records are complete and accurate. Records should be audited periodically to detect any deviations or problems in the record-keeping systems.

Written corrections or changes to any records are to be made in the following manner (Box 18-2):

- Draw a single line through the erroneous result.
- Write the correction above or beside the wrong results or answer.
- Initial the correction.
- Date the correction.

Inappropriate methods of correcting errors in blood establishments include the use of whiteout, blacking out a result, and using pencils and erasers.

If the records to be corrected or modified are computer records, the original data and the new data, along with the date and initials of the personnel entering the original data and the changed data, should be identifiable.

Because of the necessity of maintaining records of each critical step, it is important that the forms and systems used to record the information are easy to use and understand. The purpose of each form and the importance of the information it contains should be understood by all personnel using the form.

The quality assurance department should approve all manual and electronic record-keeping systems. Appropriate review and approval of validation of such a system is quality assurance's responsibility also. Quality assurance should monitor the process for reviewing records to ensure that timely reviews are occurring by the appropriate personnel. Also, quality assurance should ensure the completeness and accuracy of the records and should initiate corrective action as necessary if problems are discovered.

Records Management, Retention, and Storage

Most of the records involved in the recruitment of donors and the collection, processing, testing, labeling, storage, distribution, compatibility testing, administration, and final disposition of blood and blood products now must be retained. Examples of the records to be retained are shown in Box 18-3.

The amount of time that records are required to be retained varies from state to state, between regulating agencies, according to company-specific policies and depending on the type of record. After determining the time frames for the agencies that regulate and inspect an organization, it is best to retain records for the longest period required by any these agencies.

BOX 18-2

Proper Correction of Written Records

Jane P. Doe
MR #: 12445678
A Neg 3/1/08

BOX 18-3

Records to Retain

- Donor collection information
- Laboratory testing results
- Compatibility testing results
- Transfusion requests
- Adverse reactions
- Emergency release
- Component preparation
- Dispositions
- Storage and inspection records
- Irradiation
- Products from other, outside sources
- Old procedures
- Quality assurance records

The method of storing records varies from organization to organization. Whether records are stored in their original paper form or on microfilm or microfiche depends on the number of records to be stored and the amount of space necessary to store them. Also, the method of storage must allow relatively easy access to the records if needed at a future date and importantly ensure that records are protected from damage or destruction.

The quality assurance department should review the record management system to verify the existence of the following:

- Strict control of and access to confidential records.
- A checkout system if records are to be removed and returned to the department.
- A system of transferring records from one form of storage medium to another.
- Requested records can be retrieved within a reasonable and specified period of time.
- A system for correcting archived records.
- All production records for a specific donation number.

Nonconformance

The terminology used to describe events that are outside expected occurrences may vary from one organization to another. These events may be designated in any manner, as long as the facility has defined them for staff in an SOP. In this text, the term "nonconformance" is used generically to describe all such events and includes errors, accidents, incidents, complaints, deviations, and the like. Nonconformance should be looked at as an opportunity for improvement and should be used as learning tool. An effective nonconformance management system should be established in blood establishments and should contain processes and SOPs to accomplish the following:

- Detection
- Documentation
- Timely reporting/recall
- Investigation/root-cause analysis
- Corrective action
- Follow-up/effectiveness checks
- Communication

The nonconformance management system should apply to all departments in an organization. Nonconformance reports should be used to document internal and external problems and to find opportunities for improvements within the organization.

In some instances when the nonconformance has the potential to affect the safety, purity, potency, identity, or quality of the blood component or is an error that threatens a patient's safety, it must be reported to the FDA as part of error and accident reporting. Licensed facilities, registered and nonregistered facilities are required to report biologic product deviations (BPD) to the FDA.

As with continuous improvement, prevention of nonconformances should be a main focus of quality assurance. To prevent such events, the root cause of the nonconformance must be identified and eliminated. To accomplish this, accurate and complete records must be available for review and trending purposes. Corrective action should include short- and long-term plans, as well as improvements to the processes involved. Examples of corrective actions include, but are not limited to, retraining personnel, revising procedures, retesting samples, performing competency testing, restructuring work areas, hiring additional personnel, or buying new equipment. Caution must be exercised to ensure that unnecessary training is not done or that procedures are not "tweaked" unnecessarily. Training and procedural changes should only be embarked upon once it is determined that they will fix a root cause of a problem. Corrective action must be continuously evaluated and monitored to determine if the problem has been eliminated or corrected without creating other problems.[7]

Adverse reactions should also be investigated using written and approved procedures. Patient care personnel must be trained and competent to recognize adverse reactions in donors or recipients and to administer the appropriate intervention for a particular reaction. Timely and appropriate notification to the collection facility and the FDA must occur for fatalities related to blood collection or transfusion.[8]

Transfusion services should have procedures in place for identifying products implicated in posttransfusion disease transmission. For cases of documented posttransfusion hepatitis, human immunodeficiency virus (HIV) infection, and other diseases, the facility that collected the unit must be notified, and the patient should be followed to determine if infection has occurred.

The quality assurance department is responsible for reviewing all nonconformance reports, including those pertaining to adverse reactions. Quality assurance, along with operations, investigates and assesses the systems and processes involved to determine the root cause of the event. Corrective action can then be designed and implemented to prevent recurrence of the nonconformance in the future. Quality assurance should continue to monitor the corrective action that has been implemented to determine its effectiveness. Also, quality assurance should track nonconformance reports to look for trends and prevent nonconformances before they occur.

In some cases, blood establishments may need to hold material review boards (MRB). The purpose of the MRB is to determine if an error or issue has resulted in a potential for product impact. If this is the case, the MRB decides that product should be recalled. If no recall is deemed necessary, the rationale for that decision is documented.

Peer Review

Peer review of transfusion practice is required by various agencies and organizations as part of their accreditation or reimbursement programs, namely, AABB, CAP, the Joint Commission (TJC), and Medicare. Blood utilization review should consist of the evaluation of patient safety initiatives, appropriate and effective use of all transfusions given, the evaluation of all true transfusion reactions, and the evaluation of all cases of transfusion associated with disease transmission. The purpose of peer review is to evaluate a facility's transfusion practices and to improve the quality of patient care.

Quality Assurance Audits

An *audit* is a systematic investigation to determine if an organization's actual activities and practices are being performed according to its approved and written policies and procedures.[9] Performing audits is a important function of the quality assurance department. Audits are usually performed by staff in the quality assurance department. However, other staff members may perform audits if they have no direct responsibilities for the process being audited and have been appropriately trained to do the audit.

An audit serves as an internal self-assessment tool and provides confidence that systems and processes are in control. A focused or process audit is used to assess a specific problem. A general audit is more comprehensive and is used to assess overall operations of a department.

Audits should be used to monitor transfusion, testing, component preparation and distribution practices, and other processes, such as record reviews. Audits should be performed by people not directly involved in the activity being audited.

A schedule of which audits are to be performed, and when, should be established. This schedule should include who will conduct the audit as well as who will manage the results of the audit. Written procedures should specify how the various audits will be performed and how the results of the audit will be used.

There must be a written procedure on how to conduct an audit. This procedure should include how to develop a checklist covering the details to be reviewed during each audit. This procedure should also include a section describing the necessary documentation for each audit. This documentation should state the operation being audited, the auditors, the dates of the audit, the findings, corrective action plan, and follow-up information.

Quality assurance audits should be designed using a systems approach. The activities of any organization can be classified into major systems. Each system consists of a number of processes. The inputs and outputs of a process may affect the safety and quality of the product if the key steps in the process are not performed or functioning correctly. An input such as personnel, procedures, equipment, environment, supplies, and reagents encompass activities that must be performed correctly and consistently for the process to perform as expected and produce the expected outcome. Quality assurance audits should evaluate inputs and outputs of each process that are included in each system. See Box 18-4 for examples of systems and their associated inputs and outputs. The AABB's *The Quality Program*[4] and the FDA's *Guideline for Quality Assurance in Blood Establishments*[3] offer well-defined systems for the blood banking industry.

Every audit should be concluded with an exit interview to present the audit findings. This should be followed by a timely, written report of these findings.

An audit should be well planned with follow-up action to correct any problems discovered during the audit. Audits should be used as learning tools, not as discipline.

Quality assurance produces a written report of any audits performed. Appropriate management personnel should review and evaluate the results of

---

BOX 18-4

Examples of Systems Process: Inputs and Outputs

System: Process

Inputs		
	Compatibility testing	Donor collection
	Blood type	Donor selection
	Sample	Donor
	Reagents	Donor health screening
	Procedures	Donor history
	Equipment	questionnaire

Outputs		
	Valid blood type	Qualified donor
	ABO discrepancy	Deferred donor

all audits to ensure that they are aware of the problems and that corrective action is implemented.

Inspections

Inspections are another way to determine how an organization is performing. Inspections are performed by outside agencies, such as the FDA, TJC, and AABB or CAP, for licensing or accreditation reasons. The written inspection report is to be shared with middle and top management so they are aware of the findings of the inspection and take an active role in providing corrective action for the findings.

The key to surviving inspections by these outside agencies is always to be ready for them. Performing mock inspections is a good self-assessment tool. These mock inspections should be used to learn what activities need to be corrected to pass an official inspection.

To deal with an official inspection, a team should be formed to control the inspection process. One member of the team should stay with the inspectors throughout the inspection. When accompanying the inspectors, the team member is responsible for recording all questions asked, records examined, and copies requested. The team members should handle all inquiries and needs of the inspectors.

It is easy to see why doing things right the first time will benefit an organization during inspections. If records document appropriate information and required reviews, the chance of errors and deficiencies during an inspection is greatly reduced.

Supplier Qualification

Manufacturing of high-quality blood and blood components depends on high-quality supplies and services provided by vendors. An important part of the quality assurance program is the approval of the suppliers that will be used to provide the needed supplies and services to the blood establishment.

Depending on the organization, the responsibility for auditing suppliers may not be assigned to an individual department. There may be an organization-wide quality assurance department or the materials management department that is responsible for approving any suppliers to be used by the organization.

Each individual department should be responsible for identifying and managing the equipment, supplies, and reagents that are critical for ensuring safety and quality of their products and services. A critical equipment and supply list should be current and available on request or for referral. A written procedure should exist stating how supplies will be evaluated on receipt, tracked for appropriate storage, and inspected before use. This procedure should include

steps for documentation of the inspection steps, corrective action taken, and disposition of unacceptable supplies.

Quality assurance is responsible for ensuring that procedures exist and are followed for the receipt, inspection, approval, use, and tracking of all equipment, supplies, and reagents used in the transfusion service or blood center setting.

Facilities, Equipment, and Process Activities

To ensure accurate testing results and proper product preparation, all equipment and instruments in the blood center or transfusion service must be functioning properly. Proper equipment qualification and calibration, along with preventive maintenance, quality control, and monitoring, are necessary to ensure proper functioning.

Each piece of equipment or instrumentation used in a blood establishment should have a unique identification code and be qualified and calibrated before use, after repairs, and on a periodic basis.[8,10,11] There should be written procedures that include requirements for initial qualification, calibration, quality control, preventive maintenance, and monitoring of each piece of equipment used in manufacturing and testing. These procedures should include instructions for documentation of results of testing, actions to take for results that are unacceptable, instructions for follow-up on problems found, and instructions for documentation of corrective action taken.

Calibration, quality control, and preventive maintenance schedules should be established and described for each piece of equipment and instrument used anywhere in the blood bank. The frequency of the testing should be sufficient to ensure proper performance of each piece of equipment.

Monitoring of the results of the equipment testing should include evaluating conditions that are out of control for the potential effect on quality, safety, purity, and potency of the products produced.

Validation

Validation is defined as documented evidence providing a high degree of assurance that a process will consistently produce an acceptable result. A validation's purpose is to demonstrate that the process or equipment produce results that achieve a planned outcome. A validation protocol should be developed for all critical processes to obtain this high degree of assurance before a process is implemented. It is important to stress that processes are validated; however, equipment, is qualified or verified. There are prospective, retrospective, and concurrent validations. Prospective validations are generally used for new or revised processes prior to implementation. Retrospective validations can be used to assure and provide documentation that an existing process that was already in operation but not sufficiently tested is acceptable. Concurrent validation provides required data that cannot be obtained in a test environment. This requires extra review more frequently at predetermined intervals prior to authorization for full implementation of the process.

Processes involving computer systems and software must be validated before initial use. Such processes must be revalidated after modifications or upgrades.

Problems occurring during validation procedures should be evaluated for the need to revise and revalidate the process.

The quality assurance department is responsible for ensuring that SOPs are in place for initial validation and revalidation of processes when a change occurs, which may affect the result of the process. Quality assurance is responsible for reviewing and approving a validation protocol before a validation is begun. Quality assurance should review and approve the results of the validation testing to ensure that an adequate validation process was performed before the process is implemented. Quality assurance must also see that documentation of all validation testing and reviews is maintained.

Calibration

Calibration is a comparison of a measurement standard of known accuracy with a particular measurement on a piece of equipment to ensure the equipment's accuracy.[12] Calibration is performed on pieces of equipment that contain measurement devices. Not all equipment in the blood bank or transfusion service has a calibration requirement. Manufacturers' directions, users' manuals, and the appropriate regulations should be consulted to determine if, and what type of, calibration is required and the frequency. At a minimum, any time a piece of equipment is repaired or serviced, calibration of the measurement device of that equipment should be performed.

There must be a written procedure describing calibration, including who is to perform what, when, and how it is to be performed, and how to document the findings.

Sometimes the blood establishment has a biomedical engineering department or a metrology department that performs calibrations for it. Even though the blood bank may not perform the calibrations, it is responsible for ensuring that the calibrations are performed as scheduled, the results are acceptable, corrective actions are taken as necessary, and procedures are followed and are current.

Quality assurance is responsible for ensuring that the calibration schedules are met and that the results obtained are within the established, acceptable range. If quality assurance finds that the schedules have not been adhered to or the results of the testing are not acceptable, quality assurance may shut down the piece of equipment until the proper calibrations have occurred. An assessment of the work that was produced during the time that the equipment was out of control must be performed to evaluate the effect on the products. Products produced using improperly calibrated equipment may need to be discarded.

Quality Control

Quality control involves sampling and testing and is an important aspect of quality assurance. Quality control procedures are performed to ensure that blood bank reagents and equipment are functioning properly before using them for testing. Also, quality control procedures are performed on blood products to ensure the products at least meet the established acceptability criteria.

The technical staff understands of the reagents, equipment, and blood products they are using, why they are using them, and how they are to be used is the most important part of the quality control process.

The frequency of quality control testing and the procedure for the testing of the various reagents, equipment, and blood products are determined by reviewing the appropriate regulations and the manufacturer's instructions.

Records of quality control testing must be maintained and must include

- testing results and interpretations,
- identification of the personnel performing the tests,
- manufacturer of the reagents,
- lot numbers of the reagents tested,
- expiration dates of the reagents,
- the date of the testing,
- any corrective action required due to unsatisfactory results.

Quality assurance is responsible for auditing the quality control that is performed on reagents, equipment, and products. If quality assurance finds that the quality control requirements have not been met, it may stop the process.

An assessment of the work that was produced during the time that the quality control testing was out of control must be performed to evaluate the effect on the products. Products produced during periods of improperly performed or omitted quality control may need to be discarded. Patient testing performed in the transfusion service that provided a product or test result would also require repeat testing if quality control testing was not properly performed. Prior results would, if possible, need to be validated for accuracy.

Computers

The introduction of computer systems into blood centers and transfusion services has provided many benefits, including improved productivity and record keeping. Along with these benefits come the responsibilities of training on use of the system, validation of the software, understanding the system's capabilities, monitoring the system, and establishing procedures for operation and maintenance.

Security for any computer system is necessary to prevent unauthorized people from gaining access to the system or to particular functions in the system. This security usually consists of a password or security code system. Documentation of the security systems in place and how they are used is necessary.

Procedures must be written to describe the use and operation of the computer system. Existing procedures may need to be revised to reflect the computer interactions as software changes. Procedures on the specific uses and operations of the computer must be developed. Procedures must deal with any problems that are detected in the software. These procedures should describe how the problems are to be corrected and by whom. Corrective actions taken also should be documented. The person making changes to the software must be identified; these changes must then be monitored to make sure they have not caused problems in other areas of the software. Testing must then show that the change is working appropriately. This testing and the results should be documented. Documentation of the change is required for tracking and traceability.

Procedures for any preventive maintenance should be available to the operators of the system. These procedures should include a schedule of all preventive maintenance to be performed. A list of each piece of hardware in use, its location, and dates of any maintenance performed should be kept.

There must be a method to identify any person making changes or corrections to original records and results in the system. The original data and the person who entered this data, along with the change to the data, date of the change, and the person making the change should be documented.

As with any electronic equipment, computer systems experience times when they are not usable. During these times, there must be backup systems in place to allow the work to continue. A plan of action needs to be defined for the scheduled and unscheduled times when the computer system or other instruments that interface with the computer system are not available for use. These action plans need to address short periods of downtime (hours) versus long periods of downtime (days).[13] During downtime, continuous records of donor or patient information must be available for use. This can be accomplished by using paper records or a separate personal computer system.

All active files on the computer system should be backed up daily. These backup records should be stored off-site for future use if necessary.

After downtime, a plan to bring the system back to being functional is required. This recovery plan should include the following:

- How data will be entered into the system?
- Who will enter the data?
- Which data need to be entered before other data can be entered?
- Verify existing critical data have been maintained and unchanged.

Computer Validation

Validation is the process of testing software before it is put into use to determine if it will work consistently and reproducibly as expected. A written plan should explain how to perform the validation and how to document the results of the validation. This plan should include a definition of the process to be validated, who is to perform which piece of the validation, how the system will be challenged, the expected outcomes of each step of the validation and acceptance criteria, number of trials to be performed, and those responsible for the review and approval of this validation. These plans and any accompanying SOPs and documentation should be available for review.

Any time a new computer system is put into place or changes occur to the existing system, all affected personnel must be trained. Written procedures should explain how this training is to be accomplished. A variety of training methods can be used depending on the nature of the changes. The use of a test system is a good way to provide this training. The training procedures should specify how to document that the training occurred and the results of the training.

Monitoring the control functions of the system is necessary to ensure that the system works as expected. The control functions include the areas for which computers make decisions about the acceptability of blood products for distribution. The functions to be monitored include all of the functions involved in the storage and retrieval of data related to the collection, processing distribution, storage, and disposition of all blood products. Revalidation of these functions is necessary as changes in equipment, processes, supplies, and software occur.

Quality assurance must ensure that computer systems and software are validated and that personnel are adequately and appropriately trained in how to use the computer.

Label Control

Various steps of the manufacturing process require labeling of the blood product. In the donor room, the product is labeled according to the type of product that is intended to be made from the whole-blood unit. During component preparation, products are labeled with additional component-type labels. During the actual labeling process, the blood type and expiration date labels are applied to the components. Products can then be modified from one product type to another at the blood center or the transfusion service. Labeling process controls should be in place to ensure proper labeling of the product at each stage. Labeling controls should include

- development of label specifications,
- inspection and acceptance of labels on receipt and before release,
- storage and release of labels,
- managing defective labels,
- security of labels,
- managing discrepancies after unit labeling.

The process of labeling products should be controlled each time a product is labeled or relabeled. The process controls must ensure that the correct labels are attached to the appropriate product and that the product was maintained at its appropriate temperature during the labeling process. Relabeling of a product requires the use of the same process controls as when the product was initially labeled.

A master set of labels used in the facility should be maintained and archived following record archival procedures.

Quality assurance's role in label control is to ensure the procedures exist describing the process controls for labels and the labeling process. Also, quality assurance is responsible for ensuring that the procedures are followed and records are maintained as described.

Lot Release

Lot release requires that the record reviews be complete, accurate, and in compliance with regulations before the release of a lot for distribution. In the blood industry, a lot is defined by a single, unique unit number.[3] All of the components from the whole-blood unit bearing the same unit number are a lot of product. Any discrepancies or failures of a lot to meet the established specifications are to be thoroughly investigated.

Problem Solving

The *problem-solving* process plays a major role in a quality assurance program. As system problems arise, a defined method for investigating, analyzing, and resolving the problem is required. There are several good problem-solving methods available, and the reader is referred to the Additional Readings section for more information.

Team Building

Teamwork is important in the problem-solving process because the generation of ideas, sharing of information, and building on concepts enable a team to provide better, permanent solutions to problems. The use of teams to solve system problems is vital.

To function productively, team members need to be trained on teamwork concepts and rules, and encouraged and supported to achieve team results.

Not every problem faced in day-to-day operations requires the use of a team to solve it. However, the problem can be resolved by using the same process that the team would use.

Problem Identification

Problems that exist in any organization can be discovered from a variety of sources. Error reports, communication logs, record reviews, observation, accident reports, staff meeting minutes, staff suggestions, and customer complaints and quality indicators can all be valuable sources for identifying problems that need to be addressed.

Data Collection

To solve any problem, reliable data and facts are needed. The data collected must be relevant to the problem being investigated and must be meaningful and accurate if the problem is to be resolved successfully. Data collection may be the most important step in solving any problem.

The following items should be determined before collecting data.

- Purpose for data collection
- What data to collect

- How these data will help to meet customers' needs
- How the data will be analyzed
- How will the data be reported and to whom
- What additional data are needed

Once the necessary data have been collected, they can be used to determine the cause of the problem. Number and word data can be graphically displayed in a variety of ways to get the most out of it. This makes it easier to uncover patterns and trends within the data and immediately focus on the most important targets for improvement.

Initially, the data collected serve as the baseline against which to measure future performance. As more data are collected, the information can be analyzed against the baseline to determine the status of the performance. Evaluation of the data may then include statistical analysis and control charts.

Problem-solving tools such as flow charts, cause-and-effect diagrams, force-field analysis, control charts, histograms, and Pareto charts can be used to help evaluate and analyze the data gathered.

Corrective Action

Corrective action should be aimed at resolving the problem's root cause. This may mean eliminating the occurrence of the same kind of problem or improving the process so that the right outcome is achieved. Corrective action may be short- or long-term action or improvements to the process.

Some of the main causes of problems include lack of knowledge, defects in systems, and poor performance or behavior problems. The lack-of-knowledge issue may be addressed by developing new training sessions or revising existing training. It may be necessary to initiate new or revised competency testing programs or to revise the existing policies and procedures. Additional reference materials may need to be provided.

Defects in the systems must be addressed by revising and posting the policies and procedures so that everyone can see them and refer to them easily. Better or different equipment or supplies may be needed. Restructuring of the workflow in a particular area or developing a new maintenance schedule may be required.

Behavior or performance problems should be addressed by changing job duties, counseling, coaching, positive feedback, communication, and appropriate hiring.

A main factor in defining the right type of corrective action is to include the personnel who know the processes and tasks involved in the problem. The front-line personnel know where to look for problems that may result from solving the current problem. They will be more inclined to accept the corrective action and implement it if they have been involved in developing the action and understanding the need for the action.

There may be more than one corrective action that would resolve the problem at hand. An evaluation of the resources needed to implement each corrective action and the barriers associated with each corrective action helps determine which option best fits the organization's needs at this point in time. The team should recommend the corrective action or a number of corrective actions to upper management, along with the resources and carrier evaluation. This aids upper management in making the final decision on the corrective action to implement.

Corrective Action Plan

A plan for implementing corrective action should be developed by operations in cooperation with quality. This plan should include who or what is expected to change, who is responsible for taking the indicated action, what action is to be taken, and when the change is to occur.

Quality assurance is responsible for following up on the corrective action plan to ensure that the implementation time frame is met and that the corrective action is in place. This follow-up also involves monitoring the corrective action to see that it is effective and that other problems have not been created as a result of it.

Monitoring

Once a problem has been identified and corrective action instituted, the progress and effectiveness of the action must be formally monitored. This monitoring may show that the corrective action has effectively solved the problem or that the process must be refined further to prevent the errors or problems from recurring. Monitoring the change is necessary to measure its benefits. An important step before monitoring is to decide key points to evaluate the effectiveness of the change.

Quality assurance is responsible for auditing to see that the corrective action was implemented and monitored appropriately.

Performance Indicators

Examples of activities to use as performance indicators at a blood center or transfusion service include the following:

- Compliance with procedures
- Completeness and accuracy in documentation
- Timely delivery
- Timely and accurate reporting of results
- Results from proficiency testing

- Turnaround times
- Customer complaints
- Error reports

These indicators should be monitored only by the data that can be documented for review. These data can be collected by direct observation, record reviews, interviews, questionnaires, and prospective versus retrospective reviews. Who will collect the needed data, how to collect them, and when to collect them must be determined by quality assurance and operations.

Performance indicators should be used to monitor the critical processes in blood banks and transfusion services. A performance indicator must be measurable. Indicators may relate to administrative, technical, or results issues of the organization.[14]

Administrative issues include qualifications of personnel; inspection, audit, and customer satisfaction survey results; accident and error reports; and purchasing, billing, hiring, and clerical procedures. Technical issues include specimen quality, turnaround times, quality control, accuracy of test results, and adherence to procedures. Result issues include component utilization, outdated components, waste of components, and crossmatch-to-transfusion ratios.

When developing performance indicators, consider the types of equipment, qualifications and number of personnel and other resources in use, the procedures and technical aspects involved, and the problem, errors, or adverse effects that may occur. To monitor any of these factors, data must be collected.

The data needed to monitor an indicator usually are already available and being collected. Sources of these data include existing records and reports, such as patient and donor records; daily, weekly, and monthly statistical reports; incident reports; and departmental logbooks.

Once the type of data to collect and the source of these data has been determined, the decisions of when to collect, how often to collect, and how big the sample size needs to be should be made.

Progress on performance indicators should be shared with all departments involved in the process being monitored. The best way for the information to be distributed to the involved parties is through the organization's quality assurance department.

Examples of performance indicators in a blood bank or transfusion service are listed in Box 18-5.

Prevention

The main goal of the quality assurance process is to prevent errors and problems before they occur. Prevention techniques instead of detection techniques

---

BOX 18-5

Performance Indicators

- Resource utilization
- Patients without identification armbands
- Turnaround times
- Rh immune globulin administered within 72-hr guideline
- Charting of transfusion-related vital signs
- Transfusions started within 30 min of issuing components
- Transfusions completed within recommended time frames
- Crossmatch-to-transfusion ratio
- Autologous unit utilization
- Component waste
- Expiration of components
- Delivery times met
- Orders completed
- Repeat testing

---

are needed in blood centers and transfusion services. If problems and mistakes are prevented, the rework and production costs will decrease. Planning for this change from detection to prevention is an important part of top management's commitment to the organization.

Summary

The quality assurance process involves reviewing systems and evaluating the inputs and outputs of the related processes to determine how well they work or do not work. If problems are found, the focus should be on improving the process of the system.

Quality assurance is just one aspect of a broader process called *continuous quality improvement*. Quality assurance is the checks and tests performed to determine if a product or service meets its customers' requirements and the regulations. By incorporating some of the continuous quality improvement concepts of prevention, problem solving, and process redesign or improvement, the activities of quality assurance help improve the quality of the products and services provided to the blood center's or transfusion service's customers.

It is important to remember that quality assurance and continuous quality improvement are the responsibility of everyone in the organization, not just those in the quality assurance department. It takes training and hard work to develop the cultural climate necessary for any organization to become a continuously improving organization.

It is through this process of continuous quality improvement that the quality assurance activities of an organization can best be accomplished.

BIOSAFETY IN BLOOD ESTABLISHMENTS

All blood center and transfusion service personnel must be aware of the potential dangers of handling patient or donor blood specimens and units, as well as reagents. The primary safety goal of everyone in the workplace is to prevent accidents and injuries. Everyone is responsible for keeping the workplace safe by identifying and removing hazards to prevent accidents and injuries.

The growing concerns about the transmission of HIV and hepatitis infections through blood have increased the need for programs to train personnel in safety technique. This training is to be ongoing; it must be documented to show compliance with the various regulatory agencies' requirements, and it should be provided before workers begin any tasks or activities that may potentially expose them to biohazardous risks.[15]

The safety training programs at every health-care organization should include training in chemical, biologic, radiation, electrical, and mechanical hazards, and infection control, defensive driving, and facilities maintenance.

Regulatory Agencies

The regulatory agencies involved in the safety of health-care workers include but are not limited to the following:

- Occupational Health and Safety Administration (OSHA)
- Centers for Disease Control and Prevention (CDC)
- FDA
- Centers for Medicare and Medicaid Services (CMS)
- Environmental Protection Agency (EPA)

According to the OSHA regulation for protection from blood-borne pathogens, employers are required to[16,17]

- provide a hazard-free workplace,
- educate and train staff,
- evaluate all processes for potential exposure risk,
- evaluate each employee positions for potential exposure risk,
- implement labeling and post signs,
- supply universal precautions for handling blood and body fluids,

- provide personal protective equipment, such as gloves and other barriers,
- make hepatitis B vaccine prophylaxis available to all staff who have occupational exposure, unless previously vaccinated or immune, and provide hepatitis B immunoglobulin (HBIG) treatment for percutaneous injury.

Classification of Work Activity

Personnel positions in the blood center or transfusion service should be categorized as to their potential for exposure to blood or body fluid specimens. Each category of workers should receive infection control training specific to his or her position as well as general background information about the risks of exposure.

Each position in a blood center or transfusion service should be classified into one of the three levels, depending on the potential for exposure to blood or body fluids. These categories or biosafety levels of work as defined by the Public Health Service and listed in the AABB *Technical Manual* are as follows[5]:

Level 1: Work that involves agents of no known or of minimal potential hazard to laboratory personnel and the environment. Work is usually conducted on open surfaces and no containment equipment is needed.

Level 2: Work that involves agents of moderate potential hazard to personnel and the environment. Personnel wear laboratory coats and gloves as indicated; access to work areas is limited and containment equipment should be used for procedures likely to create aerosols. Most work with blood requires biosafety level 2 precautions. Exceptions may be appropriate if no open specimen containers will be encountered.

Level 3: Work that involves indigenous or exotic agents that may cause serious or potentially lethal disease as a result of exposure by inhalation. Requires protective clothing, decontamination of wastes, and containment equipment for all procedures.

Most activities involving work in the blood center or transfusion service fall into the biosafety level 2 guidelines.

Standard Operating Procedures and Training

SOPs should be developed for all work activities, explaining the potential for employee exposure to infectious agents and how to eliminate or reduce the risk of exposure. These procedures should be readily accessible to each employee. Also, they should be reviewed by operations and updated at least annually, or as regulations change or new positions or tasks with risks of exposure are added. All personnel should then be trained to understand these procedures and how they relate to the work requirements of each position in the organization.

Training should include the location and proper use of personal protective equipment and clothing. Personnel should be trained on the use of universal precautions, the color coding or tagging systems used to designate biohazardous materials, and on procedures to be used if they are exposed to blood or body fluids. Personnel who should receive this training include clerical, maintenance, environmental services, biomedical engineering, other support staff, and volunteers as well as all technical staff.

The OSHA recommends that employers establish initial and periodic training programs for all employees and volunteers who perform tasks with occupational exposure risk. This training should occur before an employee is asked to perform any task that puts him or her at risk for exposure. Periodic training should then be conducted to keep workers familiar with safety procedures. Training should focus on preventing exposure to potentially infectious agents.

All personnel should have access to the safety regulations and procedures.

Universal Precautions

The CDC has recommended "universal blood and body fluid precautions" to prevent exposure of health-care workers to HIV, hepatitis B virus, and other blood-borne pathogens.[17] These recommendations apply to blood, certain body fluids, or any body fluids contaminated with blood from all patients. This policy is now referred to as *universal precautions*. Using this policy for all patients is considered the safest approach because employees will take precautions when handling all specimens, regardless of whether the patient's infectious status is known. Also, it is easier for personnel to remember one set of guidelines and when to use them.

Universal precautions should be practiced with blood donors and samples from blood donors as well as with patients and patient samples. Even though healthy donors have low rates of infectious disease markers, the potential for exposure still exists.

Background infection control training should include discussion about the methods of HIV and hepatitis B virus transmission and the results of exposure to these diseases. All personnel are to be trained

on the appropriate times to use protective clothing and the types of protective clothing available for use.

The policies and procedures for each laboratory should specify the types of clothing and devices to be used and the conditions of use. The location and types of protective clothing available and how to use each piece should be spelled out in the procedures.

All people who may be in an area with **biohazards** or who are required to work with items that may be potential biohazards should receive training in the recognition, understanding, and handling of biohazards. This includes environmental services, maintenance, biomedical engineering, clerical, and volunteer personnel. All affected personnel need to understand the circumstances in which they can refuse to perform work on biohazardous items or in biohazardous areas. This training should include how to clean up potentially hazardous spills and how to report spills and possible exposure to infectious agents.

Personal Protective Equipment

It is the employer's responsibility to provide, clean, and dispose of appropriate personal protection equipment for all employees at no cost when occupational exposure is likely.[16,17] Also, the employer must see to it that employees follow the infection control procedures as written.

Clothing

Long-sleeved, protective barrier garments, such as laboratory coats (closed), gowns, or aprons, are to be worn by all staff performing tasks that may expose them to blood or body fluids. These garments are to be made of fluid-resistant material. They must protect all areas of exposed skin. Any time the covering barrier garment becomes contaminated with blood or body fluids, the barrier garment should be removed and replaced with a clean barrier garment. The contaminated barrier garments should be placed in properly labeled biohazard bags for laundering. No protective barrier garments are to be worn outside of the work area, regardless of whether they are visibly contaminated. These garments should not be worn in any administrative areas, rest rooms, break rooms, or visitor areas.

Gloves

Latex or vinyl examination gloves should be worn by all personnel who may have contact with any blood or body fluid specimen or units and when handling or in contact with contaminated items or surfaces. Gloves should be replaced as they become soiled or torn.

They must be available for all personnel who wish to use them.

The CDC recommends the following general guidelines for determining when gloves are necessary[16,17]:

- The health-care worker has cuts, scratches, abrasions, chapped hands, or other breaks in the skin.
- The health-care worker judges that hand contamination with blood may occur during a phlebotomy.
- A fingerstick or heelstick is being performed on infants and children.
- Personnel are receiving phlebotomy training.
- Personnel are handling an open blood container or specimen.
- Personnel are collecting or handling blood or body fluids from patients or donors known to be infected with a blood-borne pathogen.
- Personnel are cleaning up spills or handling waste materials.
- Potential risks of exposure cannot be assessed because of lack of experience with a procedure or situation.
- Personnel are examining mucous membranes or open lesions.
- Personnel are performing donor phlebotomy on autologous donors.

Gloves are to be removed if they become visibly contaminated, torn, or punctured, as well as after handling known high-risk specimens or donors and between patients. Gloves should be removed before handling telephones, doorknobs, faucets, pens, or computer terminals that have been designated as clean objects or areas. Also, personnel should be trained to avoid touching any parts of their face, eyes, nose, mouth, or ears with a gloved hand.

Gloves are to be removed by turning the gloves inside out as they are being removed, keeping the outsides of the gloves touching. Dispose of used gloves in a properly labeled biohazard bag. Hands are to be washed with soap and water after gloves are removed. Never wash and reuse latex or vinyl gloves; disinfectants may cause deterioration of the gloves.

Rubber gloves may be used for cleaning equipment, wiping up spills, and decontaminating the work area at the end of the day. These gloves may be disinfected and reused. However, observe carefully for any signs of deterioration, such as tears, cracks, peeling, or discoloration, and discard these rubber gloves as necessary.

Face Shields, Masks, and Safety Glasses

The face should be protected whenever the possibility of splashes, splatters, or aerosols of blood or body fluids exists. The purpose of the face shields and masks is to protect the eyes and the mucous membranes of the nose and mouth. Although many personnel do not like to wear the shields and masks, the alternative of not wearing them and risking exposure to a possibly life-threatening disease is foolish. As an alternative to wearing facial protection, permanent shields sometimes can be attached to pieces of equipment to prevent splashing.

Safety Practices

Workplace Design

To prevent the potential for accidents or injuries, the design of the workplace is an important factor. A workplace that is well laid out and allows for a smooth workflow is a must. Attention should also be paid to ergonomic factors such as location of benches, repetitive motion in performance of job tasks, and so forth. This helps to maintain a healthy workforce.

Handwashing

Handwashing is the most important action anyone can take to prevent the transmission of diseases. Specific sinks should be designated throughout the laboratory for handwashing only. These designated sinks should be kept clean from blood and body fluids. Hands should be washed immediately in the following instances:

- After contamination with blood or body fluids
- After contact with articles that may be potentially contaminated with blood or body fluids
- Whenever gloves are removed
- Any time hands become dirty
- When leaving a potentially contaminated work area
- After contact with any donor or patient
- Before eating, drinking, smoking, or applying makeup
- After using the restroom

If available, use warm water and soap to wash hands. If not available, use a waterless antiseptic hand cleanser.

Eyewash

An eyewash should be available in every laboratory and at every donor collection site. Portable, disposable eyewash bottles are available for use at a donor collection site. All employees should be trained on the location and the proper use of the eyewash equipment. The eyewash should be used any time irritants, blood, or body fluids get into the eyes. The irritant can be dust or dirt particles or chemicals that cause a person to rub his or her eyes. If hands are not clean or are gloved when they are used to rub the eyes, contamination by a blood-borne pathogen may occur.

Safety Shower

A safety shower should be located in an easily accessible part of the laboratory. The safety shower is to be used if a large portion of a person's clothing or body becomes splashed with irritants, blood, or body fluids. All employees should be trained on the location and the proper use of the safety shower.

Work Area

All work surfaces and reusable equipment should be decontaminated daily. At the end of a procedure or shift, all reusable equipment and supplies and work surfaces should be wiped down with a disinfectant. This also should be done any time spills or contamination occur. Regular household bleach, hypochlorite, is good for disinfecting work areas and reusable equipment. Bleach must be diluted daily to be effective. A ratio of 1:10 can be achieved by mixing one volume of bleach to nine equal volumes of water.

Biologic safety cabinets are to be used when working with infectious materials. Any specimen or blood units known to be positive for infectious agents should be dealt with only under the hood of a biologic safety cabinet. The National Institutes of Health has issued recommendations for the effective use of these cabinets.[19]

If carpeted areas must be used at a collection site, protect the area with a protective, absorbent covering that has waterproof backing. The site should be arranged to minimize the traffic in the actual donor processing and collection areas.

There should be well-written safety procedures with clear assignment of responsibilities for all personnel. Continuous training and monitoring of the safety practices is essential to ensure safe operations for staff, volunteers, donors, patients, and visitors.

Spills

Any time spills involving blood or body fluids occur they should be treated as potentially hazardous and cleaned up immediately. Proper training in the cleanup of spills, including the steps to take, supplies to use, and location of the supplies, is essential. The following steps should be taken whenever a spill occurs[5]:

- If an aerosol has been created, clear and leave the area for 30 minutes.

- If the spill occurs in a centrifuge, leave the lid closed for 30 minutes before opening to clean.
- Wear gloves and a protective barrier gown. If broken glass is present, the gloves should be puncture resistant.
- Eye protection should be worn if splashing can occur.
- Absorb the spill with absorbent towels.
- Clean the area with a detergent.
- Using a 1:10 dilution of freshly made bleach solution, flood the area and let it sit for at least 20 minutes.
- Wipe up the disinfectant.
- Dispose of all materials used to clean up the spill in appropriately labeled biohazard containers.

Housekeeping

A clean and orderly work area is the responsibility of all staff assigned to that work area. As with the technical staff, the environmental services or housekeeping staff should be trained specifically on the proper way to clean areas potentially contaminated with blood or body fluids. This training must identify the potential risks in these areas. To disinfect these areas, appropriate germicides, products approved by the EPA as effective against HIV, or a sodium hypochlorite solution (bleach) diluted 1:10 with water are acceptable.

Any equipment that is in need of repair should be cleaned and disinfected before it is repaired in the laboratory or biomedical engineering department or sent to the manufacturer for repairs.

Needle Precautions

To prevent injuries and exposure risks caused by needlesticks, needles should not be manipulated by hand. This means recapping, bending, breaking, or removing needles from a syringe is not allowed. Used needles and all other sharp objects used in the blood bank, such as lancets and broken test tubes, should be disposed of in puncture-resistant biohazard containers. These puncture-resistant containers should be located near the area where they are used or carried to the area where they will be used. The hospital phlebotomist should carry one of these containers on the phlebotomy tray. These containers should be available at every workstation at all donor collection sites.

Storage

Any reagents and hazardous specimen samples should be stored in areas separated from units of blood that are to be used for transfusion purposes. Although hazardous materials and blood units may have to be stored in the same refrigerator, they must be clearly separated from one another. The different storage areas in the refrigerator also must be clearly marked to indicate where reagents and blood should be stored. Maintaining clean, orderly, labeled, and sanitary storage areas and work areas helps reduce the risks of contamination.

Transportation

All samples of blood and body fluids to be transported should be placed in a well-constructed container with a tight-fitting lid to prevent leaking. The paperwork related to the samples should be enclosed in some type of sealable plastic bag to prevent contamination if a leak should occur.

Blood samples packaged for shipment by airlines, buses, taxis, and so forth should be place in sturdy, leakproof, double containers with enough absorbent padding around the sample to absorb any or all of the specimen if it spills. Consult the CDC and Department of Transportation regulations for shipping clinical and etiologic specimens.[20–22]

Transportation of blood products within a hospital or from a blood bank to a hospital does not require the same packaging as that used to transport by some type of public transportation if the staff is well trained on the handling and hazards of the products.

Any blood samples to be shipped by nonmedical carriers should be packaged according to the requirements of the shipper. In general, these requirements include wrapping the sample container in enough absorbent material to control any leaking that may occur. This wrapped sample should be placed in a plastic, sealable bag and placed in a sturdy container, usually some type of corrugated cardboard. Appropriate labels should be placed on the outside container. Biohazard labels are required on the outride of the container if the samples or units are known or suspected to be infectious.

Shipping of products or specimens on dry ice presents another set of concerns. Dry ice is classified as a hazardous material because it can cause contact burns and it gives off CO_2 gas. Insulated gloves should be worn when working with dry ice. Also, the shipping container should be sealed in such a way as to allow the CO_2 gas to escape as it is produced. Special labeling of shipments containing dry ice is also required. See CFR 49 171-3 for specifics.[22] All staff who handle dry ice must be trained in potential hazards and proper handling techniques.

Basic Safety Precautions

A biosafety manual including sections on infection control and chemical and radioactive hazards should be available and accessible to all personnel. All personnel must read this manual and attend biosafety training relevant to their particular position.

Food, drink, candy, gum, and cigarettes should not be consumed in the work areas. These items should not be stored in refrigerators containing any biologic samples. Before touching any food, hands should be thoroughly washed.

Access to the room where specimens and blood are being handled should be limited. This includes the laboratory areas and the distribution departments. AH laboratory rooms should have closable doors and "one-pass, inflow" air systems with no circulation.

Centrifuges should be used only with capped or sealed specimen tubes. Units of blood to be centrifuged should be wrapped in a plastic bag to contain any leaks that may occur during centrifugation.

Wear face shields or masks and goggles and use gauze to cover the top of any specimen tube when removing the rubber stopper. This helps to reduce the amount of aerosol produced during the uncapping process.

Never mouth-pipette. Always use rubber safety bulbs for pipetting.

All entrances to departments where blood and blood samples are handled should be labeled with biohazard signs. Refrigerators and freezers containing any blood samples or products should be labeled with these signs also.

Sinks should be designated for handwashing, and only handwashing should occur at those sinks.

Gowns and gloves are to be worn in work areas. Hands are to be washed when removing gloves. Protective clothing should be removed before leaving the work areas.

Any accidents, injuries, or potential exposures to infectious agents should be reported to supervisory personnel immediately.

Injuries and Exposures

Hepatitis B Virus Vaccination

All workers whose jobs involve participation in tasks or activities with exposure to blood or other body fluids to which universal precautions apply should be vaccinated with hepatitis B vaccine. This vaccine should be offered free to all personnel before they perform any tasks that may lead to exposure to infectious agents. Documentation of the acceptance or refusal of this vaccine should include the dates the vaccine was administered or the reason for refusal.

Exposure to Blood or Body Fluids

Exposure of personnel to blood or body fluids to which universal precautions apply is associated with a needlestick or cut, mucous membrane exposure, or contact with an open wound or nonintact skin. After an exposure occurs, the following steps should be taken[15–18,23]:

- Document the route of exposure and the circumstances surrounding the exposure incident.
- If possible, obtain a blood sample, with consent, from the person (source) from whom the exposure occurred.
- Test this sample for hepatitis B surface antigen (HBsAg) and HIV antibody.
- Collect blood from the exposed employee.
- Test the employee's blood, with consent, for HBsAg and HIV antibody.
- Counseling and treatment should be available to the person from whom the exposure originated and to the exposed person.

For exposure to a person known to be HBsAg positive, the exposed person should receive the hepatitis B vaccine series, if unvaccinated. Also, HBIG should be administered within 7 days of the exposure. If the vaccine series has been given to the exposed person, test this person for the antibody to HBsAg. If the anti-HBsAg level is inadequate, give one dose of the hepatitis B vaccine and a dose of HBIG.

If the source of the exposure is negative for HBsAg, the exposed person should be given the hepatitis B vaccine if unvaccinated.

If the HBsAg status of the source cannot be determined, hepatitis B vaccine series should be given if the exposed person is unvaccinated. HBIG should be given on the basis of whether the person from whom the exposure occurred is believed to be at high risk for HBsAg.[15–18,23]

Management of Exposure to HIV

Any person exposed to a person who is known to have acquired immunodeficiency syndrome or to be positive for the HIV antibody, or is untested, should be counseled on the potential risks from this exposure. The person should be tested for HIV infection immediately after the exposure and at 6 and 12 weeks after the exposure. He or she should be tested again 6 months post exposure if the testing remains negative. The exposed person should not donate blood or share needles and should use protection during sexual intercourse.

If the source tests negative for HIV, perform a baseline HIV antibody test on the exposed person. Repeat this testing in 12 weeks.

If the source of the exposure is unknown, testing for HIV infection should be done as requested by the exposed person.[23]

All records concerning exposure of personnel to potentially infectious agents should be kept confidential. These records are to include how the person was exposed, the source of the exposure, and the degree of adherence to the safety procedures.

Waste Management

Every blood center and transfusion service must have a well-designed waste management program. This program must include procedures for the appropriate handling of wastes and training for all personnel on the procedures and program. This waste management program must comply with all federal, state, and local regulatory requirements.

Infectious Waste

Any waste that is contaminated with blood or body fluids or would release blood or body fluids if compressed is to be considered as hazardous as the blood or body fluid itself. Biohzardous waste is to be discarded into a clearly marked biohazard container. This type of waste includes disposable equipment and supplies, such as gauze, test tubes, microtiter plates, needles, lancets, bandages, disposable pipettes, and used gloves, as well as blood and body fluids.

The biosafety manuals and training programs should include a section on the proper handling of hazardous waste. All personnel should be specifically trained on how safely to dispose of the different types of hazardous wastes.

The biohazard containers used to dispose of hazardous wastes should conform to the following:

- The word "biohazard" or the universal biohazard symbol should appear on each container.
- Red or orange plastic seamless bags are recommended.
- Double bagging is recommended.
- These plastic bags should be stored in study, protective containers during use, and transport.
- Puncture-resistant containers should be used to dispose of sharp objects, such as needles, broken glass, and glass pipettes.
- Liquids should be disposed of in leakproof, puncture-resistant containers.
- Hazardous waste should not be compacted.

The recommended final disposal method for blood samples and products and hazardous waste is incineration or autoclaving before sending to a sanitary landfill. Many liquid wastes that are only slightly contaminated with human blood may be decontaminated with equal parts of bleach and allowed to sit for 1 hour.

Any time the local trash collection agency is used for disposing hazardous wastes, the agency must be notified of the risks and the safety precautions to be taken by their personnel. A current, written contract between the trash collection agency and the facility disposing of the hazardous waste is necessary. This contract should state how the agency will handle and dispose of the waste and how the hiring facility will prepare the waste for removal from its premises.

Chemical Waste

Although the use of chemicals in the blood center and transfusion service is minimal compared with other types of laboratories, training on the use and hazards of these chemicals is required. This training should include the following:

- Location of the Material Safety Data Sheet (MSDS) for each chemical used in the laboratory
- The intended use of the chemical
- Safe handling practices
- Protective equipment to use when handling chemicals
- First aid if exposure occurs
- Routes of exposure
- Signs and symptoms of exposure
- Preventing and handling leaks and spills

Chemical waste should be removed, transported, and disposed of according to the existing regulations of the EPA, the Department of Transportation, and the state and local governments.

Radiation

In a blood center or transfusion service, radiation hazards exist during the process of irradiating units before transfusion. The Nuclear Regulatory Commission (NRC) controls the use of radioactive materials. The NRC has set licensure requirements that must be met if a facility plans to perform irradiating procedures.[24] Also, the NRC has set standards for protection against radiation hazards. The particular license issued to blood centers and hospitals requires a radiation safety officer. The safety officer is responsible for monitoring personnel for exposure to radiation and for proper handling and disposal of the radioactive materials. This monitoring is necessary to detect the amount of exposure to the radiation and to prevent further exposure and potential health problems.

Also, the license requires annual training for the personnel who handle the radioactive materials. This training is to include safety, emergency, and proper handling requirements.

SUMMARY

The safety issues involving patients, donors, volunteers, and the employees of blood centers and transfusion services are important concerns of the blood banking industry. Exposure is prevented by having employees well trained and well informed in the risks, hazards, and prevention practices associated with occupational exposure. Continuing education in the areas of biohazard safety, chemical safety, and radiation safety is essential.

Review Questions

1–6. Match the following activities with the correct function:

_____ 1. Recording daily temperatures
_____ 2. Auditing
_____ 3. Culture change
_____ 4. Making process improvements
_____ 5. Validation
_____ 6. Daily review of testing results

A. quality control (QC)
B. quality assurance (QA)
C. continuous quality improvement (CQI)

7. Define an audit.
8. The single most important component of quality assurance in a facility is the
   a. quality assurance department
   b. medical director
   c. individual
   d. supervisor

9. True or false? Record keeping should allow one to trace the history of every blood component from donor to final disposition.
10. True or false? Irradiated blood is not a licensed product and can be shipped across state lines.
11. True or false? A standard operating procedure (SOP) is required for every step involving the collection, testing, processing, component preparation, storage, and distribution of a unit of blood.

(continued)

REFERENCES

1. Deming WE. *Out of the Crisis.* Cambridge, MA: Massachusetts Institute of Technology, Center for Advanced Engineering Study; 1986.
2. Walton M. *The Deming Management Method.* New York: Putnam; 1986.
3. Food and Drug Administration. *Guideline for Quality Assurance in Blood Establishments.* Washington, DC: Food and Drug Administration; 1995.
4. Nevalainen D, Callery M. *The Quality Program.* Vols. 1 and 2. Bethesda, MD: American Association of Blood Banks; 1994.
5. Roback J, ed. *Technical Manual.* 16th ed., Bethesda, MD: American Association of Blood Banks; 2008.
6. Berte L, ed. *Transfusion Service Manual of Standard Operating Procedures. Training Guidelines, and Competence Assessment Tools.* Bethesda. MD: American Association of Blood Banks; 1996.
7. Quinley E. *GMP Fundamentals.* Raritan, NJ: Ortho Diagnostics. Inc.; 1994.
8. Code of Federal Regulations. *Title 21, Parts 600.* Washington, DC: Food and Drug Administration; 2008.
9. Klein H, ed. *Standards for Blood Banks and Transfusion Services.* 25th ed. Bethesda. MD: American Association of Blood Banks; 1996.
10. Code of Federal Regulations. *Title 21, Parts 200.* Washington, DC: Food and Drug Administration; 2008.
11. Sazama K, ed. *Accreditation Requirements Manual.* 6th ed. Bethesda, MD: American Association of Blood Banks; 1995.
12. Ortho Diagnostics Systems, Inc., and the Council of Community Blood Centers, Quality/GMP Engineering. *Train the Trainer Program.* Washington, DC: Ortho Diagnostics Systems, Inc., and the Council of Community Blood Centers, Quality/GMP Engineering; 1992.
13. *Teleconference: Current Issues in Computerization: Blood Centers.* Arlington, VA: American Association of Blood Banks; 1991.
14. Berte L. *Quality Assurance in the Transfusion Service: Beyond Blood Utilization Review. Teleconference: Specific Quality Assurance monitors for Blood Centers and Transfusion Services.* Arlington, VA: American Association of Blood Banks; 1991.
15. Centers for Disease Control. Guidelines for prevention of transmission of HIV and hepatitis B virus to health care and public safety workers. *MMWR Morb Mortal Wkly Rep.* 1989:38:S6.
16. Occupational Health and Safety Administration. Occupational exposure to blood-borne pathogens, final rule, 29 CFR 1910.1030. *Fed Regis.* 1991; 56: 64175.
17. Occupational Safety and health Administration. *Enforcement Procedures for the Occupational Exposure to Bloodborne Pathogens, OSHA Instruction CPL2-2.44D.* Washington, DC: US Government Printing Office; 1999.
18. Centers for Disease Control. Recommendations for prevention of HIV transmission in health-care settings. *MMWR Morb Mortal Wkly Rep.* 1987; 36: 2S.
19. Richmond JY. Safe practices and procedures for working with human specimens in biomedical research laboratories. *J Clin Immunoassay.* 1988; 11: 3.
20. Code of Federal Regulations. *42 CFR 72.* Washington, DC; 1996.
21. United States Postal Service. Mailability of etiologic agents. *Fed Regist.* 1989; 54: 33823.
22. Code of Federal Regulations. *49 CFR 171–3.* Washington, DC; 1996.
23. Centers for Disease Control. Universal precautions for prevention of transmission of human immunodeficiency virus, hepatitis B virus, and other blood-borne pathogens in health-care settings. *MMWR Morb Mortal Wkly Rep.* 1988: 37: 377–382, 387–388.
24. Code of Federal Regulations. *10 CFR 20.* Washington, DC; 1996.

ADDITIONAL READINGS

American Association of Blood Banks. *Quality Systems in the Blood Bank and Laboratory Environment.* Bethesda, MD: American Association of Blood Banks; 1994.

Berte LM, Managing quality in hospital transfusion medicine. *Lab Med.* 1994; 25: 118.

Centers for Disease Control and National Institutes of Health, Department of Health and Human Services. *Biosafety in Microbiology and Biomedical Laboratories. DHHS Publication No. (CDC) 88–8395.* 2nd ed.

Washington, DC: U.S. Department of Health and Human Services; 1988.

Code of Federal Regulations. *29 CFR 1910.20.* Washington, DC; 1996.

Code of Federal Regulations. *29 CFR 1904–2.* Washington, DC; 1996.

Crosby PB. *Quality Is Free: The Art of Making Quality Certain.* Markham, Ontario: Penguin; 1979.

Environmental Protection Agency. *Registered Hospital Disinfectants and Sterilants (TS767C).* Washington, DC: EPA Antimicrobial Program Branch; 1992.

Food and Drug Administration. *Guideline on General Principles of Process Validation.* Washington, DC: Food and Drug Administration; May 1987.

Harmening D, ed. *Modern Blood Banking and Transfusion Practice.* 3rd ed. Philadelphia, PA: FA Davis; 1994.

Hoppe PA, Tourault MA. Transfusion safety and federal regulatory requirements. In: Harmening D, ed. *Modern Blood Banking and Transfusion Practice.* 2nd ed. Philadelphia, PA: FA Davis; 1989: 246.

ISO Standards Compendium. *ISO 9000 Quality Management.* 6th ed. Geneva: International Organization for Standardization; 1994.

Kurtz SR, Summers SH, Kruskall MS, eds. *Improving Transfusion Practice: The Role of Quality Assurance.* Arlington, VA: American Association of Blood Banks; 1989.

Leebov W. *The Quality Quest: A Briefing for Health Care Professionals.* Chicago, IL: American Hospital Association; 1991.

Mills CA. *The Quality Audit: A Management Evaluation Tool.* New York: McGraw-Hill; 1989.

National Committee for *Clinical Laboratory Standards. Clinical Laboratory Technical Procedure Manuals.* 2nd ed. Approved Guideline. NCCLS Document GP2-A2(ISBN 1-56238-156-3). Wayne, PA: NCCLS; 1992.

Occupational Health and Safety Administration. *OSHA Instruction CPL 2-2.44B.* Washington, DC: OSHA; 1990.

Quinley ED, Caglioti TA. *GMP Fundamentals.* Raritan, NJ: Ortho Diagnostic Systems Inc.; 1995.

Rossi EC, Simon TL, Moss GL, eds. *Principles of Transfusion Medicine.* Baltimore, MD: Williams & Wilkins; 1991.

Turgeon ML. *Fundamentals of Immunohematology: Theory and Technique.* 2nd ed. Baltimore, MD: Williams & Wilkins; 1995.

U.S. Department of Health and Human Services. *Occupational Safety and Health Guidelines for Chemical Hazards.* Publication No. 89–104, Supplement II-OHG. Cincinnati, OH: HHS published; 1988.

REGULATIONS AND STANDARDS

MARY LIEB AND EVA QUINLEY

OBJECTIVES

After completion of this chapter, the reader will be able to:

1. List the agencies that regulate blood centers.
2. State what the regulatory objectives are for each agency.
3. Discuss the goals of the regulatory agency.
4. Discuss the type of accreditation each agency provides.
5. State the methods of enforcement used by each agency.

KEY WORDS

AABB

Centers for Medicare and Medicaid Services

College of American Pathologists

Food and Drug Administration

International Organization for Standardization

Joint Commission on Accreditation of Healthcare Organizations

Regulations

Sanctions

Standards

*T*he blood banking industry is one of the most heavily regulated industries in existence. In addition, a number of organizations provide voluntary *standards* to which blood banks subscribe. This chapter provides a brief overview of some of the agencies and organizations that provide either *regulations* or standards applicable to blood banks (Box 19-1). The interested reader should consult this chapter's Additional Readings section for further information.

AABB

Objectives

The AABB, formerly known as the *American Association of Blood Banks* through its Inspection and Accreditation Program, inspects blood banks and transfusion services to ensure that they meet the requirements of the *Standards*. It encourages blood establishments to develop self-assessment programs to find opportunities for improvement in operations. Box 19-2 lists some of the goals and objectives of the AABB.

Accreditation

Blood banks may be accredited by the AABB. Accreditation is voluntary and is achieved by compliance

---

BOX 19-1

Agencies That Regulate, Accredit, or Certify Blood Banks

AABB, formerly known as the American Association of Blood Banks
Food and Drug Administration (FDA)
Centers for Medicare and Medicaid Services (CMS)
Joint Commission on Accreditation of Healthcare Organizations (TJC)
College of American Pathologists (CAP)
International Organization for Standardization (ISO)
Nuclear Regulatory Commission (NRC)
Department of Transportation (DOT)
Environmental Protection Agency (EPA)
Occupational Safety and Health Administration (OSHA)

BOX 19-2

Goals and Objectives of the AABB

These goals and objectives are directed toward blood banks, plasma centers, and transfusion services.

- Accreditation
- Provision of standards
- Assessment
- Guidance
- Education
- Representation
- Publications

with the AABB's standards. Biannual assessments are conducted to ensure compliance, and facilities must address any nonconformances to retain accreditation.

Provision of Standards

The AABB provides minimal standards that blood banks must meet to be accredited. These standards are found in a publication of the organization, the *Standards for Blood Banks and Transfusion Services*. Standards for all areas of blood banking are published by AABB.

Assessment

Blood banks desiring accreditation are assessed at least biannually. Blood banks are asked to prepare a quality plan and to provide written documentation for the implementation and education of the plan. Assessors are usually individuals who are practicing blood bankers. The assessors, who are trained at least annually, serve as volunteers.

During the assessment, AABB assessors address adherence to the standards and make observations related to needed improvements or cite nonconformances in operations or quality activities of the facility.

Guidance

The AABB has staff who can provide guidance to its members in issues pertinent to blood banking. Bulletins and letters from the organization often provide direction to the membership on key issues such as testing, compliance, and the like.

Education

One of the key purposes for the existence of the AABB is to provide members with educational opportunities. The organization does this by sponsoring various seminars, programs, and teleconferences throughout the country. The organization's annual meeting also provides educational opportunities for the blood banking community.

In addition, the organization provides many different types of educational materials, such as books, web-based education, and guidance documents. The website www.aabb.org provides information, educational opportunities, and links to other industry-related websites.[1]

Representation

There are nearly 10,000 institutional and individual members, both national and international,[1] which include the fields of cellular and related biologic therapies. The AABB often represents the blood banking community in the legislative arena. In addition, the organization represents blood banking to the media and works with other blood banking professional organizations to speak on key issues related to the field of blood banking.

Publications

The organization provides a number of publications for its members, including a magazine, *AABB News*, the web-based *AABB Weekly Report*, a peer-reviewed journal (*Transfusion*), guides for various activities such as quality plan preparation, and books/proceedings from seminars or meetings.

AABB Quality Plan

As part of the requirements for accreditation, AABB requires that facilities develop and implement a quality plan that includes self-assessment activities. The AABB requires members to address Quality System Essentials (QSEs) in the quality plan and to assess these to ensure that operations are performing as expected. Box 19-3 lists the QSEs for Blood Banks and

BOX 19-3

Quality System Essentials of the AABB

Minimum elements that must be addressed in a blood bank or transfusion service quality plan

- Organization
- Resources
- Supplier and customer issues
- Process control
- Documents and records
- Deviations, nonconformances, and adverse events
- Assessments: internal and external
- Process improvement through corrective and preventive action
- Facilities and safety

Transfusion Services. These are compatible with ISO 9001 standards. Interested readers are referred to the Additional Readings section for more information on quality plans.

THE FOOD AND DRUG ADMINISTRATION

History

The *Food and Drug Administration (FDA)* is a federal agency that regulates blood establishments as manufacturers of blood and blood products. The FDA website provides information on the organization as well as updates of interest to blood establishments.[2] Box 19-4 provides a brief history of the regulation of blood and blood products by the FDA.

Objective

The objective of the FDA is to ensure the safety, quality, identity, purity, and potency of blood and blood products. The activities of the FDA fall into three major categories:

- Establishing policies and standards (rulemaking)
- Registration and licensure
- Inspection and compliance activities

The principal laws enforced by the FDA are the Federal Food, Drug, and Cosmetic Act (FDCA), and the Public Health Service Act. FDA must publish each regulation as a proposal in the *Federal Register*, allowing public review and comment. This review/comment period is a minimum of 60 days, after which the Agency reviews and responds to each type of comment, explaining FDA's position. Section 701(a) of the FDCA authorizes the FDA to promulgate regulations for the "efficient enforcement of the Act."[3] The Public Health Service Act also authorizes the FDA to promulgate standards (regulations) to ensure the safety, purity, and potency of blood products.

Blood Products Advisory Committee

The Blood Products Advisory Committee (BPAC) is the primary advisory committee to the FDA for the blood banking industry. Each BPAC meeting has a 1-hour period devoted to an "open public hearing" during which any issues of concern can be discussed. The BPAC provides opinions as to how regulations should be promulgated to best serve donors and patients.

BOX 19-4

History of Regulation of Blood and Blood Products

1902—Diphtheria epidemic in St. Louis. Manufacturer "rushing" to meet demand for antitoxin releases contaminated lots; 10 children die. Congress passes Virus, Serum, and Antitoxin Act of 1902. Establishes requirements for product and facility licensure, labeling controls, and inspection authority of the Hygienic Laboratory of the Public Health Service.

1937—First U.S. blood bank opens in Chicago.

1938—Passage of Federal Food, Drug, and Cosmetic Act (FDCA).

1944—Provisions of the 1902 Virus Act expanded and incorporated into the Public Health Service (PHS) Act.

1946—Regulation of blood banks begins with licensing of the Philadelphia Blood Bank.

1955—Biologics regulation transferred to the Division of Biologic Standards (DBS) within the National Institutes of Health.

1970—Congress makes it clear by amendment to the 1902 Act that blood products are considered a biologic product.

1972—DBS transfers biologics regulation to Food and Drug Administration (FDA) Bureau of Biologics. Also merges the regulatory requirements of the PHS Act and the FDCA, making a "biological product" (PHS Act) also a "drug" (FDCA).

1975—FDA publishes Part 606—Good Manufacturing Practices for Blood and Blood Components.

1979—FDA delegates inspection of transfusion services to Health Care Financing Administration (HCFA). HCFA incorporates FDA blood regulations for transfusion services.

1982—FDA merges Bureau of Biologics and Bureau of Drugs into the Center for Drugs and Biologics.

1988—Center for Drugs and Biologics split into the Center for Biologics Evaluation and Research (CBER) and the Center for Drug Evaluation and Research. Blood products regulated by CBER, but still treated as a biologic and drug product.

1988—CLIA Amendments passed.

1995—FDA publishes Quality Assurance Guidelines for Blood Establishments.

Regulations

Blood establishments are inspected for compliance with regulations found in 21 CFR 200, 600, and 800. The regulations in the 200 and 600 series are known as the good manufacturing practices (GMPs) are found here and the 800 series are the quality systems regulations. The 200 series contains the GMPs applicable to drug manufacturers, the 600 series contains those applicable to biologics, and the 800 series contains regulations applicable to medical devices. These regulations are legal requirements and all facilities that engage in the manufacture of blood and blood products are subject to them. They provide minimum standards for operations.

Registration

According to 21 CFR 607.7(a), all owners or operators of establishments that engage in the manufacture of blood products are required to register, pursuant to Section 510 of the FDCA. Transfusion services that receive Medicare reimbursement and are covered under **Centers for Medicare and Medicaid Services** (CMS)/FDA Memo of Understanding need not register unless they prepare components other than the following: red blood cells (RBCs), recovered plasma, pooled platelets, or cryoprecipitated antihemophiliac factor to be transfused at that facility within 4 hours of pooling.

Registration means that the establishment is subject to FDA inspection and must abide by GMPs and all other applicable requirements. It does not mean that the FDA has approved the facility's products or that the facility can participate in interstate commerce.

The FDA inspects registered or licensed blood establishments. The agreement with CMS stated that those facilities that do not routinely collect blood or do not prepare blood components are usually inspected by CMS. If units of blood are drawn on a routine basis, including autologous units, the establishments are required to register with and be inspected by the FDA.

The FDA will inspect any blood establishment that is involved in the "manufacture" of blood products. "Manufacturing" can include such operations as in-lab leukoreduction, washing, freezing, rejuvenating, and deglycerolizing RBCs as well as reconstituting RBCs with fresh frozen plasma.

Licensure

Section 351 of the Public Health Service Act requires that a license be obtained by those organizations that manufacture or prepare biologic products (including blood banks and plasmapheresis centers) to be shipped interstate for sale, barter, or exchange.[4] The licensing process actually requires the application for both an establishment license and product license(s). Product licenses must be obtained for products involved in interstate commerce.

Before any product licensure, the Center for Biologics Evaluation and Research (CBER) evaluates all aspects of the product's manufacturing: incoming component quality control, testing methods, labeling, record keeping, distribution, personnel training, and validation of all critical processes involved. The general licensing requirements for biologic products appear in parts 600, 601, and 610 of the CFR.

Inspection

Section 704(a) of the FDCA gives the FDA authority to inspect a facility at "reasonable times, within reasonable limits, and in a reasonable manner."[5] Although a facility may refuse to admit an investigator without a warrant, the Supreme Court has ruled that in "pervasively" and "closely" regulated industries, inspection without a warrant is presumed. If inspection without a warrant is denied, it can be presumed that FDA will obtain a warrant.

The investigator must first present credentials and a Form FDA 482 Notice of Inspection. The inspected firm should then ask what the purpose of the inspection is. An inspection can be a general inspection or it may focus on a specific product, process, or complaint, or serve to verify information that has been provided to FDA. FDA inspections serve as the primary means of collecting evidence for enforcement actions.[5]

The inspected company must provide the investigator access to all areas where blood products are stored or manufactured. All records associated with these activities are subject to inspection. However, records dedicated to financial data, sales figures, pricing, and personnel information (other than technical and professional qualifications) are not subject to routine inspection.

On completion of an inspection, the investigator may provide a Form FDA 483, which is a list of "observations" made during the inspection. These observations are not formal FDA notices of violations, but rather the determinations made by the investigator of possible violations. An exit conference is provided to discuss the Form 483 with top management. Form 483 reports are available to the public through the Freedom of Information Act (FOI). An establishment inspection report is prepared by the investigator back at the district office. These reports are filed with FDA headquarters and are also available through the FOI.

Enforcement

The FDA may issue a number of *sanctions* against a facility for failure to comply with regulations. These include both administrative and judicial sanctions. Box 19-5 outlines enforcement tools that may be used by the FDA as a result of noncompliance.

Administrative Tools

Warning letters are issued when the FDA makes a conclusion that a certain conduct violates a provision of the Public Health Service Act or FDCA. This notifies the facility that the FDA will take further action if the problem is not corrected. Timelines for corrective action are required by the FDA. The FDA ensures that corrective action is implemented and is working.

Product recalls are used to remove a violative product from the market and are classified according to the nature of risk to public health. A class I recall, for example, would be the recall of a product that presents a risk for death or an irreversible serious health hazard to the public.

License suspension applies to establishment or product licenses and represents a quick process to remove violative products from the market. It prevents shipment or further manufacturing of all products involved, and the FDA can proceed to revoke license or maintain suspension until compliance issues are resolved.

License revocation is a drastic action to prohibit interstate commerce of products. Violations resulting in this sanction are seen to be a health hazard to product recipients.

The FDA gives a notice of intent to revoke license, and the facility has 10 days to notify CBER of the approach it will use to achieve compliance, and 30 days to submit a detailed, comprehensive action plan, including completion dates. If the FDA perceives a danger to public health, it may revoke the license immediately without a Notice of Intent to Revoke. CBER may decline to approve any license applications or supplements until all compliance issues are resolved. Once the license has been revoked, the facility must apply for new licensure once violations are corrected. The Notice of Intent to Revoke is a public document available through FOI.

Judicial Tools

For judicial actions, all FDA enforcement litigation is brought by the U.S. Department of Justice, on recommendation by the agency's Chief Counsel. Actions that may be taken include

- Seizure
- Injunction
- Criminal prosecution
- Consent Decree of Permanent Injunction

Seizure is a civil action against violative products, not a person or company. Once products are seized, the FDA decides if the materials will be reconditioned or destroyed. The seizure may involve one or several lots of product.

An injunction is a court order, requested by FDA, used to prevent the continuance of violative behavior. This action can be brought against both corporations and individuals. It can shut down a specific area of operations or the entire business, as in the case of a repeated GMP violation history.

Criminal prosecution is generally brought against a blood establishment and its responsible individuals in instances where there is evidence of management disregard for GMPs, continuing violations, serious threat to health, or willful circumvention of the law. A "Section 305" hearing provides opportunity for the facility or individuals to present their case before initiation of criminal proceedings. This hearing, however, is not required if the FDA seeks an indictment from a grand jury. Penalties include fines for misdemeanor charges and more significant fines and imprisonment for felony charges.

The Consent Decree of Permanent Injunction is a legal document written by or on behalf of the FDA, enforced through a U.S. District Court, imposing specified sanctions against the violative firm. This sanction is used when there is an ongoing history of compliance problems identified across various systems within a firm's operations. It usually follows an FDA-filed injunction. Violative practices are described; corrective actions are prescribed and agreed to with designated time frames for completion. The district court has jurisdiction over all provisions in the decree as they apply to the firm or its individuals. The FDA (or designated qualified third party) assumes direct intervention in the firm's operations, including close monitoring of all actions, adequacy of corrective actions, and progress toward compliance. The facility agrees to provide periodic progress reports to FDA and to pay all FDA costs involved in the monitoring of the firm's actions. The FDA can take immediate enforcement actions if operations are not corrected satisfactorily within the prescribed time frames.

Centers for Medicare and Medicaid Services

The CMS formally known as the Health Care Finance Administration (HCFA) is the federal agency responsible for administering Medicare, Medicaid, HIPAA (Health Insurance Portability and Accountability Act), CLIA (Clinical Laboratory Improvement Amendments), and several other health-related programs. CMS is charged with inspection of nonlicensed blood banks.

Clinical Laboratory Improvement Amendments of 1988

In 1967, the Clinical Laboratories Improvement Act was passed in an effort to improve the quality of clinical laboratory operations. The Act was revised in 1988 (CLIA), with CMS retaining the responsibility for CLIA enforcement and certification of laboratories.

Objectives

The Clinical Laboratory Improvement Amendments of 1988 were enacted to ensure that Americans receive high-quality, reliable testing in laboratories of all types and sizes throughout the nation. In passing CLIA, Congress greatly expanded federal regulatory authority, from the 13,000 laboratories already regulated by the Department of Health and Human Services to an estimated 200,000 laboratory sites, including those located in physician offices. See Box 19-6 for a list of some of the goals of CLIA.

No laboratory, or other test site, may perform clinical tests on human specimens without a certification issued by CMS. This applies to physician office laboratories, hospital laboratories, or any site in the hospital where a test is performed (e.g., operating rooms, emergency rooms, bedside), independent testing laboratories, or even testing done at a shopping mall health fair. Tests are categorized according to complexity, as shown in Box 19-7; Table 19-1 lists the test categories.

CLIA also specifies requirements for personnel qualifications, based on test complexity level. These are listed in Table 19-2.

As of January 1, 1994, each laboratory performing high- or moderate-level tests must enroll in a CMS-approved Proficiency Testing Program for each spe-

---

BOX 19-7

Criteria for Categorization of Tests

- Knowledge required
- Training and experience required
- Level of reagent and materials preparation required
- Characteristics of the operating steps
- Availability of calibration, quality control, and proficiency-testing materials
- Test system, trouble shooting, and equipment maintenance requirements
- Level of interpretation and judgment involved in the test

---

cialty or subspecialty in which it is certified. Box 19-8 outlines proficiency testing requirements.

General Provisions

Subpart A 21 CFR 493.1 sets forth the conditions that all laboratories must meet to be certified to perform testing on human specimens under CLIA. It is applicable to all laboratories as defined under "laboratory" in 493.2 of this part. This part also applies to laboratories seeking payment under the Medicare and Medicaid programs.

"Laboratory" means a facility for the biologic, microbiologic, serologic, chemical, immunohematologic, hematologic, biophysical, cytologic, pathologic, or

---

BOX 19-6

Goals of the Clinical Laboratory Improvement Act

- Ensure safe and accurate laboratory work
- Preserve patient access to clinical tests
- Encourage continued technological innovation

TABLE 19-1 Clinical Laboratory Improvement Act Test Categories

Category	Description
Waived	~1% of all classified tests Home testing kits, spun hematocrits, HemoCue
Moderately complex	~75% of all classified tests Automated chemistry procedures requiring no operator intervention during the analytic process, hematology equipment
Highly complex	~24% of all classified tests All histocompatibility and cytology procedures, radioimmunoassays, and bacteriology serogrouping and typing automated tests that require operator intervention during the analytic process

TABLE 19-2   Personnel Requirements According to the Clinical Laboratory Improvement Act

Laboratories performing only waived tests	Minimal qualifications
Laboratories performing moderately complex tests	Qualifications specified for Laboratory Director, Technical Consultant, Clinical Consultant, and testing personnel
Laboratories performing highly complex tests	Qualifications for personnel in moderate level, plus additional requirements for Laboratory Directors, Technical Supervisors, Clinical Consultants, General Supervisors, and testing personnel

other examination of materials derived from the human body for the purpose of providing information for the diagnosis, prevention, or treatment of any disease or impairment of, or the assessment of the health of, human beings. These examinations also include procedures to determine, measure, or otherwise describe the presence or absence of various substances or organisms in the body. Facilities only collecting or preparing specimens (or both) or only serving as a mailing service and not performing testing are not considered laboratories.

CLIA and Donor Centers

The CLIA regulations require accurate and reliable laboratory testing to include

- All donor testing (ABO group, Rh type, antibody screen, human immunodeficiency virus, hepatitis, rapid plasma reagin, total serum solids)
- All applicable requirements for
  - personnel
  - quality control
  - quality assurance
  - patient test management
  - proficiency testing

The regulations do not cover the following:

- Quality control procedures performed for the purpose of ensuring proper function of equip-

---

BOX 19-8

Proficiency Testing Requirements for CLIA

- At least three testing events required per year with five samples per event
- Samples are tested with the regular workload, using routine methods, by personnel who routinely perform that testing
- Most tests require an overall score of 80% ABO/Rh compatibility testing requires 100%

---

ment being used to manufacture blood products once they have been procured from the donor and appropriately tested.

- Quality control procedures used to verify viability of the product.
- Proper performance of irradiation chambers to irradiate blood components.
- Sterility of blood components.
- All counts to assess components manufactured to meet requirements for viability determined by the FDA.

CLIA Inspection Process

Routine inspections are conducted biennially and are announced visits. Return visits may be made to determine the progress made in correcting cited deficiencies. In addition, a complaint may be made against a laboratory that could require an unscheduled inspection. Inspections are performed by trained surveyors under the CMS.

Enforcement

The CMS may impose sanctions against laboratories that are found not to meet CLIA requirements. CMS may impose the intermediate sanctions of a directed plan of correction, civil money penalties of up to $10,000 per violation or per day of noncompliance, and payment for the cost of state on-site monitoring of a laboratory that is noncompliant with CLIA condition level requirements. In addition, for any laboratory that participates in Medicare or Medicaid, CMS may suspend all or part of Medicare or Medicaid payment.

The CMS may also impose the principal sanctions of suspension, limitation, or revocation of a laboratory's CLIA certificate.

Civil actions may also be taken by CMS. The agency may enjoin a laboratory from continuing any activity that constitutes a significant hazard to the public health. CMS may also prohibit any person who had owned or operated a laboratory that had its CLIA certificate revoked from owning or operating a laboratory within 2 years of that revocation.

THE JOINT COMMISSION

Objectives

The *Joint Commission (TJC)* is committed to improving the quality of the products and services offered to health-care organizations. Spurred by the passage of CLIA in 1988, TJC saw an opportunity to improve its pathology and clinical laboratory standards for the health-care organizations it accredits.[6] The goal of TJC is to stimulate and support laboratories toward "doing the right things" and "doing them well."

Joint Commission standards are stated as performance objectives. This permits organizations and laboratory leaders to be innovative in reaching those objectives. There are six accreditation manuals, including one that contains the Standards and Scoring Guidelines for Pathology and Clinical Laboratory Services. Inclusive in the blood bank standards is the written expectation that a transfusion service is expected to follow the AABB standards even though not accredited by the AABB.

Although waived testing has no specific requirements in the CLIA regulations, TJC believes all types of patient testing are important and should be surveyed. As a result, TJC standards addressing waived testing are included.

Inspection Process

A surveyor who is a medical technologist surveys laboratories for standards in the manual for pathology and clinical laboratory services and, as applicable, either the standards for quality assessment and improvement or improving organization performance.

Compliance Issues for Blood Transfusion Services

Issues related to blood transfusion that are addressed by TJC include

- training
- written policies/procedures
- blood and blood component storage and handling
- blood supply and administration
- donor criteria and phlebotomy
- transfusion recipient sampling and labeling
- crossmatching/compatibility testing
- testing of donor and recipient
- reagent potency and reliability

- sample retention and storage
- record keeping
- adverse reactions: handling, investigation, protocols
- responsible head (director) requirements

Enforcement

The surveyed organization has 30 days on receipt of its performance report in which to submit its two-page commentary. After this 30-day period, the performance report becomes available to the public.

COLLEGE OF AMERICAN PATHOLOGISTS

Objectives

The *College of American Pathologists (CAP)* exists to improve the quality of clinical laboratory services and to ensure the accuracy and reliability of test results. Laboratory improvement is accomplished through peer review and education.[7]

Inspection Process

The CAP Laboratory Accreditation Program is an education peer review laboratory improvement program. A biennial, on-site inspection examines all aspects of quality control and safety in the laboratory. All routine inspector visits are announced.

Inspections are conducted by pathologists, medical technologists, or other qualified personnel. The CAP Laboratory Accreditation Program examines all aspects of quality assurance in the laboratory, including the following:

- Methodology
- Reagents
- Control media
- Equipment
- Specimen handling
- Procedure manuals
- Reports
- Proficiency testing
- Personnel
- Process improvement
- Safety
- Overall management principles

The CAP Laboratory Accreditation Program has been approved and granted deeming authority by TJC. This means that TJC accepts the inspection findings from the CAP Laboratory Accreditation Program and uses these findings in its own accreditation decision. In addition, the CAP Laboratory Accreditation Program meets state licensure requirements in many states.

Compliance Issues

Standards

The CAP inspects using checklists and standards, addressing the areas listed in Box 19-9.

Director and Personnel Requirements: Standard.
The pathology service shall be directed by a physician or doctoral scientist qualified to assume professional, scientific, consultative, organizational, administrative, and education responsibilities for the service. Generally, it is medically preferable that the director be a board-certified pathologist. The director shall have sufficient authority to implement and maintain the standards.

Resources and Facilities: Standard.
The pathology service shall have sufficient and appropriate space, equipment, facilities, and supplies for the performance of the required volume of work with accuracy, precision, efficiency, and safety. In addition, the pathology service shall have effective methods for communication to ensure prompt and reliable reporting. There shall be appropriate record storage and retrieval.

Quality Assurance: Standard.
There shall be an ongoing quality assurance program designed to monitor and evaluate objectively and systematically the quality and appropriateness of the care and treatment provided to patients by the pathology service, to pursue opportunities to patients by the pathology service, and to identify and resolve problems.

Quality Control: Standard.
Each pathology service shall have a quality control system that demonstrates the reliability and medical usefulness of laboratory data.

Inspection Requirements: Standard.
A pathology service that desires accreditation shall undergo periodic inspections and evaluations as determined by the Commission on Laboratory Accreditation of the College of American Pathologists.

Standards quoted in text are extracted with permission from the CAP Accreditation Checklist June 15, 2009b. College of American Pathologists, Northfield, Illinois.

Accreditation

Accreditation from CAP is received by compliance with the following:

- Agreement to provide an inspection team equal in size and complexity to that required for its own inspection.
- Successful participation in a CAP Interlaboratory Comparison Program (Surveys) for each analyte tested by the laboratory when an appropriate program is available.

Ongoing accreditation is maintained through successful participation in the appropriate CAP Interlaboratory Comparison Surveys Programs and by continued compliance with the Standards for Laboratory Accreditation as determined by the on-site inspection and interim self-inspection processes. Once initial accreditation is granted, laboratory performance for proficiency testing is reviewed periodically by the CAP Commission on Laboratory Accreditation. Responses to recurrent errors are required. Accreditation is valid for a 2-year period.

Enforcement

Laboratories that do not meet standards must respond with written documentation of corrective action within 30 days. If the response is complete and satisfactory, the regional commissioner will recommend that the laboratory be accredited. If not, accreditation is withheld.

Proficiency Test Samples

The CAP also provides proficiency test samples for laboratories. Samples are sent out to participating laboratories and results are returned to CAP for analysis and comparison with other participating laboratories CLIA accepts as providers for proficiency samples.

OTHER AGENCIES

International Organization for Standardization

The *International Organization for Standardization* (ISO) was formed in 1947. The ISO 9000 series is a set of five individual but related international standards

---

BOX 19-9

Areas Addressed by the College of American Pathologists

- Director and personnel requirements
- Resources and facilities
- Quality assurance
- Quality control
- Inspection requirements
- Proficiency testing

BOX 19-10

Benefits of International Organization for Standardization Certification

- Reduction in inspection requirements
- Reduction in rework
- Reduction in waste
- Increased customer satisfaction
- Worldwide recognition

---

on quality management and quality assurance. They are generic and applicable to any industry, including both service and manufacturing organizations. They were developed with the goal of effectively documenting the quality system within an organization. Box 19-10 lists some benefits of ISO certification. Box 19-11 lists the five standards that comprise the ISO 9000 series.

Blood banks are becoming increasingly interested in becoming certified in ISO. Most blood banks will seek certification under the ISO 9002 standards. It is not within the scope of this text to provide a full discussion of ISO standards or certification. For more information, the reader is referred to the Additional Readings section.

BOX 19-11

International Organization for Standardization (ISO)

ISO 9000 is the umbrella document. This provides (1) guidelines for selection and use of ISO 9000 standards, (2) generic guidelines for application of ISO 9001-9003, and (3) guidelines for application of 9001 to development, supply, and maintenance of software.

ISO 9001 is the broad-scope document. It deals with process conformance, from initial development through production, testing, installation, and servicing. There are 20 elements defined.

ISO 9002 standards deal with procurement, production, and installation. It is possible to be ISO 9002 certified and graduate to full ISO 9001 certification later.

ISO 9003 standards relate to production only. Formerly, it was possible to have a production process certified (an ISO 9003 certification), but this seldom happens today.

ISO 9004 is subdivided. 9004-2 covers services; 9004-3, processed materials: and 9004-4, quality improvement.

Nuclear Regulatory Commission

The Nuclear Regulatory Commission (NRC) is a federal agency that oversees and licenses organizations that receive, acquire, possess, or transfer radioactive sources. Many blood banks provide irradiated blood products, which would cause them to come under NRC jurisdiction. Because of the increased threat of terrorism, increased control and monitoring requirements have been implemented for irradiators with a radioactive source. Facilities have been required to enhance oversight and management in this area. Failure to comply can result in fines to the facility.

Department of Transportation

The Department of Transportation (DOT) provides regulations for the transport of hazardous and potentially hazardous materials. Strict rules are in place for the transportation of blood and blood products, which are considered biohazardous materials. Rules include specifics for packaging. Failure to comply can result in fines to the shipping facility.

Environmental Protection Agency

The Environmental Protection Agency (EPA) is the agency regulating waste control (hazardous and medical) and the impact of a facility's operation on the environment. Requirements for disposal of waste are to be followed by all facilities, and failure to do so could result in fines or imprisonment.

Occupational Safety and Health Administration

The Occupational Safety and Health Administration (OSHA) is a division of the Department of Labor. OSHA regulates and oversees that safe practices occur in the workplace, including laboratories. Regulations address blood-borne pathogen exposure, hazard communication, chemical safety, and personal protective equipment. Facilities are required to provide training for staff in safe work practices and to provide protective equipment, as appropriate. Failure to comply can result in large fines or criminal proceedings.

SUMMARY

Several agencies and organizations affect the operations of blood banks through regulation or accreditation. Familiarity with and understanding of the various requirements of these groups is necessary for all blood establishments. This chapter presents a brief overview of some of the most important agencies

Review Questions

1. The AABB performs which of the following activities?
   a. accreditation
   b. inspection
   c. education
   d. all of the above
2. What does TJC stand for?
3. "CLIA" is an abbreviation for the:
   a. Clinical Laboratory Improvement Act
   b. Council of Lower Intestinal Ailments
   c. Cytokine Linked ImmunoAssay
   d. Council for Laboratory Improvement and Advancement
4. Centers for Medicare and Medicaid Services certification is required for
   a. physician office clinical laboratories
   b. blood bank testing laboratories
   c. hospital clinical laboratories
   d. all of the above
5. The College of American Pathologists is a major provider of
   a. physicians to serve as inspectors
   b. diagnostic test kits
   c. proficiency tests
   d. clinical pathologists in America
6. Blood products are regulated by the Food and Drug Administration (FDA), being classified as both a _____ and a _____.
7. The Public Health Service Act requires that those organizations involved in the manufacture of blood products to be offered for sale obtain
   a. an establishment license
   b. a sales permit
   c. a psychological examination
   d. none of the above
8. A Form FDA 483 is used as
   a. a list of FDA investigator observations
   b. a Notice of Inspection by the FDA
   c. a list of the fire codes, provided by your fire department
   d. a warning to revoke your establishment license
9. The objective of the FDA is to ensure the _____, _____, _____, _____, and _____ of blood and blood products.
10. A product "recall"
    a. is used to remove violative product from the market
    b. can be issued against one or several lots
    c. is classified according to the health risk involved
    d. all of the above
11. A "seizure" is an FDA enforcement action taken against
    a. a corporation or its individuals
    b. the chief executive officer
    c. donors exhibiting adverse reactions
    d. violative products
12. A "Section 305" hearing provides an opportunity for an individual to
    a. rectify violations identified by the FDA
    b. discuss the 482
    c. present his or her case to the FDA, before initiation of criminal proceedings
    d. apply for a position as Responsible Head
13. Which series of the following International Organization for Standardization standards is most applicable to blood banks?
    a. 9001
    b. 9002
    c. 9003
    d. 9005

regulating or accrediting blood banks. The interested reader should consult the texts listed in the Additional Readings section for further information.

REFERENCES

1. AABB Website. Available at: http://www.aabb.org.
2. Food and Drug Administration Website. Available at: http://www.fda.gov.
3. Food and Drug *Administration. Guide to Inspection of Blood Banks.* Rockville, MD: Food and Drug Administration; 1994.
4. Food and Drug Administration. *FDA/CBER Workshop for Licensing Blood Establishments (Program Manual).* Rockville, MD: Food and Drug Administration; January 30–31, 1995.
5. Food and Drug Administration. *Federal Food, Drug, and Cosmetic Act, as Amended. 93–1051.* Rockville, MD: Food and Drug Administration; July, 1993.
6. Joint Commission on Accreditation of Healthcare Organizations. *Accreditation Manual for Pathology and Clinical Laboratory Services, Standards and Scoring Guidelines.* Oak-Brook Terrace, IL: The Joint Commission; 2007.
7. College of American Pathologists. *College of American Pathologists Laboratory Accreditation Program, Application Questionnaire.* Northfield, IL: CAP Commission on Laboratory Accreditation; 2008.

ADDITIONAL READINGS

College of American Pathologists. *College of American Pathologists Commission on Laboratory Accreditation Inspection Checklist.* Northfield, IL: CAP Laboratory Accreditation Program; 2007.

Food and Drug Administration. *Draft Guideline for the Uniform Labeling of Blood and Blood Components.* Rockville, MD: Food and Drug Administration; 1989.

Food and Drug Administration. *Memorandum on License Amendments and Procedures for Gamma Irradiation of Blood Products.* Rockville, MD: Food and Drug Administration; June 22, 1993.

Food and Drug Administration. *Guideline for Quality Assurance in Blood Establishments. 91N-0450.* Rockville, MD: Food and Drug Administration; 1995.

Food and Drug Administration. *Guidance for Industry: Notifying FDA of Fatalities Related to Blood Collection or Transfusion.* Rockville, MD: Food and Drug Administration; 2003.

Food and Drug Administration. *Guidance for Industry: Bar Code Label Requirements—Questions and Answers.* Rockville, MD: Food and Drug Administration; 2006.

Food and Drug Administration. *Draft Guidance for Industry: Blood Establishment Computer System Validation in the User's Facility.* Rockville, MD: Food and Drug Administration; 2007.

Food and Drug Administration. *Draft Guidance for Industry: "Computer Crossmatch" (Electronic Based Testing for the Compatibility between the Donor's Cell Type and the Recipient's Serum or Plasma Type).* Rockville, MD: Food and Drug Administration; 2007.

Food and Drug Administration. *Biological Product Deviation. Annual Summary for FY 2005 and 2006.* Rockville, MD: Food and Drug Administration; 2008.

Food and Drug Administration. *Medical Device Tracking: Guidance for the Industry and FDA Staff.* Rockville, MD: Food and Drug Administration; 2008.

Food and Drug Law Institute. *Food and Drug Law: 1991. FDLI HHS Fact Sheet.* Washington, DC: U.S. Department of Health and Human Services; February 1992.

McCurdy K. *Coping with CLIA.* Bethesda, MD: American Association of Blood Banks; April 25, 1995.

Ortho Diagnostic Systems, Inc., Council of Community Blood Centers. *Quality Engineering/GMPs II for Blood Establishments.* Raritan, NJ: Ortho Diagnostic Systems, Inc.; 1996.

Steane E.A. *ISO 9000 (Parts 1–5): Regulatory Update.* Bethesda, MD: American Association of Blood Banks; November 1994–March 1995.

Title 21, Code of Federal Regulations: Parts 210, 211, 600, 601, 606, 607,640, and 820; 2008.

Title 42, Code of Federal Regulations. Part 493; 1996.

INFORMATION TECHNOLOGY

SCOTT SCHIFTER AND SANDY HEDBERG

OBJECTIVES

After completion of this chapter, the reader will be able to:

1. Define basic information technology terms as related to blood establishments.
2. Discuss the process for developing requirements.
3. Discuss the purpose of validation and software verification.
4. Discuss at a high level implementation of information technology projects.

KEY WORDS

Blood Establishment
    Computer System
Blood Establishment
    Computer System
    Software
Functional requirements
Installation qualification (IQ)
Nonfunctional requirements
Operational qualification
    (OQ)
Performance qualification
    (PQ)
Requirements
Software verification
User validation
Validation
Worst-case scenario

*A*dvances in information technology and computer systems in general are both a blessing and a curse to blood establishments. They have brought automation to manual processes but at the same time have increased the blood establishment's burden to ensure that computer systems, including software, perform as expected. As blood establishments have moved toward automated solutions for their work, it has become more complicated to maintain systems and to be in compliance with FDA regulations, while keeping up with the constant change that hardware and software require to maintain currency. If one looks at the history of computers and how they have advanced over the past several decades, it becomes a little more evident as to why there are challenges in the area of information technology.

In the 1960s when blood establishments first started using computers to perform tasks, the computers and the tasks they performed were rather simple, really only minor functions or basic calculations. Computers were looked at as a tool and something the blood establishments were just learning how to leverage. There were few information technology departments in blood establishments. Software was not very sophisticated and did not make critical decisions. There were no packages for running equipment or for handling the complex processes that exist today. As the understanding of the power of information technology grew and capabilities were added to the basic computer, blood establishments figured out how to build programs that could provide more functionality. At this time computers were still mostly used as stand-alone systems and rarely shared any data. In the 1970s, with an expanse in the capabilities of computerization, even more opportunities to use computers in blood establishments evolved. Networking of computers became a possibility so that information could be shared. The first Ethernet was launched in 1973.

With the creation of chip technology, physical hardware changed rapidly. No longer were tubes and large circuit boards necessary; thus, the size of computers shrank. The personal computer was just around the corner. The first Apple computer was marketed in 1976.

One of the biggest issues early on was memory; it was limited and costly. The first RAM chip was developed in 1970 and the first microprocessor followed in 1971, both by Intel.[1] The race was on for smaller and faster computers. In the late 1970s, these advances led to the development of applications like word processing and spread sheets. Some companies started to use computers in unique applications such as process control and even created their own programming languages to interact with equipment in the field. A number of these were used in the chemical and pharmaceutical production environments and the FDA started to take notice. The concept of *validation* was forthcoming and those industries that were regulated, including blood banking, sought direction and guidance from the FDA.

Validation became a necessary evil and was not well understood. It was through validation, however, that blood establishments addressed the FDA's concern regarding insurance that computerization performed as intended, especially where the computer had impact on donor, patient, or recipient safety.

As the computer industry grew and the use of computers became commonplace, in the 1980s, vendors developed additional solutions for businesses. These naturally started to enter the regulated sectors of the medical and pharmaceutical industries.

The next challenge was to connect computers to each other. Developers had to ensure the integrity of the data being shared and to understand how the data was being used by a myriad of users. Because the computer was capable of making decisions, the need for good validation became even more evident, particularly in the blood banking industry. Quality assurance staff had to develop more expertise in the area of information technology, including validation plans and appropriate documentation of the execution of those plans.

By the 1990s, LANs (local area networks) and WANs (wide area networks) were common. This presented a new challenge as no longer was everything contained in one system.

Today in the blood banking world, computer systems make very complex decisions and are used to store hundreds of thousands of pieces of information such as testing records and donor information. Computers have replaced many of the manual processes in blood banking and can even perform electronic crossmatches.

REGULATORY REQUIREMENTS FOR COMPUTER SYSTEMS

Along with the expanded use of computerization in the blood banking industry came increased regulatory requirements. *Blood Establishment Computer Systems (BECS)* and the software used in such systems, known as Blood Establishment Computer Software, must be validated for intended use. 2 The FDA also requires a

510(k) clearance for computer systems used in blood establishments. 3 Guidance on how to validate the systems and how to submit a 510(k) clearance request is provided by the FDA for manufacturers of BECS and BECS software. 4 BECS software can be either home grown or manufactured by a vendor but in either case, it must be validated by the user for its intended use. The FDA considers a BECS to be equipment under Title 21 Code of Federal Regulations (CFR) 606.60 and automated electronic equipment under 21 CFR 211.68.

TERMINOLOGY

To have a working knowledge of computers, it is important to understand some "computer speak." While the intent of this chapter is not to turn the reader into a computer expert, it is important to know the basics, and they are thus presented here. BECS include computer hardware, computer software, peripheral devices, personnel, and documentation such as user manuals. Validation means confirmation by examination of provision of objective evidence that the particular requirements for the software's intended uses can be consistently fulfilled.[5] Vendors must also verify their software. *User validation* means that the user has tested the software under its conditions with its standard operating procedures and staff. Validation is discussed in more detail in a later section of this chapter. *Software verification* means confirmation by examination and provision of objective evidence that specified requirements have been fulfilled. This allows determination of whether the design outputs meet the specified requirements.

VALIDATION

As stated earlier, validation provides a high degree of assurance that the computer system is going to perform as expected in a consistent manner. Validation includes three elements: *installation qualification (IQ), operational qualification (OQ),* and *performance qualification (PQ).* The IQ provides evidence that the system is installed properly and that the environment supports it operations. For example, when installing a computer, the temperature of a room in which the computer servers are housed is considered in IQ as computers tend to perform poorly under extreme heat. The OQ determines if the system is able to perform under *worst-case scenarios* and the PQ provides evidence of the system capability under normal workflow conditions.

The level of validation work that must be done is determined by performing a risk assessment. The blood establishment must determine the risk of failure of a function and then validate accordingly. The risk assessment should include an impact analysis, probability, and detectability of a failure. If the risk is high should the computer system fail, then more validation work is needed. For example, if the computer is matching donors with recipients and fails, there is a huge risk to the patient. This function must be fully validated by assessing potential failure modes and challenging the software to ensure the system will not fail.

The Validation Protocol

Blood establishments should develop a validation protocol and a validation plan, which includes

- A description of the system to be validated
- A risk assessment
- A description of responsibilities
- A description of deviation management activities
- Data migration strategies
- Test cases, including criteria for success and failure
- A description of required documentation
- A description of approvals
- A description of change control
- A validation report format

Test cases should be established to challenge the functionality and repeated to obtain a degree of confidence that the system functions repeatedly as it should.

IMPLEMENTING COMPUTERIZATION

Implementing a new computer system or sometimes even just implementing new software is a project and can be complex. It goes beyond just the computer and its software; it involves people and procedures, and a lot of work. Unless the project is well planned, it will fail. There are a number of causes of failed information technology projects. These include but are not limited to:

- A poorly defined problem—what needs automating
- Too broad or too narrow scope
- Poorly defined requirements
- Failure to involve all stakeholders in requirements development

Some keys points to be aware of in designing an information technology project include

- Do not start with a desired finish date and crunch the project into that time frame; this will lead to problems.

- Do not push forward with a solution without knowing the detailed requirements.
- Do not begin with only a partial or unclear view of the problem; this will surely lead to many issues and missed expectations.
- Do not jump into development with minimal requirements gathering.
- Do not rely on outdated or obsolete information for requirements.
- Do not ignore existing relevant documents or institutional knowledge.
- Do not create highly customized software to reflect complex business systems releases.
- Do not try to automate a cumbersome, complex, or outdated process to make it "easier." Putting automation on top of a cumbersome, complex, or outdated process will not fix it.
- Do not limit requirements gathering to a small team of like-minded people; they tend to see things the same way. Get fresh minds and eyes to look over all deliverables.

Key elements of a successful project include:

- Early recognition that some requirements are not "good" or "valid." The best approach is to keep it simple.
- Recognition that requirements change during a project, but they must be controlled and not allowed to drift or creep.
- A reasonable time for completion. Generally if a project cannot be completed in a year, it is too big and should be broken into smaller pieces.
- Staying the course. Picking a path and sticking to it is important.

Requirements

One of the most critical steps in choosing a computer system and in developing a validation plan is to determine user requirements. Development of good requirements takes an organized approach and it takes input from all stakeholders to ensure the scope of the requirements is all encompassing.

Described below is an example of what can happen to a project that had a lot of planning but in the end did not meet the original intent and thus resulted in additional time and money to correct.

Developers started to design a bridge for the Millennium Celebration in London and the planning started in 1986. The bridge was to cross the Thames River with a length of 1,155 ft. The original cost estimate was $31 million and the project was to be completed by May 2000. The bridge was designed as a pedestrian bridge and was supposed to handle crowds of over a 100,000. What developers neglected to account for was the fact that when people walk, they tend to walk in step and have a natural sway with others around them. This natural sway set up synchronous lateral excitations; in other words it started swaying to a point it was not safe. So after only 2 days the developers had to close the bridge and figure out how to stop the swaying or limit the volume of people allowed on the bridge.

The retrofitting of the bridge would take 20 months and an additional cost of $10 million to install some 90 vertical and horizontal "shock absorbers" to control the vibrations and thus eliminate the swaying. The bridge reopened on February 22, 2002.[6]

So, failure to understand the full requirements of a foot bridge that was supposed to handle large numbers of people walking across it, the cost to fix the problem, and the time to repair it to a satisfactory performance level was almost a third of the original estimate.

Requirements are capabilities that a product must have to satisfy a specific need or to solve a problem of a business unit. They fall into two categories.

- *Functional requirements* that describe the capabilities of the product (sometimes referred to as business requirements).
- *Nonfunctional requirements* that describe the qualities that a product must have (also known as technical requirements). These requirements address performance, usability, and reliability.

If the computer system does not meet all the necessary functional and nonfunctional requirements, it may fail or at least not be viewed as successful as it should be. Common issues in establishing good requirements arise from complex and/or difficult to understand business processes, the creation of requirements by individuals who do not have the expertise, background, or experience to truly understand what is needed and failure to perform good reviews of requirements to make sure that everything is captured and accurately reflects what is needed. Failure to get all stakeholders involved can result in rework and can be very costly.

Developers may not understand the language of the business and may not interpret the requirements appropriately. This is a common problem especially in technical areas such as blood banking. These communication problems can lead to confusion and failure to meet expectations. Again, a good review of requirements will prevent problems arising from misinterpretations.

One must also ensure that requirements do not conflict. Again a good review is critical. Leadership at the blood establishment must take an active role and support the process and the decisions that are made. There is nothing worse than delivering an information technology solution and having senior management think they have backed and funded a project only to find out afterward that it is not providing the expected results or deliverables.

Every organization should have a well-defined process for the approach to establishing requirements and a detailed process for the management of this key critical step. The basic approach should include the following parts:

- Review and approval by stakeholders and sponsors
- A statement on what process is to be followed and the primary objective of the project
- A charter for how the project is to be run and a description of governance
- Standard documentation templates
- A list of deliverables and where and how they should be maintained and stored
- A description of the overall strategy and application of the life-cycle document
- An approach for managing the on going life cycle and how to address changes and approvals
- A description of reporting requirements and metrics
- A written requirements management plan
- An implementation plan
- Assumptions and constraints
- A list of stakeholders
- A document describing roles and responsibilities
- A description of required approvals

It is also important to determine all appropriate industry standards and regulations that may apply. These may need to be referenced repeatedly throughout the project and should be kept or added as appendices to the requirements document for future reference. The actual process of elicitation can take several forms, including numerous meetings, interviews, brainstorming sessions to workshops, and other forms of collaboration. This can also include observing the work force and the daily activities of the area to be impacted. Another good source of input is problem logs or other records of issues or work-arounds that might be in place. The end result of requirements gathering is a statement and capture of a common understanding of the users "expressed" needs. Good requirements management is critical (Box 20-1).

Prioritization of Information Technology Projects

One key element that must also be maintained is the overall prioritization of the project and any competing activities. Many times this will be the task of a steering committee or some form of program or project office. Budgets must always be watched and the program office or the blood establishment finance office will need to play a role here. Timelines need to be kept accurate and adjusted accordingly to ensure commitments are met and tracked efficiently.

Benefits of Requirements Management

- Opportunity to cross-train business/development staff
- Requirements for new/follow-on projects discovered
- Opportunities to align business/development goals
- Collaborative team partnership
- Engages users to help gain support and buy-in
- Prepares users for new functionality
- Helps eliminate scope creep and reduce rework
- Minimizes project "churn"
- Improves project performance
- Ensures efficient use of company resources
- More consistent stream of deliverables to business
- Establishes the ongoing costs and expectations for the future care and maintenance of the products delivered
- Creates an expectation for vendor responsibility

INFORMATION TECHNOLOGY PROCEDURES

Information technology normally has its own set of procedures. One of the key procedures is the Software Development Life Cycle that should conform to FDA Quality System regulations, 21 CFR 820. Of specific concern, 21 CFR 820.30, Design Controls help ensure that the software's design is undertaken in a controlled manner so that the design meets the requirements. These requirements are usually a more detailed account of the requirements set forth by users. These controls include elements such as

- Planning
- Establishing design requirements (inputs)
- Establishing design output
- Establishing a design review process
- Design verification and validation
- Design transfer and history files

While most blood establishments do not code their own software, they should be very familiar with the Quality System regulations as they apply to device manufacturers. Blood establishments are required to qualify their vendors and a thorough understanding of these requirements during a supplier audit may identify issues that could be better controlled at the beginning of a project than at the end.

SUMMARY

In summary, blood establishments rely heavily upon well-validated information systems in day-to-day operations and the hardware and software used have evolved into complex systems that require effective planning in order to be implemented successfully. Validation of appropriate functional requirements that is based upon risk assessments is a critical piece in ensuring information systems produce the intended results. Using a risk based approach to determine the amount of validation work ensures critical functions are fully addressed. In addition, when buying BECS, blood establishments should carefully check out their suppliers; this, if done effectively, can assist in the mitigation of issues during implementation and ultimately save the blood establishment time and dollars.

Review Questions

1. Which of the following are included in a Blood Establishment Computer System?
   a. hardware
   b. software
   c. user manuals
   d. all of the above
2. Which of the following ensures the environment in which the computer system operates is appropriate?
   a. IQ
   b. OQ
   c. PQ
   d. NQ
3. True or false? Involvement of all stakeholders is critical to developing successful requirements.

4. Testing of cases under stress conditions would be performed during which type of test?
   a. IQ
   b. OQ
   c. PQ
   d. NQ
5. Which of the following regulations would BECS software vendors be required to meet?
   a. 21 CFR 211
   b. 21 CFR 610
   c. 21 CFR 820
   d. 21 CFR 809
6. True or false? Blood establishments do not need to be familiar with the quality system regulations for medical device manufacturers.

REFERENCES

1. Bellis M. *Inventors of the Modern Computer*. Available at: http://inventors.about.com/library/weekly/aa200898.htm.
2. *General Principles of Software Validation; Final Guidance for Industry and FDA Staff*. Available at: http://www.fda.gov/cdrh/comp/guidance/938.html. Accessed January 11, 2002.
3. 510(k) Blood Establishment Computer Software. Available at: http://www.fda.gov/cber/products/510ksoft.htm.
4. *Blood Establishment Computer System Validation in the User's Facility. FDA Guidance Document*; October 2007.
5. *General Principles of Software Validation; Final Guidance for Industry and FDA Staff. FDA Guidance Document*; January 2002.
6. Strogatz SH, Abrams DM, McRobie A, et al. Theoretical mechanics: crowd synchrony on the Millennium bridge. *Nature*. 2005; 438: 43–44.

PROCESS MANAGEMENT

EVA D. QUINLEY

OBJECTIVES

After completion of this chapter, the reader will be able to:

1. Discuss the reason for process control in blood establishments.

2. List elements of process control applicable to blood establishments.

3. Discuss tools used in process control.

4. Discuss how Six Sigma and Lean can be applied in blood establishments.

KEY WORDS

Change control	5S program
Critical control points	Six Sigma
DMAIC	Statistical process control
Flowcharting	Supplier
Kaizen	Supplier qualification
Lean	System
Poka-yoke	Total process control
Process control	Value stream mapping

*O*nce processes have been validated and implemented in an organization, actions must be taken to keep them in a validated state. These actions collectively are known as *process control*. The goal is to achieve what is referred to as *total process control*, ensuring that a process is controlled and monitored at every critical phase. Total process control involves a number of things: well-written standard operating procedures, self-assessment of process performance,

monitoring of instrumentation and equipment, in-process testing, *statistical process control*, *supplier qualification*, and *change control*. This chapter provides the reader with an overview of each of these areas, but for more in-depth coverage of these topics, the reader is referred to References and Additional Readings sections of this chapter.

UNDERSTANDING PROCESSES

The first step in understanding a process is to outline the critical steps through use of *flowcharting*. This valuable tool allows one to visualize the required steps in a process and to focus on those areas critical to its successful performance. The Food and Drug Administration (FDA) and the American Association of Blood Banks (AABB) have listed systems to which blood bank processes belong.[1] By definition, a *system* is a collection of processes. Each process within a system is composed of several *critical control points*. These are important processes in a system that, if not under control, will result in system failure. For example, compatibility testing is a system defined by the FDA; sample collection is a critical control point in this system.[1] If the sample is not collected in the right tube or from the right person, for example, the system fails.

Under each critical control point are several additional activities or steps that must take place for the critical control point to produce desired results. In the example of compatibility testing, a key element under sample collection is sample identity. In each key element, there are usually checks (controls) that can be performed to ensure the key element is as it should be. Sample identity, for example, might be controlled by visual checks or barcode scans. By looking at each

TABLE 21-1	Example—Defining Systems
System	Compatibility testing
Critical control point	Sample collection
Key element	Sample identification
Control	Visual check

system and defining critical control points (Table 21-1), key elements, and controls, one can see where process control activities should be designed and implemented.

PROCESS CONTROL ELEMENTS

Standard Operating Procedures

One of the most difficult variables to control in any process is the human element. Achieving consistency in performance from individual to individual is very important in ensuring that processes are in control. Slight variations in the way in which operations are performed can lead to serious problems. Well-written standard operating procedures (SOPs) are a way in which the human variable can be more easily controlled. This is, of course, assuming that the SOP is well written and that individuals are effectively trained on the SOP. Seldom is reading, initialing, and dating an SOP sufficient to ensure complete understanding of a process so that when performed by appropriate individuals, it will produce acceptable results. SOP training should be taken seriously. Allowing individuals to make their own interpretations of SOP steps can be dangerous. Training allows an opportunity for individuals to read and understand each step of the SOP. It also allows individuals to understand the importance of the order of steps. Training should be developed as the SOP is being written and should include training tools such as checklists as well as a competence assessment instrument.

For SOPs to accomplish control, they must be readily accessible to those who are doing the work. They should therefore be placed in the areas where work is conducted. Personnel should be encouraged to consult written SOPs if they are in doubt as to how a procedure is performed or have other related questions.

SOPs must be reviewed on a regular basis, usually at least annually, to ensure that they are still applicable and meet all applicable and current standards or regulations. Outdated SOPs must be removed and one copy archived. In addition, through direct observation of individuals as they work, compliance with the SOPs should be ascertained.

Training

Training, both initial and ongoing, is crucial to maintaining control. Training programs must be developed and implemented with a great deal of thought to ensure that they are effective—in other words, to ensure the training accomplishes its objectives. Well-written objectives with measurable outcomes should be established for all training, and plans for both initial and ongoing assessment of competence should be established. Quality assurance should take a lead role in determining areas where training is needed and in ensuring that training programs meet the needs.

It is important to remember that training is not always the first solution for processes that are out of control. Often, process redesign or other measures must be taken before training is performed. Training on a bad process design or an inadequate SOP will not lead to process control.

Instrument and Equipment Monitors

All instrumentation and equipment must be monitored to ensure they are functioning before and during process performance. A system to ensure adequate ongoing monitoring of instruments and equipment using visual readouts and visual/audible alarms is essential. Quality control and adequate maintenance, including routine calibrations performed in accordance with written SOPs, are also important elements in keeping processes in a state of control. These activities can prevent major control problems. Documentation and review of these activities should be continuous.

Plans for corrective action to be taken when instrumentation or equipment is determined to be out of control should be developed. Employees should know steps to take to ensure instruments or equipment found to be out of control are not used in processes.

Review

All critical records should be reviewed for accuracy and completeness by a second individual. This review should be documented, including who did the review, the documentation of problems uncovered during review, and the implementation of corrective and preventive actions to ensure the problems will not recur.

Quality control records and quality indicators (e.g., product discards, recalls, etc.) should be reviewed for trending purposes to find opportunities to improve processes and to ward off potential out-of-control situations.

Supplier contracts should be reviewed regularly to ensure the supplier is meeting an organization's needs and quality standards. Manufacturers' package inserts (direction circulars) should be reviewed frequently for changes.

Quality Control

Quality control is defined as the operational techniques and activities such as sampling and testing that are used to fulfill requirements for quality.[2] As the definition states, this activity involves sampling and testing to ensure that reagents, equipment, and the like that are used in processes are working as expected before they are used in the process. In addition, in-process and end-product testing, which could be considered a part of quality control, help to ensure that product that is not acceptable is not distributed. Examination of quality control findings over time is important to detect potential problems that may lead to a process going out of control.

Internal Self-assessment

A crucial aspect of maintaining process control is to collect data in critical areas through the process of internal self-assessment. Ongoing self-assessment aids in prevention of problems and results in less rework and fewer regulatory problems. Plans should be incorporated in an organization's quality program that define what is to be assessed, how often it is to be assessed, how to evaluate results, and how to implement corrective actions or improvements to systems. A good internal self-assessment plan allows an organization to see the "big picture" of what is happening within the organization and allows improvements to be made in the facility's overall operations.

STATISTICAL PROCESS CONTROL

Statistical process control is a powerful tool in demonstrating control of processes as well as in finding opportunities for improvement. Using very basic statistics and meaningful data allows an organization to make decisions based on objective, not subjective, information. An important function of statistical process control is the ability to identify and characterize variations in processes, both *common cause variation* (inherent in the process itself) and *special cause variation* (attributable to specific circumstances such as personnel errors, accidents, and so forth). Good statistical process control allows distinction between process and performance problems.

Data Collection

To use statistical process control, meaningful data must be collected. There are some important guide-lines to remember in data collection. First, a plan for how the data are to be used is essential. The plan should include the following: kind of data needed, how the data are to be used, how the data will be collected and over what time period, how the data will be analyzed, and how the results of data analysis will be communicated. If these questions have not been answered, then data collection should not begin. In the actual collection of the data itself, several points must be considered.

First, who will collect the data? Will the task be assigned to those who are actually performing processes and the data collected as they are generated, or will quality assurance collect the data retrospectively? The question as to which data to collect depends on the process itself. To determine this, the process should be analyzed and critical control points determined. Data should be collected in these areas, particularly if the role of data collection is to determine if the process is in control.

The amount of data collected is also a question to be answered. Is it necessary to capture each piece of data generated, or can a sampling plan be used? If a large amount of data is generated in a short amount of time, as, for example, the number of test results generated by a large testing facility, a sample of data is more practical. For other processes, all pieces of data collected within a specific time period should be collected and analyze. Usually at least 30 pieces of data are needed for statistical analysis, but depending on the total amount of data generated, more data may be needed to get a clear picture as to whether a process is in or out of control.

The frequency of data collection must be determined. This is dictated by the criticality of the point at which the data are generated. The more critical the step, the more frequently it should be monitored to ensure control. To state this a little differently, if the impact of an out-of-control step on the successful outcome of that process is great, data should be collected more frequently.

Last, the decision as to how best to analyze the data so that they will be meaningful must be made and a logical way to communicate findings from the data must be determined. How the data are analyzed depends on whether one is comparing the process with another process, in which case statistical tools such as the chi-square or correlation coefficient may be used, or whether one is monitoring the data to determine if the process is in control, in which case the statistical mean and upper and lower limits become useful. Several tools are described in the next section that can be useful in understanding a process or in determining if a process, once implemented, is under control.

TOTAL QUALITY TOOLS

A number of tools exist for analyzing and evaluating processes and data collected from processes. The seven tools most often used are listed in Box 21-1. The following text discusses each of the tools briefly. For additional information, the reader is referred to References section.

Pareto Chart

The Pareto chart shown in Figure 21-1 is basically a bar graph that allows comparison between problems, conditions, and the like. It is helpful in determining on which problem out of several to focus corrective action. It is easy to construct a Pareto chart. Basically, a list of problems is generated by brainstorming. The occurrence of each event is tracked and tallied. A bar graph is then drawn to represent the frequency of occurrence. Normally, the vertical axis is used to denote units of measurement (e.g., frequency, percentage, dollars) and the x-axis is used for categories. A Pareto pattern appears when one of the bars drawn over a category is clearly taller (or longer, depending on graph orientation). Sometimes, it is necessary to define categories further before a clear Pareto pattern emerges. It is important to remember that this particular tool may not be applicable in all instances, but when used, it can be a valuable tool not only in problem solving but also, because it is easy to interpret, in communicating the information to others.

To create a Pareto diagram, first define the categories to be used in the diagram, sort the data into categories, make a bar graph based on the data, and observe for a Pareto pattern. A Pareto pattern is seen if one or two categories are responsible for most of the effects. Appropriate categories can be found by asking the questions what, where, when, who, why, and how.

It is important to remember that most problems require more than one Pareto diagram, each exploring a different question. The information in the Pareto diagram is useful in determining where most problems occur or where corrective action should be applied.

Flowchart

One of the most useful tools in analyzing a process is the flowchart (Box 21-2). A flowchart is a drawing that shows the steps of a work process in the sequence in which they occur. This tool allows one to visualize and analyze the steps in any process. With flowcharting, critical control points in a process can be determined and a clear picture of how a process should flow becomes evident. It is important to remember that systems are made of several processes and therefore require many different flowcharts.

Flowcharting is necessary to understand the sequence of events in any process. It can focus on just the steps of the immediate process, or can be expanded to incorporate external or simultaneous processes, such as the testing required to proceed to the next step

---

BOX 21-1

Total Quality Tools

- Pareto chart
- Flowchart
- Histogram
- Scatter diagram
- Run chart
- Control chart
- Cause-and-effect diagram

BOX 21-2

Uses of Flowcharting

- To describe the steps that reflect what is currently happening in any process
- To create a chart of how a process should be operating
- To create a diagram of how various steps in a process relate to each other
- To serve as the basis for the development of training programs, standard operating procedures, measurement point, and the like

---

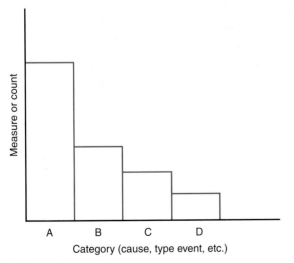

FIGURE 21-1   Pareto chart.

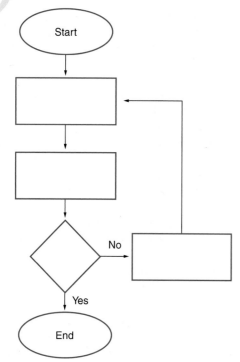

FIGURE 21-2   Flowchart.

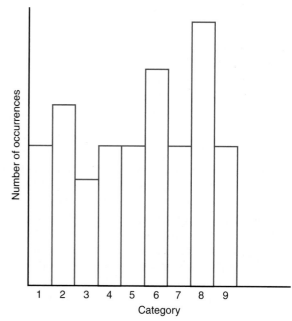

FIGURE 21-3   Histogram.

or for release of the process output. See Figure 21-2 for an example of a flowchart; Box 21-3 explains the symbology used in flowcharts.

Histograms

A histogram takes repetitive data points for *one* measurement category (e.g., temperature, time, weight deferrals) and displays the distribution of all values collected for those measurements. Because all repetitive events vary over time, the histogram reveals the amount of variation associated with the event

being studied. See Figure 21-3 for an example of a histogram.

The horizontal axis of the histogram displays the unit of measurement used in the study. The vertical axis can be expressed in terms of total frequency or, more specifically, as the frequency of the occurrence of a particular event.

Constructing a Histogram

A histogram is very easy to construct. The following steps outline how it should be done.

Determine the number of data points (*n*) already collected, or to be collected, and used in the histogram (example: *n* = 100).

Determine the range (*R*) for the entire data set by subtracting the smallest value from the largest (example: $R = [270 - 150] = 120$).

Determine the number of bars or *classes* (*K*) to be used in your histogram by using the table below:

Number of data points (*n*)	Number of bars (*K*)
Up to 35	5
36–70	6
71–125	7
126–250	8–9
Over 250	10 or more

In the example described, there are 100 data points, so we will use 7 bars (*K* = 7).

BOX 21-3

Flowchart Symbology

- ○ *Circle/oblong:* Indicates a start or stop point in the flowchart.
- □ *Square/rectangle:* Indicates an activity in the process.
- ◊ *Diamond:* Indicates the decision point.
- → *Arrow :* Indicates the direction of flow from one activity to the next (one cannot travel through the process against the direction indicated by an arrow). There can be only one output arrow from any activity box.

Determine the approximate bar width (H) (H = range of data included in the bar) by using this simple formula:

$$\text{Bar width} = \frac{\text{Range}}{\text{No. of bars}} \text{ or } H = \frac{R}{K}$$

In the example, bar width = range (120) divided by number of bars (7) = 17. Select a convenient bar width based on the calculated value—in this case, 15 or 20. Determine the boundaries of each bar by using your selected bar width. Choose the boundary value so that no data will fall directly on a boundary (usually done by applying one significant digit to data values, i.e., "0.5"). The *lower limit for each bar* is determined by adding your bar width to the lower limit of the previous bar. This process is repeated for all the bars. In the example, for the first bar, the lower limit = 150 and the upper limit = 164; for the second bar, the lower limit = (150 + 15) = 165; for the third bar, the lower limit = (165 + 15) = 180; and so forth, for the balance of eight bars.

Reading a Histogram

In reading a histogram, it is important to remember the following points:

- The greater the number of bars, the more easily visible any patterns will be.
- Some processes are naturally skewed to the left or right of your chart.
- Be suspicious if bars suddenly stop at one point without a previous decline in height (especially if at a specification limit point).

- Twin peaks may indicate data coming from two different sources (e.g., machines, shifts).

Scatter Diagrams

A scatter diagram is used to study the possible relationship between two variables. It cannot prove that one variable causes the other, but it can display whether a relationship exists and how strong that relationship is. This diagram displays the values of one variable on the horizontal (x) axis, and the values of the other variable on the vertical (y) axis. Each point in the diagram is then plotted at the location indicated by the intersection of both data values. The more the data points in a scatter diagram correspond to a straight line, the stronger the correlation between the variables. Figure 21-4 gives an example of a scatter diagram.

Constructing a Scatter Diagram

To construct a scatter diagram, follow these steps:

- Collect the data on the two variables you wish to compare (50 to 100 paired samples is appropriate).
- Construct the vertical and horizontal axes (one for each variable) so that the value of the variable increases as you move up the y-axis or to the right on the x-axis.
- Plot the x/y location for each pair of data on the diagram. If there are multiple values at the same location, the original data point should be circled as many times as necessary to represent additional, identical data points.

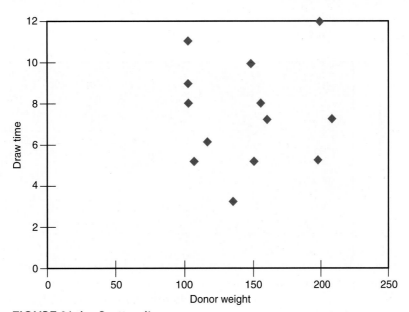

FIGURE 21-4 Scatter diagram.

Interpreting a Scatter Diagram

The more the diagram resembles a straight line, the stronger the relationship between the two variables. Box 21-4 describes the various interpretations of a scatter diagram.

Run Charts

The run chart is a simple display of trends in data collected over a specified time period. It is compiled from continuous data collected as a process is ongoing. It indicates if the long-range data average is changing. Figure 21-5 is an example of a run chart.

Constructing a Run Chart

A run chart is constructed following these steps:

- Decide which data to collect and plot.
- Collect the data on a collection sheet designed to accommodate the two categories of the axes (one of which will be a time variable).
- Construct the x-axis to accommodate the duration of time for the study, and the y-axis to fit the range of variables in the collected data.
- Plot the data on the chart *in the sequence in which they became available*.
- Connect the data points with straight lines.

Interpreting the Run Chart

The run chart is useful in determining *meaningful* trends away from an average or expected process value. Normally, in examining a run chart, an equal number of points falling above and below the average should be found. In general, nine points "running" on one side of the average statistically indicates a significant change in the process. A run of six or more points steadily increasing or decreasing is also statistically significant. The process should be investigated in either of these cases. Not all shifts from the expected average represent a problem; some process shifts can be favorable.

Control Charts

A control chart is simply a run chart with statistically determined upper and lower control limits drawn on either side of the process average (Fig. 21-6). These control limits allow the investigator to tell if the data are falling within acceptable limits established for the process.

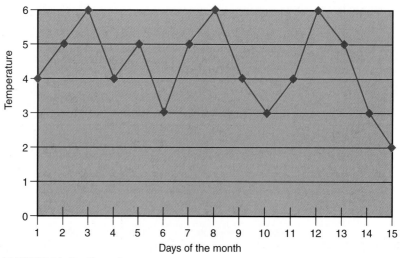

FIGURE 21-5　Run chart.

The control chart as seen in Figure 21-6 has an upper control limit (UCL) and a lower control limit (LCL). It is important to note that these limits are calculated and do not necessarily represent acceptance criteria.

Constructing a Control Chart

The control chart that has the broadest application in blood center processes is the Individual X-Moving Range (IX-MR) chart. The following construction steps are based on the control limit formula using this chart.

- Calculate the process average or mean ($\bar{x}$), for the data collected.
- Calculate the average of the moving ranges (MRs) for the data collected. The MR is the difference between two successive x values. For example, in the data 448, 460, 455, the MRs are 12 and 5.
- Calculate the control limits with these equations:
  - UCL = ($\bar{x}$) + 2.66 (average of the MRs)
  - LCL = mean ($\bar{x}$) 2.66 (average of the MRs)
- Construct a run chart.
  - Draw a horizontal line intersecting the y-axis at the value for the mean.
  - Draw the UCL and LCL as horizontal lines intersecting the y-axis at the value for each limit.
- Plot the collected data.

Additional Notes on Control Charts

An adequate number of data points (minimum 25 to 50) should be obtained before attempting to calculate control limits. Failure to do this could skew the results in an unacceptable manner.

Once the chart is constructed, compare new data values with the chart as they are generated. This provides instantaneous feedback as to whether ongoing data are deviating from established process control limits.

Levey–Jennings Control Chart

The Levey–Jennings control chart has a similar structure and function as a generic control chart. The chart received its name in 1950 when Levey and Jennings decided to use control charting to monitor the performance of control sera in their clinical laboratory. The chart is widely used to monitor laboratory test data and processes. As with any control chart, the process must first be studied by collecting data during routine runs. Statistics can then be applied to the data and the mean, control limits, and standard deviations generated.

Interpreting Control Charts

Any control chart will demonstrate changes or trends in data that *may* indicate a problem. Figures 21-6 through 21-10 show the types of trends seen in control charts.

Cause-and-Effect Diagrams

Cause-and-effect diagrams, also known as "fishbone" diagrams, are used when it is desirable to identify the possible causes of a problem. They are useful during brainstorming sessions to display the possible causes identified by the participants (Fig. 21-10).

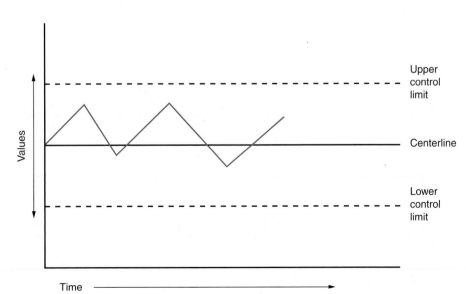

FIGURE 21-6   Control chart. Normal distribution. All values are within the control limits.

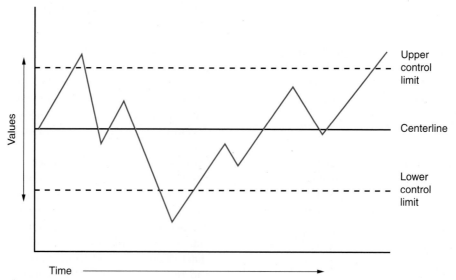

FIGURE 21-7 Control chart. Dispersion. Values fall above and below control limits. This indicates the presence of special cause variation.

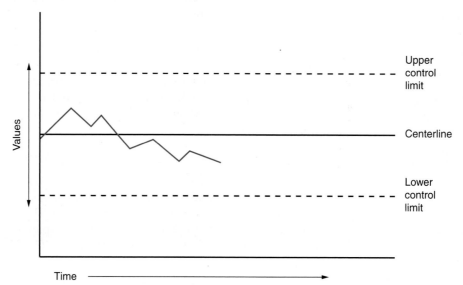

FIGURE 21-8 Control chart. Trend. Values moving slowly in a downward or upward direction.

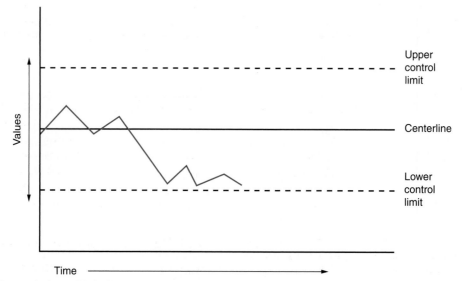

FIGURE 21-9 Control chart. Shift. Values move down or up abruptly.

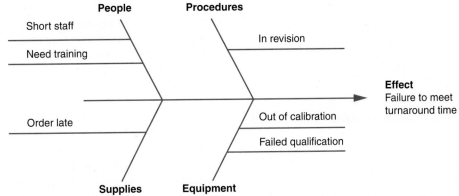

FIGURE 21-10 Cause-and-effect diagram (fishbone diagram). The fins can be designated with whatever label is desired.

Constructing a Cause-and-Effect Diagram

The steps to follow in constructing a cause-and-effect (fishbone) diagram are as follows:

- Identify the problem or "effect" for which the causes need to be identified.
- Generate a list of possible causes by brainstorming.
- Construct the cause-and-effect diagram by placing the "effect" in a box on the right and drawing a horizontal line to it.
- Add the major categories to the diagram in boxes connected to the horizontal line.
- Draw in the brainstormed ideas in their appropriate categories.
- For each cause drawn, ask "why?", and draw in responses as branching off from the brainstormed branches.

Interpreting a Cause-and-Effect Diagram

In interpreting a cause-and-effect diagram, it is necessary to look for causes that appear repeatedly. The relative frequencies of the causes must be assessed and a determination must be made as to which causes to address first.

SUPPLIER QUALIFICATION

Process controls are used to help eliminate unacceptable variations in product quality. However, challenges to product quality can be made from sources external to operations—suppliers. Success or failure in the provision of blood products relies on the quality of the products and services received from suppliers. No matter how well processes are defined, if suppliers do not meet quality standards, the overall effect is poor quality in services and products. Without adequate control over the materials and services that sup-

pliers provide to them, organizations will have a difficult, if not impossible, time in maintaining process control.

A supplier is any individual or organization that supplies a raw material, product, or service to another individual or organization. This applies to providers of a service as well.

Supplier Impact

The quality of a finished product/service is only as good as the materials provided by suppliers. The consistency of an organization's product/service quality varies with variations in the product or service quality of its suppliers. An organization's ability to plan relies on the receipt of products and services that consistently meet its established quality standards and requirements.

Supplier Qualification

Supplier qualification is the development and implementation of procedures that allow the verification of a supplier's ability to consistently provide components and services that meet established quality standards. Supplier qualification is needed because

- Continuous quality improvement extends to suppliers.
- Good manufacturing practices (GMPs) are assuming more of the International Standards Organization's approach to quality, with an emphasis on supplier qualification and preproduction quality assurance.
- The FDA *requires* supplier qualification in revised Part 820—GMPs for medical devices.

The Process of Supplier Qualification

An SOP should be written that describes the supplier qualification process in detail. Perhaps one of the

Supplier Qualification Issues to Consider

- Previous history with the supplier
- Certification by other firms
- Supplier management's commitment to quality
- Manner in which quality is incorporated into organziational structure
- Suitability of supplier's facility to manufacture
- Compliance history
- Adequacy of the supplier's training programs
- Adequacy of the supplier's quality program

most important aspects in qualifying suppliers is to define the standards and acceptance criteria that supplier products and services must meet. Standards and acceptance criteria are usually set by subject matter experts, users, and quality assurance. Once these important parameters are defined, a list of suppliers who can provide needed products or services can be compiled. The information in Box 21-5 is important in narrowing the list of suppliers.

Once the list of suppliers has been narrowed, it is important to have close dialogue with the selected suppliers. It is important to maintain open communication with selected suppliers. Constant monitoring of the supplier's ability to meet needs must be ongoing. In addition, feedback from the organization to the supplier is critical.

CHANGE CONTROL

To maintain process control within an organization, procedures for handling changes must be in place. There should be a mechanism to handle necessary changes in SOPs to ensure that the changes are validated and communicated as appropriate, and special attention must be paid to changes in computer systems. Effective training must be ensured for all changes that occur in manufacturing methods. In addition, through communications with suppliers, changes in reagents, instrumentation, or services must be noted and incorporated into organizational policies and procedures as needed.

Change control should also be a mechanism to ensure that change in an organization occurs at a manageable rate.

SIX SIGMA AND LEAN

Many blood establishments have now implemented the principles of *Six Sigma* and *Lean* into manage-

ment of their operations. Six Sigma provides a basis for solving problems and Lean principles allow one to make a process as efficient as possible. Although it is not within the scope of this text to present these topics in detail, this section will briefly discuss each.

Six Sigma

Six Sigma is a business management strategy, originally developed by Motorola, which today enjoys widespread application in many sectors of industry, including blood establishments. Six Sigma seeks to identify and remove the causes of defects and errors in manufacturing and business processes.[3] It uses a set of quality management methods, including statistical methods, and creates a special infrastructure to allow its principles to be incorporated.

Six Sigma was originally developed as a set of practices designed to improve manufacturing processes and eliminate defects, but its application was subsequently extended to other types of business processes as well. In Six Sigma, a *defect* is defined as anything that could lead to customer dissatisfaction.

Like its predecessors, Six Sigma asserts that

- Continuous efforts to achieve stable and predictable process results (i.e., reduce process variation) are of vital importance to business success.
- Manufacturing and business processes have characteristics that can be measured, analyzed, improved, and controlled.
- Achieving sustained quality improvement requires commitment from the entire organization, particularly from top-level management.

The term "Six Sigma" is derived from a field of statistics known as process capability studies. Originally, it referred to the ability of manufacturing processes to produce a very high proportion of output within specification. Processes that operate with "six sigma quality" over the short term are assumed to produce long-term defect levels below 3.4 defects per million opportunities (DPMO). Six Sigma's implicit goal is to improve all processes to that level of quality or better.

In recent years, Six Sigma has sometimes been combined with Lean manufacturing to yield a methodology named Lean Six Sigma.

Six Sigma Methodology

Six Sigma has two key methods: *DMAIC* and DMADV, both inspired by Deming's Plan–Do–Check–Act Cycle. DMAIC is used to improve an existing business process; DMADV is used to create new product or process designs.

DMAIC

The basic method consists of the following five steps:

- *Define* process improvement goals that are consistent with customer demands and the enterprise strategy.
- *Measure* key aspects of the current process and collect relevant data.
- *Analyze* the data to verify cause-and-effect relationships. Determine what the relationships are, and attempt to ensure that all factors have been considered.
- *Improve* or optimize the process based upon data analysis.
- *Control* to ensure that any deviations from target are corrected before they result in defects.

DMADV

The basic method consists of the following five steps:

- *Define* design goals that are consistent with customer demands and the enterprise strategy.
- *Measure* and identify CTQs (characteristics that are Critical to Quality), product capabilities, production process capability, and risks.
- *Analyze* to develop and design alternatives, create a high-level design and evaluate design capability to select the best design.
- *Design* details, optimize the design, and plan for design verification.
- *Verify* the design, set up pilot runs, implement the production process and hand it over to the process owners.

DMADV is also known as DFSS, an abbreviation of "Design for Six Sigma."

Roles in Six Sigma

One of the key innovations of Six Sigma is the professionalization of quality management functions. Prior to Six Sigma, quality management in practice was largely relegated to the production floor and to statisticians in a separate quality department. Six Sigma borrows martial arts ranking terminology to define a hierarchy (and career path) that cuts across all business functions and a promotion path straight into the executive suite.

Six Sigma identifies several key roles for its successful implementation.

- *Executive Leadership* includes the CEO and other members of top management. They are responsible for setting up a vision for Six Sigma implementation and empower other role holders with the freedom and resources to explore new ideas for breakthrough improvements.
- *Champions* are responsible for Six Sigma implementation across the organization in an integrated manner and act as mentors to Black Belts. The Executive Leadership draws them from upper management.
- *Master Black Belts*, identified by champions, act as coaches on Six Sigma. They assist champions and guide Black Belts and Green Belts. Apart from statistical tasks, their time is spent on ensuring consistent application of Six Sigma across various functions and departments. Six Sigma is their primary job function.
- *Black Belts* operate under Master Black Belts to apply Six Sigma methodology to specific projects. Six Sigma is their primary job function. They primarily focus on Six Sigma project execution, whereas Champions and Master Black Belts focus on identifying projects/functions for Six Sigma.
- *Green Belts* are the employees who take up Six Sigma implementation along with their other job responsibilities. They operate under the guidance of Black Belts.

Tools of Six Sigma

Six Sigma utilizes a number of tools, some of which are described earlier in this chapter (Box 21-1).

Tools of Six Sigma

- Five whys
- Failure mode and effects analysis
- Root cause analysis
- Analysis of variance
- Business process mapping
- Cause-and-effect diagram (also known as fishbone or Ishikawa diagram)
- Control chart
- Cost–benefit analysis
- Design of experiments
- Failure mode and effects analysis
- Histograms
- Pareto chart
- Process capability
- Root cause analysis
- Run charts
- SIPOC analysis (Suppliers, Inputs, Process, Outputs, Customers)

Lean Principles

Lean principles come from the Japanese manufacturing industry. For many, Lean is the set of "tools" that assist in the identification and steady elimination of waste. As waste is eliminated quality improves while production time and cost are reduced. Examples of such "tools" are *value stream mapping*, Five S, Kanban (pull systems), and *poka-yoke* (error proofing).

There is a second approach to Lean manufacturing, which is promoted by Toyota, in which the focus is upon improving the "flow" or smoothness of work. Techniques to improve flow include production leveling and "pull" production (by means of *kanban*).[4]

Lean Tools

Value stream mapping is a Lean technique used to analyze the flow of materials and information currently required to bring a product or service to a consumer. It captures and presents the whole process from end to end in a method that is easy to understand by those working the process. Through a simple to understand graphical format, future state (a diagram showing an improved and altered process) can be formulated and defined. The method encourages a team approach and through the capture of performance measurement data provides a mechanism to constructively critique activity.

As with any Lean management tool, the principle aim of value stream mapping is to improve processes. This is achieved by highlighting areas of waste within a process to enable businesses to eliminate these activities. Value stream mapping also has the benefit of categorizing process activity into three main areas— value add, nonvalue add (but necessary), and waste.

The *5s Program* is a Lean tool that allows a more efficient workflow and includes the following:

- Sort—the first step in making things cleaned up and organized
- Set in order—organize, identify, and arrange everything in a work area
- Shine—regular cleaning and maintenance
- Standardize—make it easy to maintain— simplify and standardize
- Sustain—maintaining what has been accomplished

Kanban, where kan means "visual," and ban means "card" or "board" is a concept related to Lean and just-in-time (JIT) production. It is a signaling system to trigger action. As its name suggests, kanban historically uses cards to signal the need for an item. However, other devices such as plastic markers (kanban squares) or balls (often golf balls) or an empty part-transport trolley or floor location can also be used to trigger the movement, production, or supply of a unit in a facility.

"Poka-yoke" is another Japanese term that describes efforts to make a process error proof. For example, designing something such that it will only fit in one way prevents errors. The design prevents human error.

Kaizen

Another term from the Japanese that is often heard when discussing Lean is *Kaizen*. Kaizen is a daily activity, the purpose of which goes beyond simple productivity improvement. People at all levels of an organization can participate in kaizen, from the CEO down, as well as external stakeholders when applicable. The format for kaizen can be individual, suggestion system, small group, or large group. While kaizen usually delivers small improvements, the culture of continual aligned small improvements and standardization yields large results in the form of compound productivity improvement. Hence the English usage of "kaizen" can be "continuous improvement" or "continual improvement."

This philosophy differs from the "command-and-control" improvement programs of the mid-20th century. Kaizen methodology includes making changes and monitoring results, then adjusting. Large-scale preplanning and extensive project scheduling are replaced by smaller experiments, which can be rapidly adapted as new improvements are suggested. When applied in the blood establishment, improvements can be made, which benefit all processes, from recruitment through distribution.

SUMMARY

Process management is a multifaceted activity. Processes must be validated and then monitored to ensure they remain in a validated state, producing the desired results. A wide variety of control measures exist in blood establishments, including monitors, training, SOPs, and quality control. Through the collection and analysis of meaningful data, blood establishments can maintain their processes in a controlled state.

Suppliers have a large impact on maintaining process control. Systems must be established to identify potential suppliers and then to compare the supplier's ability to meet established standards and acceptance criteria.

Change, unless handled in a systematic and logical manner, can result in serious problems in an organization's ability to maintain control. Mechanisms to monitor and handle changes in an organization must be in place, and review of the organization's processes to determine when changes are needed must be ongoing.

Lastly, utilizing Six Sigma and its tools or implementing Lean practices can vastly improve the efficiencies of processes.

Review Questions

1. A "supplier" is
   a. any individual or group that provides input into a process
   b. any person or group that receives the output of another person or group
   c. people outside your organization to whom you supply your product
   d. none of the above
2. Statistical process control refers to
   a. the use of complex mathematics to ensure maximum product quality
   b. the activities performed by your statistician
   c. the use of statistical techniques to analyze a process, or its output, so as to take appropriate actions to achieve and maintain output of designated quality
   d. the use of statistics to analyze the outputs of a process
3. Which total quality tool would you use to display the relative importance of all problems for which you have collected data?
   a. histogram
   b. fishbone diagram
   c. Pareto chart
   d. control chart
4. A diamond in a flow chart indicates
   a. an activity that is occurring
   b. a decision point
   c. a start or stop point in the process
   d. none of the above
5. A histogram is useful for
   a. displaying the frequency distribution of all data values collected for one measurement category
   b. relieving allergy symptoms
   c. determining which problem to solve first
   d. displaying the flow of a process
6. True or false? When reading a control chart, if your data points stay within your upper and lower control limits, you know you have acceptable product.
7. Supplier qualification
   a. ensures processes are in control
   b. ensures product is acceptable
   c. ensures quality input in processes
   d. none of the above
8. True or false? A Kaizen event must be a large project affecting the majority of the organization.
9. True or false? A Pareto chart is always useful in problem solving.
10. True or false? A value stream map allows organizations to see areas where waste is present in a process.

REFERENCES

1. Food and Drug Administration. *Guideline for Quality Assurance in Blood Establishments. 91N-0450.* Washington, DC: Food and Drug Administration; 1995.
2. Ortho Diagnostic Systems, Inc., Council of Community Blood Centers. *Quality Engineering/GMPs II for Blood Establishments.* Raritan, NJ: Ortho Diagnostic Systems, Inc.; 1996.
3. De Feo JA, Barnard W. *JURAN Institute's Six Sigma Breakthrough and Beyond—Quality Performance Breakthrough Methods.* New York, NY: Tata McGraw-Hill Publishing Company Limited; 2005.
4. Chalice RW. *Improving Healthcare Using Toyota Lean Production Methods—46 Steps for Improvement.* Milwaukee, WI: ASQ Quality Press; 2007.

ADDITIONAL READINGS

Carlino A, Flinchbaugh J. *The Hitchhiker's Guide to Lean.* Society of Manufacturing Engineers. Dearborn, MI: Society of Manufacturing Engineers; 2005.

Levinson WA, Rerick R. *Lean Enterprise: A Synergistic Approach to Minimizing Waste.* Milwaukee, WI: ASQ Quality Press; 2002.

Pyzdek T. *The Six Sigma Handbook: A Complete Guide for Green Belts, Black Belts and Managers at All Levels.* New York, NY: McGraw-Hill Professional; 2003.

Shainin PD. *The Tools of Quality; Quality Progress.* Milwaukee, WI: ASQ Quality Press; 1990.

PRINCIPLES OF PROJECT MANAGEMENT

ANN CHURCH

OBJECTIVES

After completion of this chapter, the reader will be able to:

1. Define a project.
2. Define project management.
3. List the nine project management knowledge areas.
4. List the key concepts to implementing project management.

KEY WORDS

Project   Project management

*S*uccessful health-care organizations are able to blend, optimize, and leverage the unique expectations of patient care, technical knowledge, quality and compliance, and business/finance. This is no small feat and underneath it all runs the current of change. Whether driven by new technology, process efficiencies, or compliance with new regulations, change is a constant element of heath care. Successful design, development, implementation, and sustainability of those changes will often set apart the good from the great. But how do you define the success of a change and how does one measure it? How do you work/develop a change to increase probability of success? Application of *project management* can address these gaps and move an organization closer to the level of excellence that patients desire and deserve.

Project management is a profession with a professional organization: the Project Management Institute. This organization certifies project managers, associate project managers, and a variety of other subspecialties within project management. Similar to the challenges

of compressing the first several chapters of this book into one chapter, this chapter cannot attempt to provide a comprehensive exploration of the project management body of knowledge (PMBOK) nor its application. It will however provide an introduction to and key elements of project management.

WHAT IS A PROJECT?

The Project Management Institute PMBOK defines a *project* as "a temporary endeavor undertaken to create a unique product, service or result."[1] This definition has two key elements embedded within it. Projects are temporary and therefore have a beginning and an end; this differentiates them from ongoing operational work. Projects create a unique outcome; this differentiates them from routine repeated execution of a process such as problem management or equipment validation, for example. It should be noted that execution of said processes or operational activities may on occasion trigger a project. Figure 22-1 displays the potential interaction between project and product life cycles while making clear that the two are distinct. Making these distinctions is key because the application of project management expectations to ongoing operations would likely be non–value-added and frustrating at best.

WHAT IS PROJECT MANAGEMENT AND WHAT IS A PROJECT MANAGER?

The Project Management Institute PMBOK defines project management as "the application of knowledge, skills, tools and techniques to project activities to meet

Project versus Product

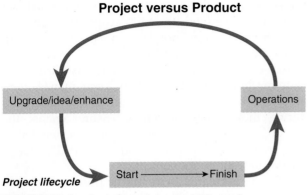

Project lifecycle

FIGURE 22-1 Project and product life cycle interaction.

the project requirements."[1] As will be seen in further sections of this chapter, the PMBOK includes numerous tools/techniques and the list of potential applicable skills is equally lengthy. To successfully implement project management (explored in subsequent sections) an organization must define the unique combination of processes, tools, techniques, and skills that are a good fit to an organizational culture and needs. These elements collectively can be referred to as the organizations project management methodology. Project management definition can therefore be restated as the consistent application of organization-specific project management methodology to meet the project requirements. This restatement highlights the reality and the inherent expectation that project management in different *organizations* is likely to look and feel different. This concept is explored further in sections later as well as in the project management literature in general.[2]

A project manager by PMBOK definition is "the person assigned by the performing organization to achieve the project objectives."[1] The practical application of this definition must go further to include the expectation that the project manager skillfully applies the project management methodology. This is similar to the highly skilled serologist that has many tests/procedures/techniques to choose from. Within the scientific principles of immunohematology, the serologist must chose which tests to perform that make the best use of a patient sample, in the least amount of time making the best use of sometimes costly reagents. Depending on the duration, complexity, or risk the project manager will need to select the appropriate tools/techniques from the project management methodology and apply them with the appropriate level of rigor. Project managers who can do this successfully will provide value-added support to the project and increase probability of project and organizational success.

This is an expectation that routinely should not be coupled with serving as the primary subject matter

expert (change lead). The change lead's role is critical to a project; it contributes in-depth knowledge of the process/area within which the change will be implemented. One person serving in both roles for moderate to highly complex projects often leads to decreased attention to the project manager role and decreased project management performance. For a more expansive discussion and details of project manager skills and competencies see the Project Management Competency Development Framework reference.[3]

OVERVIEW OF PROJECT MANAGEMENT BODY OF KNOWLEDGE: PROCESSES AND KNOWLEDGE AREAS

The keystone of project management is integration. This is evidenced throughout all aspects of the discipline and is directly seen in the manner in which the PMBOK is structured. The PMBOK is built upon 44 processes that are explored through two perspectives. The five "process groups" collectively describe the flow of a typical project: initiating, planning, executing, monitoring/controlling, and closing. Exploring the PMBOK through this perspective facilitates a how-to-do project management view. The nine knowledge areas represent the fields of study that are harnessed and leveraged to collectively create the unique discipline and profession of project management. Viewing the 44 processes from this perspective facilitates more in-depth mastery of underlying knowledge. Taken together, these two views provide an integrated foundation of how-to-do and why-to-do project management.

Processes: The Way a Project Flows

Discussion of these groups necessitates addressing them as separate entities; in reality these processes have many interactions and overlaps whose full exploration is beyond the ability of this chapter. *Initiating* is the process group that establishes the project to exist. The two processes within this group have considerable overlap to execution of portfolio management, which strives to ensure that the highest priority projects are being undertaken at the right time to bring benefit to the organization.

The *planning* process group refines and defines the project scope and goals/objectives. This group of 21 subprocesses collectively creates the plan of actions that will guide the project during execution and if successfully performed will deliver the change to the organization.

This process group is the hallmark and distinction of project management that sets it apart from other business/management approaches. Planning the work before it is performed is a discipline that brings payback and efficiency similar to the ability to build in quality upfront rather than inspect it into the back end of production. Processes within this group draw from all of the knowledge areas, explored in the following text.

Executing is the third process group and it leverages five of the nine knowledge areas. This is the area that most nonproject managers would view as the "meaty" part of the project where "the real work of the project" is done. Executing relies heavily on integration and resource management to ensure that the project planning is carried out, allowing project goals and objectives to be achieved.

The *monitoring and controlling* process group is the least discrete of the five process groups; it is utilized throughout the project life cycle. The 12 subprocesses utilize all nine of the knowledge areas and collectively measure and monitor the project progress. Routinely progress is measured by comparing actual outcomes to planned outcomes, which highlights the interaction between the planning process group and the monitoring/controlling process group. A key concept within monitoring/controlling a project is that variances between planned and actual outcomes must not be just identified but also evaluated and responded to with appropriate corrective action so that the project retains the ability to meet goals/objectives. The final process group is *closing*. This process group serves to formalize approval/acceptance of the project deliverable (service, product, result).

Knowledge Areas: The Why-To-Do Project Management

Project Integration Management

Integration permeates throughout the project life cycle and is applied in various aspects of project management. Projects must be integrated with organizational policies and processes such as resource management, change management, and reward/compensation. Integration with operational/business units must occur as well. Within a project, there needs to be integration between the project management processes; outcomes of resource planning inform cost planning and outcomes of scope planning impacts schedule planning. Seven processes collectively executed during all stages in the project contribute to this integration effort.

Project Scope Management

This knowledge area provides a framework for defining the project boundaries. What work will be done and sometimes more importantly what work will not be done is defined through scope management. Though all the nine knowledge areas and their processes are important, ineffective versus effective execution of scope management will have the most wide-reaching impact. The five scope management processes that are executed during planning and during monitoring/controlling ensure against the dreaded "scope creep": scope planning, scope definition, create work breakdown structure (WBS), scope verification, and scope control.

A WBS is created to detail the project work into smaller and manageable components. It is often anchored by the major project deliverables. Work efforts for these deliverables are then defined/decomposed until a level is reached, which represents the smallest "work package" that can be effectively assigned resources, duration, tracked, and monitored. Application of scope control continues the disciplined commitment to stay within project boundaries. Often after planning is completed and development/execution has begun, various drivers of scope change will occur. Some of these are legitimate and if appropriately managed through scope control will help ensure success of the project deliverables. However some/many will be ill advised, unjustified, and adversely impact the original intent of the project; scope control will identify these and deflect them from the project.

Project Time Management

With the WBS as a primary input, execution of the six project time management processes creates a project schedule. The six processes are activity definition, activity sequencing, activity resource estimating, activity duration estimating, schedule development, and schedule control. As is true for most of the nine knowledge areas, there is extensive literature, standards, and software tools to guide a project manager through these processes. The project schedule is a key component of the project management plan but caution and discipline must be exercised to guard against a common project pitfall; completing a project on time to the detriment of deliverable quality/performance. There are projects for which the end date is the only criteria for project success. But much more often, for the majority of projects/changes the measure of success is creating a deliverable that works, is well received, and enables sustainable change without rework. The ability to deliver this desired end point, on or before the target date, is enabled by accurate definition of the work, accurate sequencing of activities, and accurate duration estimates. Time management is therefore enabled by up-front comprehensive planning.

Project Cost Management

The three processes within cost management draw upon many finance and accounting tools and techniques. Cost management represents a key opportunity for integration between the project and the organization; linking project cost into the overall organization or department budget. Often overlooked in project cost management is that project decisions may create long-term cost consequences for the product life cycle cost. This potential highlights the need for carefully articulated measures of success for a project that go beyond project completion to product/service/result sustainability or effectiveness.

The aggregate outcome of cost management is an approved project budget that along with the project schedule and scope statement provides baseline expectations for a project. These baselines are then used to guide decisions and actions during the course of the project and provide a comparison for actual outcomes. The difference or variance between baseline expectations and actual outcomes provides an ongoing measurement system for monitoring health of the project.

Project Quality Management

This term and associated expectations should be very familiar to blood banking and transfusion medicine professionals. Per the PMBOK, project application of the quality body of knowledge leverages four key components: customer satisfaction, prevention over inspection, management responsibility, and continuous improvement. The tools and techniques to achieve this include benchmarking, design of experiments, cost of quality, quality audits, control charts, statistical sampling, and flowcharting. Their application to project quality management is measuring *during the course of the project*, whether the project/product will meet expectations. It is critical that quality measures occur during the project, not just after implementation of the deliverable. This approach increases the probability of project success and provides a more holistic in-progress view of project health. Monitoring project schedule, cost, and scope along with quality measures affords a balanced evaluation of issues/obstacles and response to variance against baseline.

Project Human Resource Management

The project application of human resource body of knowledge highlights a key reality of project management: *people work projects*. Though somewhat intuitive in nature, this reality is often overlooked while focusing on scope definition and budgeting and keeping to schedule. The ability to select, motivate, engage, and reward team members can make or break an otherwise well-planned project. The four processes within this knowledge area are human resource planning, acquire project team, develop project team, and manage project team. This area also necessitates integration with organization/department policies and practices; the act of acquiring a project team will be executed very differently in a matrix organization versus a conventional department-centered organization.

Project Communications Management

Communications as a body of knowledge is extensive and well researched. Project management leverages this area of study to provide a connection between people and information. What is communicated and when and to whom is driven by stakeholder analysis and stakeholder management tools/techniques. Project communication also calls for integration with organization-specific communication channels and vehicles. The four processes within this knowledge area are communications planning, information distribution, performance reporting, and manage stakeholders.

Project Risk Management

Executing risk management processes is especially susceptible to the pitfall of "one size fits all." Projects of high or moderate complexity will benefit from rigorous execution of all six processes: risk management planning, risk identification, qualitative risk analysis, quantitative risk analysis, risk response planning, and risk monitoring/control. Lower complexity projects may be well served by applying most of the processes and with less rigor. Project risk management is intended to decrease the probability and impact of adverse events while increasing potential for beneficial events. The tools and techniques for executing these processes vary from simple checklists to sophisticated simulation software. Integration with organizational risk threshold and tolerance is critical; a risky project in one organization may be a common element of the portfolio while in other organizations it may be a rarity.

Project Procurement Management

There are two primary perspectives from which to discuss project procurement management: your organization is the buyer of a service/product or your organization is the seller of a service/product. Both perspectives will utilize most of the six processes within this knowledge area. Because of inherent presence of a contract, procurement management must be well integrated with organizational policies such as legal, regulatory, or purchasing.

SO YOU WANT TO IMPLEMENT PROJECT MANAGEMENT?

As is true for many other business/management approaches, project management can be implemented/used in varying degrees. Table 22-1 details three levels of project management implementation: full implementation as *a way of doing business*, moderate implementation as *the way projects are managed*, and minor implementation as *a tool kit*. All three may bring value to an organization but the chosen approach must be matched to the organizational needs and culture. If an organization undertakes only low complexity changes with minimal use of cross-functional resources, then project management as a tool kit or no project management at all might be indicated. An organization that frequently needs at least moderate complexity changes and use of cross-functional teams would find value from project management as a way to manage projects and potentially from more complete implementation. Implementing project management as a way of doing business would be value-added for organizations with many simultaneous projects of high/moderate/low complexity vying for resources across departments and competing for a common pool of budget money.

In addition to the need-based assessment, the organizational culture should be considered. Implemen-

tation of project management as a way of doing business will only be successful if the culture supports integration and accountability. An organizational culture that cannot tolerate monitoring progress, accountability to forecasted outcomes, sharing lessons learned, or discipline of planning before working should likely not attempt to jump into project management as a way of doing business.

Key Concepts to Implementing Project Management

This section addresses issues and guidance associated with implementing project management as a way of doing business.

Change Management

All projects are changes but one can argue that not all changes are projects. This concept highlights the need for project management linkage to change management. A change management system that can effectively support linkage to project management would have various key elements. There should be levels or categories of changes. The change categories can be based on attributes such as complexity, cost, or duration. Categorization of changes should trigger different expectations for each level; what type of governance, what rigor of planning/reporting, and who is accountable. With a change management system of this nature, use of project management would be triggered by what category of change was

TABLE 22-1	Degrees of Project Management Implementation		
	A Way of Doing Business	**The Way Projects are Managed**	**A Tool box**
Resourcing	Dedicated project managers	Temporary project managers that return to "day job" when project is done	No project managers, tools are used by and at the discretion of change lead or team members
Processes	Centrally maintained project management methodology with defined templates, tools and expectations	Decentralized use of templates and tools	Decentralized and inconsistent use of templates
Training	Based on PMBOK and organizational project management methodology	Based on use of the templates and tools	None
Performance management	Project managers accountable for project success measures and for consistent use of project management methodology	Based on project-specific outcomes	None
Governance	Senior management execution of portfolio management	Department/business unit oversight	None

assigned. This type of approach would also ensure that project-level changes would have integration with other organizational changes.

Project Management Methodology

The definition of a *routinely used project life cycle* can be an anchor to creating a project management methodology. The PMBOK process group headings could be utilized: initiate, plan, execute, monitor/control, and close. Modification of this standard should be driven by integration with existing organization procedures/practices. An example of one such modification is initiate, design, develop, implement, and close. In this model, monitor/control would not be a distinct phase but would be embedded within each phase. Creation of a consistently used project life cycle must include definition of what general work effort is included in each phase. This will help ensure consistency across projects and enable more value-added governance (explored further in the following text).

Processes from the PMBOK should be selected for use within each project life cycle phase. It is an almost certainty that "start-up" project management efforts will not be able to sustain implementation of all 44 PMBOK processes. It is also a certainty that if core processes from each knowledge are selected, without inclusion of all nine knowledge areas, it could be questioned whether project management as defined by the professional standard is being used or not. Selection of which processes from each area to initially implement should be driven by an understanding of organizational needs. This approach can also be described as "where is the pain?" Project/change failures due to scope creep versus poor scheduling versus lack of communication versus resource management will trigger selection of a different combination of PMBOK processes. Once the initial project management methodology is implemented and measured for success, additional PMBOK processes should be added. Iteration of this approach will ensure the organization continues on a path toward project management maturity.

For each selected processes, routinely used *tools/techniques* should be identified and created. The tools/techniques should be accompanied by guidance for their use, expected outcomes, and limitations. Within each process and/or tool/technique *key terms* should be defined. The need for a common and consistently used terminology cannot be over emphasized. This is also an area where PMBOK can be leveraged many/most project management terms are provided clear definitions.

Performance Management

Project management expects that projects define expectations, measure progress toward the expectations, and be held accountable for the actual outcomes. It is therefore critical that the process of project management (as defined in the project methodology) hold itself to the same standards. Key indicators that would be monitored by all projects can be created and then evaluated from a portfolio (all projects) perspective. Selection of these key indicators should be driven by what the organization is trying to achieve through project management. Examples include project phase cycle times, actual to baseline schedule outcomes, occurrence/impact of risks, actual to baseline cost outcomes, or project deliverable effectiveness/sustainability measures. In addition to monitoring these indicators for the portfolio as a whole, they can also be monitored on an individual project manager level. Utilizing both approaches provides opportunity to identify areas for improvement at the organization level as well as individual project manager level.

Governance

Who is accountable to make decisions relative to the portfolio of projects, groups of projects, and individual projects is a key piece of successful project management. Portfolio and program management concepts are explored later. Decisions concerning individual projects are routinely linked to oversight of project progression. Once the routine project life cycle is defined (as detailed earlier) consideration should be given to the oversight/governance of how a project moves from one phase to the next. These "phase gate reviews" should be defined in terms of who performs them and what decision is being made. If a phase gate review is designed to provide technical concurrence, then it should likely be performed by individuals from that specific area. If a phase gate review is a go/no-go from a budget or strategic need perspective, then it should be performed by senior management.

WHAT IS PROGRAM AND PORTFOLIO MANAGEMENT?

As the project management discipline and body of knowledge matured, it became clear that the guidelines for project management fell short when it came to managing multiple related projects. A program as defined by PMBOK is "a group of related projects managed in a coordinated way to obtain benefits and control not available from management individually."[3] It also states that "programs may include elements of related work outside the scope of the discrete projects in the program." Program management practices focus on three themes; benefits management, stakeholder management, and program governance and is often executed at the midmanagement level of an organization. As discussed previously in this chapter, implementation of program management often follows project and portfolio management.

Portfolio management as defined by PMBOK is "the centralized management of one or more portfolios which includes identifying, prioritizing, authorizing, managing and controlling projects, programs and other related work to achieve specific strategic business objectives."[5] A key element of portfolio management is *working the right projects*. When combined with project management, which strives to *work projects right*, an organization can realize enhanced benefits from their efforts. Due to its strategic impact, portfolio management is often executed at a senior/executive level of an organization. Portfolio management routinely requires difficult decisions such as which projects/programs should be started and when, reprioritizing projects/programs based on changing organizational needs, and stopping projects/programs that no longer provide the highest priority benefits.

SUMMARY: VALUE AND PITFALLS OF PROJECT MANAGEMENT

Project management whether mature or immature, comprehensive or a tool kit, is not a silver bullet for successful change. It does increase probability of successful change. It achieves this through discipline, planning, accountability, and measurement. The cumulative affect of these key elements is visibility to the health/status of in-progress projects and effectiveness of completed projects. One can speculate that there is no greater "pain" for an organization than that of not knowing what change is underway, why it is being done, what resources the changes are using, and what benefits the change should deliver. Project management can address this pain. A recent 5-year multimillion-dollar study by Project Management Institute "Researching the Value of Project Management" has generated initial data that concludes: "Project management practices correlate highly with project outcome satisfaction, achievement of project success and organizational outcome success." The limitation of project management is linked to how it is implemented and why it is implemented. Implementation in a manner not well suited/customized to the organizations needs and culture will create non–value-added outcomes. Implemented with the correct resources, with a defined methodology, with appropriate governance and with ongoing measurements/monitoring will increase success and sustainability of change.

Transfusion medicine as well as heath care in general is constrained by the laws of nature but enabled by human ingenuity and compassion. Project management is constrained by Murphy's law but enabled by human discipline and collaborative accountability. Together, these two professions can move us closer to excellence.

Review Questions

1. The PMBOK knowledge areas include
   a. integration, time management, cost of quality
   b. communication management, cost management, human resource management
   c. scope management, quality management, cost accounting
   d. integration, procurement, scheduling
2. Portfolio is to project as
   a. transfusion is to needle
   b. nurse is to hospital
   c. whole blood is to plasma plus blood cells
   d. disease is to patient
3. A project is defined as
   a. temporary and produces costly outcomes
   b. scheduled and produces operational outcomes
   c. temporary and produces unique outcomes
   d. quality and produces scope outcomes
4. The process groups include all but
   a. integration
   b. planning
   c. closure

   d. execution
   e. monitor/control
5. Project progress is monitored in part by comparing
   a. initiation to closure
   b. planned to forecasted
   c. actual to outcomes
   d. baseline to actual
   e. none of the above
6. Creating a WBS is part of what knowledge area?
   a. integration
   b. time management
   c. scope management
   d. cost management
   e. all of the above
7. Project quality management includes
   a. designing in-progress measurements
   b. creating a WBS
   c. creating a budget
   d. activity duration estimating
   e. project charter

(continued)

REVIEW QUESTIONS (continued)

8. Manage stakeholders process is part of which knowledge area:
   a. cost management
   b. time management
   c. human resource management
   d. quality management
   e. none of the above

9. Implementation of project management should take into consideration:
   a. organizational needs and budget
   b. organizational location and needs
   c. organizational size and culture
   d. organizational needs and culture
   e. none of the above

REFERENCES

1. *A Guide to the Project Management Body of Knowledge.* 3rd ed. Newtown Square, PA: Project Management Institute; 2004.
2. Lewis PJ. *Fundamentals of Project Management.* 3rd ed. New York, NY: American Management Association; 2007.
3. *Project Management Competency Development Framework.* 2nd ed. Newtown Square, PA: Project Management Institute; 2007.
4. *The Standard for Portfolio Management.* Newtown Square, PA: Project Management Institute; 2006.
5. *The Standard for Program Management.* Newtown Square, PA: Project Management Institute; 2006.

APPENDIX

ANSWERS TO REVIEW QUESTIONS

CH. 1

1. a
2. e
3. d
4. e
5. c
6. e
7. c
8. e
9. e

CH. 2

1. a
2. b
3. d
4. c
5. d
6. a
7. c
8. a
9. d
10. d

CH. 3

1. d
2. d
3. e
4. a
5. a
6. d
7. d
8. b
9. d
10. e
11. c
12. e

CH. 4

1. b
2. d
3. b
4. c
5. b
6. a
7. b
8. c
9. a
10. c
11. False
12. False
13. True
14. False
15. True

CH. 5

1. a
2. d
3. b
4. a
5. d
6. b
7. d
8. c
9. a
10. a
11. a
12. b

CH. 6

1. d
2. c
3. True
4. True
5. False
6. True
7. There is a potential that alloantibody would be removed by the autoadsorption.
8. The red cells must lack the antigen to which the identified antibody is directed.
9. Donath-Landsteiner Test

CH. 7

1. False (DNA is **transcribed** to mRNA)
2. True
3. True
4. d
5. d
6. a
7. d
8. a
9. c

CH. 8

1. b
2. d
3. c
4. c
5. d
6. b
7. c
8. c
9. d
10. b

CH. 9

1. d
2. c
3. d
4. e
5. b
6. a
7. b
8. b
9. a
10. a
11. c
12. d

CH. 10

1. a
2. b
3. True
4. True
5. True
6. d
7. a
8. True
9. a
10. Rh immune globulin
11. B
12. P
13. N
14. B
15. N

CH. 11

1. c
2. b
3. a
4. a
5. c
6. a
7. b
8. d
9. b
10. d
11. b
12. a
13. c
14. b
15. d

CH. 12

1. True
2. Involvement in mitigating and regulating the adaptive immune response
3. c
4. a
5. True
6. False
7. b
8. b
9. True
10. Genes occur more frequently together than expected by chance
11. An antigenic determinant, the minimum structure unit with six to seven amino acids that can be perceived as foreign by T- or B-cell receptors
12. Nucleated cells
13. Avoid contamination
14. ABO, HLA
15. a
16. Complement-dependent microcytotoxicity test, flow cytometry, ELISA, Luminex technology, LABScreen antibody detection system, crossmatch
17. True
18. Graft-versus-host disease
19. TRALI
20. d

CH. 13

1. False. There is no single transfusion trigger applied to all patients. The decision to transfuse must be based on assessment of clinical factors as well as laboratory values. The TRICC trial demonstrated a restrictive transfusion policy which is at least as and possibly superior to a liberal policy in critically ill patients.
2. True. Transfusion of one unit of packed red blood cells is expected to raise the hemoglobin concentration by 1 g/dL and the hematocrit by 3%.
3. False. HLA-matched platelets are indicated for the immune cause of refractoriness due to presence of patient HLA antibodies. For nonimmune causes, there would be no benefit over transfusion of randomly selected platelets.
4. False. "Least incompatible" red blood cell units are provided in the case of the presence of autoantibodies when all alloantibodies are ruled out. Because of the broad specificity of the autoantibodies, some reactivity on crossmatch is expected with all units, since the autoantibody reacts even with the patient's own cells.
5. True. Leukocyte reduction may reduce the risk of febrile nonhemolytic reactions, CMV transmission, and HLA alloimmunization.
6. True. Lymphocytes are inactivated by irradiation at 2,500 cGy. It is indicated in directed donor components from blood relatives of the patient, bone marrow transplant recipients, immunodeficient patients, and intrauterine and neonatal transfusions as well as other conditions.
7. True. An adequate PPR is >20% when measured 10 to 60 minutes post transfusion. A CCI of 7,500 platelets × m^2 BSA per microliter is considered adequate.
8. True. Irradiation prevents graft-versus-host disease by inactivating lymphocytes, but does not affect neutrophil function. The component must be ABO and crossmatch-compatible due to the presence of contaminating red blood cells. Granulocytes must be transfused within 24 hours of collection because they undergo rapid apoptosis.
9. False. A leukocyte reduction filter would remove granulocytes from the component before transfusion to the patient.
10. False. Autologous donors may donate at a lower hemoglobin level and are not necessarily prevented from donation by various disease states that render allogeneic donors ineligible.
11. d. Platelet transfusion in TTP or HIT may fuel thrombosis. It is not indicated in ITP because it is ineffective.
12. c. Postoperative blood salvage has limited utility, and the product obtained is hemodilute, partially hemolyzed, defibrinated, and cytokine-rich.
13. F
14. C
15. G
16. A
17. D
18. B
19. H
20. E

CH. 14

1. True
2. False
3. False
4. False
5. True
6. False
7. True
8. True
9. d
10. d
11. a
12. b
13. a
14. c
15. a
16. a
17. b
18. d
19. True
20. True

CH. 15

1. d
2. a
3. c
4. d
5. b
6. c
7. a
8. d
9. d
10. c
11. d
12. b
13. d
14. c
15. d
16. d
17. b

18. d
19. d
20. b

CH. 16

1. d
2. c
3. a
4. b
5. c
6. b
7. a
8. d
9. b
10. a
11. c
12. a
13. a
14. c
15. a

CH. 17

1. a
2. a
3. b
4. c
5. c
6. a
7. e
8. c
9. True
10. a

CH. 18

1. a
2. b
3. c
4. c
5. b
6. a
7. An audit is a systematic investigation to determine if an organization's activities and practices are being performed according to its approved and written policies and procedures.
8. c
9. True
10. False
11. True
12. True
13. d

14. True
15. False

CH. 19

1. d
2. The Joint Commission
3. a
4. d
5. c
6. drug, biologic
7. a
8. a
9. safety, quality, identity, purity, potency
10. d
11. d
12. c
13. b

CH. 20

1. d
2. a
3. True
4. b
5. c
6. False

CH. 21

1. a
2. c
3. c
4. b
5. a
6. False
7. c
8. False
9. False
10. True

CH. 22

1. c
2. c
3. c
4. a
5. d
6. c
7. a
8. c
9. d

GLOSSARY

A subgroup: Division of group A based on qualitative and quantitative means. A_1 is the most common (80%), with A_2 comprising most of the rest. Subgroups such as A_3, A_x, A_m, and others occur infrequently or rarely.

AABB: An international blood banking and cellular therapy organization. The AABB issues standards for blood bank practices and cell therapy facilities, inspects, and accredits blood banking facilities.

AABB Standards: A publication of the American Association of Blood Banks. Statement of minimum requirements for blood banks in their operations.

abbreviated crossmatch: Procedures for crossmatching that do not include a complete antiglobulin test. Such procedures are acceptable for circumstances such as a recipient of blood with a negative antibody screen who has not been recently transfused.

ABO discrepancy: A difference in test results from the expected. For example, the forward grouping is interpreted as A and the reverse grouping on the same person is interpreted as O. A-positive Rh control in Rh typing is also an example of a discrepancy.

absorbed anti-A_1: Reagent made from serum of group B absorbed with A_2 red cells. Used to detect the A_1 antigen on red cells.

absorption: Process of removal of antibody from a serum; often used interchangeably with adsorption.

acquired immunodeficiency syndrome (AIDS): Clinical and laboratory evidence of infection with human immunodeficiency virus (HIV).

acquired B: Weak reaction of red cells with anti-B reagent due to (1) bacterial infection in group A individual in which acetyl group is cleaved by bacterial enzyme from *N*-acetylgalactosamine, or (2) reaction of red cells with acriflavine, the yellow dye in the anti-B reagent.

activation: The initiation of the complement cascade.

acute normovolemic hemodilution: See *preoperative hemodilution*.

additive solution: Solution used to extend the shelf life of packed red cells. Contains adenine, dextrose, and other nutritional components. Current systems extend the dating period to 42 days.

adenosine triphosphate: Multifunctional nucleotide, and plays an important role in cell biology as a coenzyme that is the "molecular unit of currency" of intracellular energy transfer.

adsorption: Process of adding specific antigen so that antibody can attach to it and be removed from a serum. The antigen adsorbs the antibody.

adverse effects of transfusion: Any unfavorable event that occurs after the transfusion of blood or blood components. Also referred to as "transfusion reaction."

agglomeration: Reversible agglutination of red cells as would occur using the reagent polybrene.

agglutination: The second stage of an antigen–antibody reaction when the antigen is particulate. This follows sensitization and is the visible stage of the reaction.

agglutinin: Another name for an antibody that agglutinates cells.

AIDS-related complex (ARC): The name given to a variety of symptoms preceding AIDS. Symptoms included persistent lymphadenopathy (swollen lymph nodes), diarrhea, and unexplained weight loss.

air embolus: A physiologic condition caused by gas bubbles in a vascular system.

alanine aminotransferase (ALT): A liver enzyme, formerly known as SGPT. Elevated in a number of circumstances, including hepatitis, consumption of alcoholic beverages, and heavy exercise. Used as a surrogate test by blood donor centers to detect presence of hepatitis not found by viral testing.

albumin: The protein found in the highest concentration in human plasma. Also used as a potentiating medium to enhance some antigen–antibody reactions.

albumin-agglutinating phenomenon: A reaction due to the presence of sodium caprylate as a preservative in albumin. The reaction occurs only when the caprylate is present.

alleles: Alternate forms of a gene that may be present at a single chromosome locus.

allo: Prefix used to denote differences within the same species. For example, anti-Kell is considered an alloantibody when produced by a K-negative individual after exposure to K-positive red cells from another individual.

alloantibody: Antibody produced by a person to an immunogen (antigen) in the same species but that is not present in that person. For example, a person who is E negative may form an anti-E (alloanti-E) if exposed to the red cells of an E-positive person.

allogeneic: Genetic dissimilarity within the same species.

alloimmunization: A condition in which the body gains immunity, from another individual of the same species, against its own cells.

allotype: Differences within the constant regions of human gamma and alpha heavy chains and kappa light chains, which are determined by allelic genes (Gm allotypes, Am allotypes, and Km allotypes). In a single person, all chains have the same allotype.

alternate pathway: Mechanism of complement activation that does not involve activation of C1, C4, C2 pathway by antigen–antibody complexes.

amniocentesis: Process of withdrawal of amniotic fluid with a needle for the purpose of analysis.

amniotic fluid: Serous fluid in the amniotic sac in which the embryo is immersed.

amorphic: Describes a gene that does not produce a serologically detectable product; a silent allele.

anamnestic response: A heightened level of immune response that occurs with the second exposure to an immunogen (antigen). The response occurs in 24 to 48 hours and normally produces a high level of IgG.

anaphylatoxin: Substance capable of releasing histamine from mast cells (i.e., C3a, C5a).

anaphylactic reaction: A hypersensitive reaction to an antigen as occurs when an IgA-deficient person is exposed to blood components containing IgA.

anemia: A condition in which there is a deficiency in red blood cells, hemoglobin, or total blood volume. Anemia may result from increased destruction of red cells, excessive blood loss, or decreased red cell production. It may also be the result of defective hemoglobin production.

antecubital: The location most frequently used for phlebotomy; found in the bend of the elbow.

antibody: The product of the humoral immune response. Antibody is produced in response to specific immunogenic (antigenic) stimulus by plasma cells, a terminal stage of B-cell proliferation.

antibody screen: An indirect antiglobulin procedure used to detect atypical antibodies (non-ABO antibodies) in serum or plasma.

anticoagulant: A substance used to prevent the coagulation (clotting) of blood.

antigen: A substance capable of reacting with the product of an immune response; often used in place of immunogen, although not all antigens are immunogens.

antigen presentation: Process in the body's immune system by which macrophages, dendritic cells, and other cell types capture antigens and then enable their recognition by T-cells.

antiglobulin: An antibody to globulins.

antiglobulin crossmatch: A crossmatch procedure where antiglobulin serum is used to detect immunoglobulin and/or complement bound to donor red cells.

antigram: An array of antigen typings on red cells used in antibody detection and identification. Normally, plus symbols (+) are used to denote the presence of an antigen on a red cell and minus symbols (–) are used to denote the absence of an antigen from a red cell. Antigrams may consist of any number of cells.

antihemophilic factor (AHF): Lyophilized form of factor VIII prepared from pools of plasma. AHF is used to treat hemophilia A.

antithetical: Term used to refer to the products of allelic genes.

anti-A₁ lectin: Plant extract prepared from *Dolichos biflorus*; agglutinates red cells that possess the A₁ antigen.

anti-H lectin: Plant extract prepared from *Ulex europeus*; agglutinates red cells that possess the H antigen.

anti-M lectin: Plant extract prepared from *Iberis amara*; agglutinates red cells that possess the M antigen.

anti-N lectin: Plant extract prepared from *Vicia graminea*; agglutinates red cells that possess the N antigen.

anti-T lectin: Plant extract prepared from *Archis hypogaea*, the peanut plant; agglutinates red cells that have exposed T antigen sites.

antepartum Rh immune globulin (RhIg): Rh immune globulin injection administered during pregnancy.

apheresis: Blood collection procedure in which whole blood is removed, a selected component separated, and the remainder returned to the donor.

atypical antibody: Antibody other than the expected ABO antibodies.

autoadsorption: The process of removing autoantibody from a person's serum or plasma using the individual's own red cells.

autoantibody: Antibody that a person makes toward self-antigens. The development of such antibody is not normal and can result in conditions such as autoimmune hemolytic anemia.

autocontrol: In serologic testing, a control composed of serum or plasma from a person and that same person's red cells; often used for comparison purposes. The autocontrol allows detection of autoantibody.

autoimmune hemolytic anemia: Type of hemolytic anemia where the body's immune system attacks its own red blood cells (RBCs), leading to their destruction (hemolysis).

autologous: Self.

autologous transfusion: A blood transfusion in which the donor and recipient are the same person.

autosome: Chromosomes other than the sex chromosomes. In humans, there are 22 pairs of autosomes.

B lymphocyte: A white blood cell which is the primary cell involved in humoral immunity. The principal functions of B cells are to make antibodies against antigens, perform the role of antigen-presenting cells (APCs) and eventually develop into memory B cells after activation by antigen interaction.

babesiosis: Malaria-like parasitic disease caused by *Babesia* which is a vector-borne illness usually transmitted by Ixodid ticks.

biphasic: Term describing a reaction that occurs in two phases. For example, the antibody in paroxysmal cold hemoglobinuria has IgG anti-P specificity and binds to red cells in the peripheral circulation, where it is colder. Hemolysis occurs when the red cells return to the warmer parts of the body.

blood component: Blood product; platelets, plasma, cryoprecipitate, granulocytes, and so forth.

Bombay phenotype: Phenotype that results from lack of the *H* gene (i.e., the person is hh). Bombay people forward group as group O and reverse as group O because of presence of a potent anti-H. Group O red blood cells, however, are highly incompatible with Bombay sera because of the anti-H.

bromelin: A proteolytic enzyme prepared from pineapple that cleaves sialic acids from red blood cells, enhancing the reactions of some antibodies and destroying the presence of certain antigens.

C3 convertase: In the classic complement cascade, an enzyme composed of activated C4a2b which cleaves C3 into C3a and C3b. In the alternate pathway, C3 convertase is composed of activated C3bBb.

C3a: A biologically active fragment of the C3 molecule; an anaphylatoxin.

C5a: A biologically active fragment of the C5 molecule; an anaphylatoxin.

categoric identification of antibodies (CIA): A systematic method of identifying serologic problems.

cell-mediated immunity: An immune response that does not involve antibodies or complement but rather involves the activation of macrophages, natural killer (NK) cells, antigen-specific cytotoxic T lymphocytes, and the release of various cytokines in response to an antigen.

Center for Biologics Evaluation and Research (CBER): Section of Food and Drug Administration to which blood banking facilities report.

Centers for Disease Control and Prevention (CDC): U.S. government agency to which certain infectious diseases are reported. The CDC makes recommendations such as those to prevent health-care workers from becoming infected with HIV.

chagas: A tropical parasitic disease caused by the flagellate protozoan *Trypanosoma cruzi.*

chemically modified antisera: Reagent antibody in which the antibody molecule has been chemically opened to span a greater distance; allows a lower-protein diluent to be used in the reagent. This reagent is useful in typing red blood cells that have a positive direct antiglobulin test (i.e., protein coats the red blood cell in vivo).

chikungunya: An insect-borne virus, of the genus, *Alphavirus,* that is transmitted to humans by virus-carrying *Aedes* mosquitoes.

chimera: A person in which a dual (mixed) cell population exists.

chloroquine diphosphate: A reagent used to dissociate IgG antibody from red blood cells. Use of chloroquine allows phenotyping of red blood cells coated with autoantibody, even when the phenotyping requires an antiglobulin procedure.

chromosome: Threads of DNA found in the nucleus of a cell. Genes are found along the strands. Humans have 23 pairs of chromosomes.

chronic hepatitis: Persistence of infection with a hepatitis virus for longer than 6 months.

circulatory overload: Blood transfusion condition that occurs due to a rapid transfusion of a large volume of blood.

classic pathway: The mechanism of complement activation initiated by antigen–antibody aggregates and proceeding by way of C1, C4, and C2.

clonal selection theory: Widely accepted model for how the immune system responds to infection and how certain types of B and T lymphocytes are selected for destruction of specific antigens invading the body.

clone: A group of identical cells **naturally** derived from a common mother cell.

closed system: System that allows manipulation of a product without exposing it to the air.

cold agglutinin disease: An autoimmune disease characterized by the presence of high concentrations of circulating antibodies directed against red blood cells.

***cis*-product antigens:** Antigens produced when two genes are on the same chromosome of a homologous pair.

citrate: Component of anticoagulants, composed of citric acid and a base. Citrate binds calcium and prevents coagulation.

***cis*-AB:** A state of inheritance where the *A* and *B* genes are linked on a single chromosome. An individual with *cis-AB* would type as an AB but could transmit the *O* gene (if the genotype is AB/O) to offspring.

citrate-phosphate-dextrose (CPD): Anticoagulant that was formerly used in routine blood collection and allowed 21-day storage.

citrate-phosphate-dextrose-adenine (CPDA-1): Anticoagulant most commonly used in routine blood collection; allows a 35-day storage period.

citrate toxicity: Condition that may develop due to the binding of calcium by citrate, resulting in tingling or tetany. Infants are particularly susceptible if they receive large amounts of anticoagulated blood.

class I antigens: HLA-A, HLA-B, and HLA-C antigens; found on all body tissue cells except the mature red blood cell. These antigens are important in rejection phenomena because of their interaction with T-cytotoxic lymphocytes.

class II antigens: HLA-DR, HLA-DQ, and HLA-DP antigens; found on the cell membranes of B lymphocytes, activated T lymphocytes, monocytes, macrophages, dendritic cells, early hematopoietic cells, and some tumor cells. These antigens interact with T-helper cells in the initial recognition of nonself antigens involved in the cell-mediated immune response.

clinically significant: Capable of reacting in the body to cause adverse reaction.

Code of Federal Regulations (CFR): Publication of the Food and Drug Administration that contains regulations by which blood banking facilities must operate. These are legal requirements.

codominant traits: Equal expression of two different inherited alleles. Most blood group genes produce codominant traits.

compatibility testing: Testing done to ensure that donor red cells are compatible with a potential recipient.

cold autoimmune hemolytic anemia (cold AIHA): Early destruction (removal from circulation) of red blood cells because of effects of complement being bound by an antibody that reacts best in colder temperatures (less than 37° C). Such antibodies are usually IgM. For example, anti-I is a cause of cold AIHA.

cold panel: Serologic testing of red blood cells with serum or plasma at 18°C or lower to detect cold-reactive antibodies.

complement: Series of proteins in the circulation that, when activated, act as enzymes and participate in a number of biologic activities, including lysis of cells, opsonization, chemotaxis, and so forth.

confidential unit exclusion: A method whereby a donor may confidentially ask that his or her blood not be used for transfusion. This may be accomplished by the use of a barcode system in which the donor privately selects an appropriate barcode stating to use or one stating not to use the donation.

constant region: The area of the immunoglobulin molecule that is composed of a relatively constant amino acid sequence.

continuous-flow pheresis: Collection and return during an apheresis procedure without interruption; involves two venipunctures with whole blood entering one line and the remainder, after removal of a component from the whole blood, returned through another line.

contraindicated: Term used to describe a case in which something (e.g., a process, administration of a particular blood component) should not be done.

Creutzfeldt–Jakob disease: A degenerative neurologic disorder (brain disease) that is very rare, incurable, and invariably fatal.

crossing-over: The exchange of genetic material during meiosis between paired chromosomes, resulting in a recombination of genetic information on these chromosomes.

cryoprecipitate: The cold insoluble portion of fresh frozen plasma that is frozen and thawed under controlled conditions. Cryoprecipitate is rich in factor VIII and also contains factor I, factor XIII, and von Willebrand factor.

cryoprotectant: A solution that, when added to cellular elements, prevents ice crystals from forming and breaking the cell membrane.

customer: The recipient of process output. Internal customers are within an organization; external customers are outside the organization.

cyanosis: Bluish or grayish discoloration of the skin resulting from lack of oxygen or carbon dioxide buildup.

cytapheresis: Apheresis procedure in which a cellular product is removed.

cytokines: A category of signaling molecules that, like hormones and neurotransmitters, are used extensively in cellular communication.

cytomegalovirus (CMV): Virus that is endemic in many areas and believed to be carried within peripheral blood leukocytes: causes a mononucleosis-like illness. Infection with CMV is problematic for neonates and immunosuppressed individuals.

cytotoxic T lymphocyte: A subgroup of T lymphocytes (a type of white blood cell) that are capable of inducing the death of infected somatic or tumor cells; they kill cells that are infected with viruses (or other pathogens), or are otherwise damaged or dysfunctional.

deferral: Prevention of donation, either temporarily or permanently, because of failure to meet donor acceptance criteria.

deglycerolization: Process of removal of glycerol from previously frozen red cells; involves thawing and washing with various solutions.

delta hepatitis: Disease caused by a small circular RNA virus. HDV is considered to be a subviral satellite because it can propagate only in the presence of another virus, the hepatitis B virus (HBV).

delayed hemolytic transfusion reaction: A type of transfusion reaction that can occur 1 to 4 weeks after the transfusion.

deletion: Condition when no allele is inherited at a locus. For example, in the Rh system, if no allele is inherited at the *Cc* locus, a person might type −De, with the (−) indicating the deletion.

dengue: Acute febrile diseases, found in the tropics, and caused by four closely related virus serotypes of the genus *Flavivirus*, family Flaviviridae.

deoxyribonucleic acid (DNA): The chemical basis of heredity. Genetic information is carried in the form of DNA for most living organisms.

derivatives: Products made from blood donor plasma.

Diamond-Blackfan anemia: A congenital erythroid aplasia that usually presents in infancy. DBA patients have low red blood cell counts (anemia). The rest of their blood cells (the platelets and the white blood cells) are normal. A variety of other congenital abnormalities may also occur.

diastolic blood pressure: The point at which the cavities of the heart dilate and fill with blood and there is the least amount of pressure in the arterial blood vessels. This is the bottom number in a blood pressure reading.

dimethylsulfoxide (DMSO): Substance used as cryoprotectant for freezing platelets.

2,3-diphosphoglycerate (2,3-DPG): Organic phosphate in red blood cells that alters the affinity of hemoglobin for oxygen. Levels of 2,3-DPG decrease as blood is stored, and the hemoglobin therefore has greater affinity for the oxygen. Once red blood cells are transfused, the level of 2,3-DPG is returned to normal.

direct antiglobulin test: Serologic test to detect the in vivo binding of antibody or complement to red blood cells; useful in cases of AIHA, drug-induced hemolytic anemia, transfusion reactions, and HDN.

directed donor: A donor chosen by the potential recipient. Such donations have been proven not to be any safer than transfusions from the general population.

disseminated intravascular coagulation (DIC): Condition in which the coagulation of blood is altered to a pathologic state. DIC results from a variety of conditions, including hemolytic transfusion reactions.

disulfide bonds: A single covalent bond derived from the coupling of thiol groups.

dithiothreitol (DTT): A sulfhydryl compound that disrupts the disulfide bonds of IgM, resulting in monomers that no longer have the reactivity of the intact molecule.

DMAIC: A problem solving method that utilizes these steps: (1) Define high-level project goals and the current process. (2) Measure key aspects of the current process and collect relevant data. (3) Analyze the data to verify cause-and-effect relationships. (4) Determine what the relationships are and attempt to ensure that all factors have been considered. (5) Improve or optimize the process based upon data analysis using techniques like design of experiments.

dominant trait: A gene product that is expressed to the exclusion of the expression of its allele. These traits are expressed in both homozygous and heterozygous states.

Donath-Landsteiner test: Test designed to identify the biphasic antibody in paroxysmal cold hemoglobinuria. The sample is kept warm after collection, cooled, and then returned to 37°C. Hemolysis in the test but not in the control is considered a positive test.

donor processing: Testing and preparation of donor blood before it is considered available for distribution, including ABO, Rh, antibody screen, and infectious disease testing.

dosage: Stronger expression due to a homozygous state of inheritance.

dyspnea: Shortness of breath.

enzyme-linked immunosorbent assay (ELISA): A serologic test using solid-phase technology in which the label is an enzyme.

eluate: The supernate resulting when an elution is performed. Antibody bound to red blood cells is released into the eluate in the elution procedure and the eluate may be used for further testing.

elution: Procedure that removes antibody bound to the red blood cell. This antibody goes into the eluate, which can be used for serologic testing.

Epstein–Barr virus: Etiologic agent of mononucleosis; may also cause viral hepatitis.

epitope: Antigenic determinant; site that stimulates immune response.

erythroblastosis fetalis: Hemolytic disease of the newborn.

erythrocytapheresis: The collection of red blood cells by automated methodology.

erythropoiesis: The process of red blood cell production within the bone marrow.

exchange transfusion: Transfusion performed postpartum in which a calculated amount of blood is removed from an infant and replaced with blood compatible with maternal serum; used in severe cases of hemolytic disease of the newborn (HDN).

expected increment: The expected increase in a blood parameter after transfusion of a blood component.

extravascular hemolysis: Removal of red blood cells from circulation by the reticuloendothelial (RE) system, also known as the mononuclear phagocytic system.

Fc receptor: A receptor on a cell surface with specific binding affinity for the Fc portion of an antibody molecule.

febrile: Fever producing.

febrile nonhemolytic transfusion reaction (FNH): Type of transfusion reaction in which fever and accompanying symptoms such as chills and nausea are the result of the interaction of white cell antigens and antibodies. No hemolysis is seen in this reaction, and it occurs most frequently in multiply-transfused or multiparous women.

fibrinogen: Also known as factor I, a protein that is produced by the liver and circulates in plasma. In the clotting process, fibrinogen becomes fibrin, which is responsible for clot formation.

ficin: Proteolytic enzyme made from the fig; used to cleave sialic acids from red blood cells in serologic testing.

Ficoll-Hypaque: Reagent used for the separation of mononuclear cells from red blood cells. Separation is based on density gradient.

Food and Drug Administration (FDA): U.S. governmental agency responsible for regulations governing blood banking practices as well as those of other manufacturers of products consumed by humans.

forward grouping: Test in which unknown red blood cells are mixed with antisera of known specificity to determine presence or absence of antigens on the red blood cells. For example, in ABO forward grouping, red blood cells are tested with reagent anti-A and anti-B. Agglutination with the reagent indicates presence of the antigen; no agglutination indicates its absence.

fresh frozen plasma (FFP): The liquid portion of whole blood that, after separation from the cellular components, is frozen within a specified time period to maintain viability of clotting factors. The product usually is about 250 mL in volume and is used to replace multiple clotting factor deficiencies.

gel test: Test system in which gel particles are used to trap red blood cells that are agglutinated because of antigen–antibody reactions.

genes: The units of inheritance.

genotype: The actual genes inherited; often can be determined only with family studies.

glycerolization: Process of adding glycerol to red blood cells as a cryoprotectant during freezing.

glycosyltransferases: Enzymes (EC 2.4) that act as a catalyst for the transfer of a monosaccharide unit from an activated sugar phosphate (known as the "glycosyl donor") to an acceptor molecule, usually an alcohol. They are involved in the formation of some blood group antigens.

good manufacturing practices (GMPs): The 200 and 600 series of the Code of Federal Regulations that regulate blood banking practices.

graft-versus-host disease (GVHD): A condition in which transfused immunocompetent cells engraft in the recipient and begin to mount response against the recipient's tissues.

granulocytes: White blood cells containing granules of biologically reactive substances in the cytoplasm.

hapten: A substance that by itself is too small to stimulate an immune response but when coupled with a protein of larger molecular weight can stimulate a response. Haptens by themselves can react with the product of an immune response.

heavy chain: The larger of the two chains that comprise the normal antibody molecule.

helper T cell: A subgroup of lymphocytes (a type of white blood cell or leukocyte) that play an important role in establishing and maximizing the capabilities of the immune system.

hematocrit: Measure of the volume of red blood cells as a percentage of the total volume of whole blood.

hemagglutinin: An antibody or other substance that causes red blood cells to agglutinate.

hemagglutination: Visible evidence of the interaction of red blood cells with antibody directed toward antigen on the red blood cells.

hematocrit: A measure of the percent of red cells in a volume of whole blood.

hemapheresis: Automated collection of blood.

hematopoietic progenitor cells: Multipotent stem cells that give rise to all the blood cell types including myeloid (monocytes and macrophages, neutrophils, basophils, eosinophils, erythrocytes, megakaryocytes/platelets, dendritic cells) and lymphoid lineages (T cells, B cells, NK cells).

hemoglobin: The iron-containing pigment in red blood cells that functions to carry oxygen from the lungs to the tissues.

hemoglobinemia: The presence of free hemoglobin in blood plasma.

hemoglobinuria: The presence of free hemoglobin in the urine.

hemolysis: The disruption of the red blood cell membrane, resulting in a release of hemoglobin into the plasma or cell suspension medium.

hemolytic transfusion reaction: Removal of red cells following transfusion either by activation of complement in the blood stream or by the reticuloendothelial system.

hemolytic disease of the newborn (HDN): Pathologic condition resulting from attachment of an IgG maternal antibody to cells of the fetus that contain the antigen to which the maternal antibody is directed. The antigen is inherited from the father and absent from the mother.

hemophilia A: Classic hemophilia, a deficiency in factor VIII activity. Also known as Christmas disease, a deficiency in factor IX activity.

hemosiderosis: Buildup of iron in tissues of the body because of excess iron. This condition is seen in multiply-transfused people such as those with thalassemia major.

heparin: An anticoagulant but not a preservative; used when blood is to be filtered for the removal of lymphocytes.

hepatitis: Inflammation of the liver caused by a variety of agents, including viruses, bacteria, and chemicals.

hepatitis B immune globulin: Antibody to hepatitis B that provides passive protection from hepatitis B virus.

hepatitis B vaccine: Vaccination that stimulates the immune system to make antibody to the surface antigen of hepatitis B. The first vaccine was made from the sera of infected individuals. Today, the commonly used vaccine is produced in yeast by recombinant technology.

hermetic seal: A seal that is impervious to air; an airtight seal.

hypogammaglobulinemia: Immunodeficiency resulting from decreased levels of gammaglobulins. Low levels of isohemagglutinins are seen in this condition.

heterozygous: Inheritance of two different alleles at a given locus (e.g., *Kk* at the Kell).

high-incidence antigen: Antigen occurring in a large percentage of the population.

high-risk donor: A donor who belongs to a particular group with lifestyles conducive to or genetic predisposition for a particular condition. For example, intravenous drug users are a high-risk group for infection with HIV.

high-titer, low-avidity antibody: An antibody that is present to a high dilution, but the strength of reaction is not higher at lower dilutions than at higher dilutions. For example, an antibody that shows agglutination with red blood cells at a dilution of 1:512, but the reaction strength in all tubes is only 1+.

hinge region: A flexible, open segment of an antibody molecule that allows bending of the molecule.

HIV positive: Refers to laboratory evidence of exposure to human immunodeficiency virus (HIV). Such people have had repeatedly reactive screening tests for HIV antibody and a reactive confirmatory test for HIV antibody (Western blot or IFA).

homologous adsorption: Use of antigen from another source other than the source making the antibody to remove that antibody from a serum; use of other than autologous cells to adsorb antibody from a serum.

homozygous: Inheritance of like genes at a chromosomal locus (e.g., *kk* at the Kell locus).

human immunodeficiency virus (HIV): Retrovirus responsible for acquired immunodeficiency syndrome. Two types (1 and 2) are currently identified.

human T-cell lymphotropic virus, type I (HTLV-I): Retrovirus associated with adult T-cell leukemia and tropical spastic paraparesia.

humoral immunity: Aspect of immunity that is mediated by secreted antibodies (as opposed to cell-mediated immunity which involves T lymphocytes) produced in the cells of the B-lymphocyte lineage (B cell). Secreted antibodies bind to antigens on the surfaces of invading microbes (such as viruses or bacteria), which flags them for destruction. Humoral immunity is called as such, because it involves substances found in the humours, or body fluids.

hybridoma: Fusion of a single antibody-producing cell with a myeloma cell to produce a rapidly dividing clone that can make monoclonal antibody. Many reagents used in blood banking are produced using such technology.

hydatid cyst fluid: Source of P1 substance.

hydroxyethyl starch (HES): Compound that will cause red blood cells to sediment faster; used to facilitate the separation of leukocytes from red blood cells in leukapheresis.

hyperkalemia: Excess potassium.

hypovolemia: Decreased blood volume.

iatrogenic blood loss: Blood loss due to physician actions (testing) or treatment.

icterus: Jaundice; yellowish color of skin, eyes, mucous membranes, and body fluids because of presence of excess bilirubin.

idiopathic: Of unknown cause or origin.

idiopathic thrombocytopenic purpura (ITP): Condition in which the number of platelets is decreased without exact known cause. Platelet antibodies may be involved.

idiotype: Portion of the immunoglobulin molecule that is the antigen combining site; found in the variable region.

immunodominant sugar: Sugar that gives a molecular specificity. For example, the addition of *N*-acetylgalactosamine gives ABO precursor substance group A specificity.

immune complex: Antigen joined with its corresponding antibody. Immune complexes circulate in some disease states.

immunofluorescent assay (IFA): A serologic test that uses a fluorochrome as a label. IFA can be used to confirm repeatedly reactive HIV antibody tests.

immunoadsorption: The removal of globulins by adsorption to appropriate antigen.

immunization: The process by which an individual's immune system becomes fortified against an agent (known as the immunogen).

immunocompetent cells: Those cells of the immune system (monocytes and lymphocytes) capable of mounting a specific immune response against a foreign substance (immunogen).

immunogen: A substance that prompts the generation of antibodies and can cause an immune response.

immunoglobulin: Proteins capable of acting as antibodies. Five classes are well studied: IgG, IgM, IgA, IgD, and IgE.

in utero: Within the uterus.

in vitro: Refers to an occurrence outside the body, as in a test tube.

in vivo: Within the body.

incompatibility: Presence of agglutination or hemolysis at any phase of testing in a compatibility procedure. Presence of antigen toward which an antibody is directed results in incompatibility.

incomplete antibody: Old term used to describe antibody that could cause agglutination of antigen suspended in saline. IgG antibodies were known as incomplete antibodies.

indirect antiglobulin test (IAT): Procedure used to detect in vitro binding of antibody or complement to antigen. The IAT has applications in antibody detection and identification, phenotyping, and compatibility tests.

infectious disease markers: Substances in the serum/plasma that indicate exposure to or presence of a particular disease.

informed consent: Refers to the requirement by law to inform blood donors of processes involved in blood donation, including testing and reporting of positive test results.

inhibition: Prevention of antigen–antibody reaction by neutralization of one of the reactants.

intermittent-flow apheresis: Procedure in which a specified amount of whole blood is withdrawn, a component separated, and the remainder returned, with these steps being repeated until the quantity of component desired is harvested.

International Organization for Standardization: Organization responsible for ISO 9000 series of quality management standards; widely known as **ISO**, it is an international standard-setting body composed of representatives from various national standards organizations.

intraoperative blood salvage: Procedure in which blood is salvaged, usually through a suction device, and reinfused with or without filtration to a patient during a surgical procedure.

intrauterine transfusion: Procedure in which blood (O-negative packed red blood cells, compatible with the mother) is administered to an unborn fetus through a needle inserted through the mother's abdomen into the baby's abdominal cavity or directly into the umbilical vein.

intravascular hemolysis: Lysis of red blood cells in the blood stream, resulting in the release of hemoglobin and red blood cell stroma.

ionic strength: Number of charged particles present in a solution.

irradiation of blood products: Exposure of blood products to gamma irradiation to prevent GVHD. The irradiation inactivates lymphocytes that could engraft in the host and cause GVHD.

ISBT: International Society for Blood Transfusion.

ISO 9000: Series of quality management standards not specific to any one industry; developed by the International Organization for Standardization. There are five sets of standards, with ISO 9001 encompassing all elements and ISO 9002 encompassing all except installation and servicing. Most blood banks would seek certification under ISO 9002.

isotype: Subclass of an immunoglobulin molecule.

isoagglutinins: ABO antibodies.

isohemagglutinin: Term used to describe ABO antibodies.

Joint Commission for Accreditation of Healthcare Organizations: A private sector U.S.-based nonprofit organization. It is the best known of a large number of active healthcare accreditation groups in the United States.

Kaizen: Japanese philosophy that focuses on continuous improvement throughout all aspects of life. When applied to the workplace, Kaizen activities continually improve all functions of a business, from manufacturing to management and from the CEO to the assembly line workers.

kernicterus: Buildup of unconjugated bilirubin in neural tissues of an infant with severe HDN that can result in irreversible damage if not treated quickly enough.

killer cell: Type of cytotoxic lymphocyte that constitutes a major component of the innate immune system. NK cells play a major role in the rejection of tumors and cells infected by viruses.

Kleihauer-Betke stain: Method for detection of fetomaternal hemorrhage. The principle of the stain is that fetal hemoglobin is resistant to elution in an acidic environment, whereas adult hemoglobin elutes from the cell. Cells containing fetal hemoglobin can then be counterstained and will be seen blue against a background of ghost cells (cells containing adult hemoglobin).

lectin: Extract of a plant, many of which are used as blood banking reagents because they bind specifically to the carbohydrate determinants of certain erythrocytes.

leukapheresis: The removal of leukocytes by apheresis.

leukoagglutinin: Antibody that is directed toward a white blood cell antigen.

leukocyte: Cells of the immune system defending the body against both infectious disease and foreign materials.

leukocyte-poor blood product: A blood product that has a reduced number of leukocytes. Such products can be produced by filtration, deglycerolization of frozen red blood cells, washing, or centrifugation.

light chain: The smaller of the two chains comprising the normal antibody molecule.

Liley graph: Graph used to interpret data from amniotic fluid studies. Three zones are present, and depending on where the absorbance at 450 nm lies, certain medical interventions are indicated.

linkage: Genes are linked together on a chromosome.

linkage disequilibrium: The occurrence of genes together more often than would normally be expected in nature (by chance alone).

locus: The site of a gene on a chromosome.

low-incidence antigen: An antigen that occurs in a low number of people in a population, usually less than 10%.

low–ionic-strength solution (LISS): A potentiating medium used in serologic testing. The reduction of the ionic strength results in a faster uptake of antibody so that incubation time can be decreased.

Lyme disease: An emerging infectious disease caused by at least three species of bacteria belonging to the genus *Borrelia*.

lymphocyte: A type of white blood cell in the vertebrate immune system.

lymphocytapheresis: Removal of lymphocytes through automated methodologies.

macrophage: White blood cell; macrophages are phagocytes, acting in both nonspecific defense (or innate immunity) as well as to help initiate specific defense mechanisms (or cell-mediated immunity) of vertebrate animals. Their role is to phagocytose (engulf and then digest) cellular debris and pathogens either as stationary or mobile cells, and to stimulate lymphocytes and other immune cells to respond to the pathogen.

major crossmatch: Serologic test in which recipient serum (plasma) is mixed with donor red blood cells in attempt to detect incompatibility, if present.

major histocompatibility complex (MHC): Complex located on chromosome 6 that contains the genes coding for the human leukocyte antigens (HLA).

malaria: Parasitic disease caused by *Plasmodium* sp. that can be transmitted by transfusion.

massive transfusion: The transfusion of blood equivalent to an individual's blood volume within a short period of time.

McLeod phenotype: Lack of Kx on the red blood cells accompanied by shortened survival and acanthocytic morphology. Reduced expression of Kell system antigens is seen. Some of these people have increased creatine phosphokinase (CPK).

meiosis: Cell division producing gametes (eggs and sperm), cells containing a haploid number (23) of chromosomes.

Mendelian: Transmission of hereditary characteristics from parent organisms to their children; it underlies much of genetics; proposed by Gregor Mendel.

membrane filtration: A technique for removing unwanted substance using a membrane to separate out the desired substance.

memory cell: Circulating cells of the immune system which "remember" a foreign antigen and quickly respond to it.

2-mercaptoethanol (2-ME): A sulfhydryl compound used to disrupt the IgM molecule into inactive monomers.

microaggregates: Clumps or aggregates of platelets and leukocytes that form during blood storage.

microlymphocytotoxicity test: Test used serologically to define HLA antigens. In this test, specific HLA antibody is in a well to which lymphocytes are added, followed by complement. If the antigen is present to which the antibody is directed, the cell is killed and a dye can enter it, which is easily seen under the microscope.

minor crossmatch: Serologic test in which donor plasma is mixed with recipient red blood cells to detect incompatibility, if present. This test is obsolete.

mitosis: Cell division that results in diploid number (23 pairs) of chromosomes. All cells except sex cells (eggs and sperm) undergo mitosis.

mixed-field agglutination: Form of agglutination in which tiny agglutinins can be seen among unagglutinated cells. This type of agglutination is seen with people who have recently been transfused (two-cell population), chimeras, and A_3 red blood cells.

mixed lymphocyte culture (MLC): Technique used to detect class II HLA antigen differences. Lymphocytes from donor and recipient are mixed in a one- or two-way test to detect evidence of proliferation, which would indicate antigenic differences. A *one-way MLC* means that either the donor or recipient cells have been treated to not respond so that if a response occurs, it is possible to know the cells responding. In a *two-way MLC*, both can respond.

mobile operation: A collection operation which is not a fixed site.

molal solution: A solution containing 1 mol/1,000 g of solvent.

molar solution: A solution containing 1 mol of solute in 1 L of solution.

monoclonal: Of a single clone; used to refer to antibody produced by a single cell line. All molecules of a monoclonal antibody are identical.

mononuclear cells: Those white blood cells with a single nucleus (i.e., monocytes and lymphocytes).

monospecific: Singular specificity as opposed to polyspecific.

monospecific antiglobulin reagent: Reagent that is specific for IgG alone or for complement alone.

monozygotic twins: Identical twins, arising from a single fertilized egg. These twins will have the same blood group.

mosaic D^a: Weakened expression of D antigen resulting from absence of a portion of the complete antigen. For example, considering the D antigen to be composed of four parts, A, B, C, and D, the D^a might be missing part B. Theoretically, a mosaic D^a can make antibody to the missing portion, which will appear to be a complete anti-D in testing.

multiparous: More than one birth.

***N*-acetyl neuraminic acid:** A sialic acid found on the red blood cell.

National Marrow Donor Program: An organized effort to establish a national registry of marrow donors.

naturally occurring: Occurring without *known* stimulus.

neocytes: Young red blood cells.

neonatal immune thrombocytopenia: Form of HDN in which maternal anti-Pl^{A1} attaches to the newborn's platelets so they are removed from circulation.

neuraminidase: Enzyme that cleaves sialic acid from the red blood cell membrane.

neutralization: Inactivation of an antibody through combination with its antigen.

non-A, non-B hepatitis: Old terminology used to describe forms of hepatitis for which hepatitis A and B were ruled out.

non–red cell stimulated: Term used to describe red blood cell antibodies that are not formed through direct stimulation by a red blood cell antigen.

normal saline: 0.9% sodium chloride solution.

nucleic acid testing: Sensitive laboratory testing which tests for DNA or RNA.

null phenotype: No expression of gene is detectable because of either inherited trait or suppression.

O variant: HIV subtype.

Occupational Safety and Health Administration (OSHA): U.S. government organization that inspects to ensure safety in the workplace.

open system: Exposed to the air.

osmolality: Measure of the osmotic concentration of a solution as determined by the amount of dissolved substances per unit of solvent.

packed red blood cells: Blood component produced when most of the plasma is removed after sedimentation or centrifugation.

paid donor: A donor who receives payment for his or her donation.

panagglutinin: Term used to describe a serum that agglutinates most normal red blood cells.

papain: Proteolytic enzyme prepared from the papaya plant used to cleave sialic acids from red blood cells in serologic testing.

paragloboside: Precursor substance for the H and P_1 antigens of the red blood cell.

parentage testing: Using genetic markers to determine parents of a child.

paroxysmal cold hemoglobinuria (PCH): Autoimmune condition in which red blood cells are lysed because of the presence of a biphasic hemolysin with IgG anti-P specificity.

parvovirus: Both a virus name and a genus of the Parvoviridae family. Parvoviruses are typically linear, nonsegmented, single-stranded DNA viruses, with an average genome size of 5 kbp. Parvoviruses are some of the smallest viruses found in nature (hence the name, from Latin *parvus* meaning *small*).

paternity testing: Testing for presence or absence of substances (e.g., antigens, enzymes) to exclude falsely accused fathers. A direct exclusion occurs when the child possesses an antigen that the alleged father should have passed to him or her.

pedigree chart: A pictorial representation of inheritance patterns.

perforin: A cytolytic protein found in the granules of CD8 T cells and NK cells.

perioral paresthesia: A tingling sensation around the mouth during apheresis procedures caused by the rapid return of citrated blood to the donor, resulting in a calcium deficit.

phagocytosis: A specific form of endocytosis involving the vesicular internalization of solid particles, such as bacteria.

phenotype: Observable expression of inherited traits.

phlebotomy: The withdrawal of blood from a person.

phthalate esters: Nonaqueous solutions of graduated specific gravities useful in the separation of young and old red blood cells.

pilot tube: Tube of blood collected from donor at time of whole-blood unit collection; used for donor processing procedures such as infectious disease testing.

plasma: The liquid portion of unclotted blood. Fibrinogen is present.

plasma cell: A cell of the immune system transported by the blood plasma and the lymphatic system. Plasma cells are formed in the bone marrow and abundant in the lymphatic liquid: they secrete large amounts of antibodies.

plasma exchange: A technique for removing plasma from a person and replacing it with donor plasma or other volume expanders. This is useful in the treatment of many diseases in which a humoral factor is believed to contribute to the disease pathology.

plasma protein fraction (PPF): Sterile pooled plasma product that can be stored in a liquid or frozen state used to replace volume; also known as Plasmanate®.

plasmapheresis: Apheresis procedure in which plasma is removed from whole blood with the remainder (cellular elements) being returned to the donor.

platelets: Cellular element of blood that is derived from the cytoplasm of the megakaryocyte. Platelets play an important role in blood coagulation, hemostasis, and blood thrombus formation.

Poka-yoke: A Japanese term that means "fail-safing," "Foolproof," or "mistake-proofing"—avoiding (*yokeru*) inadvertent errors (*poka*) is a behavior-shaping constraint, or a method of preventing errors by putting limits on how an operation can be performed in order to force the correct completion of the operation.

polyagglutination: Condition in which red blood cells are agglutinated by most normal adult sera.

polybrene: A positively charged macromolecule that causes spontaneous aggregation of red blood cells by neutralization of the negative charge at the red blood cell surface. Polybrene is useful in the identification of some antibodies, such as those of the Kidd system.

polyclonal: Term used to describe antibodies derived from more than one antibody-producing parent cell.

polyethylene glycol (PEG): Reagent useful as a potentiator in antibody detection or identification procedures.

polymerase chain reaction (PCR): A technique for the amplification of specific nucleotide sequences that is useful in detection of a conserved region of viral genome integrated into host DNA.

polymorphic: Multiple possible states for a single property.

polyspecific: Multiple specificities.

polyspecific antiglobulin reagent: Antiglobulin reagent with both anti-IgG and anticomplement specificity.

population genetics: Study of the allele frequency distribution and change under the influence of the four evolutionary processes: natural selection, genetic drift, mutation, and gene flow. It also takes account of population subdivision and population structure in space.

postoperative salvage: Procedure in which blood is salvaged from a draining wound for reinfusion. This procedure is useful in some forms of cardiac surgery.

posttransfusion purpura: A normally self-limiting thrombocytopenia that occurs mainly in multiparous women. The thrombocytopenia is usually severe, and if treatment is indicated, plasmapheresis may be used, but platelet transfusions are not usually beneficial. The exact mechanism of platelet destruction is under study, although platelet antibody is believed to be involved.

posttransfusion sample: Blood sample drawn after transfusion of blood component. Antigen typing on such samples is not reliable.

postzone: Term used to refer to the presence of excess antigen resulting in a false-negative test.

precursor substance: A substance that is converted into something else by the addition of a specific molecule. For example, paragloboside is a precursor substance that is given A specificity by the addition of the sugar, N-acetylgalactosamine.

predeposit autologous donation: Donation of one or more units of blood before a surgical procedure by a person for his or her use during or after the procedure.

preoperative hemodilution (acute normovolemic hemodilution): Procedure in which a specified amount of whole blood is removed from a patient, usually in the operating room, and replaced with volume-expanding fluids. After the surgery, the whole blood can be returned to the patient. This procedure decreases loss of red blood cells from bleeding during surgery as it dilutes the blood.

pretransfusion sample: Sample drawn before receipt of blood component transfusions.

pretransfusion testing: Serologic testing performed in vitro to ensure the safest possible transfusion. Such testing includes, but is not limited to, ABO, Rh, antibody screening, and crossmatching.

prewarmed technique: A serologic procedure in which all reactants are warmed before mixing. In red blood cell serologic testing, the red blood cells and serum are warmed before mixing and immediately incubated, followed by washing with warm (37°C) saline and subsequent addition of antiglobulin reagent.

primary immune response: First exposure of a foreign substance (immunogen) to the immune system. After the immunogen is processed by immunocompetent cells, antibody appears in 7 to 14 days and is primarily of the IgM class.

private genes: Genes found in only a few people in a population or particular family.

probability: Determination of the likelihood of an event occurring.

process: An activity that takes input and adds value to it to produce an output. A supplier provides input, and the customer is the recipient of the output of a process.

process control: All steps taken to ensure processes remain in control; elements include monitoring and maintenance of equipment, review of records, quality control, and standard operating procedures.

proficiency testing: Testing used to ensure that people performing testing or other procedures are doing so accurately and appropriately.

properdin: Stabilizing protein in the alternate pathway of complement activation. This pathway is sometimes referred to as the properdin pathway.

propositus: In a pedigree study, the propositus is the person with whom the study is initiated. Feminine form is *proposita*.

prozone: Term used to refer to the presence of excess antibody resulting in a false-negative test.

public genes: High-frequency genes, found in a large percentage of a population.

quality assurance (QA): All steps necessary to ensure that something is of as high quality as it can be. Quality control is just one aspect of QA.

quality assurance program: A program to ensure that quality assurance is in place.

quality system essentials: Those areas in blood banking for which quality systems should be in place, including record keeping, labeling, testing, and so forth.

radioimmunoassay (RIA): Very sensitive serologic test in which the label is a radioactive compound.

random donor platelets: Platelet concentrate prepared from a unit of whole blood. Each unit should contain 5.5×10^{10} platelets.

rare donor: Donor whose blood has special qualities (e.g., negative for a high-incidence antigen) not found in the general population.

rare donor file: List of donors whose blood has special qualities. Both the AABB and the American Red Cross maintain extensive rare donor files.

recessive trait: A trait that is expressed only if the gene is inherited in double dose (homozygous).

recipient: In blood banking, the person who receives a transfusion of blood or blood components.

recombinant human erythropoietin (rhEpo): Hormone produced using genetic technology that stimulates erythropoiesis. Primarily used to stimulate erythropoiesis in renal patients, it is also used to increase hematocrits in those making autologous donations.

recombinant technology: Term used to describe procedures in which DNA that will produce a specific desired product is inserted into a host, such as a yeast cell, so that the host will then produce the product for use. For example, hepatitis B vaccine is made by inserting the DNA of the virus that produces the surface antigen into a yeast cell. The yeast cell then produces surface antigen for use as a vaccine.

refractoriness: Failure to achieve the desired increment in platelets following a platelet transfusion; may result from platelet antibodies that have developed in the recipient.

rejuvenation: Process of adding a solution containing adenine, inosine, pyruvate, and other compounds to red blood cells nearing the end of their shelf life to transfuse the cells immediately or freeze them for later use. The addition of the solution increases levels of 2,3-DPG, adenosine triphosphate, or both.

retrovirus: An RNA virus that is replicated in a host cell via the enzyme reverse transcriptase to produce DNA from its RNA genome.

reverse grouping: Serologic test in which serum containing unknown ABO antibody(ies) is tested with red blood cells of known ABO group (A_1, B, and sometimes A_2 red blood cells are used). For example, if a serum reacts with the A_1 red blood cell but not with the B red blood cell, it contains anti-A and does not contain anti-B (expected reactions of a group B person).

reverse transcriptase: An enzyme found in the nucleus of RNA viruses that allows them to transfer their genetic information (carried as RNA) to the host DNA.

Rh immune globulin (RhIg): Concentrated and purified anti-D given to people who are capable of forming an anti-D (Rh negative) if exposure to the D antigen has occurred or may occur, as during pregnancy. The RhIg prevents immunization to the D antigen.

Rh$_{null}$ disease: A chronic compensated anemia that occurs in people whose red blood cells lack Rh antigens (Rh$_{null}$ cells). The cells of such people have a membrane defect that leads to their shortened survival.

ribonucleic acid (RNA): Nucleic acid that controls protein synthesis in living cells. Three types have been identified: messenger RNA (mRNA), transfer RNA (tRNA), and ribosomal RNA (rRNA). Some viruses carry their genetic information in the form of RNA.

Rosette test: Test used to determine presence of fetomaternal bleed. Fetal cells rosette around an indicator cell and can be counted.

Rouleaux: A coin-stack appearance of red blood cells that may be mistaken for agglutination. This occurs when red blood cells are sticky because of protein abnormalities or sometimes as a result of infusion of certain intravenous fluids.

routine panel: Panel of eight or more antigen-typed red blood cells that are tested under routine conditions with an individual's serum to identify an antibody.

saline antisera: Antisera prepared by diluting the antibody in a saline medium with lower protein content than routine modified antisera.

sanctions: Enforcement tools such as warning letters, fines, and the like that can be levied against a facility for failure to comply with regulations.

satellite bag: Additional bags attached to the whole-blood collection bag for the purpose of component preparation in a closed system.

score: A measure of the strength of an antibody. An antibody's score is determined by adding together points given to each positive reaction in a titer. For example, a 4+ reaction is given 12 points, a 3+ is given 10 points, and a 2+ is given 8 points. The score is more indicative of the real strength of an antibody than is the titer.

screening cells: Group O red cells used to detect unexpected antibodies in serum or plasma.

secondary immune response: Immune response that occurs as a result of antigenic memory. Antibody produced is IgG, and its titer rises very quickly.

secretor: A person who has inherited the *Se* gene in single or double dose. Such people secrete ABH substances in their body fluids.

sensitization: Initial stage of an antigen–antibody reaction in which the antibody attaches to the antigen. This is usually an invisible reaction.

sepsis: Presence of microorganisms or their toxins (poisonous products) in the bloodstream.

serologic marker: A substance in the blood detectable by serologic testing that indicates exposure to or presence of an agent. For example, anti-HBs can be detected in the blood of people who had hepatitis B; therefore, the anti-HBs is a serologic marker for hepatitis B.

serum: The liquid portion of clotted whole blood. In serum, fibrinogen has been converted to fibrin.

sex chromosome: The X or Y chromosomes that determine sex. Males inherit XY and females inherit XX.

shelf life: The period of time that a blood product is determined to be acceptable for transfusion.

sialic acids: Group of sugars attached to the red blood cell membrane that are primarily responsible for the net negative charge of the cell.

silent allele: An allele that does not produce a detectable product.

sialoglycoprotein: Combination of sialic acid glycoprotein (which is, itself, a combination of sugar and protein).

single-donor platelets: Platelets collected by cytapheresis. A single-donor platelet unit should contain 3.0×10^{11} platelets, an amount equivalent to 6 to 10 units of random-donor platelets.

Six Sigma: Business management strategy, originally developed by Motorola, that today enjoys widespread application in many sectors of industry. Six Sigma seeks to identify and remove the causes of defects and errors in manufacturing and business processes. It uses a set of quality management methods, including statistical methods, and creates a special infrastructure of people within the organization ("Black Belts," etc.) who are experts in these methods.

specific acquired immunity: Immunity that is acquired through exposure and is directed at a specific immunogen.

standard operating procedure (SOP): A statement of the exact process used to accomplish a task.

statistical process control (SPC): Use of statistics to ensure processes are in control.

sterile connecting device (sterile tube welder): A device that allows tubing to be separated and joined with other tubing without exposure to bacterial contamination. Such devices can allow entry into a blood bag without exposure to the air, which requires a change in expiration time.

storage lesion: Biochemical changes that occur in blood as it is stored.

supplier: Any individual or group that supplies input into a process.

supplier qualification: Ongoing process of ensuring suppliers meet preestablished quality and performance criteria.

suppressor gene: A gene that suppresses the expression of a trait. For example, *In(Lu)* inhibits the expression of Lutheran genes.

surface of shear: Also known as the slipping plane, the boundary of the ionic cloud surrounding red blood cells in suspension at which the zeta potential is measured.

surge: A term coined by Haemonetics to describe the elutriation of platelets from the buffy coat.

surrogate markers: Disease markers that are indicators of potential for infection with other, often more serious, infectious diseases.

syncope: Fainting, a vasovagal response.

syphilis: Sexually transmitted disease caused by a spirochete, *Treponema pallidum*.

systolic blood pressure: Blood pressure reading during which the heart is contracting to expel blood; the top number of a blood pressure reading.

tachycardia: Abnormally rapid heartbeat.

tachypnea: Abnormal rapidity of respiration.

tetany: Spasms of involuntary muscles, caused by deficiency of calcium in the blood.

thalassemia major: Congenital form of anemia found especially among Mediterranean people. The disease results from impaired synthesis of a polypeptide chain of hemoglobin.

therapeutic apheresis: Removal of blood component(s) for treatment purposes, as in the case of polycythemia.

thermal amplitude: The temperature range over which an antibody can react.

thiol reagents: Reagents that can be used to disperse agglutination caused by cold-reactive autoantibodies. Dithiothreitol (DTT) and 2-mercaptoethanol (2-ME) are examples of such reagents.

thrombocytopenia: Platelet counts below the normal level.

thrombocytopheresis: Removal of platelets using automated technology.

thrombopoietin: Hormone that stimulates platelet production.

titer: Reciprocal of the highest dilution that shows visible reaction.

toxoplasmosis: A parasitic disease caused by the protozoan *Toxoplasma gondii*.

trait: An inherited characteristic that is an expression of the actions of a gene.

traceability: The ability to trace back to a source.

transposition: Term used to refer to genes located on opposite chromosomes of a homologous pair.

transcription: The process of mRNA production from DNA, initiated by RNA polymerase.

transferase: An enzyme that adds a sugar moiety to a precursor substance.

transfusion: The administration of blood or blood components to a person, usually through an intravenous line.

transfusion reaction: Any adverse reaction after the infusion of blood or blood components.

trypsin: Proteolytic enzyme formed in the intestine used to split proteins into amino acids.

type and screen: Method of preventing unnecessary blood bank testing. A person's ABO group, Rh type, and antibody screen are performed. If the antibody screen is negative, should blood be needed, an abbreviated crossmatch can be done. If the antibody screen is positive, the antibody can be identified and antigen-negative blood crossmatched.

uniform donor history questionnaire: List of donor interview questions developed by the AABB and recommended for use in screening blood donors.

urticaria: Hives, a common sign of allergic reaction.

validation: Documented evidence providing a high degree of assurance that a process works as expected.

value stream mapping: A Lean technique used to analyze the flow of materials and information currently required to bring a product or service to a consumer.

variable region: That region of an antibody molecule in which specificity is determined by the amino acid sequence.

vasoconstriction: A tightening of blood vessels that restricts the flow of blood.

virion: A complete infective viral particle.

volunteer blood donor: A person who donates blood or blood components with no compensation readily convertible into cash.

von Willebrand disease: A congenital blood clotting disorder in which both factor VIII and platelet deficiencies are present.

warm autoimmune hemolytic anemia (WAITHA): A condition of decreased red blood cell survival that is the result of an autoantibody that shows reactivity best at 37°C.

Western blot: A specific and sensitive test for antibody to HIV, used as a confirmatory test for repeatedly reactive HIV antibody ELISA screening tests.

Wharton's jelly: A thick, gelatinous substance that coats the umbilical cord. Wharton's jelly, if present in a cord blood sample, can cause the red blood cells to stick together.

whole blood: Fluid responsible for carrying nutrients and oxygen to tissues and removing wastes and carbon dioxide, composed primarily of red blood cells, white blood cells, and platelets suspended in plasma.

window period: A period of time in serologic testing when the markers usually indicating disease are not detectable, although the disease is present. For example, in hepatitis testing, there is a period of time when neither hepatitis B surface antigen nor hepatitis B surface antibody is present, and yet the person can be infected.

X-linked: Carried on the X chromosome.

Yersinia enterocolitica: A species of gram-negative coccobacillus-shaped bacterium, belonging to the family Enterobacteriaceae. Primarily a zoonotic disease (cattle, deer, pigs, and birds), animals that recover frequently become asymptomatic carriers of the disease.

zeta potential: Net negative charge of the red blood cell, measured at the surface of shear.

zygosity: The similarity or dissimilarity of the DNA sequences in specific coding segments, or genes, on the homologous chromosomes of a zygote, or fertilized egg.

ZZAP: A reagent composed of a proteolytic enzyme and a thiol reagent that can be used to dissociate IgG molecules from red blood cells.

INDEX

Page numbers followed by *f* indicate figures; those followed by *t* indicate tables; those followed by *b* indicate boxes